Trauma-Informed and Accumulation-Aware Approaches to Child Protection

India Bryce
https://orcid.org/0000-0002-3616-8003
University of Southern Queensland, Australia

Simone Collier
https://orcid.org/0009-0008-3658-8535
University of Southern Queensland, Australia

IGI Global
Scientific Publishing
Publishing Tomorrow's Research Today

Vice President of Editorial	Melissa Wagner
Director of Acquisitions	Mikaela Felty
Director of Book Development	Jocelynn Hessler
Production Manager	Mike Brehm
Cover Design	Jose Rosado

Published in the United States of America by
IGI Global Scientific Publishing
701 East Chocolate Avenue
Hershey, PA, 17033, USA
Tel: 717-533-8845 | Fax: 717-533-7115
Website: https://www.igi-global.com E-mail: cust@igi-global.com

Library of Congress Cataloging-in-Publication Data

LCCN: 2025038332 (CIP Data Pending)
ISBN13: 9798337340647
Isbn13Softcover: 9798337340654
EISBN13: 9798337340661

British Cataloguing in Publication Data
A Cataloguing in Publication record for this book is available from the British Library.

Table of Contents

Detailed Table of Contents

relational networks and connections to communities, (7) collaborating within a multi-disciplinary care team, and (8) engaging children and young people in scalable, evidence-informed clinical and therapeutic models. The chapter advocates for aligning all elements of child protection practice with these eight principles, so that systems can move toward long-term healing.

Empathy has been described as the cornerstone of genuine human relationships and understood as an intentional and skilful act of connection. Practice with young people impacted by violence has often sought to leverage, or enhance, empathy in restorative ways. Professional training for practitioners who support this cohort has emphasised empathy as foundational to establishing safety, building rapport, and implementing relational practice. This chapter presents a critical reflection on the 'shoebox activity' from the Name.Narrate.Navigate program, an empathy-focused experiential exercise delivered with young people who have used and experienced violence, often in contexts of cumulative harm. The authors compare responses from young people with professionals being trained to deliver the activity. Through this analysis, they interrogate traditional assumptions about empathy in practice, and practice education, arguing for a more nuanced understanding of empathy as a dynamic, socially constructed, gendered and embodied phenomenon essential for trauma-informed, cumulative harm aware work.

Due to its multifaceted challenges, reunifying children in state care with their biological families is a profoundly complex and often misunderstood process. While every Australian state jurisdiction positions reunification as a legislative and policy priority, in practice, it is significantly under-resourced. This chapter will critically examine the reunification process in the Australian child protection context. The chapter focuses on the consequences of poorly supported reunification efforts, including the cumulative harm experienced by children as they navigate the child protection system. It will argue that the absence of tailored reunification therapy as a standard component of intervention and how this deepens risk and undermines the potential for safe and sustainable family restoration. This chapter will advocate for a shift toward holistic, evidence-informed approaches that consider families' individual needs and promote long-term well-being for children returning to their biological family-based care.

This chapter presents the development of the Cumulative Experiences Index – Culturally Responsive (CEI-CR) tool, an assessment tool designed to identify and measure cumulative harm experienced by First Nations children. Building on the validated Cumulative Experiences Index (CEI) tool, the CEI-CR incorporates culturally specific domains, including intergenerational trauma, cultural disconnection, systemic disadvantage, and resilience factors grounded in kinship, culture, and Country. The CEI-CR integrates historical, cultural, and structural considerations to provide a more accurate profile of risk and protective factors. Its purpose is to support early, culturally safe intervention, family preservation, and reunification, rather than justify removal. This chapter outlines the theoretical framework, co-design process with Aboriginal stakeholders, and intended application of the CEI-CR, highlighting its potential to address service gaps and improve outcomes for children experiencing chronic, layered adversity.

Betrayal trauma theory offers an important framework for preventing and responding to cumulative adverse childhood experiences. From its inception, betrayal trauma theory has highlighted the importance of the context in which trauma occurs, with applications ranging from parent-child relationships and romantic relationships to the role of institutions in shaping traumatic experiences. This chapter will address how utilizing betrayal trauma theory can support trauma-informed approaches to protecting children by contextualizing the range of diverse relationships that surround interpersonal trauma and their effects on traumatic experiences and outcomes. Furthermore, we will discuss how researchers and providers at the individual level and at the systemic level can better understand and address the accumulation of betrayals over lifetimes, beginning in childhood and perpetuated via intergenerational transmissions of trauma, through trauma-informed and multidisciplinary approaches to protecting children and their families.

Intergenerational child maltreatment, in which abuse or neglect in childhood reoccurs over generations within the same family, is a consequential yet poorly understood challenge in child protection policy and practice. Using systemic methodology, this scoping review reveals the explanatory theoretical frameworks on intergenerational child maltreatment in the literature, explores diverse intervention approaches, and finds correlations between different facets of the data.. A variety of theoretical frameworks and suggested interventions are articulated in the literature, with attachment theory being most prominent and practices focusing more strongly on various approaches to direct service provision and future research than to reflective practice and intervention at a systemic or structural level. This data, alongside correlations between different aspects of the data, holds implications for policy, practice, and research, including broadening intervention options to cater for the diversity of people seeking support and critiquing existing paradigms driving research and practice.

This chapter examines how cumulative harm influences learning through the intertwined pathways of threat, deprivation, and disrupted relational expectations. It outlines how classroom environments can unintentionally reproduce these conditions through curricular omissions, instructional habits, and unexamined assumptions. Drawing on trauma-informed, culturally responsive, and neurodevelopmental research, the chapter presents a three-phase implementation framework encompassing preparation, monitoring, and evaluation. The framework emphasises predictable routines, cultural alignment, differentiated instruction, and reflective practice as core components of safe and effective learning environments. Practical examples illustrate how educators can interpret behaviour through a developmental lens, avoid reenacting harmful relational patterns, and strengthen conditions for engagement. The chapter positions schooling as a context for repair, regulation, and identity affirmation when instructional decisions intentionally counter the effects of cumulative harm.

People's career choices are not necessarily the unfolding of normative experiences. Instead, trauma experienced throughout childhood affects developmental trajectories and career choices. Findings of the study reveal consistent themes pertaining to the meaningfulness ascribed to helping professionals' experiences of cumulative childhood trauma and re-authoring of trauma narratives through a career lens. This chapter will draw on the findings of a recent study by the author (Bryce et al., 2022; 2023) which revealed that through vocational decision making, life, career and trauma narratives converge to foster a reauthoring experience. The intention of this chapter is to collate and synthesise existing research, and the research of the authors, which explores the influence of cumulative trauma and adversity on career decision making, and trauma informed career counselling

The pervasive impact of childhood cumulative harm across the lifespan is increasingly acknowledged, yet outcomes in later adulthood are rarely examined. This chapter outlines findings of a study of older "care" leavers in Australia, individuals aged 50 years and older who spent time in childhood institutions, foster "care", or other forms of out-of-home "care" from the 1950s to the 1980s. Voices of older "care" leavers were gathered through 105 surveys and 24 in-depth interviews, which told of how their ongoing hardship reflected long-term impacts of childhood harm and adversity, and the contribution of these to relationship, housing, financial, health, and other life challenges. For some, intergenerational child removal demonstrated how the impact of cumulative harm can echo across generations. Despite enduring significant trauma, the remarkable resilience of older "care" leavers is evident.

Findings raise implications about the support needs of older "care" leavers, and the long-term consequences of institutional abuse.

Foreword

Trauma-Informed and Accumulation-Aware Approaches to Child Protection developed under the leadership of editors Dr India Bryce and Dr Simone Collier is a notable contribution to our understanding of the critical but still evolving construct of cumulative harm.

At the turn of the new millennium, when I began my research career, cumulative harm did not exist. More accurately - it was not defined in academic literature. The accumulating impacts of chronic maltreatment, trauma and adversity were clearly present, indeed prevalent, in the daily lived experience of vulnerable children.

In 1998, Felitti and colleagues published their landmark study on Adverse Childhood Experiences, finding a strong predictive relationship between the number of adverse childhood events experienced and adverse outcomes. This research catalysed a future body of work quantifying the cumulative impacts of childhood adversity.

In the early 2000s, a project focused on the characteristics and trajectories of families in which children were repeatedly reported to statutory child protection services led me to the realisation that, at that time, definitions of child abuse and neglect in both research and practice were largely framed episodically. It was as part of this research that I first proposed a definition of chronic child maltreatment, the chronic child maltreatment typology which articulated the dimensions of chronicity and the term cumulative harm (Bromfield, 2005).

Chronic child maltreatment was defined as "multiple incidents of child maltreatment occurring over a prolonged period of time." (Bromfield, 2005, p.21). The chronic child maltreatment typology (Bromfield, 2005, p.22) was conceptualised within a developmental-ecological framework with developmental perspective on the constructs of abuse and neglect and comprised the following dimensions:

1. *Frequency* - Number of incidents;
2. *Sub-type* - Number of sub-types and categorical classification of the different sub-types (physical abuse, neglect, sexual abuse, emotional abuse and witnessing family violence);

3. *Severity* - Severity of the adult behaviour and severity of harm to the child;
4. *Perpetrators* - Number of perpetrators and relationship of perpetrator to child (intra- or extra-familial); and
5. *Duration* - Period of time over which maltreatment occurred.

In relation to the potential impacts of chronic maltreatment, I proposed the term *cumulative harm* to describe the "increased risk of adverse consequences as harmful events accumulate over time" (Bromfield, 2005, p. 70).

These concepts were translated into child protection policy and practice guidance for identifying cumulative harm in the context of child abuse and neglect (e.g., Bromfield & Higgins, 2005; Bromfield & Miller, 2007; Bromfield, Gillingham and Higgins, 2007), becoming core constructs in child protection practice across Australia.

The term cumulative harm has continued to be applied and developed in research and practice over the last two decades, intertwining the two threads of foundational work into (a) the cumulative impacts of Adverse Childhood Experiences (Felitti et al, 1998) and (b) the cumulative impacts of chronic maltreatment.

This book, *Trauma-Informed and Accumulation-Aware Approaches to Child Protection,* edited by Dr Bryce and Dr Collier takes the concept of cumulative harm forward beyond these initial foundations offering further conceptual clarity and new prevalence data.

Dr Bryce and Dr Collier have for the last 10 years been at the forefront of the academic operationalisation and development of the construct of cumulative harm in research, teaching and practice. Under Dr Bryce and Dr Collier's stewardship *Trauma-Informed and Accumulation-Aware Approaches to Child Protection* brings together a combination of leading and emerging authors in the field of cumulative harm.

Trauma-Informed and Accumulation-Aware Approaches to Child Protection explores the concept of cumulative harm in different contexts, including the family court and education. It expands the concept of cumulative harm from a focus on the cumulative impacts of adversity in childhood to cumulative impacts across the lifespan.

There are few things more rewarding in academia than having an area of research that you have had some part in fostering take on a life of its own. And particularly for applied researchers, to see a theoretical construct grow and evolve, and be applied in difference contexts to make a difference to how we understand and better support those in need. *Trauma-Informed and Accumulation-Aware Approaches to Child Protection* epitomises this experience.

A quarter of a century on from proposing the term cumulative harm to describe the cumulative impacts of childhood adversity, the breadth and depth of the application of the term continues to challenge narrow and episodic framing of people and contexts, and to advance practice with a cumulative lens promoting us to see and consider the whole person, and the totality of their lived experience in context.

I commend *Trauma-Informed and Accumulation-Aware Approaches to Child Protection* for its contribution to broadening the horizons of the application of cumulative harm, and look forward to the future developments catalysed in turn by this edited volume.

Leah Bromfield
Australian Centre for Child Protection, Adelaide University, Austrailia

REFERENCES

Bromfield, L. M. (2005). *Chronic Child Maltreatment in an Australian Statutory Child Protection Sample*. Unpublished Phd thesis, Deakin University, Geelong.

Bromfield, L. M., Gillingham, P., & Higgins, D. J. (2007). Cumulative harm and chronic child maltreatment. *Developing Practice*, *19*, 34–42.

Bromfield, L. M., & Higgins, D. J. (2005). Chronic and isolated maltreatment in a child protection sample. *Family Matters (Melbourne, Vic.)*, *70*, 38–45.

Bromfield, L. M., & Miller, R. (2007). *Specialist Practice Guide: Cumulative Harm*. Victorian Government Department of Human Services.

Felitti, V. J., Anda, R. F., Nordenberg, D., Williamson, D. F., Spitz, A. M., Edwards, V., Koss, M. P., & Marks, J. S. (1998). Relationship of childhood abuse and household dysfunction to many of the leading causes of death in adults. The Adverse Childhood Experiences (ACE) Study. *American Journal of Preventive Medicine*, *14*(4), 245–258. DOI: 10.1016/S0749-3797(98)00017-8 PMID: 9635069

Preface

INTRODUCTION

This book is a true labour of love for the Authors, India and Simone. They have slaved away in the trenches of child protection and welfare for a cumulative (no pun intended) period of five decades. Their collaborative efforts began so long ago that neither of them can truly recall the origins of our partnership as passionate crusaders in the field of cumulative harm and accumulated trauma, nor our joint advocacy for its rightful and authentic implementation in child protection practice. Suffice it to say, this book represents the culmination of more than a decade of shared work to research, explore, interrogate, and implement best practice in addressing cumulative adversity across the lifespan within frontline child protection and welfare contexts.

PURPOSE

Since its public recognition in 1962 (Kempe, Silverman, Steele, Droegemueller & Silver, 1962), child maltreatment has been acknowledged in research and in practice as occurring in either isolated or repeated incidents. Bromfield and Higgins indicate "the majority of children who experience child maltreatment will have multiple incidents of maltreatment over a prolonged period of time" (2005, p.38). The Adverse Childhood Experiences (ACEs) Study concluded that there were significant correlations between adverse childhood experiences and medical, psychological and behavioural issues later in life and the more adverse experiences a child endured the greater the impact on the individual in adulthood (Felitti et al, 1998). The impact of the accumulation of ACEs has been labelled 'cumulative harm' (Bromfield, 2007). Cumulative harm is defined as "a series or pattern of harmful events and experiences that may be historical, or ongoing, with the strong possibility of the risk factors being multiple, inter-related and co-existing over critical developmental periods" (Bromfield, Gillingham & Higgins, 2007, p.1). Gilmore (2010) likens cumulative harm to global warming, in that it is a seemingly intractable problem, involving a culmination of human and environmental factors.

This volume explores the journey researchers and practitioners have taken from historical perspectives of harm to arrive at our current understanding of cumulative harm, including chronic maltreatment and re-victimisation. The valuable and insightful authors contributions will highlight the pervasive impact on the individual, behaviourally, physically and psychologically, across the lifespan and highlight additional considerations such as gender, culture, family law conflict and domestic violence. Finally, the volume will outline trauma informed prevention and intervention approaches to addressing cumulative harm as practitioners and, researchers. This book is unique as it is the only text available which specifically and comprehensively addresses the chronicity of maltreatment and victimization from a diverse range of international and multidisciplinary perspectives.

Rather than tackling the broad and diverse array of topics alone, we have called upon contacts, networks, friends, and colleagues to contribute to this text. They have provided a rich and fertile ground on which a diverse range of topics are uncovered, each within the unique perspective of the author, tempered by the aggregate literature and research. Adopting this approach, we feel that the information not only represents the best practice in each respective authors' field and region, but that it represents a global and often unified approach to deal with issues of accumulated adversity and cumulative harm. We urge the reader to take what they can from each chapter, with the knowledge and understanding that things may be different in their jurisdiction than that of the chapters' author/s. We present this current volume with the complete understanding that certain issues will differ from one location to the next, and remind the reader that concepts, terms, approaches, and legal recourse will be different from one place to the next.

We have been incredibly privileged to collaborate with the authors in this volume, whose work spans a range of international contexts, including Mexico, Singapore, and Australia. Our contributors bring new and novel research which explores cumulative adversity, risk and harm as it pertains to therapeutic practice, reunification, statutory child proection, family law, youth justice, homicide, education, aged care and higher education. However, we are most grateful for the contributions of Professor Leah Bromfield and Professor Daryl Higgins who's research (Bromfield & Higgins, 2005; Bromfield, Gillingham and Higgins, 2007) conceptualised and established our foundational understanding of cumulative harm. To have Professors Bromfield and Higgins contribute their perspectives to this volume was both humbling and exciting, as we truly felt this book would not have been complete without their insights and reflections.

This book seeks to go beyond our current understanding of what constitutes cumulative harm or accumulated risk within the child protection context, to broaden our understanding of the pervasive and far-reaching impacts of accumulation across the lifespan. This work is distinguished from the wider literature in several ways. First, this book seeks to draw attention to often overlooked or newly discovered contexts where accumulated maltreatment is relevant such as to older-care leavers, homicide victimisation, family law proceedings, and higher education and career choice. Second, impact is considered through the lens of both victimology and perpetration, focusing on chronicity, post-traumatic outcomes, and lifespan development. Third, the contributions included in this volume are recent, many of which report recent findings and evidence from exciting and controversial studies. Fourth, although empirical scholarship will inform much of the content, there will be applied material from experts and practitioners in the field - which is a significant divergence from literature most commonly provided by textbooks and academic journals. Additionally, the text provides perspectives of the international experience, rather than those of one country or jurisdiction.

CHAPTER OVERVIEWS

Chapter 1 summarises the findings from the Australian Child Maltreatment Study (ACMS), which found that 39.4% of Australians experienced multiple forms of abuse or neglect during childhood and includes that multi-type maltreatment (MTM) is a pervasive and deeply consequential reality for a significant portion of the population rather than a rare anomaly.

Chapter 2 proposes eight guiding principles for child protection practice when working with children affected by cumulative maltreatment, emphasizing long-term healing over crisis containment. Key principles include investing in workforce capability, embedding trauma-informed responses, and conducting comprehensive, functional assessments. The Author argues that while cumulative maltreatment is a globally pervasive and damaging reality for children in the welfare system, it is not a deterministic path to failure; rather, healing is possible when systems move beyond episodic interventions to provide sustained, deliberate, and evidence-informed support.

Chapter 3 critically reflects on the "shoebox activity" used in the *Name.Narrate. Navigate* program to build empathy in young people and practitioners. It identifies a disruption in expectations, where female-identifying participants often expressed intense judgment and hostility toward the "fancy-lady" shoebox, constructing narratives of maternal failure and alcoholism. The Authors suggest these responses may be adaptive survival strategies shaped by cumulative harm, where empathy is transformed into hypervigilant threat detection or “empathic resistance”. It argues that empathy is a socially constructed and gendered phenomenon influenced by social distance and the burden of emotional labour.

Chapter 4 critically examines the reunification process in Australia, characterizing it as a “wicked issue” that is frequently under-resourced despite being a statutory priority. It proposes a tripartite model consisting of Reunification Intervention, Reunification Therapy, and Post-Reunification Services to support families with complex needs. The Chapter highlights that failed reunifications—which occur in approximately 20% of cases—further compound the cumulative harm experienced by children through repeated displacements. It advocates for a specialized post-reunification support system similar to the NDIS, providing individualized, long-term care to prevent the “revolving door” of child removal.

In **Chapter 5,** the Author introduces the Cumulative Experiences Index–Culturally Responsive (CEI-CR), a tool designed to measure the unique patterns of harm faced by Aboriginal and Torres Strait Islander children. It explains that First Nations children are 11 times more likely to be in out-of-home care, often due to the layered weight of intergenerational trauma and systemic disadvantage. The CEI-CR incorporates domains like racism, geographic isolation, and disconnection from culture as specific forms of harm that standard Western tools overlook. The Chapter emphasizes a restorative, strengths-based focus that recognizes collective resilience nurtured through connections to kin, community, and Country.

Chapter 6 applies betrayal trauma theory to the study of ACEs, emphasizing that harm perpetrated by a trusted caregiver carries unique and more severe consequences due to the child's innate dependence. It introduces the concept of “betrayal blindness,” an adaptive cognitive mechanism where victims minimize or forget abuse to preserve essential attachment relationships. The Chapter extends this theory to institutional and cultural contexts, exploring how systems like the military, religious groups, and judicial systems can harm members through active commission or passive omission. It proposes group-based community interventions that integrate caregivers' own trauma histories to disrupt the intergenerational transmission of betrayal.

Chapter 7 presents a scoping review of explanatory theories for intergenerational child maltreatment, identifying attachment theory as the most dominant framework in the literature. It categorizes various perspectives, including physiological development (neurobiology), learning (social learning), and systems (ecological and current adversity). The Chapter notes a shift over time from psychodynamic theories to epigenetic and bioscientific models, reflecting broader societal changes. It highlights a significant lack of research on fathers and reflective practice, while calling for more culturally sensitive models that go beyond Western dyadic views of attachment.

Chapter 8 introduces the field of Developmental and Life-Course Victimology, which studies victimization as a dynamic process shaped by ecological and transactional dimensions. It explores the "Cycle of Violence" and intergenerational transmission, emphasizing the need to distinguish between findings of general effects versus subtype-specific mechanisms of continuity. The Chapter identifies key components such as victimization propensity, developmental cascades, and post-traumatic growth, which explain why some trajectories persist while others break the cycle. It calls for prospective longitudinal studies to better understand the permutation from victim to perpetrator and to develop more effective de-victimization interventions.

In **Chapter 9**, Authors focus on the impact of parental incarceration on children, who are often considered the "forgotten victims" of crime. It details how parental imprisonment compounds existing adversities like poverty and abuse, acting as a criminogenic risk factor that fuels intergenerational cycles of criminalization. The Chapter examines sentencing practices in South Australia, noting that while judicial officers have considerable discretion, the human rights of children are rarely explicitly considered in court. It advocates for trauma-informed, child-centric sentencing responses to break intergenerational cycles and mitigate the long-term developmental trauma experienced by these children.

The final **Chapter 10** explores the cumulative impact of Adverse Childhood Experiences (ACEs) on justice-involved youth, highlighting that over half of these individuals experience more than one ACE. It contrasts the reality of structural disadvantage—such as poverty and single-parent households—with the punitive populist narratives often promoted by media and politicians. The Chapter details how trauma disrupts brain development, leading to hypervigilance and impaired decision-making that often manifests as violent or repeat offending. It suggests that youth-justice agencies should adopt Trauma-Informed Care (TIC) and developmental crime prevention strategies rather than relying on short-term, punitive "tough-on-crime" measures.

CONCLUSION

There is no book without authors, so we acknowledge first and foremost the contributions of our authors, it takes a significant effort to contribute to a book such as this and their expertise, insight, creativity, and generosity is so very appreciated, and we thank them most sincerely. We thank our publisher, IGI Global for their support, guidance patience, and for taking a chance on this passion project. They may never know the impact they have had at a grassroots level, for vulnerable families but enabling us to create this work, for practitioners to read and consume, in order to improve their service delivery.

We thank our families and loved ones who have taken this journey alongside us, and our colleagues, which have reviewed, proofread and given their insights to this book and to the perspectives contained within.

Finally, we thank you, our readers. Without those who are willing to read our words and consider our thoughts and perspectives, the important research, theory and lived experiences contained in this volume cannot continue to grow, to be implemented, to be challenged, and to continue to gain the momentum needed to truly service our vulnerable children and families in child protection practice.

We suspect that you, as researchers, professionals and practitioners interested in informing and impacting child maltreatment in our lifetime, have more than a scholarly and practical interest in this issue. We suspect that you have the heart to protect children from those who both intentionally, and unintentionally, harm them. We suspect that your intention is to reach beyond the classroom, office, and the pages of this book to improve outcomes for children. We suspect that you want to extend your influence beyond your own children, or the children of others you hold dear. We suspect that you recognise the right of all children to live in safe, nurturing, and healthy environments. We hope this book contributes to your journey.

Introduction

PURPOSE STATEMENT

No book that seeks to explore nuanced and complex issues such as cumulative adversity and the accumulation of trauma and maltreatment in children and its impact across the lifespan would be complete without an introduction to the topic itself, before delving into the depths of its application to the many and varied contexts our valuable countries have considered. This brief introduction will summarise the various research frameworks that conceptualize cumulative harm and emphasize the importance of considering cumulative adversity and accumulation in child protection practice.

DEFINING CUMULATIVE ADVERSITY AND HARM

Cumulative harm is conceptualized as a qualitatively distinct, chronic, and escalating pattern of circumstances and events in a child's life. Rather than focusing on single incidents, this framework emphasizes the long-term developmental consequences of sustained maltreatment. Bromfield and colleagues (2007) defined cumulative harm in their foundational work on the topic as "a series or pattern of harmful events and experiences that may be historical, or ongoing, with the strong possibility of the risk factors being multiple, inter-related and co-existing over critical developmental periods" (p.1). Cumulative adversity is often ambiguous, insidious, and invisible, frequently failing to reach the legal thresholds for intervention in systems designed to respond to acute, one-off incidents. This sustained exposure diminishes a child's natural resilience and reduces their capacity to psychologically cope as the frequency, duration, and severity of the adversity manifest ongoingly. Coronial inquests in Australia have highlighted that this accumulation of "low-level" risks often leads to fatal outcomes because the totality of the harm is not recognized by protective systems (Bryce, 2024).

Accumulative adversity (often discussed in the context of "cumulative adversity" or frameworks like ACEs) refers to the clustering and count of various stressors in a child's environment. It is often understood through a dose-response lens, where the total number of adverse experiences—including both direct maltreatment and household dysfunction—is linked to long-term health and psychosocial outcomes. Accumulated adversity encompasses a broad range of experiences beyond direct abuse, such as environmental adversities (e.g., living with someone who misuses substances, experiencing neighbourhood violence, or facing economic hardship). Child maltreatment, neglect, adversity and victimisation rarely occur in isolation from these broader family and community-level adversities. For example, young people experiencing "multi-type maltreatment" alongside environmental adversities like parental mental illness are at a significantly higher risk for maladaptive behaviours, such as problematic alcohol use.

KEY DISTINCTIONS

While the terms are often used interchangeably, the research suggest a nuanced distinction in their application:

Cumulative Harm is frequently used as a practitioner and systemic lens to critique incident-based reporting and advocate for a more holistic assessment of a child's chronic experience of maltreatment.

Accumulative Adversity is often used in public health and research contexts (like the ACE framework) to screen for population-level risk based on the total "dose" or count of different types of stressors.

To distinguish the two, imagine a hiking trail. Accumulative adversity is like the total weight of the items in your backpack—the more items (adversities) you add, the harder the journey becomes. Cumulative harm is the gradual wear and tear on your body caused by carrying that weight over many miles; it isn't just about how much you are carrying right now, but how the sustained pressure has weakened your joints and exhausted your spirit over time.

CHARACTERISTICS OF ACCUMULATED ADVERSITY

Accumulated adversity is characterized by the clustering and compounding of diverse stressors that occur throughout a child's life. Rather than focusing on a single event, this concept highlights the dose relationship between the total number of adverse experiences and long-term negative outcomes.

The key characteristics of accumulated adversity include:

1. Multiplicity and Variety of Stressors
    - Diverse Categories of Harm: It involves a multiplicity of maltreatment types, including physical, sexual, and emotional abuse, along with medical, supervisory, and emotional neglect.
    - Household Dysfunction: Beyond direct abuse, it encompasses environmental stressors such as parental substance misuse, mental ill-health, criminality, and incarceration.
    - Expanded Social Context: Research now includes factors outside the family home, such as peer victimisation, community violence, racism, and systemic marginalisation, which contribute to the total trauma dose.
2. High Intensity and Chronicity
    - Frequency and Duration: Accumulated adversity is defined by the frequency and chronicity of negative experiences over an extended period.
    - Patterns of Behaviour: It is often recognized as a pattern of behaviour or a series of persistent negative experiences rather than an isolated acute incident.
    - Direct and Indirect Impact: The harm can be direct and indirect, seen and unseen, affecting a child's wellbeing even when the incidents do not meet specific legal thresholds for intervention.
3. Progressive Erosion of Wellbeing
    - Diminished Resilience: The sustained nature of these adversities diminishes any resilience a child has, reducing their ability to psychologically cope as the stressors manifest ongoingly.
    - Clinical Qualities: Cumulative adversity is characterized by the qualities of persistent *dysfunction, dysregulation, disadvantage, and disconnection* (Bryce et al., 2023). Bryce and colleagues referred to this as "quantity taking on a quality of its own".
    - Increased Vulnerability: The accumulation leads to higher risks of placement breakdowns, school disengagement, suicidal ideation, and high-level risk-taking behaviours.
4. Predictive Power
    - Dose-Response Lens: The total count or "dose" of these adversities is a stronger predictor of mortality and morbidity than any single type of abuse in isolation.
    - Fatal Consequences: Coronial evidence (Bryce, 2024) suggests that when systems fail to recognize the accumulation of risk, the results can

be fatal, with many children dying shortly after their cases were closed due to a focus on single incidents rather than the total accumulated harm.

Think of accumulated adversity like a heavy snowfall on a roof. A single snowflake (one incident) is weightless and harmless. However, as the snow continues to fall and accumulate without being cleared, the total weight creates a sustained pressure that eventually causes the structure beneath it to buckle and collapse. It is not the final snowflake that causes the damage, but the total dose of weight gathered over time.

RESEARCH FRAMEWORKS WHICH CONCEPTUALIZE CUMULATIVE HARM AND ACCUMULATED ADVERSITY

Various research frameworks conceptualise cumulative harm by moving away from viewing abuse as isolated incidents, instead focusing on the overlapping and escalating nature of adversity. These frameworks—Adverse Childhood Experiences (ACEs), Multi-Type Maltreatment (MTM), Polyvictimization, and Cumulative Harm—share the premise that harm rarely occurs in isolation and that its accumulation leads to more severe long-term consequences.

Each framework offers a different lens through which to view the patterns of childhood adversity:

Adverse Childhood Experiences (ACEs): This framework by Felitti and Colleagues (1998) uses a dose-response lens, linking the total number of adverse experiences (maltreatment and household dysfunction) to long-term health outcomes. It typically uses a simple score count to screen for population-level risk.

Multi-Type Maltreatment (MTM): MTM (Higgins & McCabe, 2004) focuses specifically on the co-occurrence and interaction of the five primary types of child maltreatment (physical, sexual, and emotional abuse, neglect, and exposure to domestic violence). It is used to identify common "constellations" of abuse and how these combinations uniquely affect psychosocial outcomes.

Polyvictimization: This model by Finkelhor and Colleagues (2007) broadens the scope to include victimisation across multiple contexts, such as school, peer groups, and the community. It defines high-risk individuals as those exposed to four or more distinct harm types, though it often lacks specific detail on the severity or timing of these events.

Chronic Maltreatment Typology: In their Chronic Maltreatment Study, Bromfield and Higgins (2005) identified that 65 percent of participants, gathered from a child protection sample, had experienced chronic maltreatment, with multiple, interrelated issues. Bromfield and Higgins (2005) indicated that many children who experience child maltreatment will have multiple incidents of maltreatment over a prolonged period. Bromfield and Higgins proposed the Chronic Child Maltreatment Typology – which included the following five dimensions: frequency– number of incidents; sub-type– number of sub-types and categorical classification of the different sub-types (physical abuse, neglect, sexual abuse, emotional abuse and witnessing family violence); severity – severity of the adult behaviour, and severity of harm to the child; perpetrators– number of per perpetrators and relationship of perpetrator to child (intra- or extra-familial); and duration– period of time over which maltreatment occurred.

Cumulative Harm: This framework conceptualised by Bromfield, Gillingham and Higgins (2007) reframed adversity as a qualitatively distinct, chronic, and escalating pattern of circumstances and events. Unlike incident-based models, it emphasizes the “existence of compounded experiences of multiple episodes of abuse or 'layers' of neglect” that diminish a child's sense of safety over time.

Dysfunction, Dysregulation, Disadvantage and Disconnection: In their 2023 study, Bryce and Colleagues contributed new knowledge to the definitions and typologies of child abuse, neglect and adversity, and draw on empirical evidence to broaden the scope of what constitutes childhood maltreatment. Their findings catalyse a paradigm shift that positioned accumulation as a distinct harm type and clarified the qualities which embody cumulative harm: persistent dysfunction, dysregulation, disadvantage and disconnection.

LONG-TERM CONSEQUENCES OF ACCUMULATION

Accumulation of harm, rather than any single event, is often the primary driver of negative outcomes (Bryce, 2004; Harris et al., 2006; Moore et al., 2024)

Mental Health Disorders: High maltreatment intensity—defined by the frequency, duration, severity, and number of perpetrators—is the most critical risk factor for mental disorders, including generalised anxiety, major depressive disorder, and PTSD. Research shows that when care-experienced individuals and non-care-experienced individuals are matched on maltreatment intensity, their odds of having a mental health disorder are equivalent, suggesting the intensity of the abuse itself is the catalyst for poor mental health.

Maladaptive Behaviours: Multi-type maltreatment is significantly associated with problematic alcohol use in young adults. This risk is further compounded by environmental adversities, such as living with someone who misuses substances or experiencing neighbourhood violence, which may normalise maladaptive coping strategies.

***Systemic Failure and Mortality*:** Coronial inquests highlight that a failure to recognise patterns of cumulative harm can have fatal consequences. These inquests reveal that repeated exposure to "low-level" neglect and abuse often goes unaddressed by systems focused on single, acute incidents, leading to a multiplicity of maltreatment types that ultimately contribute to child deaths.

***Resilience and Development*:** Sustained harm can cause persistent dysfunction, dysregulation, and disconnection. It diminishes a child's natural resilience, reducing their capacity to psychologically cope as the frequency and severity of adversity manifest ongoingly.

VULNERABLE POPULATIONS

Patterns of cumulative harm are not distributed equally across the population. Australians with gender and sexuality diverse identities are substantially more likely to experience MTM than heterosexual or cisgender individuals. Furthermore, children in out-of-home care (OOHC) typically report significantly higher maltreatment intensity, including earlier onset and more frequent exposure, than the general population.

To understand the difference between incident-based harm and cumulative harm, imagine a brick wall. An incident-based perspective looks at a single heavy brick falling and causing immediate damage. A cumulative harm perspective recognizes that even if each individual brick is light, the constant, steady stacking of bricks eventually causes the entire structure beneath it to collapse under the sustained weight.

THE IMPORTANCE OF CONSIDERING ACCUMULATION IN CHILD PROTECTION PRACTICE

Considering accumulation of adversity and cumulative harm is critical because it moves beyond viewing abuse and neglect as isolated events and instead recognizes it as a qualitatively distinct, chronic, and escalating pattern that fundamentally reshapes a child's development and long-term wellbeing. The importance of this shift in perspective is evidenced across several key areas:

***Preventing Systemic Failure and Mortality*:** Coronial inquests into child deaths (Bryce, 2024) frequently highlight that a failure to recognize patterns of cumulative harm can have fatal consequences. Systems that focus only on "acute" incidents often miss the "ambiguous, insidious and often invisible" nature of chronic neglect or low-level abuse. Analysis of 30 coronial inquests (Bryce, 2024) revealed that the multiplicity and complexity of maltreatment sustained over an extended period contributed directly to the ultimate fatality of the children involved.

Missed Thresholds: Many cases are closed during early intake or investigation because individual incidents do not meet the legal "threshold" for intervention, even when a child has been the subject of numerous notifications (Bryce, 2024; Bryce et al., 2024).

Accurately Identifying Mental Health Risks and Understanding Maladaptive Coping Mechanisms: The sources indicate that maltreatment intensity—defined by frequency, duration, severity, and the number of perpetrators—is the most critical risk factor for mental health disorders. Considering cumulative harm allows researchers to understand the interconnected pathways to problematic behaviours in young adults, such as substance misuse.

Predictive Power: Research shows that the intensity of the accumulation, and the presence of an accumulation of risk factors, rather than any single type of abuse or risk, is what drives clinical thresholds for poor lifespan outcomes, including mental and physical health (Mackenzie et al., 2011).

Resilience Erosion: Sustained exposure to harm diminishes any resilience a child has, reducing their capacity to psychologically cope as the frequency and severity of the adversity manifest ongoingly.

Social Learning: In environments of cumulative harm, maladaptive responses to stress often become normalized or serve as a social currency, making it harder to disrupt these patterns without a holistic understanding of the child's environment.

Guiding Effective Therapeutic Interventions: Focusing on the accumulation of adversity, risk and harm provides a more nuanced clinical and relational guide for healing (Harris et al., 2026). When caregivers and practitioners understand a child's unique 'maltreatment profile' (Harris et al., 2026) they can more accurately interpret adaptive stress responses and respond with greater empathy and efficacy. Recognizing cumulative harm encourages a shift toward contextual safeguarding. This means looking beyond 'bad actors' to the wider cultures and environments—such as schools, peer groups, and online spaces—where harm can accumulate (Harris et al., 2026)

To understand why cumulative harm is so important, think of a dam. An incident-based perspective only looks for a single massive flood that might crest over the top. A cumulative harm perspective, however, looks for the hundreds of tiny cracks forming over years. While no single crack causes the dam to break, the accumulation of those small fractures eventually causes the entire structure to fail, often with little warning to those who weren't looking at the pattern.

An accumulation of adversity and maltreatment, in essence, erodes an individual's sense of wellbeing, of self, and their capacity to endure. As Finkelhor and colleagues (2007) highlighted, for some, "victimization is a condition, rather than an event" (p.9). Trauma is most often cumulative and individuals, especially children, rarely experience just one or several separate incidents of victimization but rather endure repeated and multiple victimizations across different contexts (e.g., physical abuse, sexual abuse, emotional neglect, witnessing violence). This persistent and pervasive exposure to adversity, violence and maltreatment creates an enduring state—a "condition"—that fundamentally shapes an individual's development, worldview, and mental health, as opposed to a single "event" from which one might recover in a linear fashion.

Research to date, and that espoused in this volume, advocates for a fundamental shift from incident-based responses toward a comprehensive, trauma-transformative framework that actively reshapes systems, relationships, and practices to promote healing rather than mere awareness. The literature proposes a multi-layered approach to intervention and prevention, which addresses the entire ecology of a child's life. These proposals encompass systemic reforms, contextual safeguarding, and population-wide strategies. An approach which meaningfully, authentically and sustainably addresses accumulation of adversity in child protection and welfare practice requires systemic reforms to child protection thresholds, data collection, and practitioner training, using maltreatment intensity as a clinical and relational guide to provide tailored supports for children—especially those in out-of-home care—before crises emerge. Effective prevention necessitates coordinated, cross-sectoral collaboration among health, education, justice, and community services to address the clustering of direct maltreatment and environmental adversities, such as parental substance misuse. Furthermore, a contextual safeguarding lens is proposed to extend protection beyond adult-perpetrated harm to include peer environments, schools, and digital spaces, while rights-based, child-centred strategies prioritize amplifying the voices of children in policy and decision-making processes (Harris et al., 2026). Finally, interventions should strive to promote Positive Childhood Experiences (PCEs)—such as internal and external perceived safety and support—to buffer against the long-term impacts of adversity, alongside rehabilitative reforms in the youth justice system to prevent the criminalization of traumatized youth (Bryce, 2024; Moore et al., 2024).

Proposed interventions are moving from being a "firefighter"—who only shows up once a major fire (an acute incident) has already broken out—to being a "town planner or city architect". A town planner/architect looks at the whole landscape, ensuring materials are fire-resistant (resilience building), building codes are updated (threshold reform), and that the entire neighbourhood environment (contextual safeguarding) is designed to prevent a spark from ever turning into a disaster.

REFERENCES

Bromfield, L. M., Gillingham, P., & Higgins, D. J. (2007). Cumulative harm and chronic child maltreatment. *Developing Practice: The Child. Youth and Family Work Journal*, (19), 34–42.

Bromfield, L. M., & Higgins, D. J. (2005). Chronic and isolated maltreatment in a child protection sample. *Family Matters (Melbourne, Vic.)*, (70), 38–45.

Bryce, I. (2024). Revisiting cumulative harm: Reflecting on new research insights, legislative-developments and coronial evidence as a road map for next steps. *Children Australia*, *46*(2), 1–12. DOI: 10.61605/cha_3025

Bryce, I., Beccaria, G., McIlveen, P., & Du Preez, J. (2023). When quantity takes on a quality of its own: A retrospective exploration of the lived experience of cumulative harm. *Child Abuse Review*, *32*(4), e2800. DOI: 10.1002/car.2800

Bryce, I., Collier, S., Harris, L., Higgins, D., & Toohey, J. (2024). Measuring accumulation: Constructing a tool for evaluating cumulative harm in children engaged with an intensive family support service. *Child Abuse Review*, *33*(5), e2897. DOI: 10.1002/car.2897

Felitti, V. J., Anda, R. F., Nordenberg, D., Williamson, D. F., Spitz, A. M., Edwards, V., & Marks, J. S. (1998). Relationship of childhood abuse and household dysfunction to many of the leading causes of death in adults: The Adverse Childhood Experiences (ACE) Study. *American Journal of Preventive Medicine*, *14*(4), 245–258. DOI: 10.1016/S0749-3797(98)00017-8 PMID: 9635069

Finkelhor, D., Ormrod, R. K., & Turner, H. A. (2007). Poly-victimization: A neglected component in child victimization. *Child Abuse & Neglect*, *31*(1), 7–26. DOI: 10.1016/j.chiabu.2006.06.008 PMID: 17224181

Harris, L. G., Rattambige, D., Hunt, G. R., & Higgins, D. J. (2026). Accumulation of violence and victimisation: Why measuring broadly and accounting for different harm types matters. *Current Opinion in Psychology*, •••, 102260. DOI: 10.1016/j.copsyc.2025.102260 PMID: 41539030

Higgins, D. J., & McCabe, M. P. (2000). Multi-type maltreatment and the long-term adjustment of adults. *Child Abuse Review*, *9*(1), 6–18. DOI: 10.1002/(SICI)1099-0852(200001/02)9:1<6::AID-CAR579>3.0.CO;2-W

Moore, T., Vicary, D., & Bessell, S. (2024). The United Nations Convention on the Rights of the Child: Reflections on Australia's progress and challenges. *Children Australia*, *46*(2), 1–7. DOI: 10.61605/cha_3048

Chapter 1
Prevalence and Impact of Overlap in Different Forms of Child Abuse and Neglect in Australia: The Story of Multi-Type Maltreatment

Daryl John Higgins
https://orcid.org/0000-0003-0268-8243
Australian Catholic University, Australia

ABSTRACT

The concept of multi-type maltreatment, developed over 30 years ago, gained prominence through the Australian Child Maltreatment Study. It found that 39.4% of Australians aged 16+ experienced multiple forms of maltreatment, with nearly a quarter experiencing three or more types. Analyses show multi-type maltreatment is a strong predictor of mental illness and health risk behaviours—more so than single-type maltreatment. It's linked to diverse gender and sexuality, mental disorders, substance use, intimate partner violence, out-of-home care, justice system involvement, and increased health service use and costs. Odds of adverse outcomes range from 2.7× (depression) to 6.2× (cannabis dependence). Key childhood adversities—parental separation, illness, substance misuse, and economic hardship—double the risk. Controlling for co-occurring harms reveals sexual and emotional abuse as most consistently linked to negative outcomes. These findings highlight the urgent need for early intervention and comprehensive support.

DOI: 10.4018/979-8-3373-4064-7.ch001

INTRODUCTION

Child maltreatment is a pervasive and multifaceted issue that affects individuals across all demographics and life stages. Academic interest in child maltreatment—the abuse or neglect of children by parents or others with power over or responsibility for their care and wellbeing—has been gathering momentum since Kempe and colleagues' seminal 1962 article on "battered child syndrome" in the *Journal of the American Medical Association* (see Table 1). While this a well-known and often cited seminal moment in the history of child maltreatment, in this chapter, I explore the history and role of a much less celebrated concept of multi-type maltreatment, drawing on data from a recent large nationally representative dataset to highlight the overlapping nature of child maltreatment experiences and their cumulative impact on health, wellbeing, and social outcomes.

Table 1. A brief synopsis of the focus of research on child maltreatment

Era	Key advances in child maltreatment research
1960s	Kempe et al. (1962) coined the term 'Battered Child Syndrome' signalling the rise of the contemporary child maltreatment research movement.
1970s	Child maltreatment research focused primarily on physical abuse and, to a lesser extent, on neglect.
1980s	Second-wave feminism's focus on rape and sexual assault influenced the focus of attention on to child sexual abuse and paedophilia.
1990s	Many began to consider the witnessing of family violence as an independent subtype of abuse. Developmental psychopathology focused attention on the co-occurrence of different types of child maltreatment.
2000s	Greater attention was directed towards understanding the nature, prevalence and consequences of psychological (or emotional) maltreatment. The Adverse Childhood Experiences (ACEs) study that explored links between childhood abuse, neglect, and other adversities like household dysfunction, and adult health problems starts to gain traction in the clinical field, focusing attention on the issue of accumulation of adversity and its impact on wellbeing. Although understanding of the different forms of abuse and neglect increased markedly in this period, attempts to identify risk factors and outcomes specific to individual forms of maltreatment were largely unsuccessful.
2010s	Understanding the patterns of overlap and integrating different types of adversity and models to understand the unique and shared contributions to outcomes became a more widespread focus.
2020s	The concept of multi-type maltreatment is a major area of focus of the Australian Child Maltreatment study and its findings about prevalence and impact of child abuse and neglect in the first major representative study of the Australian population's exposure to all five types.

Sources: Felitti et al., 1998; Herrenkohl & Herrenkohl, 2009; Higgins, 2004a, 2004b James, 2000; Miller-Perrin & Perrin, 2007

Recently, an important shift in the focus of child maltreatment research has been the recognition of the interrelatedness of childhood experiences of victimisation, including abuse and neglect from parents and carers. Empirical evidence is now growing that points to the fact that experiences of different forms of child maltreatment seldom occur in isolation. In fact, evidence now suggests most individuals with a history of child abuse or neglect have been exposed to two or more subtypes (Arata, Langhinrichsen-Rohling, Bowers, & O'Farrill-Swails, 2005; Higgins & McCabe, 2000a; Higgins et al. 2023; Ney, Fung, & Wickett, 1994). As Price-Robertson, Higgins, and Vassallo (2013) explained:

> *"Indeed, some individual acts of violence against children involve multiple forms of maltreatment. For example, an adult who sexually abuses a child may also hit them (physical abuse) and belittle them (emotional abuse). There is also evidence to suggest that broader experiences of victimisation tend to cumulate for certain individuals or in certain environments. For instance, children who have been maltreated in a family context may be more susceptible than others to peer violence or exposure to crime, while those who have been sexually abused may be more susceptible than others to re-victimisation" (p. 1)*

A pioneer in resilience research, Garmezy (1991), emphasized how multiple risk factors—especially in disadvantaged or maltreated children—could combine to produce poor outcomes. Similarly, in her longitudinal studies (e.g., the Kauai Longitudinal Study), Werner (1996) observed that children exposed to multiple risk factors (poverty, family instability, maltreatment) were more likely to develop behavioural and emotional problems. Sameroff then formalized the concept with his "Cumulative Risk Model" in the 1980s. Sameroff and colleagues (1993) argued that the number of risk factors (rather than the specific nature of any one risk) is the best predictor of developmental outcomes. This theory is foundational in developmental psychopathology and remains influential in understanding how multiple adversities, including multi-type maltreatment, predict later difficulties.

The core idea of cumulative risk theories or models is that risk factors don't act in isolation: the more risks a person experiences, the more likely negative outcomes become. Each type of maltreatment (e.g., physical abuse, emotional neglect) adds a layer of developmental risk. These risks accumulate, creating a compounding burden that overwhelms coping systems, resulting in greater risk of developing psychopathology, substance abuse, and poor health outcomes. Similarly, the central idea behind Developmental Trauma Theory developed by van der Kolk (2005) is that repeated, interpersonal trauma during childhood disrupts normal developmental processes. When multiple maltreatment types occur—especially in the caregiving environment—they interfere with attachment formation, emotional regulation, and cognitive and identity development, which in turn contribute to higher vulnerability to outcomes such as complex PTSD, dissociation, and identity disturbances.

Alongside this shift, has been the growing recognition in the fields of traumatology and psychiatry that traditional mental health diagnoses often do not adequately capture the effects of chronic and/or multiple types of victimisations. *Complex trauma* and *cumulative harm* are both popular models that account for complexity in traumatic outcomes.

HISTORY OF INTERSECTING ADVERSITIES RESEARCH

There are several researchers who have had an important direct or indirect influence in the early development of concepts relating to overlap or intersections between maltreatment and adversity types and the importance of this conceptually for understanding impacts and addressing the consequences of harm, as well as the role of statutory child protection services in detecting and responding to harm.

Since the 1990s, Dante Cicchetti and colleagues have been prominent in conceptualizing developmental psychopathology and the co-occurrence of maltreatment types (see Cicchetti & Cohen, 2015). Their work has emphasized that children often experience multiple adversities, and these should be studied in relation to developmental outcomes. Similarly, early empirical work by Wolf and McGee (1994) showed the overlap between maltreatment types and their combined effects on mental health. McGee's work demonstrated that multi-type maltreatment is the norm, not the exception. Daro (2022) and researchers at Chapin Hall also contributed to policy-related frameworks that acknowledged the complexity of maltreatment experiences.

A leading figure in advancing the understanding of how children experience and are affected by multiple forms of maltreatment, Todd Herrenkohl's work has consistently emphasized the importance of recognizing the co-occurrence of abuse types—such as physical, emotional, and sexual abuse, as well as neglect and exposure to domestic violence—and the cumulative impact these experiences have on developmental outcomes. In their seminal paper, Herrenkohl and Herrenkohl (2009) argued that failure to account for the overlap among maltreatment types can lead to an incomplete and potentially misleading picture of a child's trauma history, thereby compromising both research validity and clinical assessment.

Herrenkohl's research also underscores the methodological challenges in measuring multi-type maltreatment, advocating for improved construct validity to ensure more accurate and consistent findings across studies. His work with the Lehigh Longitudinal Study has provided robust empirical evidence linking cumulative victimisation and life stress to long-term outcomes such as adult antisocial behaviour, substance use, and mental health problems (Herrenkohl et al., 2017). These findings have informed both policy and practice, reinforcing the need for trauma-informed, developmentally sensitive approaches in child protection and intervention services.

Three main frameworks have been developed to better understand and measure this interrelatedness: ACEs, polyvictimization and multi-type maltreatment.

ADVERSE CHILDHOOD EXPERIENCES (ACES)

Adverse Childhood Experiences (ACEs) research began with the landmark CDC-Kaiser Permanente study by Felitti et al. (1998). This seminal study, involving over 17,000 participants, revealed a strong, graded relationship between the number of adverse experiences in childhood—such as abuse, neglect, and household dysfunction—and a wide range of negative health and social outcomes in adulthood. The findings fundamentally shifted the understanding of how early life stressors contribute to long-term physical and mental health, catalyzing a global movement toward trauma-informed care and prevention strategies (Felitti et al., 1998).

Since then, ACEs research has expanded significantly, integrating insights from neuroscience, epigenetics, and public health. Hamai and Felitti (2022) have emphasized the cumulative, dose-response nature of ACEs and their intergenerational impacts, while others have critiqued the original study's limitations, including its narrow operationalization of adversity and lack of diversity in the sample (McEwen & Gregerson, 2019). The ACEs framework has also been criticized for its failure to distinguish between child maltreatment (such as abuse and neglect) and other forms of adversity (like parental separation or household substance use). This conflation is seen as both conceptually and methodologically problematic. Critics have argued that the ACEs framework treats all adversities as equivalent in impact, despite clear differences in their nature, severity, and implications. For example, Fitzgerald and Gallus (2025) contended that child maltreatment is qualitatively distinct from household dysfunction and should not be aggregated into a single cumulative score without considering context, frequency, or developmental timing. They propose that ACEs should be disaggregated into conceptually distinct subcategories to better reflect their unique contributions to developmental outcomes.

The ACEs model has also been criticised for oversimplifying complex social and psychological processes by collapsing diverse experiences into a single score. This can obscure the specific mechanisms through which maltreatment affects health and development (Racine, Bellis, & Madigan, 2025). From a measurement perspective, the ACEs checklist does not account for severity, chronicity, or timing of experiences. For instance, a child who experiences repeated sexual abuse scores the same as one who experiences a single episode of parental divorce—both count as one ACE. This lack of granularity can lead to misclassification and underestimation of risk for those who have experienced severe maltreatment. Moreover, the binary scoring system fails to capture the interactive and cumulative effects of different types of adversity. As a result, the ACEs framework may not adequately inform clinical decision-making or policy interventions that require a more nuanced understanding of trauma exposure. In terms of implications for interventions, particularly to prevent adversity, failure to differentiate between child maltreatment and other adversities may present problems if the source or nature of those harms are fundamentally different (i.e., structural or community, vs familial or parental). The types of public health initiatives that would address many of the forms of child maltreatment (such as population-wide availability of evidence-based parenting supports) may be different to the interventions to address broader adversities (such as school-based or community violence, bullying, or economic adversity or inequality. Despite these critiques, the ACEs framework remains a cornerstone in understanding the lifelong effects of childhood trauma and continues to inform policy, education, and healthcare practices worldwide (Racine, Bellis, & Madigan, 2025).

POLYVICTIMIZATION

In the US, David Finkelhor has been one of the most prominent figures in understanding children's experiences of victimization, and the overlapping nature of these experiences of victimisation. His conceptualisation of polyvictimization—the experience of multiple types of victimisation within a short timeframe—has profoundly reshaped how researchers and practitioners understand cumulative harm. Finkelhor's research has shown that children who experience multiple forms of abuse, neglect, and violence (e.g., sexual abuse, bullying, domestic violence, and community crime) are at significantly greater risk of trauma symptoms than those exposed to a single type of maltreatment (Finkelhor, Ormrod & Turner, 2007).

Through the National Survey of Children's Exposure to Violence (NatSCEV), Finkelhor and colleagues provided the first comprehensive US national data on the prevalence and impact of polyvictimization, revealing that over one in five children experience serious, multiple victimisations in a single year (Finkelhor et al., 2011; Hamby et al., 2010). His integrative framework, Developmental Victimology, offers a developmental lens for understanding how victimisation patterns evolve across childhood and adolescence, and how cumulative harm affects children differently depending on age and context (Finkelhor, 2008). His scholarship continues to be a cornerstone for trauma-informed approaches and systemic reform in child protection.

THE EVOLUTION OF MULTI-TYPE MALTREATMENT RESEARCH IN AUSTRALIA

The study of child maltreatment in Australia has undergone a significant transformation over the past three decades, evolving from a focus on isolated incidents of abuse to a more nuanced understanding of the cumulative and interrelated nature of harm experienced by children that has paralleled, but also in some ways diverged from the focus in North America. Central to this shift has been the development of the concept of multi-type maltreatment. Early work by Higgins and McCabe (1998, 2000a, 2000b, 2001a, 2001b) provided foundational evidence that different forms of maltreatment—such as sexual abuse, physical abuse, psychological maltreatment, neglect, and witnessing family violence—frequently co-occur and that this co-occurrence is associated with significantly greater adjustment difficulties in adulthood. They pioneered the concept of 'multi-type maltreatment', developed a measurement tool (adult retrospective self-report, and parent-report versions) to demonstrate empirically the frequency with which children are exposed to more than one type of harm (sexual, physical and psychological abuse, neglect, exposure to family violence), and that poorer psychological outcomes are associated with experiencing a greater range and severity of maltreatment types.

These foundational studies, using convenience, self-selected samples, nonetheless challenged prevailing assumptions that child maltreatment could be adequately understood by examining single abuse types in isolation—such as sexual abuse or physical abuse. Instead, they demonstrated that children frequently experience multiple forms of maltreatment concurrently, and that the range and severity of these experiences are critical determinants of psychological adjustment in adulthood. Drawing on retrospective self- report data, Higgins and McCabe (1998, 2000, 2001) identified that exposure to two or more types of maltreatment—including sexual abuse, physical abuse, psychological/emotional abuse, neglect, and exposure to domestic violence—was associated with poorer mental health outcomes, including depression, anxiety, post-traumatic stress, and substance misuse. These findings laid the groundwork for a paradigm shift in child maltreatment research, advocating for a cumulative harm framework that considers the interactive and compounding effects of multiple adversities.

To empirically capture the complexity of multi-type maltreatment, Higgins and McCabe (2001a) developed the Comprehensive Child Maltreatment Scale (CCMS)—a psychometrically validated instrument designed to assess the frequency, severity, and co-occurrence of different maltreatment types. The CCMS was unique in its dual-format design, offering both adult retrospective self-report and parent-report versions, thereby enabling researchers and practitioners to assess maltreatment across developmental stages and inform both clinical and policy responses. The CCMS addressed a critical gap in the field: the lack of standardised tools capable of measuring multi-dimensional maltreatment experiences. Its development was informed by earlier work (Higgins & McCabe, 1994), which emphasised the importance of capturing contextual factors such as family violence, parental mental health, and socioeconomic disadvantage. The scale has since been widely used in Australian and international studies, contributing to a more sophisticated understanding of how multi-type maltreatment predicts long-term adjustment.

A series of follow-up studies by Higgins and McCabe (2000a, b, 2001a, b) provided robust evidence confirming that multi-type maltreatment is associated with significantly worse psychological outcomes than single-type maltreatment. These studies found that individuals exposed to multiple forms of abuse and neglect were more likely to experience clinical levels of depression, anxiety, PTSD, and interpersonal difficulties in adulthood. Importantly, the research demonstrated that the number of maltreatment types was a stronger predictor of adjustment than the frequency or severity of any single type. Multi-type maltreatment had additive and interactive effects on adult functioning, and that certain combinations—such as sexual abuse and exposure to domestic violence—were particularly detrimental.

In subsequent publications, Higgins explored the differentiation between maltreatment types and the importance of degree versus type in predicting outcomes (Higgins, 2004a, b). Using cluster analysis, he identified distinct profiles of maltreatment exposure, revealing that children who experienced chronic and severe multi-type maltreatment had markedly worse outcomes than those exposed to isolated or less severe forms. In fact, the best model grouped individuals, not according to which *type* of maltreatment they had experienced—sexual abuse, physical abuse, etc.—but rather it grouped them according to the *degree* to which maltreatment behaviours were reported (higher vs lower levels). Those that were statistically grouped into the high maltreatment cluster had significantly more adjustment problems (such as trauma symptoms, anxiety and depression) than those grouped into the moderate or the low maltreatment clusters.

Then nearly a decade later, a paper compared two of the frameworks that have been developed to better understand and measure this interrelatedness: multi-type maltreatment and polyvictimization (Price-Robertson, Higgins, & Vassallo, 2013). Multi-type maltreatment provides a theoretical framework for the inclusion of five distinct forms of maltreatment: sexual abuse, physical abuse, psychological (or emotional) maltreatment, neglect, and witnessing family violence. In contrast, polyvictimization focuses not only on different forms of child maltreatment from parents and carers, but also on broader experiences of victimisation, such as bullying and exposure to neighbourhood conflicts and community violence. As well as looking at the histories and conceptual overlaps and divergence of these two frameworks and the approach to measurement that have informed them, Price-Robertson et al. also compared these frameworks empirically, to explore their utility in identifying the long-term psychosocial outcomes associated with childhood adversity. What they found was that both have different strengths that may make them preferable for particular forms of research, as outlined in Table 2. They argued that multi-type maltreatment refers specifically to interpersonal harm within caregiving relationships, whereas polyvictimization encompasses a broader range of victimisation experiences, including peer violence and community trauma. This conceptual clarity has informed the development of trauma-informed care models, risk assessment tools, and intervention strategies across child protection, mental health, and education sectors.

Table 2. Key features of research distinguishing between multi-type maltreatment and polyvictimization

Multi-type maltreatment	Polyvictimization
Developed to measure overlap in maltreatment experiences, and account for explainable variation in psychosocial outcomes associated with maltreatment	Developed to measure overlap in victimisation experiences (inc. maltreatment), and account for explainable variation in traumatic symptoms
Detailed measurement of five forms of maltreatment (i.e., sexual abuse, physical abuse, psychological maltreatment, neglect, and witnessing family violence)	Brief measurement of up to 34 forms of victimisation (e.g., conventional crime, child maltreatment, peer and sibling victimisation, sexual victimisation and witnessing and indirect victimisation)
Main measurement tool: Comprehensive Child Maltreatment Scale; adult or parent report; continuous scales	Main measurement tool: Juvenile Victimization Questionnaire; child self-report, caregiver, or adult report; dichotomous measures
Focuses on lifetime prevalence	Often focuses on 12-month incidence, although some recent studies on lifetime prevalence
Tends to focus on long-term psychosocial outcomes (e.g., internalising and externalising behaviour problems)	Tends to focus on short-term trauma symptoms (e.g., child anxiety, depressive symptoms and anger/aggression)

Source: Price-Robertson, Higgins, and Vassallo (2013).

CUMULATIVE HARM

Research led by Bromfield and colleagues has also played a seminal role in progressing the ideas of multi-type maltreatment, with a particular focus on chronic maltreatment and cumulative harm – extending it to the work of statutory child protection services (Bromfield & Higgins, 2005). In such contexts, there are numerous challenges in accurately and comprehensively identifying and responding to harm from chronic low-level abuse and neglect, that accumulates over time (Bromfield & Miller, 2012). This work highlighted the limitations of statutory child protection data in capturing the full spectrum of maltreatment experiences (Bromfield & Higgins, 2004) and called for improved measurement strategies that reflect the complexity and interrelatedness of abuse types. Reliance on administrative data obscures the true prevalence and impact of multi-type maltreatment and advocated for population-based surveys and multi-informant approaches to enhance data quality and utility.

To overcome these challenges, Bromfield's work has led to legislative reforms that direct the focus of statutory workers in their risk assessment processes way from simply looking at a discrete event, but to look at the accumulation of harm over a child's life. Her contributions have helped embed cumulative harm as a central concept in Australian child protection discourse. Her research has been used to call for reform to child protection systems, advocating for improved assessment frameworks that account for the frequency, severity, and duration of harm. Her research has highlighted the limitations of traditional definitions of maltreatment and called for a broader conceptualisation that includes chronic neglect, emotional abuse, and systemic disadvantage, and the cumulative harm from chronic exposure to child maltreatment – even if individual acts do not themselves meet the threshold (Bromfield, Gillingham & Higgins, 2007). Bromfield's work has also informed practice resources such as the Victorian Government's resource for its workers: the *Cumulative Harm Specialist Practice Resource* (Bromfield & Miller, 2012). It provides guidance for frontline child protection workers in identifying and responding to accumulation of harm over time.

Bryce and colleagues have also been instrumental in reframing cumulative harm not merely because of repeated incidents, but as a distinct form of trauma with its own typology and implications (Bryce & Collier, 2022; Bryce et al., 2024). Bryce argues that chronic exposure to adversity—across multiple domains such as abuse, neglect, dysfunction, and disadvantage—results in a unique constellation of harm that is often overlooked in episodic, incident-based child protection frameworks (Bryce & Collier, 2022). Bryce et al. (2024) developed a tool for evaluating cumulative harm in children engaged with intensive family support services, to construct a multi-dimensional assessment model. This tool incorporates indicators of maltreatment severity, chronicity, and co-occurrence, enabling practitioners to identify children at highest risk and tailor interventions accordingly. Their development of the *Cumulative Experiences Index* provides a validated tool for assessing the frequency, duration, and severity of harm, enabling practitioners to better capture the complexity of children's lived experiences (Bryce et al., 2024).

ACMS PREVALENCE AND PATTERNS OF OVERLAP

While the concept of multi-type maltreatment was developed over 30 years ago and has been adopted and used by researchers across the globe, it has achieved greatest prominence through its deployment in over 15 papers from the groundbreaking national study of all forms of child abuse and neglect across the Australian population: the Australian Child Maltreatment Study (ACMS) (see: www.acms.au). The ACMS has provided nationally representative data on the prevalence and impact of multi-type maltreatment. Findings confirm that multi-type maltreatment is common. These experiences are strongly associated with mental health disorders, substance use, and educational disruption, reinforcing the need for cross-sectoral responses that address both the individual and systemic dimensions of maltreatment. The concept of multi-type maltreatment is not new, but the ACMS provides unprecedented national-level population-representative empirical data that allows for a deeper understanding of its prevalence, patterns, and consequences. Importantly, the study reveals that multi-type maltreatment is not a rare or exceptional occurrence—it is a common experience for a significant proportion of the population.

The Australian Child Maltreatment Study (ACMS) has provided the first nationally representative data in Australia on the prevalence and impact of all five types of child maltreatment: physical abuse, sexual abuse, emotional abuse, neglect, and exposure to domestic violence. It was the first survey to measure all five forms of child maltreatment, collecting data from 8500 Australians aged 16–65 and over. One of the most striking findings from the ACMS is the high prevalence of multi-type maltreatment—the experience of more than one form of abuse or neglect during childhood (Higgins et al., 2023). The ACMS showed that 39.4% of Australians reported experiencing more than one type of child maltreatment, and 3.5% experienced all five types. These findings challenge traditional approaches that treat each form of maltreatment in isolation and underscore the need for integrated frameworks that account for the complexity of children's lived experiences.

Common patterns of overlap include:

- 5.1% experienced physical abuse, emotional abuse and exposure to domestic violence
- 5.1% experienced physical abuse, sexual abuse, emotional abuse and exposure to domestic violence
- 3.7% experienced emotional abuse and exposure to domestic violence
- 3.5% experienced all five forms (Physical abuse, sexual abuse, emotional abuse, neglect, and exposure to domestic violence)

The ACMS included an oversample of young people aged 16–24. Among this cohort of 3,500 young Australians, 40.2% experienced more than one type of maltreatment, 25.4% experienced three to five types, and 3.7% experienced all five types. Multi-type maltreatment is particularly prevalent among younger Australians. The cohort trends show that even though there are some improvements over time (e.g., a lower prevalence of child sexual abuse overall for the 16-24 year olds compared to older Australians), the problem of intersecting forms of harm from multi-type maltreatment is a problem that is increasing rather than diminishing.

The key childhood family adversities associated with more than double the likelihood of experiencing multi-type maltreatment are: parental separation/divorce, parental illness, parental substance misuse, and family economic hardship (Higgins et al, 2023). These combinations often occur in contexts of family dysfunction, and intergenerational trauma. The presence of multiple adversities amplifies the risk of long-term harm and complicates the pathways to recovery.

The ACMS data reveal that child maltreatment is often chronic and severe. For example, among those who experienced child sexual abuse: 78% reported that it happened more than once; 42% experienced it more than six times; and 11% experienced it more than 50 times. This chronicity is particularly concerning in cases of multi-type maltreatment, where repeated exposure to not just the same form of abuse or neglect, but in fact to different forms of harm can lead to complex trauma, developmental disruptions, and cumulative disadvantage.

GENDER AND DIVERSITY DIMENSIONS

Gender plays a significant role in the experience of multi-type maltreatment. The ACMS found that although boys and girls experience similar rates of physical abuse and exposure to domestic violence, girls are disproportionately affected by sexual and emotional abuse. However, gender diverse individuals reported the highest rates of multi-type maltreatment, with 90% experiencing any child maltreatment, and 66.1% experiencing more than one type (Higgins et al., 2024).

These findings highlight the intersectional nature of child maltreatment and the need for inclusive, culturally responsive approaches to prevention and intervention. Gender disparities in maltreatment experiences also reflect broader societal patterns of inequality, discrimination, and vulnerability.

Of gender diverse individuals, 81.5% experienced any child maltreatment; two-thirds (66.2%) experienced multi-type maltreatment (2+ types) and over half (51.2%) experienced severe multi-type maltreatment (3+ types). These rates are significantly higher than for men (58.4% experienced any maltreatment; 34.9% multi-type; 18.1% severe multi-type; and women (65.5% any maltreatment; 43.2% multi-type; 27.6% severe multi-type). These significantly higher rates of maltreatment—particularly multi-type maltreatment—were strongly related to experiences of mental illness and health-risk behaviours (Madzoska et al., 2024).

There were similar patterns for sexual minorities. Of sexually diverse individuals, 83.9% experienced any child maltreatment; 64.1% experienced multi-type maltreatment, and 46.8% experienced severe multi-type maltreatment (i.e., experiencing 3, 4 or 5 different child maltreatment types). In contrast, the rate for heterosexuals were 61.0% any maltreatment; 37.6% multi-type; 21.5% severe multi-type.

The youth cohort (16–24 years) had the highest prevalence of both diverse identities and multi-type maltreatment. For example, 90.5% of gender diverse youth experienced any maltreatment, and 77.5% experienced multi-type maltreatment (Higgins et al., 2024).

IMPACTS ACROSS THE LIFESPAN

The consequences of maltreatment are profound and enduring, but the particular role that multi-type maltreatment plays in understanding the relationship between maltreatment and health outcomes across life is critical. The ACMS found that individuals with histories of child maltreatment are significantly more likely to experience mental health disorders including depression, anxiety; health risk behaviours such as substance use, and self-harm, and to have higher health service utilisation, indicating a greater burden on public health systems. But across these findings, a consistent and worrying trend is the role that accumulation of harm across different types of maltreatment has in terms of its associated health-related outcomes.

These outcomes persist into middle and older adulthood, demonstrating that the effects of child maltreatment are not confined to childhood or adolescence. The cumulative impact of multi-type maltreatment can shape life trajectories, influence educational and employment outcomes, and affect relationships and parenting practices.

Those who experienced multi-type maltreatment demonstrated higher health service utilisation, indicating a greater need for medical and psychological support throughout their lives (Parcella et al., 2023). Multi-type maltreatment is associated with increased risk of chronic conditions such as cardiovascular disease, diabetes, and gastrointestinal disorders. The psychological toll of maltreatment also manifests in high rates of mental illness and disability. The ACMS also explored the relationship between childhood maltreatment and involvement in the criminal justice system. Individuals with histories of multi-type maltreatment were more likely to have had interactions with the criminal justice system, highlighting the long-term societal impacts of such experiences (Mathews et al., 2023).

Quantifying the burden of disease attributable to child maltreatment is essential for informing public health policy and resource allocation. It provides a compelling economic rationale for investing in prevention, early intervention, and trauma-informed care.

MENTAL HEALTH

Key findings on the associations between experiences of multi-type maltreatment and the risk of mental health disorders from the ACMS dataset were reported by

Scott et al. (2023). Individuals who experienced multi-type maltreatment exhibited significantly higher rates of mental health disorders compared to those who experienced single-type maltreatment or no maltreatment. Overall, young people aged 16–24 who experienced multi-type maltreatment were 2.9 times more likely to have any mental disorder. In terms of particular mental health conditions, they were 2.7 times more likely to have ever had major depressive disorder; 3.3 times more likely to have generalized anxiety disorder; 4.1 times more likely to have severe alcohol use disorder; and 5.8 times more likely to have post-traumatic stress disorder (PTSD).

Prevalence and Impact: Individuals who experienced multi-type maltreatment (two or more forms of abuse or neglect) had significantly higher rates of mental disorders than those who experienced a single type or none. For example, the prevalence of any mental disorder was 16.6% in those with no maltreatment; 27.4% in those with one type; and 45.4% in those with two or more types.

Dose-Response Relationship: The greater the number of different types of maltreatment experienced, the higher the odds of mental disorders. This pattern held across all assessed disorders: PTSD, Generalised Anxiety Disorder (GAD), Major Depressive Disorder (MDD), and alcohol use disorders. In their analysis of the ACMS subgroup of gender diverse participants, Madzoska et al. (2024) found an almost linear relationship between the number of maltreatment types experienced, and the prevalence of any mental disorders. Particularly the proportion of the population who experienced two types, or those who experienced three or more, the diverse genders grouped had the higher rate, followed by women, followed by men.

Strength of Associations: Multi-type maltreatment was associated with: 4.8 times the odds of PTSD; 3 times the odds of GAD; 2.7 times the odds of MDD; and 2.9 times the odds of severe alcohol use disorder. These associations remained strong even after adjusting for socio-economic factors and financial hardship.

Independent Effects of Each Maltreatment Type: While all five types of maltreatment were independently associated with mental disorders, multi-type maltreatment had the strongest and most consistent associations. But when accounting for the presence of other types, the two forms of abuse that had the strongest unique contribution to mental disorders were emotional abuse and sexual abuse (Scott et al., 2023).

HEALTH-RISK BEHAVIOURS

Another landmark analysis from the *Australian Child Maltreatment Study (ACMS)* examined the associations between five types of child maltreatment and six health risk behaviours and conditions: current smoking; binge drinking; cannabis dependence; obesity; self-harm and suicide attempts (Lawrence et al., 2023). Those who experienced multi-type maltreatment demonstrated higher health risk behaviours, such as 6.2 times more likely to be cannabis dependent, and 4.5 times more likely to have attempted suicide in the past 12 months. Three key findings are worth noting:

Strong relationship to health-risk behaviours: Individuals with multi-type maltreatment had significantly higher rates of all six health risks compared to those with no or single-type maltreatment.

Dose-Response Relationship: The more types of maltreatment experienced, the higher the prevalence of health risks. For example, 23.1% of those with two or more types were current smokers, compared to 17.6% with one type and 11.1% with none. Similar patterns were found for cannabis dependence, self-harm, and suicide attempts.

Independent Effects of Maltreatment Types: When all five types were modelled together (i.e., controlling for any other child maltreatment experienced), sexual abuse and emotional abuse were independently associated with nearly all health risks. Exposure to domestic violence was linked to smoking and cannabis dependence. Physical abuse was associated with suicide attempts (Lawrence et al., 2023).

CARE-EXPERIENCED AUSTRALIANS' CHILD MALTREATMENT EXPERIENCES AND MENTAL HEALTH

Harris et al. (2024, 2025a, 2025b) published several studies from the ACMS that have focused on the 5.4% who had experienced time in out-of-home care at some point during their childhood (aged 0–18). Their analysis was aimed at understanding whether the experiences of child maltreatment that this subgroup of Australians have experienced are different from those who experienced child maltreatment from the broader population (see Table 3). A key finding was the much higher frequency of multi-type maltreatment, but also unpacking the different dimensions of maltreatment that sit behind this.

Table 3. Differences between child maltreatment profiles of care-experienced and other maltreated Australians

Theme	Key findings
Higher Prevalence of Multi-type Maltreatment	• 79% of care-experienced individuals reported multi-type maltreatment • 18.5% experienced all five types • In contrast, only **37.1%** of non-care-experienced individuals reported multi-type maltreatment, and **2.6%** experienced all five types
Greater Range of Maltreatment Items	• Care-experienced individuals endorsed more items per maltreatment type, indicating broader and more varied experiences.
Earlier Age of Onset	• Child maltreatment began significantly earlier for care-experienced individuals across all types. • For emotional abuse, onset was at **5.7 years** (vs. 8.2 years for non-care-experienced).
Longer Duration	• Maltreatment lasted longer for care-experienced individuals, especially emotional abuse (average 9.8 years vs. 8.2 years).
Higher Frequency	• Physical and sexual abuse, and exposure to domestic violence occurred **more than twice as often** in the care-experienced group.
Greater number of Perpetrators	• Care-experienced individuals reported more types of perpetrators, especially for sexual and emotional abuse.
Different Perpetrator Types	• Care-experienced individuals were more likely to report both caregivers and others as perpetrators. • Notably, **15.6%** of care-experienced individuals reported sexual abuse by both caregiver and non-caregiver (vs. 2.9% in non-care-experienced).

Source: Harris et al. 2024, 2025a

Given how widespread child maltreatment is in the Australian population (62%), but yet how much smaller is the number of Australians who have come to the attention of child protection departments or been placed in out-of-home care (5.4%), Harris et al.(2025b) were interested in understanding whether care-experienced Australians greater risk of mental health issues is potentially not an artefact of them having been placed in care, but is a result of the greater intensity of maltreatment they have experienced. Using a range of maltreatment dimensions (number of maltreatment types, age of onset for each type, the range of experiences within each type, as well as their frequency and duration, and the type and number of perpetrators), they controlled for the potential confounding potential for maltreatment intensity on mental disorder outcomes, a factor that has been widely evidenced to impact long-term wellbeing. Using sophisticated propensity score matching analyses, Harris et al. (2025b) demonstrated that being care-experienced did not significantly affect the odds of developing any mental disorder once accounting for the maltreatment intensity. This suggests that the level of child maltreatment intensity, which includes multi-type maltreatment, accounts for most of the differences in mental disorders between care- and non-care-experienced groups.

This series of analyses from the ACMS by Harris et al. (2024, 2025a, b) demonstrates the value of a dimensional model of maltreatment that goes beyond type alone, and when measuring experiences of child maltreatment, the importance of incorporating timing, frequency, and perpetrator context to better understand maltreatment impacts. It also has some key implications for policymakers in the statutory child protection system, as well practitioners and managers working in child/family welfare agencies:

- Care-experienced individuals face more intense and complex maltreatment, requiring tailored and trauma-informed interventions.
- Early intervention is critical, as maltreatment often begins in early childhood.
- Multi-type maltreatment should be assumed as likely in therapeutic and support settings for care-experienced individuals.
- Parenting support and safeguarding strategies must address emotional abuse and sexual abuse risks, especially from caregivers.

PROBLEMATIC ALCOHOL USE

Using data from the youth subsample from the ACMS, Rattambige et al. (2025) examined how multi-type child maltreatment—alongside other non-maltreatment adversities—is associated with problematic alcohol use in young Australians aged 16–24. One of the key findings was that multi-type maltreatment was strongly associated with higher levels of problematic alcohol use, even after controlling for non-maltreatment adversities such as parental substance use, mental illness, separation/divorce and family economic hardship. Those who experienced multi-type maltreatment had a 55% higher rate of problematic alcohol use compared to those with no maltreatment. This shows the particular influence of multiple types. Those who had only experienced a single type of maltreatment had only 28% higher rate of problematic alcohol use. These findings suggest that there is likely a dose-response relationship between adversity and outcomes like problematic alcohol use. Not only did youth with multi-type maltreatment had significantly higher odds of alcohol use disorder compared to those with no maltreatment, but also the severity of alcohol problems increased with the number of maltreatment types experienced. This finding was not moderated by factors such as age of onset or duration of the maltreatment. The key association between problematic alcohol use in young people and experiences of multi-type maltreatment supporting cumulative risk theory. Multi-type maltreatment is a dominant risk factor for problematic alcohol use in youth. However, this does not mean that there doesn't need to be a focus on the individual contributions of each type of abuse or neglect. For example, Rattambige et al. (2025) showed that when accounting for other maltreatment types co-experienced, sexual abuse was uniquely significant and so this type of maltreatment may require targeted trauma-informed interventions due to its unique and enduring impact.

CONCLUSION AND IMPLICATIONS

Over the past several decades, the field of child maltreatment research has undergone a significant transformation—from viewing abuse and neglect as discrete, isolated incidents to recognising them as complex, overlapping experiences with cumulative developmental consequences. Early frameworks tended to categorise maltreatment by type (e.g., physical, sexual, emotional abuse, neglect), often treating each in isolation. However, empirical evidence increasingly demonstrated that children frequently experience multi-type maltreatment, and that the co-occurrence and accumulation of these harms amplify their impact.

This recognition led to the development of more nuanced constructs such as polyvictimization, which captures the breadth of victimisation across multiple domains, and cumulative harm, which emphasises the chronicity, severity, and developmental timing of adversity. These shifts prompted a move away from incident-based models toward ecological and developmental frameworks that account for the child's broader context—including family dynamics, systemic disadvantage, and exposure to violence.

Methodological innovations followed, including the creation of tools and indices to measure accumulation and chronicity, enabling researchers and practitioners to better assess the long-term effects of maltreatment. Longitudinal studies provided robust evidence linking cumulative harm to outcomes such as mental health disorders, substance use, and antisocial behaviour, reinforcing the need for trauma-informed and developmentally sensitive interventions.

In practice, these conceptual shifts have influenced child protection systems, particularly in jurisdictions that now incorporate cumulative harm into assessment protocols and policy frameworks. The integration of research into frontline practice has led to more holistic approaches that consider not just the presence of harm, but its pattern, persistence, and interaction with protective factors.

Together, these developments reflect a maturing field that increasingly recognises the complexity of children's lived experiences and the necessity of interdisciplinary, evidence-based responses. The evolution from typological to cumulative models marks a critical advancement in both scholarship and service delivery, with ongoing implications for prevention, intervention, and policy reform. The findings from a variety of analyses based on the ACMS emphasise the need for a whole-of-government response to address the high rates of multi-type maltreatment, and for better prevention and early intervention strategies to address the risk of multiple forms of abuse and neglect.

There are several key reasons by the work on accumulation of adversity and in particular multi-type child maltreatment has been so important.

- Multi-type maltreatment is particularly harmful. Harm begets harm. Prior harm is itself a risk factor for future harm. It disrupts multiple domains of functioning simultaneously (trust, safety, self-worth, autonomy, etc.). There's less opportunity for resilience if harm is coming from multiple sources (e.g., parents, environment, peers). Protective factors (supportive adult, school engagement) are more likely to be absent or undermined when harm comes from multiple sources and in multiple forms.
- Multi-type maltreatment is predictable and preventable. Family-related adversities—especially mental illness and alcohol or substance misuse—were strongly associated with multi-type maltreatment. These adversities nearly doubled the risk of experiencing multiple maltreatment types.
- Addressing multi-type maltreatment has the potential to affect multiple outcomes. Across multiple analyses conducted using the ACMS, it was one of the strongest predictors of mental illness and health risk behaviours, suggesting it as a focus as well as its costs to the community.

Implications, including the need for trauma-informed health promotion, holistic interventions, policy integration and public health approaches to prevention that cross silos of different harm types. For example, health promotion strategies must address the full extent of trauma histories, not just target behaviours. Programs should integrate mental health support, coping skills, and trauma recovery. Siloed behavioural interventions to address trauma symptoms are insufficient. Holistic psychosocial care is more effective, especially for those with complex trauma histories. Practitioners need specialised training to understand the dynamics of multi-type maltreatment and to respond effectively. This includes knowledge of trauma, attachment, developmental psychology, and cultural competence.

Preventing child maltreatment—especially multi-type maltreatment—could significantly reduce the burden of disease and improve population health. But to do this, requires system integration and/or coordination, so that child protection, mental health, and public health systems collaborate to address the cumulative and compounding effects of multi-type maltreatment. Public health strategies should target family-level risk factors, such as parental mental illness, substance misuse, and domestic violence. Universal and targeted prevention programs can reduce the incidence of maltreatment and support families before harm occurs.

Practice and policy responses to children who experience single maltreatment events may need to be different to those for children who experience multiple maltreatment events. Survivors of multiple maltreatment events are more likely to experience complex trauma and the negative effects of cumulative harm, both of which require more comprehensive intervention and treatment. Prevention strategies also need to be tailored to address the higher risk of multi-type child maltreatment for gender and sexuality diverse children and youth. For example, structured evidence-based parenting programs, and informal supports for parents though maternal and child health services, GPs, community health clinics and schools should include guidance and support for families who have children with diverse genders. All child-facing systems—including education, health, justice, and welfare—should adopt trauma-informed principles. This includes recognising the signs of trauma, avoiding re-traumatisation, and promoting safety, trust, and empowerment. Safeguarding policies in organisations must address unique vulnerabilities (e.g., sleeping arrangements, bathroom access). Finally, training for professionals (teachers, health workers, etc.) should include gender- and sexuality-sensitive practices, and prepare clinicians with awareness of the higher likelihood of multi-type maltreatment in diverse populations (and the need for comprehensive assessments), but also with skills and confidence to be inclusive and responsive to their needs.

Researchers investigating the consequences of a specific form of victimisation should account for the effects of other victimisation experiences, as well as for the effects of cumulative experiences. Analysis of the relationship of adversity to later-life outcomes can easily lead misguided attributions of 'causality' if key alternate explanations for observed relationships are not accounted for. For example, in a recent analysis of contributors to earlier age of first voluntary sexual experience, contrary to expectations, Allen (2025) found that child physical abuse emerged as an independent predictor of early sexual debut, while child sexual abuse did not after the effects of physical abuse were controlled. This shows the importance of recognising the high prevalence of multi-type maltreatment, and the importance of controlling for other adversities when understanding the potential causal links to outcomes later in life. Examining the impact of multi-type maltreatment provides a better prediction of wellbeing outcomes like mental health or health risk behaviours than measuring the effects of individual maltreatment types separately. Even if those types are experienced repeatedly, accounting for multi-type maltreatment is an important key to understanding the relationship between adversity in childhood and later outcomes.

Focusing on multi-type maltreatment also provides indications of hope. To address some of these factors associated with higher risk of multi-type maltreatment will affect safety of children and young people in multiple domains and can be a key protection against the long-term outcomes associated with child maltreatment like mental illness and health risk behaviours such as suicidal ideation and behaviours.

The history of multi-type maltreatment research in Australia is marked by a shift from fragmented understandings of child abuse to a holistic, integrated framework that recognises the cumulative and compounding nature of harm. Through the development of empirical measurement tools and the articulation of multi-type maltreatment as a distinct construct, the focus on the accumulation of harm from child maltreatment is reshaping how maltreatment is understood, measured, and addressed.

The Australian Child Maltreatment Study has fundamentally reshaped our understanding of child abuse and neglect in Australia. It gives researchers one of the richest datasets globally to understand the cumulative impact of exposure to more than one form of maltreatment. Multi-type maltreatment is not an anomaly—it is a common, complex, and deeply consequential experience. Recognising the overlapping nature of maltreatment is essential for developing effective responses that address the full spectrum of harm.

This chapter has drawn on ACMS findings to illuminate the prevalence, patterns, and impacts of multi-type maltreatment. It has argued for integrated, trauma-informed approaches that reflect the lived realities of children and adults affected by abuse and neglect. This work continues to inform efforts to prevent harm, support recovery, and build trauma-informed systems that respond to the complex realities of children's lives. As Australia moves toward generational reform in child protection, the insights from the ACMS must guide our collective efforts to prevent harm, promote healing, and build a safer future for all.

REFERENCES

Allen, B. (2025). Childhood sexual behavior as a mediator of the relationship between sexual abuse and early sexual debut: A prospective analysis. *Archives of Sexual Behavior.* , C. M., Langhinrichsen-Rohling, J., Bowers, D., O'Brien, N. (2007). Differential correlates of multi-type maltreatment among urban youth. *Child Abuse & Neglect, 31*, 393–415. https://www.sciencedirect.com/science/article/pii/S0145213407000609DOI: 10.1007/s10508-025-03228-wArata

Bromfield, L., & Miller, R. (2012). *Cumulative Harm Specialist Practice Resource.* Victorian Government Department of Human Services. https://www.cpmanual.vic.gov.au/sites/default/files/Cumulative%20harm%20specialist%20practice%20resource%202012%203014%20.pdf

Bromfield, L. M., Gillingham, P., & Higgins, D. J. (2007). Cumulative harm and chronic child maltreatment. Developing Practice: The Child [Available online.]. *Youth and Family Work Journal, 19*, 34–42.

Bromfield, L. M., & Higgins, D. J. (2004). The limitations of using statutory child protection data for research into child maltreatment. *Australian Social Work, 57*(1), 19–30. https://www.tandfonline.com/doi/abs/10.1111/j.0312-407X.2003.t01-1-00110.x. DOI: 10.1111/j.0312-407X.2003.00110.x

Bromfield, L. M., & Higgins, D. J. (2005). The course and characteristics of chronic and isolated child maltreatment. *Family Matters (Melbourne, Vic.), 70*, 38–45. https://aifs.gov.au/publications/family-matters/issue-70/chronic-and-isolated-maltreatment-child-protection-sample

Bryce, I., & Collier, S. (2022). A systematic literature review of the contribution accumulation makes to psychological and physical trauma sustained through childhood maltreatment. *Trauma Care, 2*(2), 307–329. DOI: 10.3390/traumacare2020026

Bryce, I., Collier, S., Harris, L., Higgins, D., & Toohey, J. (2024). Measuring accumulation: Constructing a tool for evaluating cumulative harm in children engaged with an intensive family support service. *Child Abuse Review, 33*(5), e2897. Advance online publication. DOI: 10.1002/car.2897

Cicchetti, D., & Cohen, D. J. (Eds.). (2015). Developmental Psychopathology *Volume Three: Risk, Disorder, and Adaptation.* Wiley.

Daro, D. (2022). Sustaining progress in preventing child maltreatment: A transformative challenge. In Krugman, R., & Korbin, J. (Eds.), *Handbook of child maltreatment* (pp. 407–427). Springer. DOI: 10.1007/978-3-030-82479-2_20

Felitti, V. J., Anda, R. F., Nordenberg, D., Williamson, D. F., Spitz, A. M., Edwards, V., Koss, M. P., & Marks, J. S. (1998). Relationship of childhood abuse and household dysfunction to many of the leading causes of death in adults: The Adverse Childhood Experiences (ACE) Study. *American Journal of Preventive Medicine, 14*(4), 245–258. DOI: 10.1016/S0749-3797(98)00017-8 PMID: 9635069

Finkelhor, D. (2008). *Childhood Victimization: Violence, Crime, and Abuse in the Lives of Young People*. Oxford University Press. DOI: 10.1093/acprof:oso/9780195342857.001.0001

Finkelhor, D., Ormrod, R. K., & Turner, H. A. (2007). Poly-victimization: A neglected component in child victimization. *Child Abuse & Neglect, 31*(1), 7–26. DOI: 10.1016/j.chiabu.2006.06.008 PMID: 17224181

Finkelhor, D., Turner, H. A., Hamby, S. L., & Ormrod, R. K. (2011). *Polyvictimization: Children's Exposure to Multiple Types of Violence, Crime, and Abuse*. OJJDP Juvenile Justice Bulletin – NCJ235504 (pgs. 1-12). Washington, DC: US Government Printing Office.

Fitzgerald, M., & Gallus, K. L. (2025). Conceptualizing and measuring childhood adversity: A comprehensive critique of the adverse childhood experiences measure and offering a new conceptualization of childhood adversity. *The American Journal of Orthopsychiatry, 95*(3), 274–287. DOI: 10.1037/ort0000785 PMID: 39298243

Garmezy, N. (1991). Resilience in children's adaptation to negative life events and stressed environments. *Pediatric Annals, 20*(9), 459–466. DOI: 10.3928/0090-4481-19910901-05 PMID: 1945543

Hamai, T. A., & Felitti, V. J. (2022). Adverse childhood experiences: Past, present, and future. In Geffner, R. (Eds.), *Handbook of interpersonal violence and abuse across the lifespan* (pp. 97–120). Springer Nature Switzerland AG., DOI: 10.1007/978-3-319-89999-2_305

Hamby, S., Finkelhor, D., Turner, H., & Ormrod, R. (2010). The overlap of witnessing partner violence with child maltreatment and other victimizations in a nationally representative survey of youth. *Child Abuse & Neglect, 34*(10), 734–741. DOI: 10.1016/j.chiabu.2010.03.001 PMID: 20850182

Harris, L., Higgins, D. J., Willis, M., Lawrence, D., Mathews, B., Thomas, H. J., Malacova, E., Pacella, R., Scott, J. G., Finkelhor, D., Meinck, F., Erskine, H. E., & Haslam, D. M. (2024). The prevalence and patterns of maltreatment, childhood adversity, and mental health disorders in an Australian out-of-home care sample. *Child Maltreatment*, •••, 1–13. DOI: 10.1177/10775595241246534 PMID: 38627990

Harris, L., Higgins, D. J., Willis, M., Lawrence, D., Meinck, F., Thomas, H. J., Malacova, E., Scott, J. G., & Haslam, D. M. (2025a). Dimensions of child maltreatment in Australians with a history of out-of-home care. *Child Maltreatment.* https://journals.sagepub.com/doi/10.1177/10775595241297944

Harris, L. G., Higgins, D. J., Willis, M. L., Lawrence, D., Mathews, B., Malacova, E., Erskine, H., Meinck, F., & Haslam, D. M. (2025b). Determining the effect of out-of-home care on mental health disorders: A propensity score-matched study of maltreatment intensity. *Child Abuse & Neglect, 167,* 107571 107571-167. DOI: 10.1016/j.chiabu.2025.107571

Herrenkohl, R. C., & Herrenkohl, T. I. (2009). Assessing a child's experience of multiple maltreatment types: Some unfinished business. *Journal of Family Violence, 24*(7), 485–496. DOI: 10.1007/s10896-009-9247-2 PMID: 20161642

Herrenkohl, T. I., Jung, H., Lee, J. O., & Kim, M. (2017). Effects of Child Maltreatment, Cumulative Victimization Experiences, and Proximal Life Stress on Adult Crime and Antisocial Behavior. Office of Justice Programs' National Criminal Justice Reference Service, US.

Higgins, D. J. (2004a). Differentiating between child maltreatment experiences. *Family Matters (Melbourne, Vic.), 69,* 50–55. http://www.aifs.gov.au/institute/pubs/fm2004/fm69/dh.pdf

Higgins, D. J. (2004b). The importance of degree versus type of maltreatment: A cluster analysis of child abuse types. *The Journal of Psychology, 138*(4), 303–324. DOI: 10.3200/JRLP.138.4.303-324 PMID: 15379008

Higgins, D. J., Lawrence, D., Haslam, D. M., Mathews, B., Malacova, E., Erskine, H. E., Finkelhor, D., Pacella, R., Meinck, F., Thomas, H. J., & Scott, J. G. (2024). Prevalence of diverse genders and sexualities in Australia and associations with five forms of child maltreatment and multi-type maltreatment. *Child Maltreatment, 30*(1), 21–41. DOI: 10.1177/10775595231226331 PMID: 38214251

Higgins, D. J., Mathews, B., Pacella, R., Scott, J. G., Finkelhor, D., Meinck, F., Erskine, H., Thomas, H., Lawrence, D., Haslam, D., Malacova, E., & Dunne, M. P. (2023). The prevalence and nature of multi-type child maltreatment in Australia. *The Medical Journal of Australia, 218*(6, Suppl), S19–S25. DOI: 10.5694/mja2.51868 PMID: 37004183

Higgins, D. J., & McCabe, M. P. (1994). The relationship of child sexual abuse and family violence to adult adjustment: Toward an integrated risk-sequelae model. *Journal of Sex Research, 31*(4), 255–266. DOI: 10.1080/00224499409551761

Higgins, D. J., & McCabe, M. P. (1998). Parent perceptions of maltreatment and adjustment in children. *Journal of Family Studies, 4*(1), 53–76. DOI: 10.5172/jfs.4.1.53

Higgins, D. J., & McCabe, M. P. (2000a). Relationships between different types of maltreatment during childhood and adjustment in adulthood. *Child Maltreatment, 5*(3), 261–272. DOI: 10.1177/1077559500005003006 PMID: 11232272

Higgins, D. J., & McCabe, M. P. (2000b). Multi-type maltreatment and the long-term adjustment of adults. *Child Abuse Review, 9*(1), 6–18. DOI: 10.1002/(SICI)1099-0852(200001/02)9:1<6::AID-CAR579>3.0.CO;2-W

Higgins, D. J., & McCabe, M. P. (2001a). The development of the Comprehensive Child Maltreatment Scale. *Journal of Family Studies, 7*(1), 7–28. DOI: 10.5172/jfs.7.1.7

Higgins, D. J., & McCabe, M. P. (2001b). Multiple forms of child abuse and neglect: Adult retrospective reports. *Aggression and Violent Behavior: A Review Journal, 6*, 547-578. DOI: 10.1016/S1359-1789(00)00030-6

James, M. (2000). *Child Abuse and Neglect: Part 1— Redefining the Issues. Trends & issues in crime and criminal justice no. 146*. Australian Institute of Criminology., https://www.aic.gov.au/sites/default/files/2020-05/tandi146.pdf

Kempe, C. H., Silverman, F. N., Steele, B. F., Droegemueller, W., & Silver, H. K. (1962). The battered-child syndrome. *Journal of the American Medical Association, 181*(1), 17–24. DOI: 10.1001/jama.1962.03050270019004

Lawrence, D., Hunt, A., Mathews, B., Haslam, D. M., Malacova, E., Dunne, M. P., Erskine, H., Higgins, D. J., Finkelhor, D., Pacella, R., Meinck, F., Thomas, H., & Scott, J. G. (2023). The association between child maltreatment and health risk behaviours and conditions throughout life in the Australian Child Maltreatment Study. *The Medical Journal of Australia, 218*(6, Suppl), S34–S39. DOI: 10.5694/mja2.51877

Madzoska, M., Lawrence, D., Higgins, D. J., Haslam, D., Mathews, B., Malacova, E., Dunne, M. P., Erskine, H., Pacella, R., Meinck, F., Thomas, H., & Scott, J. (2024). Child maltreatment, mental health disorders and health risk behaviors in people with diverse gender identities. *Journal of Interpersonal Violence, 40*(9-10), 2281–2306. DOI: 10.1177/08862605241270077 PMID: 39152737

Mathews, B., Papalia, N., Napier, S., Malacova, E., Lawrence, D., Higgins, D. J., Thomas, H., Erskine, H., Meinck, F., Haslam, D., Scott, J. G., Finkelhor, D., & Pacella, R. (2023). *Child maltreatment and criminal justice system involvement in Australia: Findings from a national survey. Trends & issues in crime and criminal justice no. 681*. Australian Institute of Criminology., DOI: 10.52922/ti77215

McEwen, C. A., & Gregerson, S. F. (2019). A critical assessment of the Adverse Childhood Experiences study at 20 years. *American Journal of Preventive Medicine, 56*(6), 790–794. DOI: 10.1016/j.amepre.2018.10.016 PMID: 30803781

Miller-Perrin, C. L., & Perrin, R. D. (2007). *Child maltreatment: An introduction* (2nd ed.). Sage.

Ney, P., Fung, T., & Wickett, A. (1994). The worst combinations of child abuse and neglect. *Child Abuse & Neglect, 18*(9), 705–715. DOI: 10.1016/0145-2134(94)00037-9 PMID: 8000901

Price-Robertson, R., Higgins, D., & Vassallo, S. (2013). *Multi-type maltreatment and polyvictimisation: A comparison of two research frameworks. Family Matters, 93, 84-98*. Australian Institute of Family Studies., https://aifs.gov.au/publications/family-matters/issue-93/multi-type-maltreatment-and-polyvictimisation

Price-Robertson, R., Rush, P., Wall, L., & Higgins, D. (2013). *Rarely an isolated incident: Acknowledging the interrelatedness of child maltreatment, victimization and trauma. CFCA Paper no. 15*. Australian Institute of Family Studies., https://aifs.gov.au/cfca/publications/rarely-isolated-incident-acknowledging-interrelatedn

Racine, N., Bellis, M. A., & Madigan, S. (2025). An introduction to twenty-five years of adverse childhood experiences: A special issue. *Child Abuse & Neglect, 168*(Part 1), 107224. Advance online publication. DOI: 10.1016/j.chiabu.2024.107224 PMID: 39730232

Rattambige, D., Higgins, D. J., Whittle, S., Cole, M., Mathews, B., Scott, J. G., Erskine, H., Meinck, F., Pacella, R., Lawrence, D., & Haslam, D. M. (2025). The impact of child maltreatment patterns and adverse childhood experiences on problematic youth alcohol use. *Child Maltreatment*. Advance online publication. DOI: 10.1177/10775595251387118

Sameroff, A. J., Seifer, R., Baldwin, A., & Baldwin, C. (1993). Stability of intelligence from preschool to adolescence: The influence of social and family risk factors. *Child Development, 64*(1), 80–97. DOI: 10.2307/1131438 PMID: 8436039

Scott, J. G., Malacova, E., Mathews, B., Haslam, D. M., Pacella, R., Higgins, D. J., Meinck, F., Dunne, M. P., Finkelhor, D., Erskine, H., Lawrence, D., & Thomas, H. (2023). The association between child maltreatment and mental disorders in the Australian Child Maltreatment Study. *The Medical Journal of Australia, 218*(6, Suppl), S26–S33. DOI: 10.5694/mja2.51870

van der Kolk, B. A. (2005). Developmental Trauma Disorder: Toward a rational diagnosis for children with complex trauma histories. *Psychiatric Annals, 35*(5), 401–408. DOI: 10.3928/00485713-20050501-06

Werner, E. E. (1996). Vulnerable but invincible: High risk children from birth to adulthood. *European Child & Adolescent Psychiatry, 5*(S1), 47–51. DOI: 10.1007/BF00538544 PMID: 9010664

Wolfe, D. A., & McGee, R. A. (1994). Dimensions of child maltreatment and their relationship to adolescent adjustment. *Development and Psychopathology, 6*(1), 165–181. DOI: 10.1017/S0954579400005939

Chapter 2
Responding to Maltreatment Accumulation Across the Child Protection Continuum

Lottie Harris
https://orcid.org/0009-0000-6084-3593
Institute of Child Protection Studies, Australian Catholic University, Australia

ABSTRACT

This chapter introduces eight guiding principles for child protection practice with children who have experienced cumulative maltreatment. These principles include (1) investment into the child protection workforce, (2) embedding trauma-informed responses as core components of care across all domains, (3) engaging children and young people in comprehensive maltreatment-sensitive functional, behavioural and health assessments, (4) proactive planning to address maltreatment related issues, (5) supporting safety and wellbeing through enhanced stability, (6) strengthening relational networks and connections to communities, (7) collaborating within a multi-disciplinary care team, and (8) engaging children and young people in scalable, evidence-informed clinical and therapeutic models. The chapter advocates for aligning all elements of child protection practice with these eight principles, so that systems can move toward long-term healing.

DOI: 10.4018/979-8-3373-4064-7.ch002

INTRODUCTION

This chapter offers a practice-oriented lens for practitioners and sector leaders at the tertiary end of the child protection continuum, where maltreatment has already occurred and services are actively involved. Though the ultimate goal is always to prevent harm before it happens, the reality is that high rates of maltreatment persist globally (Moody et al., 2018). Many children and families only come to the attention of services after maltreatment has already occurred, i.e., once maltreatment has been reported or substantiated (Slack & Berger, 2020). In these contexts, practitioners are entrusted with responding to complex and often cumulative experiences of maltreatment. Their decisions can profoundly shape the trajectories of children's lives (Benbenishty et al., 2015), either through direct intervention, or by supporting caregivers to address the maltreatment risk factors present in their ecosystem (Belsky, 1993).

In this chapter, child protection services refer generally to the full spectrum of interventions aimed at safeguarding children and young people conducted by child and family welfare systems. These typically include a variety of services dependent on the needs and severity of concerns, ranging from early intervention and less intensive family support programs designed to prevent further maltreatment, to intensive family preservation services, and statutory responses such as care and protection orders and out-of-home care (OOHC). In most high-income countries, statutory child protection involvement is triggered when the assessed risk of harm is such that no less intrusive intervention is likely to keep the child safe, acknowledging the challenges associated with standardised risk assessing (Darlington et al., 2010). Although child protection systems are designed to protect children from harm and promote recovery, research on their effectiveness is mixed (Isokuortti et al., 2020, Lima et al., 2019, MacMillan et al., 2009; Russell et al., 2018). Additionally, many children who experience intensive and cumulative maltreatment do not enter the "pointy end" of the system given the high severity threshold for entry to OOHC (Biehal et al., 2018). Instead, the majority are likely to be engaged through early intervention or family preservation services, often without formal statutory involvement. These children may have experienced similar levels of harm and adversity as those at the statutory end (Harris et al., 2025), though their needs are less likely to be recognised or addressed with equal intensity and therapeutic focus. This is partly because less intensive services tend to focus on parental behaviour change rather than the child's wellbeing.

Cumulative maltreatment demands consistent, evidence-informed responses across all tiers of child protection, not only in statutory contexts. Practitioners working in early intervention and family support services must also be equipped to recognise and respond to the long-term impacts of cumulative maltreatment, even when statutory thresholds are not met. This requires a dual focus of addressing the child's immediate needs while actively disrupting cycles of harm and disadvantage. Importantly, there are core practice approaches, described in this chapter, that are grounded in developmental science, trauma-informed care, and relational safety principles that are applicable to all children who have experienced maltreatment (Cox et al., 2021; Timmer et al., 2022). These approaches provide a common foundation for supporting healing and resilience, whether a child is in OOHC, receiving family support, or engaged through early intervention programs.

The practice principles outlined in this chapter are grounded in several critical assumptions that shape how maltreatment is understood and addressed in child protection settings. The first underlying assumption is that maltreatment is highly prevalent among children and young people involved in child protection services, yet its cumulative nature frequently goes unrecognised. Second, past experiences of maltreatment can have as much, if not a greater long-term impact on a child's development and day-to-day functioning than their current environment, necessitating practitioners to have a foundational understanding of maltreatment and its impacts. The third assumption for working with this cohort is that practitioners can play a pivotal role in disrupting cycles of harm and disadvantage when they are equipped with evidence-based frameworks tailored to the needs and contexts of their clients. And finally, healing from cumulative maltreatment is possible, but requires a combination of interpersonal and systemic responses that are consistent, deliberate, and extend beyond episodic or crisis-driven intervention.

The purpose of this chapter is to translate best-practice evidence into actionable guidance for practitioners working with children and young people who have experienced cumulative maltreatment. In particular, this chapter focuses on guidance for practitioners within high-income child protection systems actively working with children who have experienced maltreatment. It aims to strengthen practice knowledge and skill development in responding to cumulative maltreatment, and to support practitioners in navigating the complex realities of frontline work with clarity and confidence. Additionally, the practice principles serve a broader purpose in so far as they guide sector leaders, service designers, and policymakers in creating the conditions that enable effective practice across child protection systems. These principles reflect a shared responsibility for change, recognising that while practitioners are pivotal agents of positive outcomes, sustainable reform requires alignment across all levels of the system. When applied collectively, the principles offer a structured foundation for responding to cumulative maltreatment in ways that are therapeutically impactful, operationally feasible, and systemically supported.

To support this aim, the chapter is structured in three parts. First the chapter addresses the four conceptual assumptions that are foundational to effective child protection responses to cumulative maltreatment. Next it identifies eight evidence-informed principles for working directly with children, young people, and families. For each principle there are a series of action statements provided for practitioners and for sector leaders. The chapter concludes with a summary of the need for integrating these principles into a wider service structure within child protection systems.

1. ASSUMPTIONS THAT UNDERPIN CHILD PROTECTION RESPONSES TO CUMULATIVE MALTREATMENT

1.1 Cumulative maltreatment is highly prevalent in children and young people involved with child protection services.

Childhood maltreatment is a globally pervasive issue (Moody et al., 2018; Stoltenborgh et al. 2015) and experienced at high rates among children and young people involved in child protection systems (Harris et al., 2024). Of those who experience any childhood maltreatment, cumulative maltreatment is a common pattern (Kim & Drake, 2019; Zeanah & Humphreys, 2018). Cumulative maltreatment is particularly damaging and is strongly associated with significant impacts on children's developmental experience (Annerback et al., 2012; Bryce & Collier, 2022; Vizard & Bentovim, 2022). Recognising that the pattern of cumulative maltreatment is the norm rather than the exception, is essential for practitioners seeking to understand and respond to the full spectrum of harm.

Historically, research and policy responses have focused on discrete categories of abuse or neglect, particularly physical and sexual abuse, without accounting for the frequent co-occurrence of maltreatment types (Wamser-Nanney, 2016; Villodas et al., 2021). Since the landmark Adverse Childhood Experiences (ACE) study (Felitti et al., 1998), researchers have increasingly recognised that children rarely experience just one form of maltreatment (Descartes et al., 2020). Instead, the more common pattern is to endure multiple types including physical abuse, sexual abuse, emotional abuse, neglect, and exposure to domestic violence, either concurrently or sequentially during childhood (Higgins et al., 2023; Warmingham et al., 2019; Witt et al., 2016). Early studies highlighted cumulative maltreatment patterns (Higgins & McCabe, 2000), and subsequent research has confirmed that cumulative maltreatment is associated with more severe and enduring health and social outcomes than single-type maltreatment (Descartes et al., 2020; McLaughlin et al., 2021). Some evidence suggests that exposure to more than on type of maltreatment may have a greater impact on outcomes than repeated incidents of the same type (Cyr et al., 2012; Obsuth et al., 2018), though debate continues about whether this reflects dose-response effects or the distinct psychological toll of each maltreatment type (Cecil et al., 2017). Regardless, it is widely accepted that focusing on a single type of maltreatment risks oversimplifying the broader spectrum of harm and may distort our understanding of its impact (Gabrielli & Jackson, 2019).

Although definitions and data collection methods vary across countries, international prevalence data reinforces the scale of the issue. Population studies from Australia, Canada, China, Israel, and Vietnam report prevalence rates ranging from one-third to over 80% of children and adolescents having experienced at least one form of maltreatment (Afifi et al., 2014; Fu et al., 2018; Lev-Weisel et al., 2018; Mathews et al., 2023; Tran et al., 2017). Meta-analyses further estimate global rates of emotional abuse at 36%, physical abuse at 23%, and neglect between 16% and 18%, with sexual abuse disproportionately affecting girls (Stoltenborgh et al., 2015; Moody et al., 2018). Children and young people involved in child protection systems are especially likely to have experienced cumulative maltreatment. Studies from Australia, the UK, the U.S., and Finland show that the vast majority of children entering OOHC have endured multiple forms of maltreatment prior to placement (Åsen et al., 2024; Baldwin et al., 2019; Conn et al., 2013; Harris et al., 2024; Salazar et al., 2013). Importantly, cumulative maltreatment is also prevalent among children engaged through early intervention and family preservation services, even when statutory thresholds are not met. Across service tiers, cumulative maltreatment often spans critical developmental periods and is strongly associated with long-term mental and physical health challenges (Baldwin et al., 2023; Kisely et al., 2018; Seker et al., 2022).

Despite its prevalence and impact, cumulative maltreatment frequently goes undetected. Unlike single-type maltreatment, which may be easier to document, cumulative maltreatment can be obscured by fragmented service records, narrow assessment tools, and siloed systems. In Australia, for example, child protection systems tend to document only the most severe cases, potentially underestimating the true prevalence at the population level (Moore et al., 2015). Child welfare administrative data systems tend to only capture data on incidents of maltreatment that have been reported or disclosed which presents a small fraction of the spectrum of maltreatment a child may have experienced (Gilbert et al., 2009; Kim et al., 2017). Where there are inconsistent definitions of maltreatment, data is also likely to remain fragmented and unreliable, weakening the evidence base for policy and practice (Daro et al., 2015; Jud et al., 2021; Higgins & Hunt, 2024; Mathews et al., 2020). Low disclosure rates compound this issue given that maltreatment often occurs in private, and children face significant barriers to reporting, relying on others to identify and respond to their needs (Mehta et al., 2021). These limitations not only obscure cumulative maltreatment but also risk overestimating the impact of single-type maltreatment while disregarding the more complex and enduring effects of cumulative exposure. Unlike discrete forms of maltreatment, cumulative maltreatment has a compounding effect that presents as deeply individualised.

Recovery then requires more than procedural compliance or crisis containment but demands sustained, trauma-informed engagement that honours the complexity of the child's lived experience.

For practitioners, this assumption has direct implications. Assuming that cumulative maltreatment is common is not just a theoretical stance but allows for a practical shift away from narrow, incident-based assessments toward holistic, developmentally attuned approaches that account for the full spectrum of adversity. It also requires practitioners to anticipate the complexity of cumulative maltreatment even when it is not immediately visible or known, and to respond with consistent, evidence-informed strategies that support recovery, relational safety, and long-term wellbeing. By recognising cumulative maltreatment as the baseline, practitioners are better equipped to meet children where they are and not where systems assume they should be.

1.2 Cumulative maltreatment critically impairs outcomes.

The existing evidence shows that cumulative maltreatment is consistenly strongly associated with more pervasive and often compounding disruptions to a child's daily functioning, relational capacity, and developmental trajectory (Lueger-Schuster et al., 2018; Scott-Storey, 2011; Steine et al., 2017; Rosenzweig & Sundborg, 2022), beyond the impact of single-type maltreatment (Arata et al., 2005; Bijlsma et al., 2023). While single-type maltreatment may trigger acute distress, cumulative maltreatment can become embedded within the child's developmental bio-psycho-social make-up, shaping how they interpret relationships and navigate everyday life (Bryce & Collier, 2022; Carr et al., 2020; Doyle & Cicchetti, 2017; Hu et al., 2024; Wong, 2016). These effects are not always immediately visible, but they manifest in persistent challenges with trust, safety, learning, and emotional wellbeing (Eiberg et al., 2024). Children with accumulated maltreatment histories often require therapeutic caregiving, relational consistency, and long-term recovery-oriented support, not just crisis intervention (Hughes, 2004; Kagan, 2014; MacMillan et al., 2009).

For practitioners, recognising cumulative maltreatment as a distinct and pervasive pattern that substantially influences outcomes, is essential. It enables more accurate assessment, deeper empathy, and more responsive planning. By understanding a child's full maltreatment history, practitioners can better anticipate long-term needs, tailor interventions, and support healing in a way that is developmentally attuned and trauma informed. This assumption is foundational to effective practice but may require rethinking approaches, timeframes and case planning goals, particularly in family services where the parents, rather than the children themselves, are typically the recipients of short-term services.

1.3 Child protection systems are transformative when practice is resourced, relational and supported by effective structures.

Child protection systems are tasked with both preventing further harm and to be agents of recovery, wellbeing, and developmental repair (Berger & Slack, 2014). This potential is especially critical in cases of cumulative maltreatment where recovery does not begin and end with the removal of immediate danger. Instead, it requires sustained, deliberate efforts to address the long-term impacts of adversity that must be embedded within the system itself. Therefore, understanding the nature and consequences of maltreatment is foundational to effective practice by informing intervention design, fostering empathy among practitioners, and strengthening stakeholder advocacy efforts. When practitioners grasp the developmental and relational impacts of cumulative maltreatment, they are better equipped to interpret behaviours, tailor support, and build trust. Conversely, overlooking these impacts can lead to misdiagnosis, inappropriate responses, and missed opportunities for healing (Harris et al., 2026).

Practitioners play a pivotal role in redirecting trajectories shaped by cumulative maltreatment. But their capacity to do so depends on several interdependent conditions. First the system must be resourced properly. Practitioners need access to evidence-informed frameworks, therapeutic tools, and adequate time to engage meaningfully with children and families. Chronic under-resourcing undermines innovation, limits service reach, and forces reactive rather than proactive responses that limit real, relational work (Russ et al., 2024). Second, the system can be transformational when it centres relational practice with all children and young people (Cleese et al., 2025; Ruch, 2005). When practitioners are supported to build trust-based relationships, even in contexts of involuntary engagement, change can occur. This requires time, consistency, and organisational cultures that value relational depth over procedural compliance (Morley, 2022). Finally, to make change practitioners must be supported by coherent systems that enable continuity of care, cross-sector collaboration, and long-term planning (Munro, 2005). Fragmented services, crisis-driven mandates, and compliance-heavy environments erode the conditions needed for therapeutic work.

When these constraints are addressed, systems can become powerful platforms for healing and transformation. For practitioners and decision-makers, this assumption may offer both optimism and direction. It affirms that meaningful change is not only desirable but achievable. It gives agency to those working within the system, reminding them that their efforts matter, and that with the right support, they can create extraordinary outcomes for children and families who have experienced cumulative maltreatment. It also places responsibility where it belongs: on leaders, funders, and policymakers to build systems that are not just reactive, but restorative.

1.4 Healing from cumulative maltreatment is possible.

Cumulative maltreatment does not guarantee a lifetime of poor outcomes. Although the pathway from early adversity to later challenges is well-established, it is not deterministic (Ungar, 2013). A proportion of children and young people will go on to thrive, demonstrating resilience, adaptability, and growth in the face of profound harm (Ioannidis et al., 2020; Mohr & Rosén 2017). This reality offers a powerful counter-narrative that healing is not only possible, but achievable when the right supports are in place. For this reason, it is essential that practitioners understand how to support healing beyond just preventing further harm. Across the continuum of child protection involvement, responses must be tailored to the child's specific developmental and relational needs, rather than focusing solely on family circumstances or parental behaviour. In family preservation contexts, for example, interventions must address the psychological and emotional consequences of maltreatment exposure rather than focusing only on promoting behavioural change in caregivers. Similarly, in OOHC, therapeutic work must begin early and be sustained over time to mitigate the long-term effects of complex trauma. Research continues to identify protective factors that can buffer the impacts of maltreatment (Afifi & MacMillan, 2011; Meng et al., 2018). Stable relationships, safe environments, cultural connection, and access to trauma-informed care all play a critical role in promoting recovery for all children and young people who have experienced maltreatment. This requires a whole-of-system response, supported by policy frameworks that acknowledge the prevalence and impact of cumulative maltreatment.

This assumption matters because it affirms that the work of child protection is about transformation more than just containment. It reminds practitioners and decision-makers that their efforts can disrupt entrenched pathways and create new ones where healing is possible, but requires coordinated, intentional, and well-resourced action. Investing in the wellbeing and future outcomes of children affected by cumulative maltreatment is both a moral and strategic imperative.

2. PRINCIPLES FOR ADDRESSING AND RESPONDING TO CUMULATIVE MALTREATMENT

The following principles form a foundational framework for practitioners and decision-makers working across the child protection continuum to impact the healing journey of children and young people who have experienced cumulative maltreatment. They are not isolated strategies or optional enhancements, but a cohesive, interdependent system of practice and policy principles that must be enacted collectively to support the wellbeing of maltreated children and young people. Each principle should be understood as holding equal weight. Future research may further delineate their individual impacts, but current evidence underscores their interconnectedness where no single principle is sufficient in isolation. Clinical interventions, for example, rely on relational trust, stability depends on collaboration, and healing requires both everyday attuned caregiving and targeted therapeutic intervention. These principles must be embedded across all levels of engagement, from frontline interactions to systemic design. These principles offer a roadmap for collective action, providing guidance on how practitioners perceive, interpret, and prepare for each child's unique needs. The first set of principles (1-3) focus on building workforce knowledge and preparation skills ahead of engaging in any specific interventions, establishing the foundations of understanding how to support children and young people. The last 5 principles (4-8) focus on the practical application of child protection work, or the 'doing' of maltreatment-sensitive practice.

Practice Principle 1. Invest in a capable and sustained workforce for responding to cumulative maltreatment

Whether working in early intervention, statutory child protection, or OOHC, practitioners' capacity to support healing and development hinges on the depth of their knowledge, the stability of their teams, and the culture of their organisations. Yet globally, child protection workforces remain under-resourced, overstretched, and often ill-equipped to meet the psychological and relational needs of the children and young people they serve (Blome & Steib, 2008; Murphy, 2023). High turnover rates, limited trauma-informed training, administrative burdens and reactive service models undermine the consistency and quality of care (Lonne et al., 2020). These conditions not only compromise practitioner wellbeing but also destabilise the relationships that children rely on for safety and recovery.

To improve outcomes for maltreated children, the child protection sector must invest in a skilled, empowered, and sustainable workforce across all service touch-points. This includes targeted recruitment and retention strategies that prioritise values alignment, cultural competence, and long-term commitment. Rigorous training and ongoing professional development in trauma-informed care, the latest maltreatment research, therapeutic engagement and reflective supervision must be delivered to all child protection practitioners. Equally, fair compensation and workload management should be considered essential to ensure practitioners are resourced to do the heavy relational lifting their roles require.

Child protection teams, comprising both professionals and caregivers, are often tasked with navigating complex service systems (e.g., mental health, disability and education) on behalf of the children and young people they support. Their ability to do so effectively depends on having timely, accurate information about available services, as well as a deep understanding of trauma symptoms, physical and mental health disorders, and the broader child protection context (Bunger et al., 2021; Hambrick et al., 2016). Studies have shown that when care teams lack this expertise, children's mental health needs are frequently misunderstood, overlooked, or mismanaged, leading to delayed or ineffective interventions (Modderman et al., 2023). Although mental health literacy has not traditionally been expected of child protection practitioners, emerging evidence suggests that even a foundational understanding of distress indicators, such as suicidal ideation or trauma-related behaviours, is essential for early identification and responsive care (Pollock et al., 2024; Russell et al., 2021). Without this, care and health planning becomes fragmented, and outcomes are compromised.

This principle reinforces the need for systemic investment in workforce development, ensuring that all care teams are equipped to meet the complex and evolving needs of children and young people who have experienced cumulative maltreatment. Equally important is the creation of safe, supportive organisational cultures. Specialists in therapeutic approaches, reflective supervision, and trauma-informed leadership are essential to building resilience among practitioners and preventing burnout. A stable workforce translates directly into safer, more secure experiences for children and young people and into systems that are capable of sustaining healing over time.

For Practitioners:

- Engage in reflective practice and trauma-informed supervision to build resilience and deepen understanding of children's experiences.
- Advocate for training and support that aligns with the realities of cumulative maltreatment and relational care.
- Prioritise curiosity-driven inquiry into children's histories and behaviours, resisting quick-fix approaches in favour of meaningful engagement
- Strengthen mental health literacy by developing foundational knowledge of distress indicators, trauma-related behaviours, and common mental health presentations in children and young people.
- Actively seek out cross-disciplinary learning to improve navigation of other systems and enhance collaboration with clinical teams and caregivers.
- Model relational consistency by maintaining predictable, attuned engagement with children, even amidst systemic pressures and organisational instability.
- Contribute to team stability by mentoring new colleagues, sharing practice wisdom, and fostering a culture of psychological safety and mutual support.
- Document and communicate children's needs holistically, ensuring that behavioural observations are contextualised within trauma-informed frameworks.

For Decision-Makers and Sector Leaders:

- Invest in workforce capability across the continuum through standardised, evidence-informed training and development strategies.
- Stabilise the workforce by addressing organisational safety, remuneration, and vicarious trauma through targeted retention strategies.
- Collaborate with educational institutions to align pre-service training with the demands of trauma-informed, relational child protection work.
- Reduce administrative burdens and restructure systems to enable practitioners to focus on child-centred, therapeutic engagement.
- Embed trauma-informed leadership practices at all levels of the organisation to foster relational safety, emotional regulation, and reflective decision-making.
- Mandate ongoing professional development in trauma, maltreatment, and therapeutic engagement as a core requirement for all child protection roles.
- Fund specialist roles in reflective supervision, therapeutic consultation, and trauma-informed practice to support frontline teams and prevent burnout.
- Develop workforce planning strategies that prioritise long-term sustainability, including succession planning, career pathways, and leadership development.
- Ensure mental health literacy is embedded in workforce standards, job descriptions, and performance expectations across the child protection continuum.
- Establish feedback loops between frontline practice and policy, enabling practitioners to inform system design and reform based on lived experience and relational insight.
- Create mechanisms for shared care planning that integrate child protection, mental health, and education systems to reduce fragmentation and improve outcomes.

A well-supported and skilled workforce is a prerequisite for effective child protection intervention. When practitioners and caregivers are equipped, valued, and sustained, they are better able to build trust, respond to trauma, and promote healing, including implementing the other principles in this chapter. This principle calls for a shared commitment across practice, policy, and leadership to ensure that those caring for maltreated children are themselves cared for, prepared, and empowered to make a lasting difference.

Practice Principle 2. Embed a strong, trauma-informed foundation across all aspects of practice

Trauma-informed care is widely recognised as a foundational principle in child protection, particularly when working with children and young people who have experienced cumulative maltreatment (Bath, 2008; Wall et al., 2016). Trauma-informed care acknowledges the pervasive impact of trauma on development, behaviour, relationships, and health and responds with practices that prioritise safety, empowerment, and healing (Kimberg & Wheeler, 2019). Trauma-informed approaches also enhance treatment success, stabilise placements, and foster more attuned, compassionate responses to children's needs (Menschner & Maul, 2016). These approaches also help children and young people make sense of their own experiences, reducing shame and promoting emotional regulation and resilience. Trauma-informed care is not a therapeutic technique, rather it is a systemic orientation. It shifts the question from "What's wrong with you?" to "What has happened to you?" and embeds this understanding across all levels of service delivery. Evidence-based models such as TF-CBT, EMDR, Theraplay®, and Therapeutic Foster Care demonstrate how trauma-informed principles can be operationalised to repair developmental disruptions and support recovery (Delfabbro & Osborn, 2020). Recent evidence suggests that trauma-informed care interventions positively affect the emotional and behavioural wellbeing of children involved with the child welfare system (Zhang et al., 2021).

Maltreatment, particularly when chronic or cumulative, can profoundly disrupt a child's neurodevelopment, attachment systems, and capacity to engage with support. Systems risk misinterpreting behaviours as defiance, pathologising adaptive coping mechanisms, and retraumatising children if they are not based on trauma-informed responses. The consequences of trauma-unaware systems are far-reaching. Children may be labelled as "difficult" or "non-compliant," and behavioural symptoms such as withdrawal or hypervigilance may be treated in isolation, without recognising their roots in trauma leading to exclusion from services or placement breakdowns. This contributes to service fragmentation, with children cycling through multiple systems including justice, mental health, and education, without coordinated care. It also places immense strain on professionals, who may experience burnout or compassion fatigue when trauma responses are misunderstood as personal attacks or failures.

Trauma-informed care offers a critical practice and theoretical lens. It recognises trauma as a root cause of many presenting issues, rather than a peripheral concern. It creates environments of psychological safety, where children and young people can feel seen, heard, and protected. It also builds relational trust, which is essential for healing and engagement, and supports regulation and recovery. This orientation is especially vital for children who have experienced complex trauma from cumulative maltreatment. These children require integrated, multi-disciplinary that recognise how trauma intersects with identity, community, and systemic disadvantage. For practitioners, trauma-informed care also demands robust training and reflective supervision, enabling them to respond with attunement rather than reactivity (Bunting et al., 2019). Trauma-informed care must extend beyond clinical settings, informing all aspects of child protection practice, from processes such as assessment and screening, placement and goal setting decisions, daily caregiving, community engagement and policy and system design.

For Practitioners

- Interpret behaviours (e.g. aggression, withdrawal, hypervigilance) as potential trauma responses, not defiance or pathology.
- Prioritise psychological safety in every interaction to ensure children feel seen, heard, and protected.
- Apply trauma-informed principles in assessments, placement decisions, goal setting, and case planning.
- Connect children and young people to evidence-based approaches such as TF-CBT, EMDR, Theraplay®, and Therapeutic Foster Care where appropriate.
- Build attuned, compassionate relationships that foster emotional regulation and resilience.
- Avoid control-based responses; focus on co-regulation and empowerment.
- Ensure trauma-informed language and understanding are shared across multidisciplinary teams.

For Decision-Makers and Sector Leaders:

- Embed trauma-informed principles into sector and organisational policies, procedures, and service design.
- Ensure all levels of service delivery reflect an understanding of trauma's impact.
- Provide ongoing, high-quality training in trauma-informed care for all staff, including non-clinical roles and caregivers.
- Fund and prioritise reflective supervision models that support practitioner wellbeing and trauma-informed care capacity.
- Create environments that promote safety, trust, and dignity for children, families, and staff and avoid punitive or compliance-driven approaches that re-traumatise or disempower.
- Develop cross-sector protocols that support shared understanding and coordinated care for children with complex trauma.
- Implement indicators that assess the quality and impact of trauma-informed care across services.

- Use feedback from children, families, and practitioners to refine and improve trauma-informed approaches.

Practice Principle 3. Engage every maltreated child in comprehensive, trauma-informed assessment

Comprehensive assessment is a cornerstone of effective child protection practice but goes beyond initial risk assessing. For children and young people who have experienced maltreatment, functional assessments offer a critical opportunity to understand both the immediate and long-term impacts of maltreatment across all domains and subsequently inform clinical or therapeutic formulation (Haune et al., 2024; Lockhart et al., 2021; Luke et al., 2014; Verbist et al., 2020). When conducted regularly and with a trauma-informed lens, assessments help practitioners and systems move beyond reactive responses and toward proactive, tailored support (Manuscript under review).

Annual, multidisciplinary assessments should be standard practice across the child protection continuum. These assessments must go beyond surface-level screening to explore maltreatment histories, developmental disruptions, and emerging needs. They should be holistic to evaluate wellbeing as a combination of behavioural, neurocognitive, physical, mental health, and social functioning. They should also be developmentally attuned to the child's age and stage. Importantly, assessments must be trauma-informed, ensuring that the process itself promotes emotional safety and does not retraumatise the child or young person. Although comprehensive assessments are relatively common in OOHC settings, they are far less routine in other child protection contexts, particularly in early intervention or family support services. This gap means that many children and young people with significant needs may not receive the tailored support they require. To address this, assessments should be initiated as soon as a child becomes involved with any formal child protection service. Early assessment provides practitioners with a clear, shared understanding of the child's individual needs, strengths, and risks, enabling more targeted and effective support from the outset.

Research consistently shows that early and ongoing assessments improve outcomes by identifying complex needs and informing appropriate referrals and care planning (Bunger et al., 2021; Haune et al., 2023; Lockhart et al., 2021). However, many systems still rely on fragmented or crisis-driven assessments, leading to unmet needs and missed opportunities for early intervention. Inconsistencies in assessment practices remain a significant barrier to effective care. Standardised, validated tools designed for child protection contexts are urgently needed to ensure consistency and quality. Effective assessment is also not a one-off event. Rather, it must be embedded into case planning and revisited regularly to reflect the evolving needs of the child or young person. This includes gathering information from multiple sources including direct engagement with the child, input from caregivers, educators, health professionals, and any adults with critical insight into the child's history and current environment. Where health services lead the assessment process, child protection systems must establish clear pathways and shared responsibilities to ensure findings are translated into action.

Critically, assessment alone is not enough. As cautioned by the Royal Australian College of Physicians (2023), the value of assessment lies in its follow-through. Recommendations must be implemented, monitored, and integrated into the child's broader care plan. Without this, assessment risks becoming a procedural formality rather than a meaningful tool for change. Given the known impacts of maltreatment and the complexity of needs within this cohort, comprehensive assessment should be treated as a priority, not an optional task or just a diagnostic tool. Conducting and using the data from assessments should be seen as a relational and strategic practice that sets the foundation for healing, enabling practitioners to see the full picture, respond with precision, and support children and young people in ways that are attuned to their lived experiences. It is a foundational practice that enables systems to respond with precision, compassion, and accountability.

For Practitioners:

- Initiate comprehensive, trauma-informed assessments as soon as a child enters any formal child protection or support service.
- Engage children and young people in an initial assessment that explores both historical and current needs, with follow ups depending on the length of time-of-service delivery.
- Use assessments to inform proactive case planning, therapeutic referrals, and relational strategies.
- Engage children and young people in the process, ensuring their voice and experience shape the understanding of their needs.
- Treat assessment as a relational process, using it to build trust, understand lived experience, and guide tailored support from the outset.
- Revisit the outcomes of assessments regularly to reflect the child's evolving needs, developmental changes, and emerging risks or strengths.
- Apply assessment tools that go beyond surface-level screening, to explore physical, emotional, behavioural, neurocognitive, and social functioning.
- Ensure assessments are developmentally appropriate, adapting methods and language to suit the child's age and, importantly, developmental stage.
- Avoid re-traumatisation by conducting assessments in emotionally safe, child-centred ways that respect autonomy and dignity.

- Incorporate input from caregivers, educators, health professionals, and others with insight into the child's history and current environment.
- Translate assessment findings into actionable care plans that reflect the full picture of the child's needs and strengths.
- Use assessment data to inform referrals, therapeutic interventions, and relational strategies that support healing and development.
- Advocate for consistency in assessment practices across teams and jurisdictions to reduce fragmentation and improve outcomes.

For Decision-Makers and System Leaders:

- Mandate annual, multidisciplinary assessments across all child protection service tiers, not just OOHC.
- Standardise assessment procedures across services, ensuring tools are validated for child protection contexts and developmentally appropriate.
- Embed assessment into organisational policy as a core function of care and not as a reactive or optional task.
- Ensure cross-sector collaboration in assessment processes, with clear responsibilities and pathways for implementation of recommendations.
- Embed assessment as a core component of case planning, with clear protocols for initiation, review, and follow-through.
- Ensure tools are trauma-informed, culturally responsive, and developmentally attuned.
- Provide training and guidance to practitioners on how to use these tools effectively and sensitively.

Practice Principle 4. Adopt proactive approaches to understanding and addressing cumulative maltreatment

A proactive, maltreatment-responsive child protection system can prevent harm from becoming entrenched if it is designed to anticipate, identify, and respond to the full spectrum of impacts early and consistently. Children and young people who have experienced maltreatment often carry complex, transdiagnostic impacts that reach far beyond immediate safety concerns. These psychological, relational, emotional, behavioural, and social effects may not be immediately visible, but they shape how children engage with caregivers, peers, education, and support systems. Waiting for issues to become visible often results in mismatched assessments, delayed treatment, and missed opportunities for early support (Beal et al., 2022). Waiting for symptoms to escalate before responding risks entrenching harm and missing critical windows for healing (Devlin et al., 2022; Lockhart et al., 2021). The child protection system must operate proactively, with maltreatment-responsive planning embedded across all levels of engagement.

A proactive system anticipates the likely consequences of cumulative maltreatment, even before formal diagnoses or acute presentations emerge. This means recognising early indicators such as emotional dysregulation, attachment disruption, social withdrawal, developmental delays, and behavioural adaptations that may reflect trauma. It also requires equipping practitioners, caregivers, educators, and allied professionals with the knowledge and tools to interpret these signs and respond with sensitivity and consistency. Proactive planning must begin at the point of engagement and not be deferred until stability is achieved. In early intervention and family preservation services, this means integrating therapeutic support into casework from the outset, rather than focusing solely on parental behaviour or risk mitigation. In statutory child protection, it means designing recovery-oriented plans that address the child's developmental needs alongside safety concerns from the beginning with referral pathways that are accessible, timely, and not contingent on formal diagnoses.

Importantly, proactive systems must look beyond clinical symptoms. Children who have experienced maltreatment often struggle with trust, identity, belonging, and relational safety. Their behaviours may reflect unmet emotional needs rather than pathology. A truly proactive approach requires a holistic lens that considers the full spectrum of maltreatment-related impacts and engages children, caregivers, and support networks in planning for recovery.

For Practitioners:

- Embed maltreatment-responsive planning into casework from the outset, anticipating both visible and invisible impacts.
- Engage children and caregivers in early conversations about emotional well-being, relational needs, and developmental support.
- Use a non-diagnostic lens to identify early signs of distress and refer to appropriate services before crisis thresholds are met.
- Integrate mental health and therapeutic supports into early intervention and family preservation as core components.
- In statutory child protection, co-design plans that reflect the child's lived experience and anticipate cumulative maltreatment.
- In OOHC, treat mental health care as a core function, not a crisis response, with proactive planning from entry into care
- Recognise early indicators of trauma (e.g. emotional dysregulation, attachment disruption, social withdrawal) even without formal diagnoses.
- Interpret behavioural adaptations through a trauma-informed lens, distinguishing survival strategies from defiance or pathology.

- Initiate therapeutic support at the point of engagement and not only after stability is achieved or symptoms escalate.

For Decision-Makers and System Leaders:

- Redesign referral pathways to prioritise early engagement with mental health and therapeutic services, regardless of formal diagnosis.
- Allocate funding to support therapeutic integration in early intervention and statutory services.
- Remove diagnostic requirements from access to critical services i.e., disability, education or health for children in care.
- Embed proactive planning into organisational policies, ensuring it is treated as a core function of care.
- Invest in training and tools that help carers and professionals recognise and respond to the full spectrum of maltreatment-related impacts.
- Develop interagency protocols that prioritise early support and recovery planning for maltreated children.
- Support co-design processes that include children, families, and frontline practitioners in shaping service responses.

Practice Principle 5. Prioritise stability across all domains of a child's life

Stability across life domains is foundational to recovery from cumulative maltreatment. For children and young people who have experienced cumulative maltreatment, stability is a therapeutic necessity. The cumulative impacts of maltreatment are often exacerbated when children face instability across key domains of life including where and with whom they live, relationships, education, health care, and community connections. Practitioners must therefore prioritise stability as a core component of recovery-oriented practice across the entire child protection continuum, not just within OOHC.

Research consistently shows that early, sustained, and well-matched care arrangements significantly improve social, emotional, and mental health outcomes for children and young people in OOHC (Conn et al., 2015; Frederico et al., 2017; Tarren-Sweeney, 2021). However, placement instability remains endemic in OOHC systems globally, often triggering a cascade of disruptions that extend beyond the home environment such as with trusted adults, therapists, teachers, coaches etc. Such instability can disrupt access to critical information sharing between stakeholders, for example relating to assessment, planning, and treatment (Devlin et al., 2022; Hambrick et al., 2016). The current mismatch between placement demand and culturally appropriate care options is a growing concern (Smart et al., 2022), and practitioners must advocate for systemic reforms that address this gap.

Importantly, instability is not confined to OOHC. Children engaged through early intervention or family preservation services may also experience frequent changes in caregivers, schools, caseworkers, and service providers. These disruptions compound the effects of maltreatment and erode the consistency needed for healing. Practitioners must therefore adopt a whole-of-system lens that recognises stability as a priority across all service tiers. For First Nations children and young people, stability must also include cultural continuity and connection to Country, kin, and community. Stability alone however cannot resolve complex maltreatment-related issues, though it is a critical enabler of therapeutic progress. Without a reasonable level of stability, even the most sophisticated interventions risk being undermined by inconsistency and fragmentation. Practitioners must therefore treat stability as both an outcome to be achieved after crisis resolution, and as a guiding principle from the outset of engagement.

For Practitioners:

- Minimise unnecessary disruptions by maintaining consistent relationships with children, even across changes in casework or service settings.
- Facilitate warm handovers between professionals and services to ensure continuity of therapeutic care, education, and support.
- Document and share critical health and developmental information to prevent loss of knowledge during transitions and enable accurate planning.
- Engage caregivers in understanding trauma-related behaviours and equip them with strategies to respond predictably and support relational safety.
- Coordinate with schools and community services to promote educational and social stability, including consistent routines and peer relationships.
- Advocate for cultural continuity for First Nations children and young people, including connection to Country, kin, and community.
- Use reflective supervision to identify risks to stability and plan proactively for relational and environmental consistency.

For Decision-Makers and System Leaders:

- Invest in placement matching systems that prioritise therapeutic fit, cultural safety, and long-term permanency over speed of placement.
- Fund and embed continuity-focused roles (e.g., transition coordinators, cultural connectors) to support stable relationships across service tiers.
- Establish integrated data systems that track placement history, health records, and relational networks to inform decision-making and prevent fragmentation.

- Mandate stability-focused planning in casework protocols, care plans, and review processes across early intervention, statutory, and OOHC services.
- Support workforce retention and consistency through fair remuneration, trauma-informed supervision, and career development pathways.
- Ensure access to trauma-informed training for all professionals and caregivers involved in child protection, with a focus on relational and developmental stability.
- Create policy frameworks that embed stability as a core outcome.
- Monitor and report on stability indicators (e.g., placement changes, school transitions, therapeutic continuity) as part of system performance metrics.

Practice Principle 6. Strengthen relational networks and supportive communities around every child

A maltreatment-responsive child protection system must embed relational care and community connection as a core principle of practice. Children and young people who have experienced maltreatment require more than safety; they need enduring, nurturing relationships and access to diverse communities that foster belonging, identity, and healing as a prerequisite to feeling safe. Children and young people who have experienced cumulative maltreatment experience fractured attachments and disrupted caregiving relationships. Practitioners and research alike emphasise the importance of secure, attuned, and trauma-aware caregiving, whether from statutory carers or parents. These relationships must be predictable and responsive, offering persistent safety and emotional availability. To achieve this, investment in caregiver support is critical. Supporting caregivers' wellbeing and capacity enhances their ability to provide consistent, therapeutic care and reduces the risk of instability and disruption (Appleyard & Osofsky, 2003; Cyr & Alink, 2017; Monson et al., 2021). Caregivers must also be recognised as central partners in the care team, with their insights and relational role actively integrated into planning and decision-making.

The practice of supporting children and young people to build safe and meaningful relationships extends beyond just professionals in the care team. Children and young people benefit profoundly from mentorship programs, peer networks, and relationships with cultural advisors, community leaders, and trusted adults outside the child protection system (Chesmore et al., 2017). These connections offer social acceptance, identity affirmation, and opportunities for normative development. This could include facilitating engagement with interest-based, faith-based, and cultural communities, connecting children to peers with shared lived experiences or supporting participation in hobby groups, sports clubs, and community events. For First Nations children and young people connection to cultural healing practices such as storytelling, yarning, music, and dance are a critical part of building trusted relationships through communities.

Young people often face an abrupt loss of support and connections once they are transitioned out of child protection services, particularly a concern for those in statutory OOHC. Practitioners must be actively building into plans mechanisms to establish and maintain positive relationships and communities that advocate for and support young people into adulthood. This includes extended family, former caregivers, mentors, and community groups. Family networks, especially extended family such as aunts, uncles, cousins, and former foster siblings, are instrumental in reducing isolation and providing stability to children who have experienced cumulative maltreatment. This is particularly salient as connection to community is a well-evidenced protective factor for mental health (Cheung et al., 2017; Jean-Thorn et al., 2023). These connections also serve as social capital, supporting resilience, wellbeing and even material support into adulthood (Leve et al., 2012; McPherson et al., 2014; Mendes & Chaffey, 2024). A relationally focused approach to child protection practice is cultivated through a deliberate focus on supporting relationships, belonging, and community. Child protection systems must enable practitioners and caregivers to act with urgency and intentionality to ensure that every child and young person has access to the relational ecosystems they need to thrive.

For Practitioners

- Prioritise the development of warm, predictable, trauma-aware relationships with children and young people from the first point of engagement.
- Actively support caregivers (statutory carers and parents) to provide attuned, therapeutic care through coaching, reflective supervision, and wellbeing support.
- Recognise and respond to relational disruptions caused by placement changes or staff turnover, and advocate for continuity wherever possible.
- Identify and connect children and young people to interest-based, cultural, faith-based, and peer communities that reflect their identity and interests.
- Engage First Nations children and young people in cultural healing practices such as storytelling, yarning, music, and dance.
- Support participation in mentorship programs and peer networks, especially those involving lived experience of maltreatment and child protection involvement.
- Map and activate extended family networks (e.g. aunts, uncles, cousins, former foster siblings) as part of care planning and transition support.
- Prepare families to support the child or young person's maltreatment-related needs, especially in anticipation of reunification or transition from services.

- Use tools like life story work and cultural action plans to reinforce identity and relational continuity.

For Decision-Makers and System Leaders:

- Formalise relational care and community connection as core components of child protection policy, standards, and practice frameworks.
- Ensure relational consistency is treated as a therapeutic intervention, not a discretionary feature.
- Integrate caregiver wellbeing and support and reflective practice infrastructure to enhance relational capacity, into system-level planning and funding models.
- Fund mentorship programs, peer networks, and community-based initiatives that foster belonging and identity for children and young people.
- Remove structural barriers that prevent children in OOHC from participating in community groups due to care status or administrative restrictions.
- Prioritise cultural connection for First Nations children and young people through dedicated funding and partnerships.
- Recognise caregivers as essential partners in the care team and embed their voices in decision-making processes.
- Develop policies that support continuity of care and reduce placement disruptions.

Practice Principle 7. Collaborate meaningfully with stakeholders across all facets of the child's life

Children and young people who have experienced maltreatment often navigate a complex web of systems including child protection, education, health, mental health, disability, housing, and justice. Each holds partial responsibility for their wellbeing, yet too often, these systems operate in isolation, resulting in fragmented care, siloed information, and inconsistent therapeutic support (Bertram, 2018; Devlin et al., 2022; Vasileva & Petermann, 2017). Cross-sector and interagency collaboration is another foundational requirement for effective practice to address maltreatment-related concerns (Firmin et al., 2022; Herbert & Bromfield, 2019). While much of this evidence emerges from the OOHC context, its implications extend across the entire child protection continuum, from early intervention and statutory investigation through to reunification, kinship care, and post-care support.

Practitioners working within child protection systems are uniquely positioned to act as mediators given their proximity to the child or young person's lived experience, and their role in coordinating responses which places them at the nexus of multiple systems. However, this integrative function cannot be fulfilled in isolation. It demands deliberate, structured collaboration with other stakeholders in the child or young person's life, including mental health professionals, educators, cultural advisors, disability workers, housing providers, caregivers, and critically, the child or young person themselves. The wellbeing of children and young people is a shared societal responsibility, and many others must be actively involved. Multi-disciplinary teams are essential, not only for their breadth of expertise but for their capacity to hold a shared understanding of the child's needs and coordinate responses that are holistic, trauma-aware, and culturally grounded (Alfandari & Taylor, 2022). These teams must be supported by system-level structures that compel collaboration. Formal institutional agreements, shared planning protocols, and interagency liaison roles are all mechanisms that move collaboration from discretionary practice to structural expectation.

Collaboration must also be embedded as a shared knowledge system and a set of tangible practices. This includes joint assessment protocols, shared treatment planning, multi-disciplinary meetings, and mechanisms for cultural consultation. Child protection practitioners are expected to co-created care plans that were holistic, individualised, and continuously monitored with all stakeholders who can support the child or young person. However, the current landscape is marked by systemic barriers to collaboration. Information about diagnoses, medication, and therapeutic progress is often held separately by child protection and mental health services, for example, leading to substandard care and fractured treatment pathways. If the intrinsically differing theoretical orientations and practice paradigms are not explicitly negotiated, they can further disrupt coordinated responses *(manuscript under review)*. Practitioners must therefore be equipped not only with clinical or statutory expertise, but with the relational and strategic skills to navigate these complexities and equally, be supported by institutional agreements that formalise collaboration, so that this collaboration can be captured meaningfully. When participation is prioritised through shared decision-making, transparent communication, and respectful engagement, interventions are more likely to improve outcomes, therapeutic relationships are strengthened, and young people are likely to feel more empowered in child protection decision-making. Therefore, child protection practitioners must lead efforts to convene multi-sector teams and ensure that care plans reflect the collective expertise of all stakeholders. This includes recognising the limits of their own sector and actively engaging others to fill those gaps.

For Practitioners

- Initiate and maintain regular communication with professionals across health, education, mental health, housing, and justice sectors involved in the child's life.

- Facilitate multi-disciplinary planning meetings that include caregivers, cultural advisors, educators, and mental health clinicians.
- Share relevant information (e.g. assessments, diagnoses, medication plans) with other sectors to ensure continuity and quality of care.
- Actively involve children and young people in decisions about their mental health care, using age-appropriate, trauma-informed engagement strategies.
- Ensure that care plans reflect the child's voice, preferences, and cultural identity, and are revisited regularly with their input.
- Advocate for youth participation even when systems do not mandate it, recognising its therapeutic and ethical importance.
- Use shared tools and protocols to coordinate care planning across sectors, including joint assessments and collaborative treatment plans.
- Engage in cross-sector training to build mutual understanding of trauma, cultural safety, and sector-specific constraints.
- Identify and escalate gaps in collaboration, such as siloed information or conflicting treatment approaches, to team leaders or system navigators.
- Embrace a structural mindset, recognising that no single practitioner or team can meet all needs in isolation.

For Decision-Makers and System Leaders:

- Establish formal interagency agreements that mandate collaboration across child protection, mental health, education, and other sectors.
- Create and fund intersectoral liaison roles to coordinate care and bridge gaps between systems.
- Require shared planning protocols and joint accountability for outcomes across sectors.
- Mandate child and youth participation in mental health care planning across all relevant systems.
- Develop policies and tools that support meaningful engagement, including co-designed care plans and feedback mechanisms.
- Monitor and report on participation rates to ensure accountability and continuous improvement.
- Fund multi-disciplinary teams that include cultural advisors, clinicians, educators, and lived experience practitioners.
- Support cross-sector training initiatives that build shared language, trauma literacy, and collaborative capacity.
- Ensure that funding models allow for time and infrastructure to support collaboration (e.g. joint meetings, shared documentation systems).

- Invest in integrated data systems that allow for safe, ethical information sharing across sectors.
- Align theoretical frameworks and practice models across child protection and other related service systems to reduce conflict and duplication.
- Evaluate and reform policies that inadvertently reinforce siloed practice or limit collaborative flexibility.

Practice Principle 8. Engage with evidence-informed clinical approaches tailored to maltreatment experiences

In contemporary child protection practice, clinical and therapeutic interventions must be recognised as critically important mechanisms for recovery and wellbeing. Children who have experienced maltreatment often carry complex emotional, behavioural, and relational wounds that cannot be addressed through caregiving alone. While safe and nurturing relationships are foundational for some children, they must be complemented by evidence-based interventions that directly engage children in healing processes tailored to their developmental stage, trauma history, and lived experience. To effect meaningful outcomes, child protection systems must move beyond reactive models and embed therapeutic engagement as a proactive, standardised component of care. This requires a shift in practice culture that sees clinical intervention not as a specialist referral for crisis cases, but as a routine part of supporting children's recovery. Practitioners must be equipped to identify trauma-related needs early, facilitate access to appropriate services, and advocate for sustained therapeutic involvement regardless of placement type or formal diagnosis.

Evidence shows that interventions grounded in trauma-informed, attachment-focused principles—such as Parent-Child Interaction Therapy (PCIT), Attachment and Biobehavioral Catch-Up (ABC), and the Family Thriving Program—can significantly improve emotional regulation, relational capacity, and long-term mental health outcomes (Valentino, 2017; Van der Put et al., 2018). However, for these interventions to be effective, children must be actively engaged in the process. This means designing services that are developmentally attuned, culturally safe, and flexible enough to accommodate the realities of children's lives including placement changes, family dynamics, and systemic barriers.

Therapeutic engagement should not be siloed within mental health services but integrated across care teams, case planning, and everyday interactions. Practitioners need training in recognising trauma symptoms, understanding intervention pathways, and supporting children's participation in formal, clinical treatment. This includes building trusting relationships, preparing children for therapeutic work, and ensuring that interventions are not disrupted by system transitions.

Importantly, therapeutic engagement must be framed as a right. All children who have experienced maltreatment deserve access to interventions that support their healing, not just those who meet diagnostic criteria or are placed in certain care settings. This calls for investment in scalable, evidence-informed models that can be embedded across statutory, community, and clinical services. It also requires a commitment to monitoring outcomes, learning from practice, and continually improving the therapeutic landscape within child protection.

For Practitioners:

- Identify trauma-related needs early through structured assessment and observation, even in the absence of formal diagnoses.
- Normalise therapeutic support by introducing clinical interventions as part of routine care planning, not just in crisis.
- Facilitate access to specialised programs such as PCIT, ABC, or trauma-focused CBT, advocating for child inclusion regardless of placement or service type.
- Prepare children for therapeutic engagement by building trust, explaining the process in developmentally appropriate ways, and supporting emotional readiness.
- Collaborate across sectors to ensure therapeutic plans are integrated into case management and not siloed within mental health, disability or other services.
- Monitor engagement and progress by maintaining regular communication with clinicians and adjusting care plans based on therapeutic feedback.
- Champion culturally safe practices by ensuring interventions are responsive to the child's identity, community, and lived experience.
- Support continuity of care during transitions (e.g., placement changes, reunification) to prevent disruption of therapeutic relationships.

For Decision-Makers and System Leaders:

- Position therapeutic and clinical engagement as a core component of child protection practice, not an ancillary service.
- Fund and scale evidence-based interventions that are tailored to maltreatment-related needs and accessible across diverse child protection settings.
- Develop cross-sector protocols that integrate therapeutic services into statutory pathways, case planning, and review processes.
- Invest in workforce development to ensure practitioners are trained in trauma-informed practice, therapeutic referral pathways, and child engagement strategies.

- Establish outcome monitoring systems to track therapeutic engagement, effectiveness, and long-term recovery trajectories.
- Create flexible service models that accommodate placement instability, family complexity, and systemic barriers to engagement.
- Champion a shift in practice culture that values healing and relational repair as central to child protection, not secondary to safety and risk management.

3. CONCLUSION

To respond meaningfully to the effects of cumulative maltreatment, child protection systems must evolve beyond crisis-driven models and embrace relationally driven trauma-informed therapeutic engagement as foundational to practice. Children who have experienced cumulative maltreatment require more than safety, but caregiving, practice and interventions grounded in evidence that support healing. This chapter has argued that clinical and therapeutic supports must be embedded across statutory, community, and clinical services, not reserved for those who meet diagnostic thresholds or are placed in formal care settings. Practitioners must be equipped to recognise cumulative maltreatment symptoms early, through proactive case work and engagement with multi-disciplinary teams to facilitate access to specialised programs, assessments and support children's active participation in treatment. Sector leaders must invest in scalable, evidence-informed models and champion a culture that values healing as central to protection for children, and stability and security as pivotal for a sustainable workforce. By integrating trauma-informed principles, fostering cross-sector collaboration, and prioritising continuity of care, child protection practice can move from containment to transformation. This shift is essential not only for individual wellbeing but for disrupting intergenerational cycles of disadvantage and building a more equitable, responsive child protection system.

REFERENCES

Afifi, T. O., & MacMillan, H. L. (2011). Resilience following child maltreatment: A review of protective factors. *Canadian Journal of Psychiatry*, *56*(5), 266–272. DOI: 10.1177/070674371105600505 PMID: 21586192

Afifi, T. O., MacMillan, H. L., Boyle, M., Taillieu, T., Cheung, K., & Sareen, J. (2014). Child abuse and mental disorders in Canada. *Canadian Medical Association Journal*, *186*(9), E324–E332. DOI: 10.1503/cmaj.131792 PMID: 24756625

Alfandari, R., & Taylor, B. J. (2022). Community-based multi-professional child protection decision making: Systematic narrative review. *Child Abuse & Neglect*, *123*, 105432. DOI: 10.1016/j.chiabu.2021.105432 PMID: 34922154

Annerbäck, E. M., Sahlqvist, L., Svedin, C. G., Wingren, G., & Gustafsson, P. A. (2012). Child physical abuse and concurrence of other types of child abuse in Sweden—Associations with health and risk behaviors. *Child Abuse & Neglect*, *36*(7-8), 585–595. DOI: 10.1016/j.chiabu.2012.05.006 PMID: 22854707

Appleyard, K., & Osofsky, J. D. (2003). Parenting after trauma: Supporting parents and caregivers in the treatment of children impacted by violence. *Infant Mental Health Journal*, *24*(2), 111–125. DOI: 10.1002/imhj.10050

Arata, C. M., Langhinrichsen-Rohling, J., Bowers, D., & O'Farrill-Swails, L. (2005). Single versus multi-type maltreatment: An examination of the long-term effects of child abuse. *Journal of Aggression, Maltreatment & Trauma*, *11*(4), 29–52. DOI: 10.1300/J146v11n04_02

Åsen, M. E., Schalinski, I., Lehmann, S., Lydersen, S., Von Oertzen, T., & Greger, H. K. (2024). Child maltreatment in young adults with residential youth care background: Prevalence and post-placement trends. *Child Abuse & Neglect*, *157*, 107. DOI: 10.1016/j.chiabu.2024.107074 PMID: 39395227

Baldwin, H., Biehal, N., Cusworth, L., Wade, J., Allgar, V., & Vostanis, P. (2019). Disentangling the effect of out-of-home care on child mental health. *Child Abuse & Neglect*, *88*, 189–200. DOI: 10.1016/j.chiabu.2018.11.011 PMID: 30537620

Baldwin, J. R., Wang, B., Karwatowska, L., Schoeler, T., Tsaligopoulou, A., Munafò, M. R., & Pingault, J. B. (2023). Childhood maltreatment and mental health problems: A systematic review and meta-analysis of quasi-experimental studies. *The American Journal of Psychiatry*, *180*(2), 117–126. DOI: 10.1176/appi.ajp.20220174 PMID: 36628513

Bath, H. (2008). The three pillars of trauma-informed care. *Reclaiming Children and Youth, 17*(3), 17–21.

Beal, S. J., Ammerman, R. T., Mara, C. A., Nause, K., & Greiner, M. V. (2022). Patterns of healthcare utilization with placement changes for youth in foster care. *Child Abuse & Neglect, 128*, 105592. DOI: 10.1016/j.chiabu.2022.105592 PMID: 35334304

Belsky, J. (1993). Etiology of child maltreatment: A developmental ecological analysis. *Psychological Bulletin, 114*(3), 413–434. DOI: 10.1037/0033-2909.114.3.413 PMID: 8272464

Benbenishty, R., Davidson-Arad, B., López, M., Devaney, J., Spratt, T., Koopmans, C., Knorth, E. J., Witteman, C. L. M., Del Valle, J. F., & Hayes, D. (2015). Decision making in child protection: An international comparative study on maltreatment substantiation, risk assessment and interventions recommendations, and the role of professionals' child welfare attitudes. *Child Abuse & Neglect, 49*, 63–75. DOI: 10.1016/j.chiabu.2015.03.015 PMID: 25935254

Berger, L. M., & Slack, K. S. (2014). Child protection and child well-being. In *Handbook of child well-being* (pp. 2965–2992). Springer., DOI: 10.1007/978-90-481-9063-8_120

Biehal, N., Baldwin, H., Cusworth, L., Wade, J., & Allgar, V. (2018). In-home support or out of home care? Thresholds for intervention with abused and neglected children. *Children and Youth Services Review, 89*, 263–271. DOI: 10.1016/j.childyouth.2018.04.041

Bijlsma, A. M., Assink, M., Overbeek, G., van Geffen, M., & van der Put, C. E. (2023). Differences in developmental problems between victims of different types of child maltreatment. *Journal of Public Child Welfare, 17*(2), 408–429. Advance online publication. DOI: 10.1080/15548732.2022.2044429 PMID: 36896409

Blome, W. W., & Steib, S. (2008). An examination of oversight and review in the child welfare system: The many watch the few serve the many. *Journal of Public Child Welfare, 1*(3), 3–26. DOI: 10.1300/J479v01n03_02

Bryce, I., & Collier, S. (2022). A systematic literature review of the contribution accumulation makes to psychological and physical trauma sustained through childhood maltreatment. *Trauma Care, 2*(2), 307–329. DOI: 10.3390/traumacare2020026

Bunger, A. C., Maguire-Jack, K., Yoon, S., Mooney, D., West, K. Y., Hammond, G. C., & Kranich, C. (2021). Does mental health screening and assessment in child welfare improve mental health service receipt, child safety, and permanence for children in out-of-home care? An evaluation of the Gateway CALL demonstration. *Child Abuse & Neglect*, *122*, 105351. DOI: 10.1016/j.chiabu.2021.105351 PMID: 34628151

Bunting, L., Montgomery, L., Mooney, S., MacDonald, M., Coulter, S., Hayes, D., & Davidson, G. (2019). Trauma informed child welfare systems—A rapid evidence review. *International Journal of Environmental Research and Public Health*, *16*(13), 2365. DOI: 10.3390/ijerph16132365 PMID: 31277339

Cecil, C. A., Viding, E., Fearon, P., Glaser, D., & McCrory, E. J. (2017). Disentangling the mental health impact of childhood abuse and neglect. *Child Abuse & Neglect*, *63*, 106–119. DOI: 10.1016/j.chiabu.2016.11.024 PMID: 27914236

Chesmore, A. A., Weiler, L. M., & Taussig, H. N. (2017). Mentoring relationship quality and maltreated children's coping. *American Journal of Community Psychology*, *60*(1-2), 229–241. DOI: 10.1002/ajcp.12151 PMID: 28792079

Cheung, K., Taillieu, T., Turner, S., Fortier, J., Sareen, J., MacMillan, H. L., Boyle, M. H., & Afifi, T. O. (2017). Relationship and community factors related to better mental health following child maltreatment among adolescents. *Child Abuse & Neglect*, *70*, 377–387. DOI: 10.1016/j.chiabu.2017.06.026 PMID: 28750346

Conn, A. M., Szilagyi, M. A., Franke, T. M., Albertin, C. S., Blumkin, A. K., & Szilagyi, P. G. (2013). Trends in child protection and out-of-home care. *Pediatrics*, *132*(4), 712–719. DOI: 10.1542/peds.2013-0969 PMID: 24062369

Conn, A. M., Szilagyi, M. A., Jee, S. H., Blumkin, A. K., & Szilagyi, P. G. (2015). Mental health outcomes among child welfare investigated children: In-home versus out-of-home care. *Children and Youth Services Review*, *57*, 106–111. DOI: 10.1016/j.childyouth.2015.08.004

Cox, A., Frederico, M., Mosse, H., Radford, L., Ambry, D., & Ryan, C. (2021). Australian maltreated infants and young children can achieve positive relational health with neurodevelopmentally-and trauma-informed interventions provided within relationally-positive and stable environments. *Frontiers in Psychiatry*, *12*, 680343. DOI: 10.3389/fpsyt.2021.680343 PMID: 34393846

Cyr, C., & Alink, L. R. (2017). Child maltreatment: The central roles of parenting capacities and attachment. *Current Opinion in Psychology*, *15*, 81–86. DOI: 10.1016/j.copsyc.2017.02.002 PMID: 28813275

Cyr, K., Chamberland, C., Lessard, G., Clément, M. È., Wemmers, J. A., Collin-Vézina, D., Gagné, M.-H., & Damant, D. (2012). Polyvictimization in a child welfare sample of children and youths. *Psychology of Violence*, *2*(4), 385–400. DOI: 10.1037/a0028040

Darlington, Y., Healy, K., & Feeney, J. A. (2010). Approaches to assessment and intervention across four types of child and family welfare services. *Children and Youth Services Review*, *32*(3), 356–364. DOI: 10.1016/j.childyouth.2009.10.005

Daro, D., Donnelly, A. C., Huang, L. A., & Powell, B. J. (Eds.). (2015). *Advances in child abuse prevention knowledge: The perspective of new leadership*. Springer International Publishing., DOI: 10.1007/978-3-319-16327-7

Delfabbro, P., & Osborn, A. (2020). Therapeutic approaches to children and families in child protection contexts. In *Child Protection and the Care Continuum* (pp. 134–148). Routledge. DOI: 10.4324/9781003121305-8

Descartes, C. H., Maharaj, P. E., Quammie, M., Mills, J., Ramesar, M., & Pulwarty, H. (2020). It's never one type: The co-occurrence of child abuse and neglect among children living in community residences in Trinidad. *Journal of Child & Adolescent Trauma*, *13*(4), 419–427. DOI: 10.1007/s40653-019-00293-x PMID: 33269042

Devlin, R., Jairam, R., Asghari, M., & Eapen, V. (2022). Does assertive mental health care make a difference to children in out-of-home care? A pilot study. *Developmental Child Welfare*, *4*(1), 73–93. DOI: 10.1177/25161032211064644

Felitti, V. J., Anda, R. F., Nordenberg, D., Williamson, D. F., Spitz, A. M., Edwards, V., & Marks, J. S. (1998). Relationship of childhood abuse and household dysfunction to many of the leading causes of death in adults: The Adverse Childhood Experiences (ACE) Study. *American Journal of Preventive Medicine*, *14*(4), 245–258. DOI: 10.1016/S0749-3797(98)00017-8 PMID: 9635069

Firmin, C., Lefevre, M., Huegler, N., & Peace, D. (2022). Improving interagency collaboration. In *Safeguarding young people beyond the family home* (pp. 43–52). Policy Press., DOI: 10.2307/j.ctv2zjz6z3.8

Frederico, M., Long, M., McNamara, P., McPherson, L., & Rose, R. (2017). Improving outcomes for children in out-of-home care: The role of therapeutic foster care. *Child & Family Social Work*, *22*(2), 1064–1074. DOI: 10.1111/cfs.12326

Fu, H., Feng, T., Qin, J., Wang, T., Wu, X., Cai, Y., Lan, L., & Yang, T. (2018). Reported prevalence of childhood maltreatment among Chinese college students: A systematic review and meta-analysis. *PLoS One*, *13*(10), e0205808. DOI: 10.1371/journal.pone.0205808 PMID: 30321243

Gabrielli, J., & Jackson, Y. (2019). Innovative methodological and statistical approaches to the study of child maltreatment: Introduction. *Child Abuse & Neglect, 87*, 1–4. DOI: 10.1016/j.chiabu.2018.12.001 PMID: 30551809

Gilbert, R., Widom, C. S., Browne, K., Fergusson, D., Webb, E., & Janson, S. (2009). Burden and consequences of child maltreatment in high-income countries. *Lancet, 373*(9657), 68–81. DOI: 10.1016/S0140-6736(08)61706-7 PMID: 19056114

Hambrick, E. P., Oppenheim-Weller, S., N'zi, A. M., & Taussig, H. N. (2016). Mental health interventions for children in foster care: A systematic review. *Children and Youth Services Review, 70*, 65–77. DOI: 10.1016/j.childyouth.2016.09.002 PMID: 28496286

Harris, L. G., Higgins, D. J., Willis, M. L., Lawrence, D., Mathews, B., Malacova, E., Erskine, H. E., Meinck, F., & Haslam, D. M. (2025). Determining the effect of out-of-home care on mental health disorders: A propensity score-matched study of child maltreatment intensity. *Child Abuse & Neglect, 167*, 107571. DOI: 10.1016/j.chiabu.2025.107571 PMID: 40532408

Harris, L. G., Higgins, D. J., Willis, M. L., Lawrence, D., Mathews, B., Thomas, H. J., Malacova, E., Pacella, R., Scott, J. G., Finkelhor, D., Meinck, F., Erskine, H. E., & Haslam, D. M. (2024). The Prevalence and patterns of maltreatment, childhood adversity, and mental health disorders in an Australian out-of-home care sample. *Child Maltreatment, 0*(0). Advance online publication. DOI: 10.1177/10775595241246534 PMID: 38627990

Harris, L. G., Higgins, D. J., & Willis, M. L. (2026). Practitioners' perspectives on enablers of improved mental health outcomes for children and young people in out-of-home care: Beyond a "scattergun approach". *Child Protection and Practice, 100283*. Advance online publication. DOI: 10.1016/j.chipro.2026.100283

Haune, M., Christiansen, Ø., Heiervang, E. R., & Haavind, H. (2024). "Great day! But now what?" Adolescents' and foster carers' experiences of a comprehensive health assessment for children in out-of-home care. *Children and Youth Services Review, 158*, 107464. DOI: 10.1016/j.childyouth.2024.107464

Herbert, J. L., & Bromfield, L. (2019). Multi-disciplinary teams responding to child abuse: Common features and assumptions. *Children and Youth Services Review, 106*, 104467. DOI: 10.1016/j.childyouth.2019.104467

Higgins, D. J., & Hunt, G. R. (2024). Child, parent and contextual factors associated with child protection system involvement and child maltreatment in the family: A rapid evidence review. *The Australian Journal of Social Issues, 59*(2), 358–400. DOI: 10.1002/ajs4.306

Higgins, D. J., Mathews, B., Pacella, R., Scott, J. G., Finkelhor, D., Meinck, F., Erskine, H. E., Thomas, H. J., Lawrence, D. M., Haslam, D. M., Malacova, E., & Dunne, M. P. (2023). The prevalence and nature of multi-type child maltreatment in Australia. *The Medical Journal of Australia, 218*(S6), S19–S25. DOI: 10.5694/mja2.51868 PMID: 37004183

Higgins, D. J., & McCabe, M. P. (2000). Multi-type maltreatment and the long-term adjustment of adults. *Child Abuse Review, 9*(1), 6–18. DOI: 10.1002/(SICI)1099-0852(200001/02)9:1<6::AID-CAR579>3.0.CO;2-W

Hughes, D. (2004). An attachment-based treatment of maltreated children and young people. *Attachment & Human Development, 6*(3), 263–278. DOI: 10.1080/14616730412331281539 PMID: 15513268

Ioannidis, K., Askelund, A. D., Kievit, R. A., & Van Harmelen, A. L. (2020). The complex neurobiology of resilient functioning after childhood maltreatment. *BMC Medicine, 18*(1), 32. DOI: 10.1186/s12916-020-1490-7 PMID: 32050974

Isokuortti, N., Aaltio, E., Laajasalo, T., & Barlow, J. (2020). Effectiveness of child protection practice models: A systematic review. *Child Abuse & Neglect, 108*, 104632. DOI: 10.1016/j.chiabu.2020.104632 PMID: 32818821

Jean-Thorn, A., Tremblay-Perreault, A., Dube, V., & Hebert, M. (2023). A systematic review of community-level protective factors in children exposed to maltreatment. *Trauma, Violence & Abuse, 24*(4), 2827–2842. DOI: 10.1177/15248380221117234 PMID: 36047717

Jud, A., Mitrovic, T., Portmann, R., Gonthier, H., Fux, E., Koehler, J., Kosirnik, C., & Knüsel, R. (2021). Multi-sectoral response to child maltreatment in Switzerland for different age groups: Varying rates of reported incidents and gaps in identification. *Child Abuse & Neglect, 111*, 104798. DOI: 10.1016/j.chiabu.2020.104798 PMID: 33213853

Kagan, R. (2014). *Rebuilding attachments with traumatized children: Healing from losses, violence, abuse, and neglect*. Routledge., DOI: 10.4324/9780203822319

Kim, H., & Drake, B. (2019). Cumulative prevalence of onset and recurrence of child maltreatment reports. *Journal of the American Academy of Child and Adolescent Psychiatry, 58*(12), 1175–1183. DOI: 10.1016/j.jaac.2019.02.015 PMID: 30851398

Kim, K., Mennen, F. E., & Trickett, P. K. (2017). Patterns and correlates of co-occurrence among multiple types of child maltreatment. *Child & Family Social Work, 22*(1), 492–502. DOI: 10.1111/cfs.12268 PMID: 29225485

Kimberg, L., & Wheeler, M. (2019). Trauma and trauma-informed care. In *Trauma-informed healthcare approaches: A guide for primary care* (pp. 25–56). Springer International Publishing., DOI: 10.1007/978-3-030-04342-1_2

Kisely, S., Abajobir, A. A., Mills, R., Strathearn, L., Clavarino, A., & Najman, J. M. (2018). Child maltreatment and mental health problems in adulthood: Birth cohort study. *The British Journal of Psychiatry*, *213*(6), 698–703. DOI: 10.1192/bjp.2018.207 PMID: 30475193

Leve, L. D., Harold, G. T., Chamberlain, P., Landsverk, J. A., Fisher, P. A., & Vostanis, P. (2012). Practitioner review: Children in foster care–vulnerabilities and evidence-based interventions that promote resilience processes. *Journal of Child Psychology and Psychiatry, and Allied Disciplines*, *53*(12), 1197–1211. DOI: 10.1111/j.1469-7610.2012.02594.x PMID: 22882015

Lima, F., Maclean, M., & O'Donnell, M. (2019). *Exploring outcomes for young people who have experienced out-of-home care*. Telethon Kids Institute.

Lockhart, G., Atkins, L., & King, A. (2021, March). *Children in Care Evidence-Based Clinical Review & Practice Guide*. NHS England South East, Clinical Delivery and Networks. CiC_Evidence_Based_Clinical_Review_and_Practice_Guide.pdf

Lonne, B., Higgins, D., Herrenkohl, T. I., & Scott, D. (2020). Reconstructing the workforce within public health protective systems: Improving resilience, retention, service responsiveness and outcomes. *Child Abuse & Neglect*, *110*, 104191. DOI: 10.1016/j.chiabu.2019.104191 PMID: 31543276

Lueger-Schuster, B., Knefel, M., Glück, T. M., Jagsch, R., Kantor, V., & Weindl, D. (2018). Child abuse and neglect in institutional settings, cumulative lifetime traumatization, and psychopathological long-term correlates in adult survivors: The Vienna Institutional Abuse Study. *Child Abuse & Neglect*, *76*, 488–501. DOI: 10.1016/j.chiabu.2017.12.009 PMID: 29276971

Luke, N., Sinclair, I., Woolgar, M., & Sebba, J. (2014). *What works in prevention and treating poor mental health in looked after children?* REES Centre. https://www.education.ox.ac.uk/wp-content/uploads/2019/06/What-Works-in-Preventing-and-Treating-Poor-Mental-Health-in-Looked-After-Children.pdf

MacMillan, H. L., Wathen, C. N., Barlow, J., Fergusson, D. M., Leventhal, J. M., & Taussig, H. N. (2009). Interventions to prevent child maltreatment and associated impairment. *Lancet*, *373*(9659), 250–266. DOI: 10.1016/S0140-6736(08)61708-0 PMID: 19056113

Mathews, B., Pacella, R., Dunne, M. P., Simunovic, M., & Marston, C. (2020). Improving measurement of child abuse and neglect: A systematic review and analysis of national prevalence studies. *PLoS One*, *15*(1), e0227884. DOI: 10.1371/journal.pone.0227884 PMID: 31990913

Mathews, B., Pacella, R., Scott, J. G., Finkelhor, D., Meinck, F., Higgins, D. J., Erskine, H. E., Thomas, H. J., Lawrence, D. M., Haslam, D. M., Malacova, E., & Dunne, M. P. (2023). The prevalence of child maltreatment in Australia: Findings from a national survey. *The Medical Journal of Australia*, *218*(S6), S13–S18. DOI: 10.5694/mja2.51873 PMID: 37004184

McLaughlin, K. A., Sheridan, M. A., Humphreys, K. L., Belsky, J., & Ellis, B. J. (2021). The value of dimensional models of early experience: Thinking clearly about concepts and categories. *Perspectives on Psychological Science*, *16*(6), 1463–1472. DOI: 10.1177/1745691621992346 PMID: 34491864

McPherson, K. E., Kerr, S., McGee, E., Morgan, A., Cheater, F. M., McLean, J., & Egan, J. (2014). The association between social capital and mental health and behavioural problems in children and adolescents: An integrative systematic review. *BMC Psychology*, *2*(1), 1–16. DOI: 10.1186/2050-7283-2-7 PMID: 25566380

Mehta, D., Kelly, A. B., Laurens, K. R., Haslam, D., Williams, K. E., Walsh, K., Baker, P. R. A., Carter, H. E., Khawaja, N. G., Zelenko, O., & Mathews, B. (2021). Child maltreatment and long-term physical and mental health outcomes: An exploration of biopsychosocial determinants and implications for prevention. *Child Psychiatry and Human Development*, •••, 1–15. DOI: 10.1007/s10578-021-01258-8 PMID: 34586552

Mendes, P., & Chaffey, E. (2024). Examining the Mental Health Care Needs and Outcomes of Young People Transitioning from Out-of-Home Care (OOHC) in Australia. *Institutionalised Children Exploration and Beyond*, *11*(1), 103–124. DOI: 10.1177/23493003231182474

Meng, X., Fleury, M. J., Xiang, Y. T., Li, M., & D'arcy, C. (2018). Resilience and protective factors among people with a history of child maltreatment: A systematic review. *Social Psychiatry and Psychiatric Epidemiology*, *53*(5), 453–475. DOI: 10.1007/s00127-018-1485-2 PMID: 29349479

Menschner, C., & Maul, A. (2016). Key ingredients for successful trauma-informed care implementation. Center for Health Care Strategies. https://www.fredla.org/wp-content/uploads/2016/04/Trauma-informed-care-implementation-1.pdf

Modderman, C., Sanders, R., Cordon, E., Hocking, C., Wade, M., & Vogels, W. (2023). Integrating health systems for children and young people in out of home care: Challenging the nature of siloed service delivery in rural Australia. *The Australian Journal of Rural Health, 31*(4), 670–679. DOI: 10.1111/ajr.12991 PMID: 37129555

Mohr, D., & Rosén, L. A. (2017). The impact of protective factors on posttraumatic growth for college student survivors of childhood maltreatment. *Journal of Aggression, Maltreatment & Trauma, 26*(7), 756–771. DOI: 10.1080/10926771.2017.1304478

Monson, K., Herrman, H., Moeller-Saxone, K., Humphreys, C., & Harvey, C. (2021). How can mental health practitioners collaborate with child welfare practitioners to improve mental health for young people in out of home care? *Early Intervention in Psychiatry, 15*(6), 1768–1776. DOI: 10.1111/eip.13118 PMID: 33474788

Moody, G., Cannings-John, R., Hood, K., Kemp, A., & Robling, M. (2018). Establishing the international prevalence of self-reported child maltreatment: A systematic review by maltreatment type and gender. *BMC Public Health, 18*(1), 1–15. DOI: 10.1186/s12889-018-6044-y PMID: 30305071

Morley, L. (2022). Contemporary practitioner experiences of relational social work: The case of child welfare. *Australian Social Work, 75*(4), 458–470. DOI: 10.1080/0312407X.2021.2001831

Munro, E. (2005). Improving practice: Child protection as a systems problem. *Children and Youth Services Review, 27*(4), 375–391. DOI: 10.1016/j.childyouth.2004.11.006

Murphy, C. (2023). How learning from the lived experiences of child protection social workers can help us understand the factors underpinning workforce instability within the English child protection system. *Journal of Social Work Practice, 37*(2), 263–276. DOI: 10.1080/02650533.2023.2185213

Obsuth, I., Mueller Johnson, K., Murray, A. L., Ribeaud, D., & Eisner, M. (2018). Violent poly-victimization: The longitudinal patterns of physical and emotional victimization throughout adolescence (11–17 years). *Journal of Research on Adolescence, 28*(4), 786–806. DOI: 10.1111/jora.12365 PMID: 29193435

Pollock, C., Grenyer, B. F., & Townsend, M. L. (2024). Responding to suicidal behaviour in children and young people with a child maltreatment history: A scoping review. *Children and Youth Services Review, 166*, 107927. DOI: 10.1016/j.childyouth.2024.107927

Rosenzweig, J. M., & Sundborg, S. A. (2022). The neurobiology of toxic stress. In Rapp-McCall, L., Corcoran, K., & Roberts, A. R. (Eds.), *Social Workers' Desk Reference* (pp. 278–289). Oxford University Press.

Ruch, G. (2005). Relationship-based practice and reflective practice: Holistic approaches to contemporary child care social work. *Child & Family Social Work, 10*(2), 111–123. DOI: 10.1111/j.1365-2206.2005.00359.x

Russ, E., Stonehouse, D., Reimer, E. C., Hitchcock, C., & McPherson, L. (2024). Supporting staff wellbeing in child welfare services. DOI: 10.25918/report.353

Russell, D. H., Trew, S., & Higgins, D. J. (2021). Vulnerable yet forgotten? A systematic review identifying the lack of evidence for effective suicide interventions for young people in contact with child protection systems. *The American Journal of Orthopsychiatry, 91*(5), 647–659. DOI: 10.1037/ort0000555 PMID: 34383517

Russell, J. R., Kerwin, C., & Halverson, J. L. (2018). Is child protective services effective? *Children and Youth Services Review, 84*, 185–192. DOI: 10.1016/j.childyouth.2017.11.028

Salazar, A. M., Keller, T. E., Gowen, L. K., & Courtney, M. E. (2013). Trauma exposure and PTSD among older adolescents in foster care. *Social Psychiatry and Psychiatric Epidemiology, 48*(4), 545–551. DOI: 10.1007/s00127-012-0563-0 PMID: 22898825

Scott-Storey, K. (2011). Cumulative abuse: Do things add up? An evaluation of the conceptualization, operationalization, and methodological approaches in the study of the phenomenon of cumulative abuse. *Trauma, Violence & Abuse, 12*(3), 135–150. DOI: 10.1177/1524838011404253 PMID: 21511684

Seker, S., Boonmann, C., Gerger, H., Jäggi, L., d'Huart, D., Schmeck, K., & Schmid, M. (2022). Mental disorders among adults formerly in out-of-home care: A systematic review and meta-analysis of longitudinal studies. *European Child & Adolescent Psychiatry, 31*(12), 1963–1982. DOI: 10.1007/s00787-021-01828-0 PMID: 34169369

Slack, K. S., & Berger, L. M. (2020). Who is and is not served by child protective services systems? Implications for a prevention infrastructure to reduce child maltreatment. *The Annals of the American Academy of Political and Social Science, 692*(1), 182–202. DOI: 10.1177/0002716220980691

Steine, I. M., Winje, D., Krystal, J. H., Bjorvatn, B., Milde, A. M., Grønli, J., Nordhus, I. H., & Pallesen, S. (2017). Cumulative childhood maltreatment and its dose-response relation with adult symptomatology: Findings in a sample of adult survivors of sexual abuse. *Child Abuse & Neglect, 65*, 99–111. DOI: 10.1016/j.chiabu.2017.01.008 PMID: 28131947

Stoltenborgh, M., Bakermans-Kranenburg, M. J., Alink, L. R., & van IJzendoorn, M. H. (2015). The prevalence of child maltreatment across the globe: Review of a series of meta-analyses. *Child Abuse Review*, *24*(1), 37–50. DOI: 10.1002/car.2353

Tarren-Sweeney, M. (2021). A narrative review of mental and relational health interventions for children in family-based out-of-home care. *Journal of Family Therapy*, *43*(3), 376–391. DOI: 10.1111/1467-6427.12341

Timmer, S. G., Hawk, B. N., Washington, A. M. L., & Urquiza, A. J. (2022). Trauma-Informed Care for Maltreated Children: Evidence-Based Treatments from a Developmental Perspective. In Krugman, R. D., & Korbin, J. E. (Eds.), *Handbook of Child Maltreatment. Child Maltreatment* (Vol. 14). Springer., DOI: 10.1007/978-3-030-82479-2_25

Tran, N. K., Alink, L. R., Van Berkel, S. R., & Van Ijzendoorn, M. H. (2017). Child maltreatment in Vietnam: Prevalence and cross-cultural comparison. *Journal of Aggression, Maltreatment & Trauma*, *26*(3), 211–230. DOI: 10.1080/10926771.2016.1250851

Ungar, M. (2013). Resilience after maltreatment: The importance of social services as facilitators of positive adaptation. *Child Abuse & Neglect*, *37*(2-3), 110–115. DOI: 10.1016/j.chiabu.2012.08.004 PMID: 23260114

Valentino, K. (2017). Relational interventions for maltreated children. *Child Development*, *88*(2), 359–367. DOI: 10.1111/cdev.12735 PMID: 28138967

Van der Put, C. E., Assink, M., Gubbels, J., & Boekhout van Solinge, N. F. (2018). Identifying effective components of child maltreatment interventions: A meta-analysis. *Clinical Child and Family Psychology Review*, *21*(2), 171–202. DOI: 10.1007/s10567-017-0250-5 PMID: 29204796

Verbist, A. N., Winters, A. M., Collins-Camargo, C., & Antle, B. F. (2020). Standardized assessment domains as predictors of prescription of trauma-focused treatment for youth in out-of-home care. *Children and Youth Services Review*, *118*, 105401. DOI: 10.1016/j.childyouth.2020.105401

Villodas, M. T., Morelli, N. M., Hong, K., Duong, J., Evans, M. C., Elson, D., Rose, E., Picci, G., & Fishbein, D. (2021). Differences in late adolescent psychopathology among youth with histories of co-occurring abuse and neglect experiences. *Child Abuse & Neglect*, *120*, 105189. DOI: 10.1016/j.chiabu.2021.105189 PMID: 34273863

Vizard, E., Gray, J., & Bentovim, A. (2022). The impact of child maltreatment on the mental and physical health of child victims: A review of the evidence. *BJPsych Advances*, *28*(1), 60–70. DOI: 10.1192/bja.2021.10

Wall, L., Higgins, D. J., & Hunter, C. (2016). *Trauma-informed care in child/family welfare services*. Australian Institute of Family Studies.

Wamser-Nanney, R. (2016). Examining the complex trauma definition using children's self-reports. *Journal of Child & Adolescent Trauma*, *9*(4), 295–304. DOI: 10.1007/s40653-016-0098-8

Warmingham, J. M., Handley, E. D., Rogosch, F. A., Manly, J. T., & Cicchetti, D. (2019). Identifying maltreatment groups with patterns of maltreatment type and chronicity: A latent class analysis approach. *Child Abuse & Neglect*, *87*, 28–39. DOI: 10.1016/j.chiabu.2018.08.013 PMID: 30224068

Witt, A., Münzer, A., Ganser, H. G., Fegert, J. M., Goldbeck, L., & Plener, P. L. (2016). Experience by children and adolescents of more than one type of maltreatment: Association of different classes of maltreatment profiles with clinical outcome variables. *Child Abuse & Neglect*, *57*, 1–11. DOI: 10.1016/j.chiabu.2016.05.001 PMID: 27254375

Zeanah, C. H., & Humphreys, K. L. (2018). Child abuse and neglect. *Journal of the American Academy of Child and Adolescent Psychiatry*, *57*(9), 637–644. DOI: 10.1016/j.jaac.2018.06.007 PMID: 30196867

Zhang, S., Conner, A., Lim, Y., & Lefmann, T. (2021). Trauma-informed care for children involved with the child welfare system: A meta-analysis. *Child Abuse & Neglect*, *122*, 105296. DOI: 10.1016/j.chiabu.2021.105296 PMID: 34478999

Chapter 3
Empathy Disrupted?
Reflections on the "Fancy-Lady" Shoebox

Tamara Blakemore
https://orcid.org/0000-0002-2562-5416
University of Newcastle, Australia

Louise Rak
University of Newcastle, Australia

Chris Krogh
https://orcid.org/0000-0003-1378-082X
University of Newcastle, Australia

ABSTRACT

Empathy has been described as the cornerstone of genuine human relationships and understood as an intentional and skilful act of connection. Practice with young people impacted by violence has often sought to leverage, or enhance, empathy in restorative ways. Professional training for practitioners who support this cohort has emphasised empathy as foundational to establishing safety, building rapport, and implementing relational practice. This chapter presents a critical reflection on the 'shoebox activity' from the Name.Narrate.Navigate program, an empathy-focused experiential exercise delivered with young people who have used and experienced violence, often in contexts of cumulative harm. The authors compare responses from young people with professionals being trained to deliver the activity. Through this analysis, they interrogate traditional assumptions about empathy in practice, and practice education, arguing for a more nuanced understanding of empathy as a dynamic, socially constructed, gendered and embodied phenomenon essential for trauma-informed, cumulative harm aware work.

DOI: 10.4018/979-8-3373-4064-7.ch003

POSITIONALITY STATEMENT

The authors of this chapter simultaneously hold numerous identities: mother, daughter, father, son, social worker, counselor, manager, chairperson, carer, partner, survivor, advocate, and ally. Readers will note that our writing style intentionally embraces a conversational and reflective voice. We choose this approach to honor the trauma-informed and culturally responsive aims of our work, recognizing that knowledge sharing, like healing, happens best through genuine connection and shared understanding. We pay our respects to the traditional owners of the Awabakal, Worimi, Darkinjung, Bundjalung, and Yaegl lands on which we work.

EMPATHY DISRUPTED? REFLECTIONS ON THE "FANCY-LADY" SHOEBOX

The Disruption Begins

Empathy, with its origins in the philosophy of aesthetics, has been defined and operationalized differently across disciplines and fields of study (Howe, 2016). It has been described as the cornerstone of genuine and reciprocal human relationships (Bons et al., 2013), involving both the ability and inclination to recognize, understand, and vicariously share the emotional state and experience of another (Decety & Moriguchi, 2007; Eisenberg et al., 2006). Today, empathy is deeply embedded in society's understanding of connection and care—familiar, popularized, and positioned as both a natural capacity and a teachable skill. This appreciation of empathy is central to our work with young people who use and experience violence, and the workers who support them.

While not all young people who experience violence will use violence, many young people who use violence have simultaneously also experienced violence (Baglivio et al., 2018). Adverse childhood experiences (ACEs), including the experience of violence, may synergistically disrupt the development of skills for empathy and increase risk for offending. These experiences exist not as separate problems requiring separate interventions but as interrelated developmental impacts of cumulative harm (Narvey et al., 2021). From a psychological perspective, meta-analytic evidence suggests low empathy correlates with antisocial, aggressive, and delinquent behavior (Joliffe & Farrington, 2006), while higher empathy serves as a protective factor for these behaviors (Broidy et al., 2003). From the same lens, research on ACEs has found that each additional ACE increases the risk of using violence from 33% to 144% among high school students (Duke et al., 2010), and cumulative adversity—encompassing childhood neglect, abuse, victimization, and deprivation—has been associated with empathy deficits (Simons et al., 2002; Zhang et al., 2024). These findings suggest both a challenge and an opportunity for intervention. Research by Narvey et al., (2021) examined whether empathy-building could interrupt this cycle among adjudicated serious juvenile offenders in residential treatment. Their findings confirmed that higher ACEs predicted lower empathy and higher recidivism; however, their study also revealed that empathy remains modifiable even in high-risk populations. When young people in the study experienced substantial improvements in empathy during treatment, the effects of ACEs on recidivism were no longer significant.

Empathy-building interventions typically conceptualize empathy as a developmental skill that progresses from emotion recognition through perspective-taking to emotion replication (Marshall et al., 1995). Experiential learning approaches—activities designed to help young people deeply appreciate another's perspective through direct engagement with curated scenarios or objects—have been found to be especially effective (Chan et al., 2021). Examples such as letter writing, perspective-taking role-plays, and object-based reflection and projection activities have all been cited for their capacity to stimulate empathy in young people who use and experience violence (Calley & Gerber, 2008). These "empathy tools" (Pratte et al., 2021) target both cognitive empathy (understanding another's internal state) and affective empathy (feeling what another feels), with the expectation that this empathic response will translate to prosocial behavior.

Yet the efficacy of these intervention tools rests on dual assumptions that warrant examination. First, as Pratte et al. (2021) highlight, empathy-building activities typically assume universal responses—that "stepping into someone else's shoes" will reliably produce understanding and compassion across all participants. Second, and perhaps more fundamentally, these approaches assume that practitioners possess both the empathic capacity and the practice-based skills needed to facilitate such interventions. Delivering empathy-building interventions requires practitioners who themselves embody empathic practice. The significance of practitioner empathy has long been established in social work theory and research (Gerdes & Segal, 2009, 2011; Raines, 1990), with empathy understood as involving not only affective responses and cognitive perspective-taking but also demonstrating understanding of the other's emotional experience through active listening, validation, and accurate reflection of feeling and content (Gerdes & Segal, 2009; King, 2011). For trauma-informed practice, an empathic stance is foundational to creating safety and therapeutic connection. Consequently, training practitioners to deliver empathy-focused work involves cultivating self-awareness of their own empathic capacity alongside equipping them with intervention skills.

Theoretical confidence in empathy—as a capacity and skill, and as the focus of intervention—has shaped our approach as we developed the Name.Narrate.Navigate

(NNN) program. With input from a stakeholder consortium of Aboriginal elders and community members, frontline practitioners, peak body representatives, and young people, facilitated through a community-based participatory action research project, we have embedded empathy-building activities in our intervention for young people who use and experience violence and in the training curriculum for the workers who support them. Yet as experienced practitioner-researchers who have worked across the fields of violence, abuse, and trauma for much of our careers, we have come to question this confident familiarity. We thought we intuitively understood what empathy was, what its presence or absence looked like, and what it felt like in our work. But confronted with the experience of what we came to recognize were potential gaps in our understanding of empathy, our discomfort has forced us to contemplate a difficult question: What if empathy itself is more contingent and contextual than we have assumed to date?

What We Saw Versus What We Expected

These contemplations were triggered by an experiential activity involving curated shoeboxes delivered separately to young people and workers. Both groups were asked to look at the shoeboxes with their peers and imagine who the contents belonged to, what was happening in that person's life, and how they felt about them. One particular shoebox—dubbed the "fancy-lady" shoebox—drew our attention. In our practice observations, this box seemed to elicit responses that were more intense and divisive than those elicited by the other shoeboxes. Anecdotally, we perceived that this box triggered expressions of negativity, judgment, and antagonism, notably from female-identifying participants and workers. To us, these reactions felt counter to our understandings and assumptions about empathy.

From the existing evidence base, we were aware that gender has been suggested to influence empathy. Studies have reported that females score higher on indices and tests of empathy than males (Baron-Cohen & Wheelwright, 2004), with perceptible differences between male and female experiences of empathy also confirmed by some neurophysiological studies (Rueckert & Naybar, 2008). While we anticipated gendered responses to the activity, we had not expected them in this direction.

In attempting to make sense of our observations, we considered studies showing that while young women are, overall, more empathic, there appears to be greater variability in their ability to resonate with and sit with the emotional distress of another person than in their ability to appreciate and understand another person's emotional state (Dinic et al., 2016). Other research reporting that young women who use violence score highly on personal distress—indicating heightened emotional responses and greater sensitivity to affective cues (Lindsey et al., 2001; Jonason

& Kroll, 2015)—made us wonder whether cumulative harm had, either directly or indirectly, disrupted empathy expression.

Wrestling with these observations created tension on multiple levels. We were uncomfortable positioning women as potentially less empathetic toward another woman, particularly in the context of direct or indirect experiences of gender-based violence. We also questioned whether our own lens—shaped by experience, positionality, and theoretical leanings—had narrowed our gaze, obscuring alternative interpretations. Confronting this discomfort thus became the focus of this chapter.

This Chapter

This chapter explores whether what appeared as empathy disruption might actually reveal something about our understanding of empathy. It considers what disruption might teach us about empathy beyond a psychological frame, as contextual, embodied, and shaped by experience. We situate our work by describing the NNN program and the shoebox activity (Section 2), before outlining what we thought we knew about empathy from the existing literature (Section 3). Our methodology (Section 4) and findings (Section 5) detail our learnings from the "fancy-lady" box, while the discussion (Section 6) reframes these observations, informing recommendations (Section 7) for more contextually informed, gender-responsive, and accumulation-aware understandings of empathy.

THE NNN PROGRAM AND THE SHOEBOX ACTIVITY

Since its inception in 2018, the NNN program has evolved as a community-engaged response to an unmet need for trauma-informed and culturally safe interventions for young people aged 12–18 years who use and experience violence, as well as for accessible specialist training for the workers who support them. NNN has a dual focus of working with young people and practitioners toward mutual goals of self-awareness, self-regulation, and skills for connection (Blakemore et al., 2024).

Working from a trauma-informed and culturally sensitive ethos, the theory of change underpinning NNN recognizes that young people need skills to recognize, regulate, and communicate emotions and needs; empathy to respond to others and themselves; an understanding of power, control, and shame; and opportunities to explore what positive change might look like in their lives. NNN posits that new knowledge, skills, and behaviors, along with greater confidence, coping skills, and connection, can improve life circumstances, well-being, and safety. The aim of NNN is to enhance these factors to drive and sustain change toward better, safer outcomes.

NNN is informed by a broad body of evidence-based learning and practice approaches, including Kolb's (2015) experiential learning model, universal design for learning (Rose & Meyer, 2006), dialectical behavior therapy (Linehan, 2015), and Photovoice (Fitzgibbon & Healy, 2019; Fitzgibbon & Stengel, 2018; Wang, 1999). NNN minimizes reliance on dominant literacies by focusing instead on expression and exploration as a way of knowing and being known. It foregrounds the importance of story, visual representation, and creative methods to explore concepts, experiences, meaning, and impact.

Empathy is the focus of the third session in the NNN program. Building on prior content, activities in this session explore the experience and expression of empathy. Key amongst these is the "shoebox activity." The design and delivery of this activity adopt an experiential learning approach. Experiential learning is defined by Chan et al. (2021) as a process that "facilitates learners to transform and create knowledge, skills, attitudes and ways of thinking" (p. 2).

In the activity, young people (and practitioners being trained to deliver it) are presented with curated shoeboxes themed to different stereotypical or heteronormative genders and life stages. Each shoebox contains a pair of shoes and an assortment of found objects representing the miscellanea of everyday life. The "fancy-lady" shoebox is displayed in Figure 1. Contents of the box include a pair of animal-print high heels, a fascinator and a pair of sunglasses, a foldable tourist map, an aged photo of a beach scene, a lip gloss and eyelash brush, a packet of instant coffee, a curled ribbon, one Christmas earring, and a "to do" list that reads: "buy milk, call Damien, hairdresser at 5 pm, find the key to the back gate."

Figure 1. The "fancy-lady" shoebox

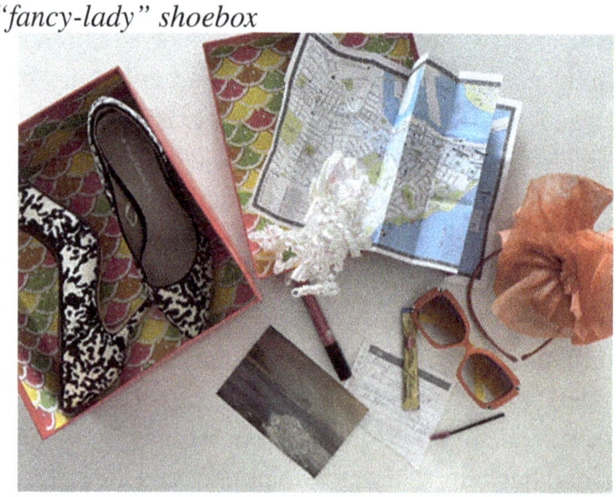

The activity situates young people (and practitioners) at the center and seeks to better understand, with greater sensitivity, their experiences and perspectives. Participants are encouraged to inspect, play with, and try on the contents of the shoeboxes. Facilitators provide conversation prompts to explore ideas about the imagined owners of these shoes, considering what might be happening in their lives and what types of feelings the imagined owner might elicit. These prompts are consistent with Marshall et al.,'s (1995) conceptualization of empathy as a developmental task involving four sequential components: emotion recognition, perspective taking, emotion replication, and response decision. The intent of this activity is to provide young people and practitioners with opportunities for exposure, experience, and exploration of different life narratives and to imagine themselves in lives they understand as different from their own (Adelman et al., 2016).

To date, the activity has been delivered to over 500 young people who have participated in the NNN program and to over 200 practitioners trained as NNN facilitators. It has also been used in teaching activities with social work and human services students and in trauma-awareness training delivered to domestic violence, out-of-home care, education, and justice sector workers. While both young people and practitioners engage deeply with this activity—with narratives emerging that explore ingroup/outgroup identities, heteronormative gender and age-related stereotypes, and the experience of violence across the life course—the "fancy-lady" shoebox stands out for its perceived capacity to provoke responses that challenge our assumptions and expectations.

LITERATURE REVIEW: WHAT WE THOUGHT WE KNEW

Empathy occupies familiar ground in our work with young people who use and experience violence and the professionals who support them. Dominant theoretical frameworks from psychology and neuroscience have been influential in shaping our understanding of empathy as a measurable, predictable capacity—one with identifiable determinants and developmental trajectories. This evidence base presents empathy as largely known and knowable, even as debates continue about its precise mechanisms and manifestations across different populations and contexts.

Understanding Empathy

Commonly described as "the ability to put oneself into the shoes of another," empathy is a part of the human experience, a capacity and a process involving both experience and behavior. Foundational to the helping work that is human services and social work practice (Blakemore & Rak, 2024), empathy has been contemplated and written about for centuries. It is apparently simple to talk about, as though we all agree on what it means, yet it remains a highly complex concept, without clear agreement on its conceptualization (Alexander & Alessi, 2024). Academic disciplines such as medicine, psychology, social work, and the social sciences (Berardi et al., 2020) have each contributed to its study and to understanding its importance. The emerging field of neurosociology is applying transdisciplinary empirical research integrating neuroscience and sociology to better understand empathy's social and biological intersections (Auriemma, 2023).

Commonly, empathy is considered to cover cognitive, affective, and behavioral dimensions. The cognitive aspect includes the ability to understand what another person is thinking, feeling, or believing about their situation at any particular moment and how that shapes their behavior (Blakemore & Rak, 2024). Cognitive empathy is associated with "theory of mind," the learned skill initiated in earliest childhood by which people recognize differentiation between their own and others' representations of the world and see the link between these representations and others' behavior (Rakoczy, 2022). Theory of mind, aligned with the notion of mentalization, is integral to much social cooperation and can be applied reflectively by an individual to their own mental states and behavior (Rakoczy, 2022).

As Mauroy et al. (2025) discussed, integral to cognitive empathy is empathic accuracy, the degree to which our inferences about another's mental state are accurate to the way the other understands their experience. Distinct from cognitive empathy is affective empathy, which is an involuntary, autonomic response to the emotions of the other (Stevens & Woodruff, 2018b). Affective empathy orients one's attention to the emotions of the other and provides a congruent response to their experience. Silke et al., (2018) distinguished the supportive-responding aspect of affective empathy as "prosocial behavior." Prosocial behavior is an example of behavioral empathy, which recognizes that empathy is a process involving not only thinking and feeling (internal processes) but also acting in response, a feature particularly important in helping professions such as social work.

More recently, neurobiological understandings of empathy have gained prominence (e.g., Stevens & Woodruff, 2018a). These understandings demonstrate the evolutionarily shaped neural foundations of empathic experiences and responses. One finding of this research is the role of "mirror neurons," which facilitate the ability to share or mirror the experience of others while maintaining a degree of flexibility in the response—that is, just because we share the experience of another does not mean we have to act on it (Iacoboni, 2009). A particular implication of this finding, and important for our work in NNN, is that empathy is an embodied experience. As such, it is likely to be influenced by intra- and interpersonal experiences and the socio-political, historical, and cultural contexts in which they arise.

Skills for empathy are sparked in the earliest parent–child interactions and develop through childhood and adolescence (Silke et al., 2018; Stevens & Woodruff, 2018b), learned and shaped by relationships with significant others across developmental trajectories (Mauroy et al., 2025). Empathy may be impacted by the relational proximity of the other (i.e., someone related, familiar, or a stranger), levels of stress in the observer, and the degree to which the emotional experience is expressed by the other (expression of emotion that is experienced as too little or too much may lead to disengagement by the observer; Flasbeck et al., 2018). Empathy is also likely to be shaped by the same circumstances that shape development, such as autistic spectrum disorder (Marchetti et al., 2019), schizophrenia and borderline personality disorder (Flasbeck et al., 2018), adverse childhood experiences, attachment disruption, and trauma (Levy et al., 2019).

Cumulative Harm and Empathy

Conceptualizations of cumulative harm recognize that early-life experiences of adversity frequently co-occur and have compounding impacts that can diminish children's sense of safety, stability, and well-being (Miller, 2007). Understanding the association between cumulative harm and empathy is particularly critical for our work with young people in NNN, where histories of multiple, co-occurring adversities are common.

A substantial body of work suggests that childhood adversity, including neglect, abuse, victimization, and deprivation, may diminish empathy development (Cerqueira & Almeida, 2023; Meidan & Uzefovsky, 2020; Satapathy et al., 2022; Simons et al., 2002; Zhang et al., 2024). Narvey et al. (2021) found that adversity predicted lower empathy among juvenile offenders, and Wang et al. (2021) demonstrated associations between childhood maltreatment and cognitive empathy specifically, but not affective empathy. Other research has identified positive associations between experiences of harm and empathy. Greenberg et al. (2018) found trauma severity positively associated with various empathy dimensions, while childhood maltreatment has been linked to greater emotional sensitivity and dispositional empathy (Ozdemir & Sahin, 2020; Staub & Vollhardt, 2008).

Explanations for whether and how adversity may impact empathy have focused on both the toll and type of harm experienced. While cumulative harm describes the compounding developmental impacts of multiple adverse experiences, much research has relied on *cumulative risk approaches* in its methodology. Cumulative risk approaches tally adversities to create risk scores, assuming that adverse experiences influence development through a dose–response pattern, where more adversities produce proportionally worse outcomes (McLaughlin & Sheridan, 2016). The prevailing mechanism proposed within cumulative risk frameworks is allostatic load, in which chronic activation of stress-response systems is thought to disrupt the brain architecture of the hippocampus, amygdala, and prefrontal cortex (Bromfield et al., 2007), areas thought to be critical for empathy.

Dimensional approaches, by contrast, suggest that adversity and empathy may be linked through learning processes. Rather than counting adversities, dimensional frameworks distinguish between *threat* (experiences involving harm or threat of harm, such as abuse or witnessing violence) and *deprivation* (absence of expected or required inputs, such as neglect or poverty). Threat experiences are argued to disrupt emotional learning processes, with impacts on emotional regulation that may particularly affect affective empathy. Deprivation, by contrast, is suggested to compromise executive function and pattern learning, potentially affecting the self–other awareness central to cognitive empathy (Kahhale et al., 2025; McLaughlin & Sheridan, 2016).

Gender and Empathy

Research has also explored the association between adversity, harm, and empathy, highlighting gender differences consistent with longstanding societal assumptions that females exhibit greater empathy than males (Komatsu et al., 2024). These assumptions are supported by research reporting gender differences in empathic expression and ability. In these studies, female participants consistently performed higher than male participants on diverse measures of empathy (Garaigordobil, 2009; Löffler & Greitemeyer, 2023; Mestre et al., 2009; Pang et al., 2023), with some findings indicating that these differences were particularly marked for, or limited to, affective empathy (Eisenberg et al., 2005; Jolliffe & Farrington, 2006; Van der Graaff et al., 2014). Studies have similarly reported gendered differences in social abilities and tasks associated with empathy, with significant differences between the capacities of female and male participants to demonstrate both compassion and empathy, as well as a higher likelihood for female participants to engage in prosocial volunteering and donations (Schurz et al., 2023).

Gendered differences in prosocial, sympathetic, and empathetic behaviors are suggested to emerge in childhood and widen in adolescence (Lam et al., 2012; Rose & Rudolph, 2006). In a comprehensive review of evidence regarding gender and empathy, Christov-Moore et al., (2014) argued that the developmental stability of gender differences suggests they are unlikely to be caused exclusively by experience alone but rather reflect some evolutionary important difference that is present, at least in some form, from birth. The authors drew on evidence from psychological and behavioral studies to suggest that the basic neural networks involved in affective empathy are more developed for females compared to males (e.g., Cheng et al.,

2009; Takeuchi et al., 2013), while social, contextual, and cultural influences may foster observed behavioral differences.

These broader influences are of interest in our work, particularly for the role they may play in explaining observations that appear contrary to the evidence presented. For example, research has found that the accuracy of empathy exhibited between genders may be influenced by motivational and contextual factors. Klein and Hodges (2001), for instance, found increased female empathic capacity specifically when female participants were presented with scenarios in which an empathic response was elicited based on a target person. However, when both female and male participants were presented with financial motivation, empathic responses increased for both groups. Other research has questioned whether differences in measures of empathy between males and females might, in fact, reflect gendered differences in self-assigned or socially prescribed roles, given the reliance on self-report in many studies (Baez et al., 2017; Löffler & Greitemeyer, 2023; Pang et al., 2023). Rather than being merely an artefact of measurement differences, this observation may provide insight into how females conceive what is expected of them in social situations and raises questions about the risks and rewards of empathy.

Professionals and Empathy

The pivotal role empathy plays in fostering and maintaining effective therapeutic relationships has long been acknowledged (Cochran & Cochran, 2015). Carl Rogers's (1951) seminal work *Client-Centred Therapy* is suggested to have established empathic engagement as the cornerstone of therapeutic practice (Watson et al., 2022), significantly influencing psychology, social work, and occupational therapy. In practice, empathy toward another is often demonstrated through communication behaviors. Lynch et al. (2019) studied social work child protection practice in England by reviewing transcripts of professional conversations with parents. They found that social workers with the highest empathy levels interacted with parents with curiosity, accurately understood the other person, and focused on feelings, whereas the inverse behaviors were demonstrated by 80% of practitioners in their study who had lower empathy scores.

Research conducted with helping professionals has identified that empathy can have positive and protective effects for their well-being. Consistent with findings reported by Wagaman et al., (2015), an Australian study of social workers and psychologists found that higher rates of recorded empathy were related to lower risks of acquiring secondary stress symptoms (Rayner et al., 2020). In the field of medicine, empathic responding has been shown to increase the likelihood that patients follow directions, be more satisfied, and litigate less often (Hojat, 2009), while in business, empathy has been noted to improve customer experiences, create solutions to problems, and expand operations (Sarantou & Miettinen, 2022). The gendered dimension of empathy for professionals has also been examined, with studies outside the helping context finding that females consistently contribute to higher levels of empathetic work across organizations, and that this work is viewed as both intrinsically motivated and socially expected (Hsu et al., 2022).

This gives pause for considering the potential emotional, psychological, and occupational challenges that might be associated with empathy for professionals. Vial and Cowgill, (2022) highlighted that expectations on females in leadership positions frequently include prosocial leadership styles marked by empathy and altruism. The authors noted that when female leaders do not show these traits or lapse in consistently accommodating the feelings of others, they risk social and career consequences. These expectations and potential consequences can create a double-edged sword for female leaders who must manage not only task-oriented objectives but also relational expectations (Vial & Cowgill, 2022).

Research has also suggested that empathy in therapeutic contexts may negatively affect health professionals' well-being (Grynberg & Konrath, 2020; Klimecki & Singer, 2012; Leiberg et al., 2011). Evidence from brain imaging studies showing that affective empathy can activate the brain's pain matrix (Decety & Lam, 2006) has informed suggestions that continual activation of empathy for pain responses may lead to empathic distress, defined as "a strong aversive and self-oriented response, accompanied by the desire to withdraw from a situation in order to protect oneself from negative feelings" (Singer & Klimecki, 2014). Over time, empathetic distress has been suggested to diminish the capacity for empathic engagement and increase negative emotional states (Klimecki & Singer, 2012).

Some workers may be more susceptible to challenges associated with the effective use of empathy than others. In a study of professionals working in counselling roles, Watson et al., (2025) found that participants who reported drawing on their own lived experiences enhanced their ability to empathize with their clients' situations, but they also recognized that this could elicit strong emotional responses. The authors noted that these responses were often heightened when clients shared similar life experiences with workers. Evidence of the high rates of helping professionals—particularly females—with lived experience of cumulative harm associated with adverse childhood experiences (e.g., Elliott & Guy, 1993; Pope & Feldman-Summers, 1992) suggests that empathy may be a complex experience for some professionals.

METHOD

The work presented in this chapter emerged from practitioner reflexivity. We sought to understand, with greater sensitivity and objectivity, our anecdotal observations of how participants—particularly women—engaged with the "fancy-lady" shoebox and what insights from the activity might contribute to our understanding of empathy.

Research Design

Our observations initially suggested a research question: Might the direct or indirect experience of cumulative harm shape women's expression of empathy, particularly toward other women? However, tensions raised by our observations suggested a more pertinent and primary research question: What does the "fancy-lady" box contribute to our understanding of empathy? The iterative process of observation, disruption, and reconceptualization described here reflects what Schön (1983) calls reflection-in-action, or the capacity of practitioners to critically reflect on their work while they are doing it.

Participants

Our analysis draws on data from two participant groups: young people who participated in the NNN program and professionals trained to deliver the program.

Young People

Data from young people were drawn from 16 NNN groups delivered between 2018 and 2023, involving 150 participants aged 12–18 years. Of these, 39 young women took part in female-only groups delivered across community, on-country, and education settings, while 21 young men participated in male-only groups delivered across community, custodial, and education settings. The remaining 90 young people participated in mixed-gender groups delivered in educational settings.

Professionals

Data from professionals were drawn from 19 deliveries of NNN training delivered between 2023 and 2025, involving 171 participants. Participants included those identifying with she/her pronouns ($n = 103$), he/him pronouns ($n = 63$), and they/them pronouns ($n = 5$). Ages ranged from 19 to 68 years (mean = 40 years), and participants held diverse roles, including caseworkers ($n = 10$), youth justice caseworkers ($n = 5$), student support officers ($n = 5$), youth workers ($n = 3$), team leaders/managers ($n = 2$), academics ($n = 2$), program coordinators ($n = 2$), family workers ($n = 2$), and a range of other positions across community services, education, and therapeutic settings.

Professional experience ranged from six weeks to 42 years, spanning youth justice, child protection, education, out-of-home care, family support, and community services, with a median of 8.0 years and a mean of 10.6 years. Notably, 59% of participants reported six or more years of professional experience. Female-identifying practitioners were, on average, 4.4 years older and had 3.4 more years of professional experience than male-identifying practitioners, with 63% of female-identifying participants reporting six or more years of experience compared to 49% of male-identifying participants. Female-identifying participants were also more likely than male-identifying participants to report holding management roles.

Data Collection

Three distinct types of data inform our analysis: practitioner reflection forms, written responses to survey prompts, and observations from the field. Each data source captures different aspects of responses to the "fancy-lady" shoebox.

Practitioner Reflection Forms (Young People's Sessions, 2018–2023)

Following each NNN session delivery, facilitating practitioners completed structured reflection forms documenting their observations of young people's engagement with program activities, including the shoebox exercise. These forms captured immediate impressions of participant responses, notable interactions, and facilitator reflections on session dynamics. Practitioners also participated in reflective conversations with NNN team members focused on implementation learnings and practice support. In some instances, reflections were gathered through social yarning (Bessarab & Ng'andu, 2010), an Aboriginal practice for sharing knowledge and building belonging through story.

Pre-training Survey Responses (Professionals' Training, 2023–2025)

Training participants completed a pre-training survey designed to capture demographic characteristics of attendees and their baseline understanding and perceptions of core content. The survey included a photograph of the "fancy-lady" shoebox (Figure 1) alongside three open-ended questions: (a) Who owns these shoes? (b) What might be happening for them? (c) How do you feel toward the owner of these shoes? Later in the training session, participants handled the actual shoebox and discussed their responses with peers, with field observations made during this interactive aspect of the training.

Observations From the Field (Young People's Sessions and Practitioner Training, 2018–2025)

Throughout the delivery of both young people's sessions and practitioner training, members of the NNN team (and authors of this chapter) shared observations of participant responses during the shoebox activity. These observations were more informal and were captured through post-session and post-training debriefs and shared reflections among the research team.

Rationale for Multiple Data Sources

These different data types captured empathic responses at different levels: practitioner observations (what facilitators noticed in practice), self-report (what workers undertaking training articulated), and field observations (what facilitators witnessed and experienced). Triangulation across these sources—and particularly the comparison between written and embodied responses—became central to our analysis.

Data Analysis

Thematic analysis (Guest et al., 2011) was undertaken for all data sources, with analytical approaches tailored to each data type. This analysis was collaborative throughout, with all authors reviewing data and interrogating emerging patterns.

Analysis of Practitioner Reflection Forms and Field Observations

Qualitative data from practitioner reflections on young people's sessions—including reflections gathered through social yarning and field observations—were analyzed thematically. Written notes were divided among the authors, who analyzed them for core themes using open coding. The team then met to compare and discuss prominent findings as well as the connections and comparisons that emerged from the data relating to young people's experience of the activity (axial coding). Analytical notes taken during this meeting were then amalgamated, and a final set of themes was discussed, refined, and agreed upon by the authors. This analysis was reflexive, with the authors examining their own assumptions and emotional responses to the data. This autoethnographic dimension (Chang, 2008; Ellis & Bochner, 2000) positioned us as both observers and participants, acknowledging that our surprise and discomfort at observed responses constituted relevant data in their own right.

Analysis of Pre-Training Survey Responses

Written responses to the three survey questions were initially examined by all authors using an Excel spreadsheet to identify evident themes (open coding). Data were then coded in NVivo, with the question "How do you feel toward the owner of these shoes?" receiving focused attention. From this, fifteen codes emerged, which clustered into three parent codes: neutral responses, emotional (affective) responses, and cognitive responses. To preserve context, coded data were transferred back to Excel spreadsheets so that each participant's complete set of responses could be examined together alongside demographic information. Data were then reorganized by parent code and examined for patterns within and across response types.

Comparative Analysis

Responses were compared across participant groups (young people versus practitioners) and, for practitioners, between their written pre-responses and their observed embodied reactions. Throughout the analysis, we maintained reflexive attention to our own interpretive assumptions, particularly regarding gendered expressions of empathy and the potential role of cumulative harm.

Ethical Considerations

Ethics approval was obtained from the University of Newcastle Human Research Ethics Committee (H-2023-0205) for the use of practitioner training data, and from the Australian Institute of Aboriginal and Torres Strait Islander Studies (E0107-1402019) for the delivery of the NNN program and use of non-identifying data from the program. All participants provided informed consent, with young people's consent obtained alongside parental/guardian consent where required.

Multiple ethical considerations shaped our research approach. First, the dual relationship inherent in studying our own practice required reflexivity about power dynamics and interpretation. As program developers, facilitators, and trainers, we acknowledged our investment in NNN's success and actively interrogated assumptions that might bias our analysis. Second, working with young people who had used and experienced violence demanded trauma-informed research practices. We relied on practitioners' professional judgment about which observations to document, avoided re-traumatizing inquiry, and maintained strict confidentiality. All data were de-identified, with pseudonyms used for any illustrative quotes. Third, cultural safety was foundational, given Aboriginal young people's participation in NNN. Cultural protocols were embedded throughout, including the use of social yarning as a culturally appropriate data-gathering method, guidance from the Cultural Advisory Group, and attention to cultural safety in how we interpreted and presented findings. Finally, we recognized the ethical complexity of presenting findings that might appear critical of participants' responses—particularly young women and female practitioners. Our analysis aimed to interrogate our own frameworks rather than pathologize participants, maintaining respect for all responses as contextually meaningful.

FINDINGS: THREE DISRUPTIONS TO OUR UNDERSTANDING

Findings from the analysis of the data described above are organized into three sections. The first presents practitioner reflections and field observations from NNN sessions with young people, with particular attention to the "fancy-lady" shoebox. The second section reports field observations from training sessions with cross-sector workers learning to deliver the activity in NNN. The third section examines written survey responses from these workers, capturing their reflections on the "fancy-lady" shoebox prior to their experiential training.

Before presenting the findings, we clarify key terms. *Facilitators* refers to trained practitioners who delivered the NNN program to young people across various sites. *Young people*, *young women*, *young men*, or *participants* refers to those who attended NNN groups and engaged with program activities, including the shoebox activity. *Professionals* describes adults from diverse service contexts and professions who participated in NNN training, potentially to deliver the program in the future. *Workers* refers to practitioners who attended NNN groups in specific settings to support young people, but who were not trained to deliver the program.

First Disruption: Young Women and the "Fancy Lady"

Thematic analysis of practitioner reflections and field observations from NNN program delivery found that the shoebox activity was generally well received, with notable gendered patterns emerging. Delivery to a large mixed cohort of young men and women suggested the activity "worked well" but "seemed to engage boys more," with "stories told about the boxes pretty gendered" (group 14). In other settings, some young women found the activity difficult due to concerns about boundaries and safety. These participants were quick to remark, "you can't tell someone else's story" (group 3) and explicitly linked the storytelling intent of the activity to "snitching" (group 3), which they had previously explained as a serious social infraction with real consequences for their personal safety. Facilitators observed that this gender divergence was particularly visible in responses to the "fancy-lady" shoebox, where young men and young women constructed interconnected narratives about who owned the shoes, what was happening in her life, and how they felt about her, revealing possible fractures along gender lines.

"Stuck Up" and "Not Like Me"

Participants offered narratives about the "fancy lady" that alternated between suggestions that she came from a position of privilege or disadvantage. Assumptions about socioeconomic status shared in the group setting sometimes escalated quickly and were tied to moral judgements about the owner's character. For example, in delivery to a mixed group, when asked if they thought they would like her, one participant said she was "stuck up," and in response, another said she "drove a Mercedes," while "others agreed" (group 13). Facilitators noted that this sequence was revealing: When asked about liking her—an emotional and relational question—participants immediately invoked markers of presumed socioeconomic status and presumed social distance.

"Stuck up" here might position her as arrogant due to perceived privilege, while "drove a Mercedes" might assign specific wealth, marking her as "not like me" (group 13). The collective agreement suggests this was not just one participant's opinion but became shared group positioning. When other groups were "told some groups think she is stuck up, there was definite agreement" (group 13), solidifying a sense of outgroup positioning. This meta-commentary could indicate that, while participants seemed to recognize that others imagined the owner would be "stuck up" and could see why, they did not always assign a moral judgment to it. For example, young men in one group said the shoes looked like they belonged to "a model. Probably rich. Maybe poor (because of the fake glasses)" (group 9). Participants in this group noticed contradictory evidence, trying to reconcile fancy items with those that might be fake or inauthentic. The "fake glasses" became evidence that the imagined owner might not be genuinely wealthy, suggesting participants were actively reading social markers as indicators of her socioeconomic position rather than making snap judgments.

Interestingly, the phrase "not like me" was explicitly introduced by a female worker attending a group for young men when characterizing the imagined owner of the "fancy-lady" shoebox. This distancing language—establishing what one is by asserting what one is not—was not observed to be sufficient to elicit group sentiment. Facilitators noted that while this distancing was modeled by the female worker, "the boys weren't negative toward the box" (group 12), perhaps suggesting they were not invested in establishing difference as grounds for judgment.

"Drunk" Incapable Mothers

Perhaps most striking—and disruptive—to facilitators' sense of empathy in the group was a pattern of evidence-free assumptions about motherhood, drinking, and incompetence that seemed to emerge in response to the "fancy-lady" shoebox. These narratives, constructed primarily by young women (but also introduced by some female workers), appeared to be triggered by specific objects in the shoebox: the fascinator, the single Christmas-themed earring, the shoes (their style and height), and the to-do list. For some women, these items seemed to prompt assumptions linking privilege, socializing, excessive drinking, and moral failure.

Female workers attending a boys' group suggested "frankly, she's been on the drink" and "she's forgetful, she's lost her keys and an earring" (group 12). Participants associated the fascinator with "going to the Melbourne Cup" (group 11) and "going to the races to get smashed" (group 6). This projected link between the fascinator and drinking appeared to make some young women wary of the imagined owner, suggesting "you'd need to stay clear of her" because she might be associated with "drama" (group 16). The intensity of some young women's condemnations is illustrated by a comment from one young woman: "...look at this slut, out drinking when she should have been home with her kids...why does she even need a list to remember milk...and she's lost her keys, stupid bitch" (group 7). The to-do list—mentioning "buy milk" and "call Damien," with no reference to children—was interpreted as evidence of maternal inadequacy. This young woman seemed to weaponize it as proof of the owner's assumed incompetence ("why does she even need a list to remember milk"), while citing the missing earring and lost keys as further evidence of irresponsibility.

Practitioner reflections noted that initial facilitator attempts to redirect conversations or reframe participants' judgmental commentary often met with resistance. Young women maintained their negative characterizations of the imagined owner even when facilitators pointed out the absence of evidence for their assumptions (group 10). Other reflections suggested that when one participant expressed hostile commentary, others frequently joined in or amplified these judgments (group 15). Facilitators suggested that the collective nature of these responses created sessions in which antagonism toward the "fancy-lady" box became a shared group stance.

Yet despite examples of hostility toward the "fancy lady," some of these same young women were drawn to the items in the box. Facilitators observed in one group that "participants were drawn to the 'fancy-lady' shoebox"—despite previous negative sentiments—and noted that "one participant wore the shoes and tried on hat" (group 3). In another group, facilitators recorded that one participant "tried on the stilettos and found it very hard because she had never worn any before," whereas another participant commented "that she could run in them" (group 13).

These differing experiences of the objects in the shoebox, and participants' familiarity or comfort with them, meant that the patterns observed above were not universal or unchallenged. In one mixed cohort, a participant intervened, suggesting that the others were "stereotyping her and it looked like she had her life together" (group 13). Facilitators noted that this challenge opened space for a conversation about possible reasons for differences in how males and females reacted to the shoebox. One participant suggested it was because "guys were easier going," and facilitators observed that the discussion demonstrated "awareness that judgment was occurring and that it varied by gender" (group 13).

Consistent reflections suggested that young men "did not have any negative attitude toward the owner of the [fancy-lady] shoes" (group 1) or had "no strong feelings about her. None really felt they would like her particularly, but not many negative reactions to her" (group 11). They described her as "going to a party, enjoying dressing up, going out" (group 9). While they associated her with similar scenarios—attending a social event, potentially drinking, dressing up—these narratives were not conveyed in ways that implied moral judgment. The "fancy-lady" shoebox reminded young men of "people in their lives, sisters, friends, etc." (groups 9, 12); in this way, she was familiar rather than foreign, recognized rather than rejected as an outgroup influence.

Experienced facilitators reported that perceived gendered patterns across NNN deliveries were surprising. They were struck not only by the hostility young women directed toward the imagined owner but also, in some instances, by how other female workers themselves participated in constructing and reinforcing judgments that appeared to disrupt the empathy-building intent of the activity.

Second Disruption: Female Professionals' Responses

Cross-sector professionals learning to deliver NNN participate in training activities as if they were program participants themselves. The findings in this section draw from facilitator field observations made during these training sessions. For clarity, in this section, *facilitators* refers to those delivering the training, while *professionals* refer to those undertaking it.

As with young people's groups, facilitators found that cross-sector professionals actively engaged with the shoebox activity. The activity often provoked intense reactions, depending on the associations professionals made with different box contents. However, field observations revealed an unexpected pattern: Some female-identifying professionals expressed responses to the "fancy-lady" shoebox strikingly similar to those observed among young women, sometimes mirroring the antagonistic reactions described in the previous section.

"High-Maintenance" and "Not Like Me"

Field observations from training sessions found that professionals across gender identities sometimes identified the "fancy-lady" box as the one they felt least warm toward, least familiar with, or least able to connect with. However, those expressing these sentiments were more often female-identifying, and they explicitly positioned the imagined "fancy-lady" persona as "not like them" or "not like me." When characterizing the "fancy lady," these professionals commonly used terms such as "high maintenance" and "hard work." Facilitators noted that professionals often delivered these descriptions with exhausted or exasperated tones, their body language signaling distance or disdain.

The imagery professionals used to describe the "fancy lady" proved particularly revealing. Several professionals across different training sessions spontaneously referenced intoxicated women at the Melbourne Cup, specifically invoking the image of women "in the bushes with their shoes in their hands." One professional explicitly referenced the popular Australian television comedy series *Kath and Kim* and its satirical take on this vignette. Facilitators observed that, for some professionals, the racing imagery and its associations with privilege and conspicuous consumption triggered responses rooted in distaste or discomfort with visible markers of socio-economic difference.

Facilitators noted that some female-identifying professionals appeared hesitant to articulate negative characterizations of the "fancy lady," lowering their voices, qualifying their statements, or openly acknowledging discomfort in voicing their assumptions. This suggested to facilitators an awareness that these reactions might conflict with those held by others in the room, or with their espoused values. One facilitator observed that "when given permission to explore or extend on this conceptualization," these professionals elaborated in more detail and were often joined by others who said, "I thought that too but didn't want to say…"

Ingroup/Outgroup Polarity

Facilitators felt that what was central to professionals' responses to the "fancy lady" was how well they identified with her. They wondered whether middle-aged women could see themselves in the "fancy lady," recognizing her in their own lives, priorities, and challenges reflected in the box's contents. In contrast, they questioned whether professionals who could not identify with her—those who saw her as "not like me" because of differences in age or values—were more likely to default to more dismissive or critical characterizations.

The polarity that seemed to emerge around the "fancy-lady" shoebox was observed by facilitators as quite distinct from the other shoeboxes. They noted that while professionals reported varying degrees of connection or distance with other personas represented in the activity, it was the "fancy lady" that uniquely generated a sense of needing to defend one's position. One professional commented, "Aside from the shoes and the fascinator, everything in that box is in my bag right now," almost seeming to defend herself against the claims leveled at the imagined shoebox owner. From this perspective, facilitators felt there seemed to be a projective aspect to this box, perhaps revealing female-identifying professionals' internalized beliefs about socioeconomic status, femininity, aging, and what women could and should be doing.

The responses of male-identifying professionals in the room provided a telling contrast to this polarization. Consistent with observations of young men participating in NNN groups, they were observed to demonstrate notably less emotional investment in the "fancy lady." Their comments, when offered, remained relatively neutral and speculative, often focusing on practical questions or curiosity. One male professional suggested she might be preparing for a "romantic rendezvous," while others questioned her age or identity, seemingly without the morally charged assumptions observed in some female professionals' responses.

The perceived parallel between young women's responses and female-identifying professionals' responses provoked a second disruption in our understanding of empathy. It prompted us to consider whether the workers undertaking the training might share common experiences with young women, either through direct or indirect experiences of cumulative harm or broader gendered socialization. In the spirit of reflexive inquiry, we also considered the potential for facilitators to influence the embodied, in-the-moment dynamics of group and training deliveries and the meaning derived from them. The following section examines this disruption by analyzing professionals' written survey responses.

Third Disruption: Expressed Versus Embodied Responses

The themes presented in the previous sections emerged from *embodied* encounters—young people and professionals physically handling the contents of the "fancy-lady" shoebox, responding in real time to group settings, and navigating social dynamics as they unfolded. These observations captured how participants engaged with the "fancy-lady" shoebox while together in the room, experiencing the activity as it was designed and within the context of scaffolded, facilitated reflective learning. These findings prompted us to question whether the responses we observed were inevitable reactions to the contents of the "fancy-lady" shoebox or were shaped by group dynamics, facilitator presence, or the visceral experience of handling the objects as part of the activity.

To explore this question, we examined a third data source: written survey responses that professionals provided as part of a pre-training questionnaire. These responses were elicited using a photograph of the "fancy-lady" shoebox and its contents, alongside questions about who they thought owned the shoes, what might be happening for them, and how they felt toward them. These data offered a natural comparison point: the same population and the same stimulus, but without the embodied and social elements that characterized the training room observations.

Presenting a third disruption to our understanding, we found that professionals expressed responses painted a notably different picture from their observed embodied experience. Written data did not show the distinct differentiation between male and female perspectives observed by facilitators, and direct negative characterizations of the "fancy lady" were outliers across the dataset. Instead, analysis indicated that professionals were curious, willing to acknowledge that assumptions should be treated with caution, and expressive of both cognitive and affective constructions of the "fancy lady" and her reality.

Thinking About the "Fancy Lady"

Almost a quarter of professionals (46 of 171) provided responses that focused primarily on the cognitive task of imagining who the "fancy lady" was and what might be happening to her. The vast majority of these professionals—almost two-thirds of whom identified as female—constructed positive, generous, or multi-dimensional narratives of the imagined owner. One wrote, "I think they are a positive, friendly person." Another actively interpreted visual evidence to build a coherent, sympathetic story: "I feel she is busy and is hoping to get a rest on a holiday, hence the photo of the beach." One professional offered a sophisticated construction: "I feel like she's busy, maybe a little aloof. Nostalgic but sociable. Independent and slightly unorganized. Affectionate and likeable," holding multiple, even contradictory qualities together and recognizing the imagined owner's complexity and humanity. Others expressed positive curiosity about the owner: "I want to know them. They seem really interesting," and "I feel interested to hear this person's story and find out a little bit more about them."

The use of the phrase "I feel," followed by clearly cognitive content, was notable, perhaps reflecting how thinking and feeling interweave in constructing a response. Some professionals remained in a state of active wondering, without rushing to definitive narratives: "curious," "I feel intrigued," and "I find myself curious about the owner of the shoes' career, lifestyle, and interests." These responses suggested that professionals were willing to sit with not-knowing, remain curious, and avoid assumptions about the owner's identity and experience.

Within this predominantly positive cognitive engagement with the "fancy lady," distinct subgroups emerged. A small subset of respondents constructed narratives specifically around socioeconomic difference and assumptions of privilege. Some made straightforward observations: "This person isn't poor." Others positioned the owner's assumed privilege in more problematic ways: "They hold power and control. They have money and use this to their advantage." One professional constructed the narrative: "May not have experienced poverty, social isolation, being looked at as different to others, well resourced, therefore may find it challenging to understand unless they have had experience working alongside others who are disadvantaged," inferring not just the imagined owner's circumstances but also their capacity for understanding others based solely on visual cues about presumed wealth.

Some professionals connected the shoebox contents to "the races," which appeared to serve as a reference point that triggered negative associations: "It looks like they are going to the races—so not great." Yet one response demonstrated reflexivity about this very reaction: "Initially, I felt this person was well-off, and I felt slightly judgmental about them attending the races. However, looking more closely, it appears there might be more to her story." The professional's capacity to notice their initial judgement, reconsider, and revise their interpretations might reflect the more deliberate, unhurried engagement with the photograph that this method allowed.

A few other cognitive responses offered narratives that were concerned or critical. One imposed a story of maternal failure despite no evidence in the photograph: "The mother is not present in the young person's life; young person longs for understanding and love." Another expressed concern about physical discomfort: "I think their feet will hurt wearing those shoes." A very small group (n = 4) responded to the actual shoes rather than imagining who owned them: "Would not be comfortable to explore a new place," "I used to wear them, not now though," and "old school."

Feeling for the "Fancy Lady"

Only one response expressed overt rejection of the "fancy lady": "A bit of disgust, I suspect that the person is very superficial." This singular dismissive response appeared as an outlier in the dataset. Instead, the largest proportion of professionals (82 of 171) responded to the emotional reactions evoked by the "fancy-lady" shoebox, describing how they felt toward the imagined owner. The predominant tone of these responses was notably warm. Professionals expressed excitement for the imagined owner's experiences: "Happy for her—that she had a good time out," "Warm, affectionate," "I'm excited for her. This looks like fun in a box," and "I hope they had a fun day at whatever event they are attending." Others expressed worry or concern ($n = 11$): "I feel sorry for her. It looks as if she works hard but needs a break when she can," "I feel concerned about how safe they will be out in Newcastle," "Compassion—their feet are going to hurt." These responses, imagining vulnerability and expressing worry or concern, were proportionally less present in female-identifying professionals' responses compared to male-identifying professionals.

Nine professionals expressed envy toward the imagined owner: "How lucky are they, jealous of her freedom to have plans," "jealous," "envious," and "envious, I need a holiday." One professional explicitly connected their cognitive construction of the imagined owner with their affective response: "I feel like she is successful and has lots of friends. I feel some envy of her position because from the picture, her life seems so perfect." This response revealed how the narrative construction about the imagined owner's life circumstances—seeing her life as "perfect"—connected to feelings of "envy." Responses citing envy were roughly split between female- and male-identifying professionals.

Relational Positioning: "Worlds Apart" or "Similar Enjoyments"

What seemed particularly revealing across affective response was how professionals positioned themselves relationally to the imagined owner—whether they located connection, distance, or centered their own experience. Of the 82 affective (or feelings-based) responses, the majority ($n = 64$) foregrounded the imagined owner's experience, focusing on her well-being or circumstances: "Excited for her, hoping she has a great time away/celebrating," "Concern or empathy for what is going on in their life." Eight responses indicated points of connection or identification with the imagined owner: "A positive vibe as I have similar enjoyments," "Go on her. I want to go with," "She's my favorite cousin." In these responses, professionals appeared able to see themselves, their experiences, or people they knew in the "fancy lady," and these positions were entirely positive.

Ten responses were self-referential, centered on the professionals' own reactions or feelings: "Envious, I need a holiday," "I like them and wish my old knees would allow me to also wear them." Other responses, by contrast, articulated social distance: "I feel worlds apart," "They may not socialize in the same circles as me. Prioritize looks." These responses positioned the imagined owner as "not like me"—occupying different social worlds or holding different values. The pattern of relational positioning seemed significant. Professionals who located relational connections—who saw "similar enjoyments" or wanted to "go with her"—expressed positive regard, whereas those who positioned the imagined owner as socially distant ("worlds apart," "different circles") or as holding problematic power ("They hold power control. They have money and use this to their advantage") were more likely to construct critical narratives or express disconnection.

Gender and Neutrality

Perhaps most striking was what the written survey responses did not show. There were no significant differences between the responses of male- and female-identifying professionals, with both reporting a spread of responses across neutral, cognitive, and emotive categories proportional to their representation in the overall cohort. Nearly a quarter of professionals (41 of 171) explicitly declined to take an emotional or cognitive position about the imagined owner.

The largest subgroup in this category stated they did not have a feeling response ($n = 17$): "I don't have any feelings regarding the owner," "I'm neutral. I don't know them and I have not met them to determine any way I might feel towards them," "no feelings really—I haven't made any assumptions about who they may be." Others ($n = 4$) were specific about withholding judgment: "No judgment," "Calm, interested, non-judgmental." Three professionals stated they did not know or were unsure. These responses suggested deliberate choices not to project onto or construct narratives about the person based on the photograph provided.

Narrative Themes Across Disruptions

Analysis of three data sources describing young people's and professionals' engagement with the "fancy-lady" shoebox identifies both common and distinct narrative themes that are instructive—and at times disruptive—to our understanding of empathy and the value of the activity. Common across the data were narratives emphasizing relational aspects of empathy. How participants "related to" or "identified with" the "fancy lady" appeared to influence—and often amplify—their expressed thoughts and feelings about her, both positive and negative.

Across data sources, the "fancy lady" was considered in different ways. She was constructed alternately as vulnerable, fun, successful, neglectful, or to be avoided. These interpretations were often qualified by markers of social proximity, indicating closeness or distance between the participants' identities and that of the imagined "fancy lady." Markers of social distance, including phrases such as "not like me," were commonly associated with less positive regard, whereas markers of social closeness—either to participants' own identities or to someone familiar to them—were usually linked with more positive sentiments of warmth, generosity, excitement, and curiosity.

However, this was not true in all cases. Narratives that constructed the "fancy lady" as a mother were a particularly striking example. These narratives were more commonly offered by young people, especially young women, compared to professionals, who almost entirely avoided this interpretation. When this narrative was presented by female-identifying professionals, consistent with observations from young women, it cast the mother as neglectful. While this finding was not universally endorsed, it is notable because it suggests that expressions of empathy can be contextual or conditional and are likely shaped by prior experiences and their impacts.

As foregrounded, cumulative harm exists as both a common and complex experience shaping our work. Young people who participate in the NNN program, particularly young women, frequently present with concurrent experiences of cumulative harm. For these young people and the professionals who support them, cumulative harm provides a context in which interventions are delivered and may influence their effects. While not explicitly referenced in participant or professional narratives associated with the "fancy lady," a reflexive perspective acknowledges the variability of human experience, strength, and survival. We should not overlook the potential influence of cumulative harm on young people's engagement with the activity. Likewise, we cannot ignore evidence that many helping professionals—most of whom are female-identifying—have their own direct experiences of harm, as well as indirect exposure to cumulative harm through their work, which may also shape their engagement.

Attention to context is also important for understanding how the shoebox activity operates. Analysis of the collective data reveals that the activity was experienced as deeply engaging, inviting complex and rich responses from both young people and adults. While grounded in material objects, the activity functions as an imaginative trigger to projective storytelling, in which participants construct and narrate an imagined "other," creating their character (Who owns the shoes?), developing a plot (What might be happening for them?), and positioning themselves relationally to them (How do you feel toward them?). Triangulation of data related to the activity suggests that its delivery format may have significantly influenced the responses elicited and the meanings made from them.

The divergence between professionals' written and embodied responses to the "fancy-lady" shoebox suggests that engaging with the activity in situ may stimulate or situate particular kinds of response. Considering this, we are drawn to notice the intra- and interpersonal dynamics of embodied experience and to attend to the socialized expectations implicit in the activity, particularly along gendered lines.

DISCUSSION: WHAT OUR DISRUPTIONS TAUGHT US

The findings presented in this chapter emerged from the discomfort we felt as practitioner-researchers in response to some reactions to the "fancy-lady" shoebox, particularly among young women and female-identifying practitioners engaged in the NNN program. The gaps between what we expected to see, what we thought we witnessed, and what was recorded in the data became a critical focus of our inquiry. The reflexive nature of this research allows us to diverge from conventional academic writing practices, introducing new literature and theoretical perspectives to discuss our findings and what they reveal about empathy as a contextual, embodied, and socially constructed phenomenon, likely shaped by gender, power, and lived experience.

Empathy, Relational Proximity, and Ingroup/Outgroup Dynamics

Our findings suggest that expressions of empathy may depend on relational proximity and identification. The "fancy-lady" shoebox uniquely appeared to activate ingroup/outgroup boundaries, particularly when experienced in person. Social identity theory (Tajfel & Turner, 1979) posits that individuals categorize themselves and others into social groups to establish positive social identity, with assumed ingroup/outgroup status shaping perception, emotional response, and behavior. Participants who positioned the "fancy lady" within their ingroup (as "like me" or "like someone I know or care for") expressed warmth and curiosity toward her. These responses align with evidence that empathy operates more readily toward ingroup members (Cikara & Fiske, 2011). Conversely, responses positioning the "fancy lady" as outgroup ("not like me," "worlds apart," or "different circles") were associated with less positive regard.

Attributions of privilege ("rich," "has money," "stuck up") served as a common form of social distancing. Consistent with evidence that differences in feelings toward other social groups can be triggered by visually salient cues to their categorization (Avenanti et al., 2010), these attributions were often made in reference to the fascinator and the idea that the "fancy lady" was attending the races. While empathic feelings and thoughts may be broadly human traits, expressions of empathy appear to be heavily influenced by social context. "Empathy rules" are the socially informed, internalized norms regarding what, when, and how expressions of empathy are appropriate, as well as which people are deemed acceptable recipients of empathic responses (Strauss, 2004). Historical examples of socially acceptable empathy responses to women involved in highly publicized murder trials—such as Lindy Chamberlain, Kelly Laine, or Erin Patterson—illustrate this point. The cultural symbolism attached to "the races" in Australia was both implicitly and explicitly referenced in negative reflections on the "fancy lady" made by professionals, perhaps reflecting a values-based stance against racing or conspicuous consumption.

The gendered dimension of these dynamics was particularly salient. Young women's and some female-identifying professionals' responses to the "fancy lady" might reflect intragroup competition, consistent with research showing that peer responses vary depending on whether the target of empathy is considered a rival (Cikara et al., 2011) or has a higher perceived status (Feng et al., 2016). Strauss (2004) notes that gender differences in empathy appear more pronounced in individualist nations than in collectivist countries, suggesting biocultural rather than purely biological explanations. The tendency of young women, compared to adult professionals, to distance themselves from the "fancy lady" may reflect that her assumed activities are outside their experience or beyond the norm for adults they feel familiar with and favorable toward. Research on adolescent empathy confirms that young people find it easier to feel empathy for someone they know and respect, with empathic action more likely toward those relationally closer (Silke et al., 2024).

While empathy has often been conceptualized as an innate and somewhat unidimensional capacity, our practice observations, consistent with emerging research, suggest it is more nuanced, influenced by proximity, familiarity, and identification. Young people in the study by Silke et al. (2024) indicated that empathy is shaped by interpersonal relationships—with parents, peers, and other family members—as well as external factors such as social media. Importantly, young people perceived social norms, including the notion of empathy as a weakness, as influential in the expression of empathy (Silke et al., 2024). Gender norms were particularly significant, with females seen as more empathic and males often not given permission to express empathy. Miklikowska et al. (2022) find that adolescents tend to associate with peers who are similar in empathic propensity, and these relationships influence the development (or stagnation) of empathy. This contingent nature of empathy may be an important consideration for practice.

Gender, Socialization, and Empathic Labor

The perceived gendered dimensions of our findings cannot be understood without examining how patriarchal socialization shapes expectations and expressions of empathy. While neuroscience suggests that gender differences have ontogenetic and phylogenetic foundations (Christov-Moore et al., 2014), the behavioral expression of empathy is likely influenced by social expectations, social learning, and cultural constructs (Sanchis-Sanchis et al., 2020). It has long been recognized that the gendering process is applied differently to children whose sex is female or male, with caregivers responding in contrasting ways to the emotional expressions of girls and boys from infancy (Gansen & Martin, 2018). These differential response processes likely frame how empathy is expressed, under what circumstances, and toward whom

(Chaplin et al., 2005). In this way, the gendered expression of empathy becomes socially constructed.

Social constructivist theories highlight the importance of contextual societal expectations in the expression of internalized behaviors, with men and women expressing their emotions and empathy in line with specific social contexts (Sanchis-Sanchis et al., 2020). The social construction of empathy is produced and reproduced within power dynamics that regulate which empathic expressions are acceptable and whose emotions are deemed deserving of empathic regard. Tension between felt and expressed emotions regularly surfaced in our findings, perhaps revealing the complex monitoring work female participants, in particular, perform around empathic expression. When female professionals characterized the "fancy lady" as "high maintenance" or "hard work," facilitators noted they often delivered these descriptions with exhausted or exasperated tones, their body language signaling distance or disdain, yet they simultaneously lowered their voices, qualified their statements, or openly acknowledged discomfort in voicing their assumptions. One facilitator observed that "when given permission to explore or extend on this conceptualization," these professionals elaborated with more detail, often joined by others who would say, "I thought that too but didn't want to say." This pattern may reveal the surveillance women maintain over their expressions—performing the emotional labor of monitoring whether their authentic reactions align with professional or gender-prescribed expectations about appropriate empathic response.

First coined by Arlie Hochschild in 1983, emotional labor refers to the management of feelings and expectations required to fulfill the emotional demands of a task or job. Emotional labor involves surface acting—producing or displaying an emotion without authentically feeling it—and deep acting—authentically attempting to feel the emotions one is expected to display in a specific context (Hochschild, 2012). Emotional labor carries risks, one being emotional dissonance, the psychological strain that can occur when felt and expressed emotions diverge, potentially leading to burnout or dissociation from authentic feelings (Hochschild, 2012; Wharton, 2009). Beauregard (2024) argues that empathic labor exists within hierarchical, patriarchal systems that inequitably allocate the burden of unrecognized emotional work toward women. Studies of American cohorts suggest that women are assigned higher levels of emotional labor compared to men, including hermeneutic labor, where women are tasked with maintaining relationships and interpreting the emotions of others (Anderson, 2023). This type of gendered allocation of empathic responsibility, which ensures social functioning, is often invisible.

The defensive quality of responses to the "fancy lady," when participants identified with the imagined owner, may illuminate how this burden operates. One professional's statement—"Aside from the shoes and the fascinator, everything in that box is in my bag right now," was offered almost as self-protection against judgments directed at the imagined owner. Facilitators noted that the professional seemed compelled to defend herself against assumptions about the "fancy lady" being superficial, high-maintenance, or irresponsible. This projective dimension suggests the activity activated anxieties about being judged for markers of femininity, busyness, and everyday self-care that many participants perceived the shoebox to represent: the coffee packet for staying alert, the to-do list for managing responsibilities, and the photo of a beach for longing for rest.

A growing understanding of the costs of emotional labor, most often described as a duty assigned to women, positions it as a dynamic that functions as an apparatus producing and maintaining inequality (Beauregard, 2024; Gabriel et al., 2023). These insights are supported by research extending the conceptualization of emotional labor from work contexts to intimate partner relationships. Oschatz et al.'s (2024) findings are particularly significant because they challenge narratives that frame gendered emotional capabilities as inherently favorable rather than burdensome.

It may be that for helping professionals, these dynamics of emotional labor are intensified. Our observations revealed these pressures in action when facilitators attempted to redirect hostile judgments. Young women maintained their negative characterizations of the "fancy lady" even when facilitators pointed out the absence of evidence for their assumptions: the box contained no alcohol, no evidence of children, and no proof of wealth beyond the shoes. This resistance may reflect not defiance but exhaustion with constant expectations to perform empathy, particularly empathy that requires suspending one's own perspective or distress. The professional women in our study likely navigate these pressures regularly, and the stark divergence between their written and embodied responses may illustrate this. In written surveys, nearly half the cohort provided predominantly warm emotional responses to the "fancy lady." Yet some of these same professionals, when engaging with the physical shoebox in training groups, expressed markedly different sentiments, some describing the imagined owner as "high maintenance," and spontaneously invoking images of an intoxicated woman "in the bushes with their shoes in their hands." The social context of group observation appeared to shift what people felt comfortable expressing. Once a negative sentiment was voiced by one person, the rest of the group felt freer to share the sentiment, sometimes amplifying it further in more detail. It frequently seemed as though a sense of relief emerged, with professionals suspending a tightly held expectation of empathy to speak freely once it appeared safe to do so.

When Empathy Becomes Strategic: Competition and Conditional Care

Patriarchal socialization practices are also relevant to understanding contexts in which empathic responses may be strategically deployed (Berke et al., 2018). Gender roles are engendered through cultural practices and institutions via operant learning processes (Berke et al., 2018), operating within hierarchical systems where emotional labor expectations reflect power differentials (Hochschild, 1983). Patriarchal systems and structures can create scarcity conditions in which women, consciously or otherwise, compete for access to and control over resources—social and financial capital, relationships, or safety—with the underlying competition affecting empathic dynamics (Reynolds & Palmer-Hague, 2022). The "fancy-lady" shoebox, with its markers of leisure, femininity, and presumed socioeconomic status, appeared to activate resource-competitive frameworks. For young people, the narratives they created about the imagined owner of the shoes often linked presumed financial resources to negative character traits ("drove a Mercedes," "stuck up"), sentiments that gained wider endorsement and often created sessions where antagonism toward the "fancy lady" became an established group stance. Notably, this competitive dynamic was not universal or unchallenged. When conceptualizations were challenged by some as "stereotyping," young people themselves recognized the gendered dimensions of their responses, even as they participated in them.

Resources associated with relationships are not limited to those arising in intimate partner relationships but also include peer relationships. Research on female friendships finds that women report friendship violations or hurts more often than men, and that this kind of disjuncture can damage female-to-female social standing through furtive competitive processes (Reynolds & Palmer-Hague, 2022). Across social discourse, female friendships have been typified by mutual mistrust; however, feminist scholars argue that when not constrained by competitive constructs, female friendships can be powerful and life affirming (Kelner & Gavriel-Fried, 2023). Few young women engaged with the "fancy-lady" shoebox in ways that suggested she might be considered as a relational resource or friend. Rather, her presumed privilege marked her as "not like me," an attribution that seemed to socially distance themselves from her. This competitive dynamic was not observed for young men, who constructed similar narratives around presumed wealth or privilege ("probably rich") but, when noticing contradictory evidence ("maybe poor because of the fake glasses"), described her position rather than assigning emotional value.

Consideration of gender in relation to competition and contextual empathy must recognize intersectional experiences. Culture and socioeconomic status can influence opportunities for female friendship, with women from marginalized communities often encountering restrictions that impinge on curating broader social circles (Kelner

& Gavriel-Fried, 2023). Contemporary sociological opinion argues that friendship schemas situated in gender determinism inevitably influence experiences in gendered ways (Fox, 2024). Where competition between women exists, it should be recognized through the many intersecting identities that influence resource access, shaping when emphatic responses are intentionally withheld or extended (Kelner & Gavriel-Fried, 2023). The young women in our study, many with cumulative harm histories and marginalization experiences, may have recognized the "fancy lady" as possessing resources they themselves lacked or struggled to access. Yet this recognition remained complex and contradictory. Despite hostile commentary, facilitators observed that young women were simultaneously drawn to the box's contents. This simultaneous attraction and repulsion suggest the "fancy lady" may have represented both aspiration and threat—embodying a femininity that was desired yet felt dangerous or unattainable.

Cumulative Harm, Hypervigilance, and Empathy as Survival Strategy

Perhaps most crucial for accumulation-aware practice is reframing what appeared as empathy deficits as potentially adaptive responses to cumulative harm. The paradoxical relationship between empathy and trauma is substantially absent from research into emotional labor, particularly considering that for some people who have experienced trauma, empathic responses can be both protective tools and sources of vulnerability and threat. Research by Sanchis-Sanchis et al. (2020) suggests trauma may affect emotional regulation, which in turn may contribute to hypervigilant empathic scanning and enhanced sensitivity to the emotional states of others. In turn, this may act as a type of survival mechanism for some who have experienced trauma. This is particularly the case for people who experienced childhood adverse experiences, where understanding and anticipating the emotions of negligent caregivers became a protective system, with empathy becoming less about placing oneself in the shoes of another and more about threat detection and safety (Sanchis-Sanchis et al., 2020). For the young women in NNN who frequently present with cumulative harm experiences, the hostile responses to the "fancy lady" may reflect this transformation of empathy from connection into threat detection. The immediate leap to assumptions about privilege can be understood as hypervigilant scanning for markers of danger or difference. The "stuck up" attribution positions the imagined owner not just as different but as potentially threatening, that is, someone who might judge, reject, or harm. This protective wariness toward those positioned as "other" in class and status hierarchies represents adaptive threat assessment rather than empathy failure.

However, as noted by Gabriel et al. (2023), this transformation of prosocial empathic capability into empathic hypervigilance can carry a cost for the user, as the consistent monitoring of others' emotional states depletes emotional and cognitive resources and can lead to emotional exhaustion. For some people who have experienced trauma, especially those from marginalized groups who face intersectional and compounding social expectations, the cost may intensify into significant personal risk (Beauregard, 2024). The intensity and speed of young women's hostile reactions might reflect the exhaustion that accompanies constant vigilance. These rapid moral judgments may indicate depleted cognitive resources, where young women lack the capacity for the slower, more complex cognitive-empathy work of imagining alternative narratives. The collective amplification of hostile responses—"when one participant expressed hostile commentary, others frequently joined or amplified these judgments"—might reflect a shared experience of empathic exhaustion within the group.

If we contextualize empathy as a survival strategy, we may reframe what can, on face value, appear to be empathic resistance as self-preservation. When some people who have experienced trauma—especially those who experienced trauma in childhood—seem to withhold or avoid empathic engagement, we can understand this not as defiance but as a form of boundary setting and regulation that prioritizes survival over civic compliance (Sanchis-Sanchis et al., 2020). The finding that young women maintained their negative characterizations even when facilitators pointed out the absence of evidence for their assumptions might illustrate this protective boundary setting. Similarly, young women's resistance to the activity (out of fear of snitching) might represent not stubbornness but self-protection. For these young women, allowing empathic connection to the "fancy lady" might have required vulnerability that felt too dangerous. For young women navigating cumulative harm, extending empathy toward someone who appeared safe, resourced, and free from consequences they themselves faced daily may have felt like betraying their own experience or exposing themselves to further harm.

For many females who experience trauma, dominant gendered socialization can intersect with trauma-based adaptations, placing them in situations were refusing socially desired or expected responses can carry personal, social, or professional costs (Oschatz et al., 2024). The expectation that females naturally exhibit empathic responses is especially harmful when society pathologizes trauma-based adaptive responses as dysfunctional, oppositional, or unfeminine instead of understanding them as self-protective. Recognizing that empathic resistance may be adaptive challenges the existing discourse that empathy is innately female and desirable and instead acknowledges that for people who have experienced trauma, empathic resistance may be an attempt to navigate complex situations where connection may ignite a sense of threat (Beauregard, 2020).

For young women with cumulative harm experiences, withholding empathy from the "fancy lady" may represent sophisticated risk assessment rather than an empathy deficit. If extending empathy has previously resulted in exploitation, betrayal, or harm, strategic withdrawal of empathic engagement becomes a learned protective behavior. The activity inadvertently asked these young women to practice the very vulnerability—open-hearted connection to an unknown other—that their survival has required them to resist. High rates of helping professionals with lived experience of cumulative harm (Elliott & Guy, 1993; Pope & Feldman-Summers, 1992) likewise suggest that some professionals in our study may share these adaptive patterns. The divergence between written and embodied responses becomes particularly significant through this lens. Written responses, completed individually in private, showed professionals capable of sophisticated empathic work: constructing multi-dimensional narratives, expressing warmth and curiosity, and acknowledging complexity. Yet in group training contexts, some of these same professionals expressed hostility or withdrew empathic engagement. This shift may not represent hypocrisy but the activation of trauma-based protective mechanisms in social contexts where vulnerability feels unsafe.

Reflexive Disruption: Interrogating Our Own Lens

Implicit, but perhaps understated, in the discussion of our findings so far is that our findings emerged through interpretive frameworks shaped by our own positions as facilitators, practitioners, and researchers embedded in the knowledge generation process. Practitioner reflections and field observations were interpreted through the lens of our experiences, biases, and theoretical leanings. We noticed what "disrupted" us. These disruptions may themselves reveal as much about our own acculturated assumptions as about participants' actual empathy. Our commitment to reflexivity demands that we question whether the responses we experienced as disruptive were genuinely anomalous or whether we noticed and amplified them because they deviated from gendered scripts, we had unconsciously internalized.

The divergence between written responses and embodied responses to the activity poses a particular point of reflection. While written responses occurred outside our facilitative influence, embodied responses occurred within group contexts we facilitated, shaped by our presence, prompts, and reactions. This raises difficult questions: Did our facilitation inadvertently activate particular dynamics? Did our own discomfort with certain responses become visible, influencing group interactions? Did the permission we gave to "explore assumptions" open space for expressions that participants might otherwise have monitored? We cannot know definitively whether the patterns we observed represent participants' authentic responses or co-constructed performances shaped by complex group dynamics, including our own participation.

What we can say is that the activity functions as more than a neutral stimulus; it operates within relational, social, and power-laden contexts that include facilitator presence, expectations, and interpretations. Acknowledging this embeddedness does not invalidate our findings but enriches them, positioning the "disruptions" as data about the entire empathy-building enterprise—how we design, deliver, and interpret empathy work—rather than simply about participants' capacities.

CONCLUSION: EMBRACING DISRUPTION AS DATA

This chapter began with our discomfort, a productive unease sparked by observing responses to the "fancy-lady" shoebox that challenged our assumptions about empathy in trauma-informed practice. What we initially perceived as disruptions became, through reflexive inquiry, an invitation to interrogate our own theoretical frameworks and practice assumptions. Our findings reveal empathy as a contextual, embodied, and profoundly social phenomenon, shaped by gender, power, life experience, circumstance, and the very conditions under which it is invited or demanded.

Key Contributions

This work makes several meaningful contributions to accumulation-aware and gender-responsive practice. First, it highlights that empathic responses cannot be understood outside relational and social contexts. The stark divergence between professionals' written and embodied responses to the "fancy-lady" shoebox reveals how group dynamics, social expectations, and facilitator presence likely shape what participants feel safe to express. What appears as empathy—or its absence—may often reflect complex negotiations between felt experience and social performance, particularly for women navigating the burden of emotional labor.

Second, this work reframes apparent empathy deficits as potentially adaptive responses to cumulative harm. When participants positioned the "fancy lady" as threatening or withdrew empathic engagement, they may have been demonstrating sophisticated risk assessment rather than empathy failure. For those whose survival has required hypervigilant monitoring of threat, strategic withholding of empathy can function as boundary-setting and self-protection. This challenges deficit-based interpretations and the pathologizing of responses that actually reflect hard-won survival strategies. The intragroup dynamics we observed among young women and female-identifying professionals highlight complex relational networks where identification, competition, and safety concerns intersect to shape empathy. Recognizing these dynamics moves us beyond gender-blind interventions toward accumulation-aware practice that accounts for how gender shapes both empathic capacity and its strategic deployment.

Finally, the shoebox activity itself represents a methodological contribution to experiential learning in trauma-informed contexts. Despite—or perhaps because of—the disruptions it provoked, the activity demonstrated a remarkable capacity to engage participants across age groups, professional backgrounds, and settings. Its strength lies in accessibility: it requires no dominant literacy skills, invites tactile and embodied exploration, and creates psychological distance through projection onto imagined others. The curated objects function as what we might call "empathy probes," that is, material artifacts that invite storytelling while allowing participants to regulate their own emotional proximity to the content. Critically, the activity served dual purposes: as an intervention tool engaging participants in empathic practice, and as a research instrument revealing otherwise invisible dynamics around identification, social positioning, and contextual empathy.

Limitations and Future Research Directions

Limitations of the work presented in this chapter are inseparable from its reflexive methodology. Our findings emerged through interpretive frameworks shaped by our own positions as facilitators, practitioners, and researchers. The reliance on practitioner observations and field notes means our data captures facilitators' interpretations rather than participants' unmediated experiences. We cannot definitively disentangle participants' authentic responses from co-constructed performances shaped by group dynamics and our own facilitative influence.

The study's scope presents additional constraints. We lacked systematic measures of participants' cumulative harm experiences, instead inferring these from program eligibility criteria and anecdotal knowledge. The young people's data came primarily through practitioner reflections rather than direct participant accounts, limiting our access to their own meaning-making. Sample sizes for gender-specific groups were small, and the predominance of female-identifying professionals in our training cohorts prevented robust comparison across gender identities. The retrospective nature of some data collection and potential selection bias in what facilitators chose to document further qualify our findings.

Future research might address these limitations in several ways. Systematic measurement of adversity exposure, coupled with validated empathy assessments, would strengthen inferences about the relationships we observed. Participatory research methods that center young people's own interpretations of their responses would complement practitioner observations. Investigation of facilitator effects on group dynamics could clarify the extent to which observed patterns reflect participant characteristics versus social co-construction. Cross-cultural replication would test whether findings extend beyond the Australian context, where patriarchal, colonial, and socioeconomic dynamics take particular forms.

Methodologically, future work might employ multiple response formats—written, verbal, and embodied—simultaneously rather than sequentially, directly examining divergence within participants rather than across data sources. Comparative research examining responses to different shoebox personas could clarify whether the patterns we observed are specific to the "fancy lady" or reflect broader dynamics. Finally, intervention research testing accumulation-aware, gender-responsive modifications to empathy-building activities could move from observation to action, developing and evaluating practice innovations informed by these findings.

Implications for Accumulation-Aware, Trauma-Informed Practice

The lessons from our disruptions challenge assumptions that empathy-building interventions operate universally or neutrally. The "fancy-lady" activity generated different responses depending on participants' histories, gender, group composition, and delivery format. This suggests empathy work requires careful assessment of readiness, safety, and contextual appropriateness rather than standardized application.

Our findings suggest that accumulation-aware practice should not automatically interpret empathic resistance or hostility as deficits requiring remediation. Instead, practitioners might ask: What protective function might this response serve? What experiences taught this young person that empathic engagement carries risk? What resources or safety measures would need to be present for them to risk vulnerability? This reframing shifts practice from correcting perceived deficits to supporting adaptive capacity while creating conditions where connection can emerge safely.

Similarly, gender-responsive practice should consider emotional labor dynamics, recognizing that expectations for empathic performance fall disproportionately on women and may intensify for those with trauma histories. Creating a safe space for women navigating harm to prioritize their own well-being over empathic responsiveness represents recognition of survival needs.

Practitioners themselves require support in navigating these complexities. Training should prepare facilitators to recognize adaptive trauma responses, emotional labor exhaustion, or legitimate resistance to emotional demands. Facilitators need permission not to redirect or correct these responses reflexively, instead holding them as meaningful data about safety, readiness, and what the activity is actually asking of participants. Supervision should create space to examine facilitators' own discomfort with responses that deviate from expected empathic expression, interrogating whose comfort is centered in these moments.

Final Reflections

The "fancy-lady" shoebox taught us that disruption itself is data, not noise to be explained away but a signal revealing the limitations of our frameworks. By sitting with discomfort rather than rushing to resolution, we discovered empathy to be far more complex, contingent, and consequential than we had appreciated. This work invites practitioners to embrace similar disruptions in our own practice, treating moments when clients do not respond as expected not as implementation failures but as invitations to deeper understanding.

Moving forward requires humility about what we thought we knew. Empathy cannot be reduced to a teachable skill or a measurable capacity divorced from relational context, lived experience, and social positioning. For young people navigating cumulative harm, empathy work must proceed with acute sensitivity to how we ask them to be vulnerable, with whom, and at what cost. The goal becomes not universal empathic expression but supporting each person's capacity to connect safely, on their own terms, when conditions permit.

We close with appreciation for the young people and professionals whose responses disrupted our certainty. Their willingness to engage authentically—whether with warmth, hostility, curiosity, or withdrawal—generated the very data that challenged and ultimately enriched our understanding. In honoring their responses as meaningful rather than deficient, we move toward practice that is responsive to the complex realities of those who navigate trauma, survival, and the ongoing work of healing in contexts not always safe enough for the vulnerability that empathy demands.

REFERENCES

Adelman, M., Rosenberg, K. E., & Hobart, M. (2016). Simulations and social empathy. *Violence Against Women*, *22*(12), 1451–1462. DOI: 10.1177/1077801215625850

Alexander, L. H., & Alessi, E. J. (2024). A critical review of the conceptualization of empathy: Toward a deeper understanding for clinical social work practice. *Clinical Social Work Journal*, *52*(3), 300–309. DOI: 10.1007/s10615-023-00912-z

Anderson, E. (2023). Hermeneutic labor: The gendered burden of interpretation in intimate relationships between women and men. *Hypatia*, *38*(1), 177–197. DOI: 10.1017/hyp.2023.11

Auriemma, V. (2023). *Empathy: The contribution of neuroscience to social analysis*. Palgrave Macmillan., DOI: 10.1007/978-3-031-38860-6

Avenanti, A., Sirigu, A., & Aglioti, S. M. (2010). Racial bias reduces empathic sensorimotor resonance with other-race pain. *Current Biology*, *20*(11), 1018–1022. DOI: 10.1016/j.cub.2010.03.071

Baez, S., Flichtentrei, D., Prats, M., Mastandueno, R., García, A. M., Cetkovich, M., & Ibáñez, A. (2017). Men, women… who cares? A population-based study on sex differences and gender roles in empathy and moral cognition. *PLoS One*, *12*(6), e0179336. DOI: 10.1371/journal.pone.0179336

Baglivio, M. T., Wolff, K. T., Jackowski, K., & Greenwald, M. A. (2018). A multilevel examination of risk/need change scores, community context, and successful reentry of committed juvenile offenders. *Youth Violence and Juvenile Justice*, *15*(1), 38–61. DOI: 10.1177/1541204015596052

Baron-Cohen, S., & Wheelwright, S. (2004). The empathy quotient: An investigation of adults with Asperger syndrome or high functioning autism, and normal sex differences. *Journal of Autism and Developmental Disorders*, *34*(2), 163–175. DOI: 10.1023/B:JADD.0000022607.19833.00

Beauregard, P. (2024). Emotional labor in decision making: Gender, race, and relational practices in the White House. *Presidential Studies Quarterly*, *54*(3), 691–712. DOI: 10.1111/psq.12884

Berardi, M. K., White, A. M., Winters, D., Thorn, K., Brennan, M., & Dolan, P. (2020). Rebuilding communities with empathy. *Local Development & Society*, *1*(1), 57–67. DOI: 10.1080/26883597.2020.1794761

Berke, D. S., Reidy, D., & Zeichner, A. (2018). Masculinity, emotion regulation, and psychopathology. *Clinical Psychology Review*, *66*, 106–116. DOI: 10.1016/j.cpr.2018.01.004

Bessarab, D., & Ng'andu, B. (2010). Yarning about yarning as a legitimate method in Indigenous research. *International Journal of Critical Indigenous Studies*, *3*(1), 37–50. DOI: 10.5204/ijcis.v3i1.57

Blakemore, T., & Rak, L. (2024). Empathy expressed and experienced. In Blakemore, T., Rak, L., Krogh, C., McCarthy, S., & Stuart, G. (Eds.), *Working with youth violence: The Name.Narrate.Navigate program* (pp. 194–219). Routledge.

Blakemore, T., Rak, L., Krogh, C., McCarthy, S., & Stuart, G. (Eds.). (2024). *Working with youth violence: The Name.Narrate.Navigate program*. Routledge.

Bons, D., van den Broek, E., Scheepers, F., Herpers, P., Rommelse, N., & Buitelaaar, J. K. (2013). Motor, emotional, and cognitive empathy in children and adolescents with autism spectrum disorder and conduct disorder. *Journal of Abnormal Child Psychology*, *41*(3), 425–443. DOI: 10.1007/s10802-012-9689-5

Broidy, L., Cauffman, E., Espelage, D. L., Mazerolle, P., & Piquero, A. (2003). Sex differences in empathy and its relation to juvenile offending. *Violence and Victims*, *18*(5), 502–516. DOI: 10.1891/vivi.2003.18.5.503

Calley, N. G., & Gerber, S. (2008). Empathy-promoting counselling strategies for juvenile sex offenders: A developmental approach. *Journal of Addictions & Offender Counseling*, *28*(2), 68–85. DOI: 10.1002/j.2161-1874.2008.tb00034.x

Cerqueira, A., & Almeida, T. C. (2023). Adverse childhood experiences: Relationship with empathy and alexithymia. *Journal of Child & Adolescent Trauma*, *16*(3), 559–568. DOI: 10.1007/s40653-023-00520-6

Chan, H. H.-K., Kwong, H. Y., Shu, G. L., Ting, C. Y., & Lai, F. H. Y. (2021). Effects of experiential learning programmes on adolescent prosocial behaviour, empathy, and subjective well-being: A systematic review and meta-analysis. *Frontiers in Psychology*, *12*, 709699. Advance online publication. DOI: 10.3389/fpsyg.2021.709699

Chang, H. (2008). *Autoethnography as method: Developing qualitative inquiry*. Left Coast Press.

Chaplin, T. M., Cole, P. M., & Zahn-Waxler, C. (2005). Parental socialization of emotion expression: Gender differences and relations to child adjustment. *Emotion (Washington, D.C.)*, *5*(1), 80–88. DOI: 10.1037/1528-3542.5.1.80

Cheng, Y., Chou, C. H., Decety, J., Chen, I. Y., Hung, D., Tzeng, O. J. L., & Lin, C.-P. (2009). Sex differences in the neuroanatomy of human mirror-neuron system: A voxel-based morphometric investigation. *Neuroscience*, *159*(2), 713–720. DOI: 10.1016/j.neuroscience.2008.10.026

Christov-Moore, L., Simpson, E. A., Coudé, G., Grigaityte, K., Iacoboni, M., & Ferrari, P. F. (2014). Empathy: Gender effects in brain and behavior. *Neuroscience and Biobehavioral Reviews*, *46*, 604–627. DOI: 10.1016/j.neubiorev.2014.09.001

Cikara, M., Botvinick, M., & Fiske, S. T. (2011). Us versus them: Social identity shapes neural responses to intergroup competition and harm. *Psychological Science*, *22*(3), 306–313. DOI: 10.1177/0956797610397667

Cikara, M., & Fiske, S. T. (2011). Bounded empathy: Neural responses to outgroup targets' (mis)fortunes. *Journal of Cognitive Neuroscience*, *23*(12), 3791–3803. DOI: 10.1162/jocn_a_00069

Cochran, J. L., & Cochran, N. H. (2015). *The heart of counseling: Counseling skills through therapeutic relationships*. Routledge, Taylor & Francis Group.

Decety, J., & Lam, C. (2006). Human empathy through the lens of social neuroscience. *TheScientificWorldJournal*, *6*(280363), 1146–1163. DOI: 10.1100/tsw.2006.221

Decety, J., & Moriguchi, Y. (2007). The empathic brain and its dysfunction in psychiatric populations: Implications for intervention across different clinical conditions. *BioPsychoSocial Medicine*, *1*(22), 1–21. DOI: 10.1186/1751-0759-1-22

Dinic, B. M., Kodzopeljic, J. S., Sokolovska, V. T., & Milovanovic, I. Z. (2016). Empathy and peer violence among adolescents: Moderation effect of gender. *School Psychology International*, *37*(4), 359–377. DOI: 10.1177/0143034316649008

Duke, N. N., Pettingell, S. L., McMorris, B. J., & Borowsky, I. W. (2010). Adolescent violence perpetration: Associations with multiple types of adverse childhood experiences. *Pediatrics*, *125*(4), e778–e786. DOI: 10.1542/peds.2009-0597

Eisenberg, N., Cumberland, A., Gurthrie, I. K., Murphy, B. C., & Shepard, S. A. (2005). Age change in prosocial reasoning and moral reasoning in adolescence and early adulthood. *Journal of Research on Adolescence*, *15*(3), 235–260. DOI: 10.1111/j.1532-7795.2005.00095.x

Eisenberg, N., Spinrad, T. L., & Sadovsky, A. (2006). Empathy related responding in children. In Killen, M., & Smetana, J. (Eds.), *Handbook of moral development* (pp. 517–549). Erlbaum.

Elliott, D. M., & Guy, J. D. (1993). Mental health professionals versus non-mental-health professionals: Childhood trauma and adult functioning. *Professional Psychology, Research and Practice*, *24*(1), 83–90. DOI: 10.1037/0735-7028.24.1.83

Ellis, C., & Bochner, A. (2000). Autoethnography, personal narrative, reflexivity: Researcher as subject. In N. Denzin & Y. Lincoln (Eds.), *Handbook of qualitative research* (2nd ed.). Sage Publications.

Feng, C., Li, Z., Feng, X., Wang, L., Tian, T., & Luo, Y.-J. (2016). Social hierarchy modulates neural responses of empathy for pain. *Social Cognitive and Affective Neuroscience*, *11*(3), 485–495. DOI: 10.1093/scan/nsv135

Fitzgibbon, W., & Healy, D. (2019). Lives and spaces: Photovoice and offender supervision in Ireland and England. *Criminology & Criminal Justice*, *19*(1), 3–25. DOI: 10.1177/1748895817739665

Fitzgibbon, W., & Stengel, C. M. (2018). Women's voices made visible: Photovoice in visual criminology. *Punishment & Society*, *20*(4), 411–431. DOI: 10.1177/1462474517700137

Flasbeck, V., Gonzalez-Liencres, C., & Brüne, M. (2018). The brain that feels into others: toward a neuroscience of empathy. In L. C. Stevens & C. C. Woodruff (Eds.), *The neuroscience of empathy, compassion, and self-compassion* (pp. 49–93). Elsevier Science & Technology. https://ebookcentral.proquest.com/lib/newcastle/detail.action?docID=5434360

Fox, E. (2024). Toward a sociological perspective on the gender and sexuality of friendship. *Sociology Compass*, *18*(8), e13263. DOI: 10.1111/soc4.13263

Gabriel, A. S., Diefendorff, J. M., & Grandey, A. A. (2023). The acceleration of emotional labor research: Navigating the past and steering toward the future. *Personnel Psychology*, *76*(2), 397–440. DOI: 10.1111/peps.12576

Gansen, H. M., & Martin, K. A. (2018). Becoming gendered. In Risman, B. J., Froyum, C. M., & Scarborough, W. J. (Eds.), *Handbook of the sociology of gender* (pp. 83–93). Springer International Publishing., DOI: 10.1007/978-3-319-76333-0_6

Garaigordobil, M. (2009). A comparative analysis of empathy in childhood and adolescence: Gender differences and associated socio-emotional variables. *Journal of Psychology and Psychological Therapy*, *9*(2), 217–235.

Gerdes, K., & Segal, E. A. (2011). Importance of empathy for social work practice: Integrating new science. *Social Work*, *56*(2), 141–148. DOI: 10.1093/sw/56.2.141

Gerdes, K. E., & Segal, E. A. (2009). A social work model of empathy. *Advances in Social Work, 10*(2), 114–127. DOI: 10.18060/235

Greenberg, D. M., Warrier, V., Allison, C., & Baron-Cohen, S. (2018). Elevated empathy in adults following childhood trauma. *PMC*, Article 6169872.

Grynberg, D., & Konrath, S. (2020). The closer you feel, the more you care: Positive associations between closeness pain intensity rating, empathic concern and personal distress to someone in pain. *Acta Psychologica, 201*, 103175. Advance online publication. DOI: 10.1016/j.actpsy.2020.103175

Guest, G., MacQueen, K. M., & Namey, E. E. (2011). *Applied thematic analysis.* Sage Publications., DOI: 10.4135/9781483384436

Hochschild, A. R. (1983). *The managed heart: Commercialization of human feeling.* University of California Press.

Hochschild, A. R. (2012). *The managed heart: Commercialization of human feeling.* University of California Press. DOI: 10.1525/9780520951853

Hojat, M. (2009). Ten approaches for enhancing empathy in health and human services cultures. *Journal of Health and Human Services Administration, 31*(4), 412–450. DOI: 10.1177/107937390903100403

Howe, D. (2016). *Empathy: What it is and why it matters.* Palgrave MacMillan.

Hsu, N., Newman, D. A., & Badura, K. L. (2022). Emotional intelligence and transformational leadership: Meta-analysis and explanatory model of female leadership advantage. *Journal of Intelligence, 10*(4), 104. DOI: 10.3390/jintelligence10040104

Iacoboni, M. (2009). Imitation, empathy, and mirror neurons. *Annual Review of Psychology, 60*(1), 653–670. DOI: 10.1146/annurev.psych.60.110707.163604

Jolliffe, D., & Farrington, D. (2006). Development and validation of the basic empathy scale. *Journal of Adolescence, 29*(4), 589–611. DOI: 10.1016/j.adolescence.2005.08.010

Jonason, P. K., & Kroll, C. H. (2015). A multidimensional view of the relationship between empathy and the dark triad. *Journal of Individual Differences, 36*(3), 150–156. DOI: 10.1027/1614-0001/a000166

Kahhale, I., Byrd, A., & Hanson, J. (2025). Early life adversity and empathy: A scoping review of past research and recommendations for future directions. *Clinical Child and Family Psychology Review, 28*(2), 275–321. DOI: 10.1007/s10567-025-00516-8

Kelner, J., & Gavriel-Fried, B. (2023). "The relationship changed because I had changed": Experiences and perceptions of friendships between women treated for substance use disorder in women-only residential programs. *Feminism & Psychology, 33*(4), 647–667. DOI: 10.1177/09593535231176349

King, S. H.Jr. (2011). The structure of empathy in social work practice. *Journal of Human Behavior in the Social Environment, 21*(6), 679–695. DOI: 10.1080/10911359.2011.583516

Klein, K. J., & Hodges, S. D. (2001). Gender differences, motivation, and empathic accuracy: When it pays to understand. *Personality and Social Psychology Bulletin, 27*(6), 720–730. DOI: 10.1177/0146167201276007

Klimecki, O., & Singer, T. (2012). Empathic distress fatigue rather than compassion fatigue? Integrating findings from empathy research in psychology and neuroscience. In Oakley, B., Knafo, A., Madhavan, G., & Wilson, D. (Eds.), *Pathological altruism* (pp. 368–383). Oxford University Press.

Kolb, D. A. (2015). *Experiential learning: Experience as the source of learning and development.* FT Press.

Komatsu, A. V., Costa, R. C., Buoso, F. P., Dos Santos, P. V., Caetano, L. A. O., & Bazon, M. R. (2024). Psychosocial adaptation under adverse experiences: A study on the role of empathy with adolescents from vulnerable contexts in Brazil. *Child Abuse & Neglect, 150*, 106298. DOI: 10.1016/j.chiabu.2023.106298

Lam, C. B., Solmeyer, A. R., & McHale, S. M. (2012). Sibling relationships and empathy across the transition to adolescence. *Journal of Youth and Adolescence, 41*(12), 1657–1670. DOI: 10.1007/s10964-012-9781-8

Leiberg, S., Klimecki, O., & Singer, T. (2011). Short-term compassion training increases prosocial behavior in a newly developed prosocial gam. *PLoS One, 6*(3), e17798. Advance online publication. DOI: 10.1371/journal.pone.0017798

Levy, J., Goldstein, A., & Feldman, R. (2019). The neural development of empathy is sensitive to caregiving and early trauma. *Nature Communications, 10*(1), 1–10. DOI: 10.1038/s41467-019-09927-y

Lindsey, R. E., Carlozzi, A. F., & Eells, G. T. (2001). Differences in the dispositional empathy of juvenile sex offenders, non-sex-offending delinquent juveniles, and nondelinquent juveniles. *Journal of Interpersonal Violence, 16*(6), 510–522. DOI: 10.1177/088626001016006002

Linehan, M. M. (2015). *DBT skills training manual* (2nd ed.). The Guilford Press.

Löffler, C. S., & Greitemeyer, T. (2023). Are women the more empathetic gender? The effects of gender role expectations. *Current Psychology (New Brunswick, N.J.)*, *42*(1), 220–231. DOI: 10.1007/s12144-020-01260-8

Lynch, A., Newlands, F., & Forrester, D. (2019). What does empathy sound like in social work communication? A mixed-methods study of empathy in child protection social work practice. *Child & Family Social Work*, *24*(1), 139–147. DOI: 10.1111/cfs.12591

Marchetti, A., Miraglia, L., & Di Dio, C. (2019). Toward a socio-material approach to cognitive empathy in autistic spectrum disorder. *Frontiers in Psychology*, *10*(10), 2965.

Marshall, W. L., Hudson, S. M., Jones, R., & Fernandez, Y. M. (1995). Empathy in sex offenders. *Clinical Psychology Review*, *15*(2), 99–113. DOI: 10.1016/0272-7358(95)00002-7

Mauroy, A., Galdiolo, S., Meillerais, S., Verhofstadt, L. L., & Gaugue, J. (2025). Empathic Accuracy Across Childhood, Adolescence, and Within Parent-Child Interactions: A Systematic Review. *Personal Relationships*, *32*(1), e70000. DOI: 10.1111/pere.70000

McLaughlin, K. A., & Sheridan, M. A. (2016). Beyond cumulative risk: A dimensional approach to childhood adversity. *Current Directions in Psychological Science*, *25*(4), 239–245. DOI: 10.1177/0963721416655883

Meidan, A., & Uzefovsky, F. (2020). Child maltreatment risk mediates the association between maternal and child empathy. *Child Abuse & Neglect*, *106*, 104523. Advance online publication. DOI: 10.1016/j.chiabu.2020.104523

Mestre, M. V., Samper, P., Frias, M. D., & Tur, A. M. (2009). Are women more empathetic than men? A longitudinal study in adolescence. *The Spanish Journal of Psychology*, *12*(1), 76–83. DOI: 10.1017/S1138741600001499

Miklikowska, M., Tilton-Weaver, L., & Burk, W. J. (2022). With a little help from my empathic friends: The role of peers in the development of empathy in adolescence. *Developmental Psychology*, *58*(6), 1156–1162. DOI: 10.1037/dev0001347

Miller, R. (2007). *Cumulative harm: A conceptual overview*. Victorian Government.

Narvey, C., Yang, J., Wolff, K. T., Baglivio, M., & Piquero, A. R. (2021). The interrelationship between empathy and adverse childhood experiences and their impact on juvenile recidivism. *Youth Violence and Juvenile Justice*, *19*(1), 45–67. DOI: 10.1177/1541204020939647

Oschatz, T., Piemonte, J. L., & Klein, V. (2024). The intimate and sexual costs of emotional labor: The development of the Women's Sexual Emotional Labor Assessment. *Archives of Sexual Behavior*, *54*(1), 117–138. DOI: 10.1007/s10508-024-03061-7

Ozdemir, N., & Sahin, S. (2020). The impact of childhood traumatic experiences on self-esteem and interpersonal relationships. *Psychiatry and Behavioral Sciences*, *10*(4), 185–191. DOI: 10.5455/PBS.20200502025907

Pang, C., Li, W., Zhou, Y., Gao, T., & Han, S. (2023). Are women more empathetic than men? Questionnaire and EEG estimations of sex/gender differences in empathic ability. *Social Cognitive and Affective Neuroscience*, *18*(1), nsad008. DOI: 10.1093/scan/nsad008

Pope, K. S., & Felman-Summers, S. (1992). National survey of psychologists' sexual and physical abuse history and their evaluation of training and competence in these areas. *Professional Psychology, Research and Practice*, *23*(5), 3530361. Advance online publication. DOI: 10.1037/0735-7028.23.5.353

Pratte, S., Tang, A., & Oehlberg, L. (2021). Evoking empathy: A framework for describing empathy tools. In *Proceedings of the Fifteenth International Conference on Tangible, Embedded and Embodied Interaction (TEI '21)*. DOI: 10.1145/3430524.3440644

Raines, J. C. (1990). Empathy in clinical social work. *Clinical Social Work Journal*, *18*(1), 57–72. DOI: 10.1007/BF00759070

Rakoczy, H. (2022). Foundations of theory of mind and its development in early childhood. *Nature Reviews Psychology*, *1*(4), 223–235. DOI: 10.1038/s44159-022-00037-z

Rayner, S., Davis, C., Moore, M., & Cadet, T. (2020). Secondary traumatic stress in related factors in Australian social workers and psychologists. *Health & Social Work*, *45*(2), 122–130. DOI: 10.1093/hsw/hlaa001

Reynolds, T. A., & Palmer-Hague, J. (2022). Did you hear what she did to me? Female friendship victimization disclosures offer reputational advantages. *Journal of Experimental Social Psychology*, *101*, 104311. DOI: 10.1016/j.jesp.2022.104311

Rogers, C. (1951). *Client-centred therapy: Its current practice, implications and theory*. Houghton Mifflin.

Rose, A. J., & Rudolph, K. D. (2006). A review of sex differences in peer relationship processes: Potential trade-offs for the emotional and behavioral development of girls and boys. *Psychological Bulletin*, *132*(1), 98–131. DOI: 10.1037/0033-2909.132.1.98

Rose, D., & Meyer, A. (2006). *A practical reader in universal design for learning*. Harvard Education Press.

Rueckert, L., & Naybar, N. (2008). Gender differences in empathy: The role of the right hemisphere. *Brain and Cognition*, *67*(2), 162–167. DOI: 10.1016/j.bandc.2008.01.002

Sanchis-Sanchis, A., Grau, M. D., Moliner, A. R., & Morales-Murillo, C. P. (2020). Effects of age and gender in emotion regulation of children and adolescents. *Frontiers in Psychology*, *11*, 946. Advance online publication. DOI: 10.3389/fpsyg.2020.00946

Sarantou, M., & Miettinen, S. (2022). Introduction. In Sarantou, M., & Miettinen, S. (Eds.), *Empathy and business transformation* (pp. 1–12). Routledge., DOI: 10.4324/9781003227557-1

Satapathy, S., Choudhary, V., Behera, C., Swain, R., Sharma, R., & Sagar, R. (2022). Adverse childhood experiences, aggression, empathy, and psychopathology in adult males accused of rape. *Indian Journal of Psychological Medicine*, *44*(5), 466–473. DOI: 10.1177/02537176221106278

Schön, D. (1983). *The reflective practitioner: How professionals think in action*. Basic Books.

Silke, C., Brady, B., Boylan, C., & Dolan, P. (2018). Factors influencing the development of empathy and pro-social behaviour among adolescents: A systematic review. *Children and Youth Services Review*, *94*, 421–436. https://www.sciencedirect.com/science/article/pii/S0190740918301889. DOI: 10.1016/j.childyouth.2018.07.027

Silke, C., Brady, B., Dolan, P., & Boylan, C. (2024). Empathy rules, maps and paths: A qualitative exploration of the factors that facilitate or inhibit empathy and prosocial responding among youth. *Journal of Community Psychology*, *52*(2), 326–343. DOI: 10.1002/jcop.23106

Simons, D., Wurtele, S. K., & Heil, P. (2002). Childhood victimization and lack of empathy as predictors of sexual offending against women and children. *Journal of Interpersonal Violence*, *17*(12), 1291–1307. DOI: 10.1177/088626002237857

Singer, T., & Klimecki, O. (2014). Empathy and compassion. *Current Biology*, *24*(18), R875–R878. DOI: 10.1016/j.cub.2014.06.054

Staub, E., & Volhardt, J. (2008). Altruism born of suffering: The roots of caring and helping after victimization and other trauma. *The American Journal of Orthopsychiatry*, *78*(3), 267–280. DOI: 10.1037/a0014223

Stevens, L. C., & Woodruff, C. C. (Eds.). (2018a). *The neuroscience of empathy, compassion, and self-compassion*. Elsevier Science & Technology.

Stevens, L. C., & Woodruff, C. C. (2018b). Where caring for self and others lives in the brain, and how it can be enhanced and diminished: Observations on the neuroscience of empathy, compassion, and self-compassion. In L. C. Stevens & C. C. Woodruff (Eds.), *The neuroscience of empathy, compassion, and self-compassion*. Elsevier Science & Technology.

Strauss, C. (2004). Is empathy gendered, and if so, why? An approach from feminist psychological anthropology. *Ethos (Berkeley, Calif.)*, *32*(4), 432–457. DOI: 10.1525/eth.2004.32.4.432

Tajfel, H., & Turner, J. C. (1979). An integrative theory of intergroup conflict. In Austin, W. G., & Worchel, S. (Eds.), *The social psychology of intergroup relations* (pp. 33–47). Brooks/Cole.

Takeuchi, H., Taki, Y., Thyreau, B., Sass, Y., Hashizume, H., Sekiguchi, A., Nagase, T., Nouchi, R., Fukushima, A., & Kawashima, R. (2013). White matter structures associated with empathizing and systemizing in young adults. *NeuroImage, 77*, 222–236. DOI: 10.1016/j.neuroimage.2013.04.004

Van der Graaf, J., Branje, S., De Wied, M., Hawk, S., Van Lier, P., & Meeus, W. (2014). Perspective taking and empathic concern in adolescence: Gender differences in developmental changes. *Developmental Psychology*, *50*(3), 881–888. DOI: 10.1037/a0034325

Vial, A. C., & Cowgill, C. M. (2022). Heavier lies her crown: Gendered patterns of leader emotional labor and their downstream effects. *Frontiers in Psychology, 13*, 849566. DOI: 10.3389/fpsyg.2022.849566

Wagaman, M. A., Geiger, J. M., Shockley, C., & Segal, E. (2015). The role of empathy in burnout, compassion satisfaction, and secondary traumatic stress among social workers. *Social Work*, *60*(3), 201–209. DOI: 10.1093/sw/swv014

Wang, C. C. (1999). Photovoice: A participatory action research strategy applied to women's health. *Journal of Women's Health*, *8*(2), 185–192. DOI: 10.1089/jwh.1999.8.185

Wang, Y.-L., Guo, J.-N., Yin, X.-B., Zhang, Q., Dong, L.-Y., Wang, K., & Wang, Y.-Y. (2021). The role of empathy in the relationship between childhood trauma and borderline personality tendencies in male offenders. *Journal of Forensic Psychiatry & Psychology*, *32*(5), 679–696. DOI: 10.1080/14789949.2021.1886314

Watson, T., Hodgson, D., Watts, L., & Waters, R. (2022). Historiography of empathy: Contributions to social work research and practice. *Qualitative Social Work: Research and Practice*, *21*(4), 714–730. DOI: 10.1177/14733250211033012

Watson, T., Waters, D., Watts, L., & Hodgston, T. (2025). Exploring the challenges of empathy in a therapeutic context: An interpretative phenomenological analysis. *Qualitative Health Research*, *0*(0), 1–14. DOI: 10.1177/10497323251331460

Wharton, A. S. (2009). The sociology of emotional labor. *Annual Review of Sociology*, *35*(1), 147–165. DOI: 10.1146/annurev-soc-070308-115944

Zhang, H., Gao, X., Liang, Y., Yao, Q., & Wei, Q. (2024). Does child maltreatment reduce or increase empathy? A systematic review and meta-analysis. *Trauma, Violence & Abuse*, *25*(1), 166–182. DOI: 10.1177/15248380221145734

KEY TERMS AND DEFINITIONS

Affective Empathy: An involuntary, autonomic emotional response that involves feeling congruent emotions with another person's experience, orienting attention to their emotions and providing an emotional response consistent with their state.

Cognitive Empathy: The intellectual capacity to understand what another person is thinking, or feeling and how that shapes their behavior, involving perspective-taking and theory of mind abilities.

Emotional Labour: The process of managing feelings and expressions to fulfill the emotional requirements of a task or role, involving surface acting (displaying emotions without authentically feeling them) and deep acting (authentically attempting to feel expected emotions), often associated with gendered implications for who bears this burden.

Experiential Learning: A pedagogical approach that facilitates learners to transform and create knowledge, skills, attitudes and ways of thinking through direct engagement with curated trigger activities, scenarios or objects, allowing participants to explore concepts through concrete experience.

Ingroup/Outgroup Dynamics: Social identity processes through which individuals categorize themselves and others into groups, shaping empathic responses based on perceived similarity or difference, with empathy operating more readily toward those positioned as "like me" versus "not like me."

Relational Proximity: The degree of perceived closeness, familiarity, or identification between individuals that influences empathic capacity and expression, recognizing that empathy is contingent on social positioning rather than being universally applied.

Trauma-Informed Practice: An approach to service delivery that recognizes the widespread impact of trauma, understands potential paths for recovery, and creates environments of safety while avoiding re-traumatization.

Chapter 4
A Wicked Issue: Reunification and Its Relationship to Cumulative Risk and Harm

Simone Collier
https://orcid.org/0009-0008-3658-8535
University of Southern Queensland, Australia

ABSTRACT

Due to its multifaceted challenges, reunifying children in state care with their biological families is a profoundly complex and often misunderstood process. While every Australian state jurisdiction positions reunification as a legislative and policy priority, in practice, it is significantly under-resourced. This chapter will critically examine the reunification process in the Australian child protection context. The chapter focuses on the consequences of poorly supported reunification efforts, including the cumulative harm experienced by children as they navigate the child protection system. It will argue that the absence of tailored reunification therapy as a standard component of intervention and how this deepens risk and undermines the potential for safe and sustainable family restoration. This chapter will advocate for a shift toward holistic, evidence-informed approaches that consider families' individual needs and promote long-term well-being for children returning to their biological family-based care.

INTRODUCTION

Child Protection systems across Australia and internationally are initially concerned with children's safety. Efforts over the decades have shifted from immediate child removal to approaches focused on safety planning and placing children with known, safe adults who can care for and protect them without statutory intervention.

DOI: 10.4018/979-8-3373-4064-7.ch004

However, there remain significant concerns about the long-term outcomes for children and their connections to their biological families following such interventions.

Reunification is the process through which children in statutory state care systems are returned to the care of their parents or primary family members once it is determined it is safe and appropriate to do so. Within the state child protection system, reunification is regarded as the preferred permanent outcome, reflecting the principle that children have a fundamental right to be raised within their family of origin wherever this can occur without compromising their safety and wellbeing. Decisions regarding reunification are made within a complex framework of legal mandates, developmental considerations and the broader goals of state child protection legislation.

Reunification typically occurs when the risks that precipitated the child's removal –such as abuse, neglect, parental substance misuse, parental mental health concerns, family violence, or incarceration – have been sufficiently reduced or resolved. Parents are generally expected to demonstrate not only a willingness to change but also a sustained capacity to provide safe, stable, and nurturing care. Child protection authorities monitor this progress through engagement with targeted interventions, family support services, and ongoing risk assessments and safety planning. Importantly, the decision to pursue reunification is not based solely on the remediation of parental difficulties; it must also consider the child's developmental needs, attachment relationships, cultural identity, and long-term stability.

The timing of reunification is shaped by statutory requirements and developmental considerations. For younger children, permanency decisions are often made within shorter timeframes in recognition of the critical importance of early stability for healthy attachment and development. For older children and adolescents, greater flexibility may be afforded, particularly where family connections remain strong and the risks associated with reunification can be effectively mitigated through wraparound supports.

Ultimately, reunification is supposed to occur when the balance of evidence suggests that returning a child to their family will not only preserve their safety but also promote their identity, belonging, and continuity of cultural and familial relationships. While reunification is not always achievable, its pursuit reflects a commitment to both the protective and restorative aims of the child protection system.

MAIN FOCUS OF THE CHAPTER

Reunification is internationally recognised as a preferred permanency outcome in child protection, reflecting children's fundamental right to grow up within their family of origin wherever it can be achieved safely (Bromfield & Holzer, 2008;

Delfabbro et al., 2019). This chapter examines the current processes of reunification within Australian state child protection systems, with particular attention to the challenges and risks that emerge for families attempting to navigate a system that is often complex and difficult to understand. At present, there is no consistent, evidence-informed framework to guide practitioners in safely supporting the return of children to their families. In response to this gap, this chapter proposes a structured framework designed to assist practitioners and clinicians in working effectively with families who present with multiple and complex needs, with the overarching aim of facilitating safe and sustainable reunification.

The circumstances precipitating child removal are seldom the product of a single factor; rather, they represent a confluence of complex and cumulative harms (Bromfield & Higgins, 2005). These harms may include domestic and family violence, parental mental health difficulties, intergenerational trauma, involvement with the criminal justice system, parental substance misuse, child maltreatment and neglect, disability, educational disengagement, geographical isolation, language and cultural barriers, and entrenched poverty (Kezelman & Stavropoulos, 2012; Higgins et al., 2007).

Moreover, when children are removed from their family home due to extreme risk or harm, the experience is profoundly traumatic for all parties involved. The acute stress response triggered in such moments frequently overwhelms the capacity for clear thinking and can significantly impair, or even entirely disable, prefrontal cortex executive functioning (Herman, 1992; Cloitre et al., 2011). This neurobiological reality is well recognised within trauma research yet is often overlooked in statutory child protection practice.

In the Australian context, across the different states and territories there are complex legal practices and child protection system methodological tactics that appear to favour the foster and kinship care sector. Despite the multifaceted nature of the harms and the impacts of stress outlined above, biological parents are frequently provided with little support to navigate the labyrinth of interagency systems – legal, health, education, disability, and welfare – that are ostensibly designed to assist them (Osborn & Bromfield, 2007). Consequently, many parents struggle to build the capacity required to meet statutory expectations for reunification, with systemic gaps in service provision perpetuating cycles of disadvantage, family fragmentation, and ongoing statutory involvement (Cashmore & Parkinson, 2008).

In the context of child protection and reunification, the term "statutory requirements" refers to the legal obligations and timeframes set out in legislation or policy that child protection authorities must follow when making decisions about children in state care. Such decisions include timeframes for decision-making. In Queensland, for example, under the *Child Protection Act 1999* Child Safety must work within permanency planning timeframes and make decisions within set periods about whether reunification, long-term guardianship, or adoption is the most appropriate goal; for children under three years of age, decisions need to be made within a twelve-month period. In New South Wales, under the *Children and Young Persons (Care and Protection) Act 1998* when a child is removed into care child protection authorities must quickly establish a structured care plan, assess reunification potential, and present a permanency plan to the court. If reunification remains the goal, it must be pursued proactively, often through Short-Term Custody Orders capped at 24 months. Case planning and reviews continue at defined intervals (90 days, 6 or 12 months) according to the child's case plan goal, ensuring that reunification remains realistically examined and that permanence is pursued without undue delay, particularly for very young children. An overview of the statutory reunification or permanency timeframes by Australian state/territory jurisdiction can be seen in the below table. This equates to hard caps existing in Victoria and New South Wales (and effectively in Queensland via order durations). These statutes force earlier decisions about whether reunification is realistic and set maximum windows to achieve it. South Australia, Western Australia, the Australian Capital Territory, the Northern Territory, and Tasmania rely on case-specific assessments and reviews, with no legislated month-count for reunification.

Reunification / Permanency Timeframes by Jurisdiction (Australia)

Statutory and policy settings that shape timelines for restoration/reunification decisions once a child is removed into care.

Table 1.

Jurisdiction	Governing Act	Statutory/Policy Timeframes Affecting Reunification	Key References (sections/policy)
New South Wales (NSW)	*Children and Young Persons (Care and Protection) Act 1998* (NSW)	Court-approved permanency plan must consider whether restoration is a realistic possibility within a reasonable period. Short-Term Care Orders (STCOs) can allocate parental responsibility to the Minister for up to 24 months while restoration/other permanency is pursued. Permanency plans involving restoration must be reviewed at the end of the active restoration period or within 12 months; case planning uses scheduled reviews.	s 83; s 85A; DCJ STCO Guidance (Oct 2020)
Victoria (VIC)	*Children, Youth and Families Act 2005* (Vic)	Family Reunification Orders (FRO) may run up to 12 months initially. Cumulative time caps: if out of home care (OOHC) <12 months, FRO cannot extend beyond 12 months; if OOHC 12–<24 months, cap 24 months. Reunification permanency objective generally applies where cumulative OOHC is <12 months and safe reunification is likely.	s 287; s 287A; s 167(3)
Queensland (QLD)	*Child Protection Act 1999* (Qld)	Short-term custody/guardianship orders have statutory duration limits (orders must state a period; subsequent orders generally capped by the 2-year rule relative to the prior order). Permanency principles embedded; case plans must include permanency goals with timeframes and use concurrent planning.	s 62; Child Safety Practice Manual (case planning)
South Australia (SA)	*Children and Young People (Safety) Act 2017* (SA)	Before seeking final orders, the Chief Executive must assess the likelihood of reunification and, if likely, the period within which it is likely to occur. No fixed statutory month-cap; timeframes are case-specific.	s 50(4)
Western Australia (WA)	*Children and Community Services Act 2004* (WA)	Care plans must be reviewed at intervals not exceeding 12 months. No fixed statutory reunification cap: planning principles emphasise prompt decision-making and early consideration of returning the child to parents.	s 90 (review ≤12 months); s 9(g), (h)
Tasmania (TAS)	*Children, Young Persons and Their Families Act 1997* (Tas)	No fixed statutory timeframe for reunification. Case and care planning is reviewed per practice guidance; permanency framework and stability planning guided by policy rather than a legislated month-cap.	Act in force; Case & Care Planning guidance (Dept. TAS)

continued on following page

Table 1. Continued

Jurisdiction	Governing Act	Statutory/Policy Timeframes Affecting Reunification	Key References (sections/policy)
Australian Capital Territory (ACT)	*Children and Young People Act 2008* (ACT)	Care plans are developed under the Act and reviewed via Care Teams; annual review reports must be prepared at least annually. No fixed statutory reunification month-cap.	CYPS Case Management Framework (s 457 context); Annual review provisions
Northern Territory (NT)	*Care and Protection of Children Act* 2007 (NT)	No fixed statutory reunification timeframe. NT Reunification Policy states the process commences when a child enters care; permanency options (e.g., Permanent Care Orders) pursued if restoration is not viable.	NT Reunification Policy; Act in force

Notes: Some jurisdictions (NSW, VIC, QLD) embed explicit order durations or statutory decision requirements that constrain reunification timeframes. Others (SA, WA, TAS, ACT, NT) rely on case-specific assessments and review cycles without a fixed month-cap in statute. Always read the current Act/policy and local court practice.

Given that reunification is embedded in every Australian child protection statute, a more explicit policy and practice conversation is required about safely returning children to their families. This entails elevating reunification from a peripheral consideration to a core statutory objective in each jurisdiction, rather than defaulting to sustaining out-of-home care (OOHC). The emphasis should shift toward the conditions that make reunification viable, timely risk remediation and parental capacity building, clear timeframes and concurrent planning, and coordinated cross-sector supports while maintaining the paramount consideration of the child's safety, well-being, and stability as the priority.

BACKGROUND

Child maltreatment is a significant social issue across the world, including Australia where 45,500 children were found to have been subjected to maltreatment in 2020–21 (Australian Institute of Health and Welfare, 2023a) and rates of child protection removals continue to spiral (Australian Institute of Health and Welfare, 2023; Bywaters et al., 2018). Despite this, across Australia there is a lack of nationally agreed definitions and language explaining reunification and the processes involved with reunification services, therapy, and interventions. There are varying legal orders across the Australian states and territories, which can promote permanency for children and young people or counteract it. The resulting instability in the foster and kinship care system impacts children in many ways, particularly when interstate transfers occur, and particularly in the kinship carer arena.

Kinship Care in the Australian Context

Kinship care involves children being placed with grandparents, relatives, or individuals who share a significant pre-existing relationship with the child, whereas foster care refers to placements with carers who have been formally recruited, trained, and authorised by statutory or non-government agencies (in some states), and who usually have no prior relationship with the child (Australian Institute of Family Studies, 2022). In Australia, kinship care has now overtaken foster care as the most common form of OOHC, with the majority of children removed from their biological parents being placed with relatives or extended family members rather than agency-recruited foster carers (Australian Institute of Health and Welfare, 2023).

The policy shift towards kinship care reflects recognition of the benefits of preserving familial, relational, and cultural continuity, particularly for Aboriginal and Torres Strait Islander children, for whom the *Aboriginal and Torres Strait Islander Child Placement Principle (ATSICPP)* mandates prioritising kinship or community placements to maintain cultural identity and belonging (SNAICC, 2017). Emerging evidence suggests that children in kinship care often experience more stable placements and stronger identity development than those in foster care (DCJ, 2023).

These benefits notwithstanding, recent Australian research (DCJ POCLS 2023; Australian Institute of Family Studies 2022) demonstrates that, on average, relative/kinship carers are older, have lower incomes, report poorer physical health, and exhibit higher rates of psychological distress than foster carers. Many kinship carers assume caring roles suddenly, with little preparation or training, and often receive inadequate financial and therapeutic support compared to foster carers (Australian Institute of Family Studies, 2022; Kiraly, 2024). These inequities create significant pressure, with carers frequently navigating poverty, housing instability, and intergenerational trauma while attempting to meet the complex needs of children in their care (Childhood Foundation, 2022).

From a reunification perspective, kinship placements can both enable and complicate outcomes. On one hand, they maintain relational proximity, making it easier to sustain parent–child contact and preserve family identity. On the other hand, unresolved family conflict, ongoing exposure to violence, or entrenched disadvantage can limit the viability of reunification and exacerbate systemic barriers. As current research emphasises, reunification planning must account for these differences and ensure that kinship carers receive adequate preparation, financial support, and therapeutic services if long-term family reunification is to be achievable (Australian Institute of Family Studies, 2022; Kiraly, 2024).

Interstate Transfers for Children in Statutory Care

As an experienced clinician in the child protection reunification field, I have observed the fragmentation of child protection systems, both nationally and across individual states, creating significant challenges when facilitating the interstate transfer of children for reunification. A lack of national cohesion, with each state and territory operating under separate legislation, processes, and oversight bodies, creates significant instability for children in OOHC, particularly when interstate transfers are involved. In the context of kinship care, this becomes especially problematic; there is no nationally consistent protocol for recognising kinship carers across jurisdictions, meaning there are often delays in assessment, approval, and funding, leaving children in limbo. Recognition of guardianship or custody orders is often inconsistent across state borders, and this can result in breaks in legal care arrangements and disruption to a child's sense of safety and belonging. Children may lose access to vital support services (e.g., trauma therapy) because systems are not automatically transferred or recognised interstate and often the historical narratives about what bought the children into care are not shared between the statutory bodies in the different state offices, and this can affect decision making relating to informed reunification decisions and safety of the children. Interstate moves often interrupt schooling, health care, and attachment relationships, compounding the trauma already experienced by children in care. Carers often feel unsupported and disoriented, wondering how to navigate unfamiliar bureaucracies without guidance, leading to placement breakdown or re-entry of children into more formal foster or residential care systems.

The Statutory Care System in Australia

Many carers report feeling undervalued, misunderstood, and overwhelmed, with volunteer carers often feeling mistreated by the broader system as a result of financial hardship, lack of adequate support, and misalignment between expectations and systemic resources. This disillusionment is driving foster carers out of the system in increasing numbers and placing Australia's statutory care system is under significant strain. Victoria saw a 5.2% drop in active foster-carer households in a single year (Foster Care Association of Victoria, 2024; Australian Broadcasting Corporation, 2024), while NSW experienced a 13% decrease in authorised foster carers between 2021 and 2024 (Australian Institute of Health and Welfare, 2023b; DCJ POCLS, 2023). Nationally, over 1,500 foster carers exited the system in 2022–23 alone (EQT, 2024). However, no jurisdiction routinely publishes disaggregated exit counts for foster versus kinship carers, and the absence of consistent administrative reporting on exits obscures the true scale and distribution of attrition across care types at a time of growing demand. The only three states for which comparable data is available are NSW, Victoria and Queensland, as shown in Figure 1.

Figure 1. Percentage decline in carer numbers by state (2021–2024) (QFCC & PeakCare, 2024)

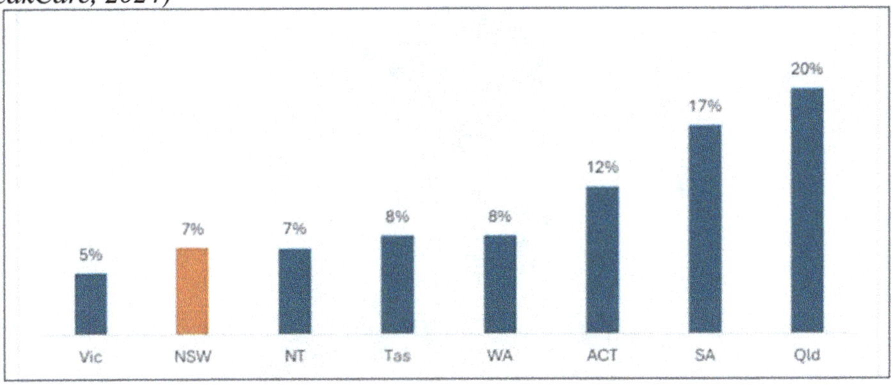

Nationally, 45,393 children were in OOHC on 30 June 2022 (Australian Institute of Health and Welfare, 2023c), with 32% of these children aged 10–14 years, 42% of Aboriginal and Torres Strait Islander descent, and 29% living with a disability (Australian Institute of Health and Welfare, 2023a). With the distinct shortage of foster carers, many children and young people have been placed into residential care, particularly in Queensland and NSW, with children – including infants – being left in residential care for significant periods of time due to a lack of foster care placements and a lack of investment in the biological parents to support the reunification process. Queensland has the highest proportion of children residing in residential care, with 2200 in state residential care as of December 2024 (Parnell, 2024) (see Figure 2).

Figure 2. Children aged 0–17 years in OOHC: Proportion of children aged 0–17 in residential OOHC by jurisdiction, 2023–24 (Productivity Commission, Report on Government Services 2025, Part F, 16: Child protection services data tables)

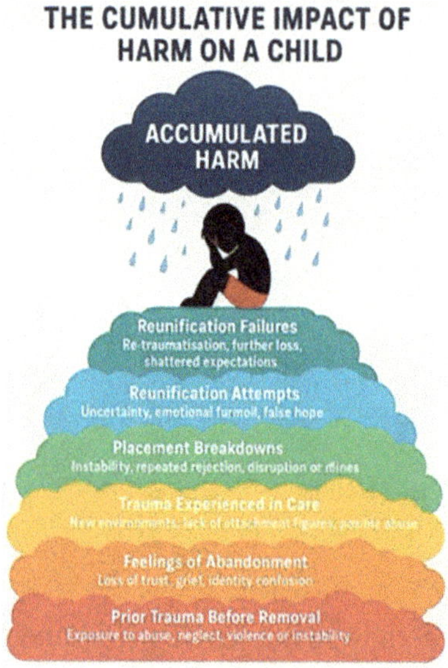
THE CUMULATIVE IMPACT OF
HARM ON A CHILD
ACCUMULATED
HARM
Reunification Failures
Re-traumatisation, further loss,
shattered expectations
Reunification Attempts
Uncertainty, emotional turmoil, false hope
Placement Breakdowns
Trauma Experienced in Care
Feelings of Abandonment
Loss of trust, grief, identity confusion
Prior Trauma Before Removal
Exposure to abuse, neglect, violence or instability

As a result of the shortage of residential homes in Australian states to support the number of children who need OOHC, Coote and Shams (2023) report there are often crises with children accommodated in motel rooms for up to a year.

Cumulative Risk

The removal of a child from their biological family unit is itself evidence that the child has been exposed to an accumulation of adverse experiences, almost always including some combination of emotional, psychological, or physical harm. The consequences of these cumulative adversities are well established; exposure to multiple adverse experiences has a dose–response relationship with later outcomes, including heightened risk of substance use disorders, mental illness, social and relational difficulties, criminality, physical health problems, and the likelihood of revictimisation across the lifespan (Felitti et al., 1998; Edwards et al., 2003; Hughes et al., 2017; Bryce & Collier, 2022). Importantly, cumulative harm does not always arise from a single, catastrophic event. Rather, it is often the persistent, "low-level" adversities, such as chronic neglect that exert the most pervasive and damaging effects on children's development (Bryce, 2018; Bromfield & Higgins, 2005). Recognising this, child protection practitioners may determine that the threshold of harm has been exceeded, prompting removal into statutory care in order to arrest further damage.

Once a child is removed, however, each Australian jurisdiction's Child Protection Act places a statutory responsibility on the relevant department to begin planning for reunification as early as possible, provided it is safe to do so. Ideally, reunification should be guided by a structured case planning process in which service providers, independent of statutory authorities, support parents to address the issues that led to removal. Intensive therapeutic intervention should focus on reducing cumulative risk and breaking entrenched cycles of harm, while simultaneously building protective factors to sustain safe caregiving. However, the reality across Australia diverges sharply from this ideal. No state or territory currently offers a consistent, intensive reunification service model for biological parents following child removal. Statutory authorities may choose whether or not to commission the non-government sector to provide such services. Where services are provided "in-house," the therapeutic alliance between statutory caseworkers and parents is often compromised. Parents frequently perceive child protection departments as adversarial actors, given their direct role in child removal, and the resulting mistrust undermines the possibility of authentic engagement or sustained behavioural change (Kertesz et al., 2021).

In practice, statutory caseworkers are primarily tasked with compliance activities, risk assessments, safety planning, and documentation to satisfy legislative and policy frameworks. While these functions are critical, they rarely address the complex therapeutic needs of parents whose capacity to provide "good enough" care has been compromised by trauma, disadvantage, and systemic exclusion. As a result, the broader structural work required to reduce cumulative risk, such as addressing housing insecurity, poverty, mental health, and substance misuse is left underdeveloped. This gap reflects a systemic failure to operationalise the intent of child protection legislation, which mandates reunification planning, but does not resource or enforce intensive supports to achieve it.

Children, meanwhile, continue to experience trauma through the process of removal itself. Separation from parents, siblings, and familiar environments constitutes an additional layer of adversity, further compounding cumulative risk (Fernandez & Lee, 2013). This underscores the urgency of investing in early, intensive reunification supports that can expedite safe restoration to family care, where appropriate, and prevent the long-term harms associated with extended out-of-home care. Without such investment, opportunities to mitigate cumulative risk are missed, and intergenerational cycles of harm are perpetuated.

Factors Affecting Reunification

Families who have endured the traumatic removal of their children due to chronic maltreatment and accumulated harm often present with entrenched intergenerational disadvantage, socio-economic deprivation, and systemic exclusion. These parents are rarely equipped with the knowledge, skills, or capacity to initiate meaningful change without intensive therapeutic and structural support. This trend is widely recognised in Australian research (Bromfield & Higgins, 2005; Fernandez & Lee, 2013), yet there is no consistent investment targeted at reunification services at the point of removal, during early planning, or after children return home. Instead, statutory systems overwhelmingly direct resources toward sustaining out-of-home care placements rather than addressing the root causes of harm and building parental capacity (Australian Institute of Health and Welfare, 2023b).

For example, contemporary research, such as the *Australia's Welfare 2023* report (Australian Institute of Health and Welfare, 2023c) identifies housing instability and homelessness as risk factors strongly associated with child protection involvement. Similarly, the *Crisis Accommodation in Australia* study (Australian Housing and Urban Research Institute, 2023) illustrates how families living in temporary or insecure accommodation face ongoing risks to health, safety, and stability. Regional analyses further demonstrate that housing shortages and affordability crises in non-metropolitan areas amplify vulnerabilities for families already at risk (Beer et al., 2024).

Housing instability also impacts the reunification process. Parents whose children have been removed are increasingly being expected to demonstrate parenting capacity while experiencing significant housing insecurity. Clinicians in the field report cases where parents, often single parents, are engaging in reunification processes while residing in highly precarious and unsafe arrangements such as tents, caravans, or short-term leases at showgrounds. Despite persistent efforts by service providers to secure stable housing through creative means, state child protection authorities have frequently failed to provide meaningful housing support. This results in untenable situations in which parents are judged against statutory reunification benchmarks while their most basic physiological and safety needs remain unmet.

For parents in such unstable conditions, chronic stressors, such as the threat of eviction, inability to refrigerate food, or exposure to theft, create constant hypervigilance. This heightened cognitive load diminishes their capacity to meet the needs of children who are themselves often dysregulated and traumatised. Reunification expectations in these contexts reflect a systemic disconnect between policy intent and lived reality. Unless stable housing is addressed as a prerequisite for reunification, parents are effectively set up to fail, and cycles of removal, homelessness, and intergenerational disadvantage are perpetuated (Australian Institute of Health and Welfare, 2023b; Australian Housing and Urban Research Institute, 2023, 2024).

The absence of intensive reunification services creates a contradiction between legislative mandate and practice reality. Every state and territory Child Protection Act emphasises reunification "as soon as safely possible", yet there is no structured intervention point to operationalise this goal. Placement instability and repeated disruptions consume vast fiscal resources across the child protection, health, housing, education, and justice systems, while families remain unsupported in addressing the adversities that led to removal. Without early, well-resourced interventions, the statutory system risks perpetuating cycles of disadvantage rather than breaking them.

The likelihood of successful reunification is shaped by multiple intersecting factors:

- **Parental risk factors**, such as mental illness, substance misuse, and exposure to family violence.
- **Socio-demographic factors**, including poverty, housing instability, and intergenerational trauma.
- **Child characteristics**, such as age, developmental delays, or complex trauma histories.
- **Systemic factors**, such as placement instability due to foster carer shortages and the unmet needs of kinship carers.

The interplay of these factors creates cumulative risk, often making reunification less likely for children who have experienced chronic neglect, emotional abuse, or exposure to complex family harms (Cunningham et al., 2021; Fernandez, 2013). Research consistently shows that children exposed to cumulative harm or placed in contexts where parental challenges remain unresolved face markedly reduced prospects of returning home.

What emerges is a systemic contradiction: while legislation prioritises reunification, fiscal policy and service structures prioritise placement. Without significant investment in early intervention and intensive reunification supports, delivered by providers independent of statutory authorities, parents remain unsupported, carers remain overstretched, and children remain vulnerable to further harm in care. Addressing these gaps requires governments to not only legislate reunification but also resource and enforce practice models capable of sustaining safe reunification, thereby reducing both cumulative risk and the long-term reliance on OOHC.

Failed Reunification and Its Impacts

According to Cunningham et al., (2021), reunification in Australia is defined as successful when a child or young person does not return to OOHC within the

12-month period after reunification takes place; this is despite international data demonstrating that reunification breakdown continued to occur 12–24 months following reunification (Chambers et al., 2019).

In terms of failure rates, Farmer (2014) found in a UK study that of 180 child participants, 37% had experienced two or more failed reunification experiences and had alternated between the care sector and being at home. In the USA, the rate of failed reunification within the first 12 months is approximately 24% (Teague, 2017). There is limited data in Australia on the rates of failed reunification, although in one Queensland study of 2509 children, it was found that one in five children reported they had experienced one or more failed reunification attempts (Teague, 2017).

Failed reunification has both direct an indirect economic impacts. The Queensland Family and Child Commission (2017) reports that in 2017 the annual cost of a failed reunification per child was A$110,000. The *Cost of Late Intervention (COLI) Report 2024* (O'Connell, 2025) highlights the significant consequences of delayed government action in child protection and youth justice. The report argues that strategic investment in early intervention services, delivered through tailored, individualised, and well-supported approaches for each family, is likely to generate substantially greater returns, both socially and economically. The report notes that while the number of children in care since 2019 in Australia has remained relatively stable, the costs of later intervention have grown by 40%, with an increase from $5.9 billion spent on child protection services in Australia in 2019 to $10.3 billion in 2024 (O'Connell, 2025).

Moreover, following failed reunification children will re-enter OOHC, having suffered further maltreatment in the home in the interim. The cumulative impact of the trauma experienced before the initial removal, the feelings of abandonment, dislodgement, and displacement from biological family, any trauma experienced while in care, placement breakdowns, reunification attempts, and reunification failures will impact and further contribute to an accumulation of harm, as depicted in Figure 3 below:

Figure 3. The cumulative impact of harm on a child

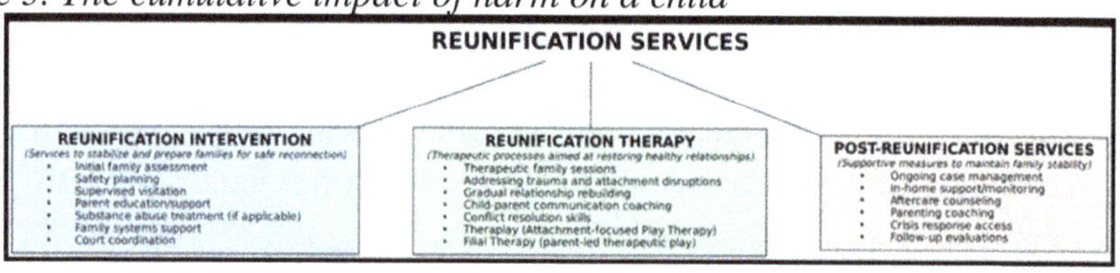

REUNIFICATION SERVICES
REUNIFICATION INTERVENTION
(Services to stabilize and prepare families for safe reconnection)
Initial family assessment
Safety planning
Supervised visitation
Parent education/support
Substance abuse treatment (if applicable)
Family systems support
Court coordination
REUNIFICATION THERAPY
(Therapeutic processes aimed at restoring healthy relationships)
Therapeutic family sessions
Addressing trauma and attachment disruptions
Gradual relationship rebuilding
Child-parent communication coaching
Conflict resolution skills
Theraplay (Attachment-focused Play Therapy)
Filial Therapy (parent-led therapeutic play)
POST-REUNIFICATION SERVICES
(Supportive measures to maintain family stability)
Ongoing case management
In-home support/monitoring
Aftercare counseling
Parenting coaching
Crisis response access
Follow-up evaluations

In the 2015 report *The Cost of Unresolved Childhood Trauma and Abuse in Adults in Australia*, Dr Cathy Kezelman and colleagues estimate that unresolved childhood trauma costs the Australian economy approximately $16.1 billion annually. This figure encompasses both direct and indirect costs associated with the long-term impacts of childhood trauma:

Direct Costs:

- **Healthcare Expenditures:** Increased demand for medical and mental health services due to trauma-related conditions such as depression, anxiety, and PTSD.
- **Justice System Costs:** Higher rates of criminal justice involvement among trauma survivors, leading to increased policing, court, and incarceration expenses.
- **Welfare and Social Services:** Greater reliance on social welfare programs, including unemployment benefits and housing assistance.

Indirect Costs:

- **Lost Productivity:** Reduced workforce participation and productivity losses due to chronic health issues and disability stemming from unresolved trauma.
- **Education Impacts:** Lower educational attainment among survivors, leading to decreased earning potential and economic contribution.
- **Intergenerational Effects:** The perpetuation of trauma-related issues across generations further burdens social and economic systems.

The report emphasises that addressing unresolved childhood trauma through early intervention and trauma-informed care could lead to significant economic benefits. Specifically, it suggests that a minimum of $9.1 billion could be saved annually by implementing effective strategies to support adult survivors of childhood trauma. This then has a flow-on effect for adult survivors of childhood abuse and their families when they are faced with reunification with their children following removal.

THE REUNIFICATION PROCESS

The remainder of this chapter critically examines the reunification process, with particular attention to the evidence base and practical implications of implementing reunification services comprehensively across three phases: Reunification Intervention, Reunification Therapy, and Post-Reunification Services. Reunifying children is reflected in child protection legislation and policy frameworks across Australian states and territories, and this proposed tripartite model underscores the importance of a structured, therapeutic, and sustained approach to restoring and maintaining safe family connections. The following sections will explore each phase in detail, highlighting the mechanisms, supports, and systemic considerations necessary to ensure enduring and safe reunification outcomes for children and families.

Based on the research literature and professional experience of working extensively on a multitude of reunification cases, this section will explore the factors that affect the success of reunification within the three entities.

Reunification Intervention

Reunification intervention encompasses many non-therapeutic tasks necessary to ensure accurate measurement and evaluation of the intervention and therapeutic process for children, parents, and families. This approach is fundamentally designed to prioritise the safety and protection of the child while simultaneously providing a mechanism for evaluating the effectiveness and appropriateness of the intervention. It serves to inform both clinical practice and accountability to funding bodies by assessing whether their investment in the family system is achieving the intended outcomes.

The collection and analysis of relevant data is essential to determine:

- whether the intervention has been sufficiently individualised to meet the specific developmental and psychosocial needs of the child;
- the level and type of support required by parents or caregivers, and whether this support needs to be increased, decreased, or adjusted;
- the broader support requirements of the family unit, including consideration of more suitable or diverse therapeutic modalities in response to contextual complexity; and
- the fidelity and integrity of the intervention model as implemented.

Systematic evaluation ensures that service delivery remains responsive, evidence-informed, and aligned with the best interests of the child, particularly in families presenting with multifaceted needs.

This is the focus of structured assessments and decision-making tools, which need to be used by experienced and expert child protection practitioners who have not been involved in the removal of the children. From the time of initial assessment, a therapeutic alliance needs to be developed with the family members given that assessments, while data driven, are also diagnostic in that they give practitioners an evidence base for risk assessment and informed decision making (Choate, 2009; Kirk, 2010; Kirk, 2015b; Reed-Ashcraft, Kirk & Fraser, 2001), which is then further cemented by professional judgement and practice knowledge (Fish & Hardy, 2015).

There are numerous standardised tools available and careful consideration is needed to ensure sufficient tools are used without families being over-assessed. Baseline data is essential, and both midway and closing data are needed to evaluate individual progress and family functioning to accurately inform the post-reunification recommendations. Throughout the literature, and certainly in the author's experience, the most commonly employed and most useful tool is the North Carolina Family Assessment Scale (NCFAS), a validated reunification assessment tool used to support the assessment of family functioning and inform interventions and decision making in child protection settings (Kirk, 2015a; Reed-Ashcraft, Kirk & Fraser, 2001). The author has made use of the NCFAS-R, the Reunification-specific Scale, and has found it particularly useful in reunification work with families with highly complex needs.

Alongside the NCFAS-R, the author uses the Attachment Style Interview (ASI) and Parenting Role Interview (PRI) throughout the intervention. Effective reunification planning in child protection contexts requires a nuanced understanding of both relational dynamics and broader systemic factors influencing parenting capacity. While no single tool can fully capture the complexities inherent in high-risk family systems, integrating the ASI, the PRI, and the NCFAS-R offers a comprehensive framework that supports relational assessment, psychological insight, and evidence-informed planning.

The ASI is a semi-structured interview used to assess adult attachment representations and behaviours in close relationships (Bifulco et al., 2002). In reunification contexts, the ASI provides critical insights into the parents' ability to establish trust, regulate emotional closeness, and remain attuned to the child's relational needs. These insights are essential for re-establishing safe and consistent bonds following OOHC. The ASI also identifies how unresolved trauma or disorganised attachment strategies may undermine parenting readiness and stability (Bifulco & Thomas, 2013).

The PRI complements the ASI by exploring parental mentalisation and caregiving representations. It assesses reflective functioning, emotional responsiveness, and caregiving role identity, all of which are linked to attachment security in children (Brennan et al., 2016). This tool is especially valuable for understanding how parents interpret their child's trauma-related behaviours and whether they can respond with sensitivity, coherence, and appropriate boundaries.

The NCFAS-R has emerged as a widely used tool for assessing family functioning in the context of reunification. It provides a structured ecological framework across multiple domains—including environment, parental capabilities, family interactions, family safety, child well-being, caregiver/child ambivalence, and readiness for reunification—allowing practitioners to identify both risks and protective factors, measure change over time, and guide decision-making (Kirk et al., 2005; Nelson & Landsman, 2006). International research demonstrates its utility. For example, an Australian study found that improvements in NCFAS-R domain scores at case closure significantly increased the likelihood of reunification, with domains such as *Parental Capabilities* and *Readiness for Reunification* being particularly predictive of positive outcomes (National Family Preservation Network, 2008).

More recent international evidence highlights the ongoing relevance of structured family assessment tools. A psychometric validation of the NCFAS in Ecuador confirmed its reliability and internal consistency in assessing family functioning in culturally distinct settings, underscoring its adaptability across diverse populations (Pérez-Villalobos et al., 2023). In the United States, the National Quality Improvement Center on Family-Centered Reunification (2023) has recently developed a *Family-Centered Reunification Best Practice Assessment Tool*, which builds on principles similar to NCFAS-R by prioritising readiness, ambivalence, and ecological family dynamics, but integrates these with a stronger emphasis on post-return supports.

Collectively, this international evidence suggests that structured tools such as NCFAS-R remain critical in reunification planning. They not only provide a systematic method for identifying family strengths and challenges but also highlight where targeted interventions are most needed. However, tools alone are insufficient; as the evidence on re-entry demonstrates, the predictive power of assessment must be paired with ongoing supports in housing, mental health, financial stability, and family relationships if reunification is to be both successful and sustainable.

Together, these tools create a multidimensional approach for reunification assessments:

- The ASI and PRI deepen understanding of relational and psychological readiness for reunification.
- The NCFAS-R contextualises these relational insights within broader family functioning and systemic stressors.
- Their combined use enables more accurate, child-centred planning that addresses trauma, risk, and resilience holistically.

This integrative framework promotes evidence-based and ethically sound reunification decision-making that recognises the complexity of family recovery, attachment disruption, and systemic involvement.

A significant barrier to successful reunification lies in the inconsistency and subjectivity of decision-making by individual child protection workers, which can create uncertainty and distress for biological parents. Collings et al., (2024) describe this phenomenon as "shifting goalposts", where initially agreed-upon case plan expectations, perceived as achievable, are later reinterpreted or redefined by new caseworkers, legal representatives, or the court. This shifting interpretation can undermine the parent's progress and contribute to a sense of futility. For many parents, especially those with cognitive or emotional vulnerabilities, this repeated moving of the goalposts becomes overwhelming and demoralising, eroding their ability to remain engaged in the reunification process.

The consequences extend beyond the parent, with children often unaware of the systemic dynamics and instead internalising narratives of parental abandonment or lack of care. This contributes to further emotional harm, including compounded attachment trauma and deteriorating mental health for both the child and the parent.

Strong relationships are a potent key factor in the success or otherwise of the reunification process. As mentioned in the introductory section of this paper it is unfair on the family, the children, and the case worker to try to establish a therapeutic alliance following removal and then journey through the logistics of the many difficult conversations and relationship ruptures that occur as the change process begins and continues and the biological family learns "new ways" to parent, to operate a home, to abstain from alcohol and drug misuse and learn healthier coping strategies, to emotional regulate and to manage relationship dynamics. The tenacity and robustness of this therapeutic relationship cannot be sustained with a caseworker who removed their children, implements rules around contact between a parent and their children, and warns that contact will be even more restricted if they fail. Sadly, however, this is the reality of the relationship for many parents. Strong relationships with biological parents are required to weather the ruptures that occur as the stages of change are navigated. This is supported by Cunningham et al., (2021) who state:

> *Relationships with workers emerged as a significant theme in the literature and were identified as a critical factor for reunification to occur. Studies indicated that when meaningful partnerships are formed between practitioners and families, better reunification outcomes are achieved. Successful reunification is also associated with practitioners working collaboratively with children, young people and families in the implementation and review of case plans (p 48).*

The Role of Parent–Child Contact during Reunification

Parent–child contact during periods of OOHC has long been recognised as a critical predictor of reunification success. Early work by Davis et al., (1996), involving 925 children in foster care, demonstrated that regular contact visits significantly increased the likelihood of children returning to their biological families. More recent studies have reinforced and extended these findings. McWey and Cui (2021), analysing children in non-kinship foster care, found that both the frequency and quality of contact with birth parents were strongly associated with higher odds of reunification and shorter durations in care. Similarly, Oosterman and Schuengel (2023) highlight that consistent, positive contact not only preserves relational bonds but also supports children's attachment security, emotional adjustment, and behavioural regulation, which in turn facilitates more stable reunification outcomes. These findings underscore the dual function of contact visits: they maintain parental commitment and relational continuity, while also providing practitioners with an ongoing opportunity to observe parenting behaviours, assess safety, and inform case planning. Importantly, the literature cautions that the benefits of contact are contingent on quality; visits that are conflictual, sporadic, or poorly supported may exacerbate children's stress and undermine reunification efforts. Taken together, the evidence suggests that when embedded within a structured reunification framework, frequent and meaningful parent–child contact operates as a key protective factor, significantly improving the prospects of safe and sustainable family reunification.

Parental Psychoeducation & Support

Parental psychoeducation and capacity building are recognised as core foundations of any effective reunification intervention. This component of the intervention is necessarily intensive and adopts a coaching, hands-on, and action-oriented style, requiring parents to actively replace maladaptive or neglectful caregiving practices with more adaptive and responsive care strategies. These strategies encompass the establishment of day-to-day routines and household structures that provide children with safety, stability, and predictability, alongside parenting education tailored to supporting children's behavioural, emotional, cognitive, and developmental needs (Bronson et al., 2008; Macdonald et al., 2018).

Contemporary practice highlights the importance of delivering in-home, real-time support during peak stress points in family life. Intervention is most impactful when staff are present during critical daily transitions, such as before school, after return from school, mealtimes, and bedtimes, when routines are being tested and relational strain is most likely to emerge (Chambers et al., 2019; Jones et al., 2021). During the early phases of a child's return home, these highly structured and practical supports aim to re-establish routines, behavioural expectations, and consistent caregiving practices that contrast with pre-removal patterns of instability or neglect. The emphasis is not only on technical skills but also on creating a relational climate that is safe, responsive, and emotionally attuned, thereby fostering both child well-being and parental confidence.

Best practice also suggests that reunification should be guided by a collaborative, continuity-focused model. This requires deliberate consultation with foster or kinship carers, who can share strategies, routines, and regulatory practices already effective for the child (Fernandez & Lee, 2013; Testa & Poertner, 2020). Integrating these existing strategies into the biological family's caregiving repertoire ensures continuity, reduces the risk of dysregulation, and supports smoother adjustment.

Such continuity is particularly important for children with histories of trauma or attachment disruptions, whose capacity for regulation is often fragile.

Parental capacity building during this phase must be both targeted and therapeutic. Training should explicitly focus on behaviour management strategies, emotional attunement, and co-regulation techniques, as well as the practical application of trauma-informed and attachment-based principles in daily routines (Dozier & Bernard, 2019; Oosterman & Schuengel, 2023). Emphasis should be placed on "pressure points" in family life—mornings, transitions, and bedtimes, where relational strain and conflict most frequently occur. Embedding therapeutic learning into these everyday contexts ensures that parents are not simply absorbing information but are actively practising new skills in real time, with guided feedback from practitioners.

Ultimately, the goal of psychoeducational and in-home support is to maintain a strong relational focus, positioning connection and co-regulation as the foundation of restored parent–child relationships. By providing parents with intensive, context-specific support during the transition back to family care, service providers can reduce the risk of placement breakdown, promote stability, and foster long-term emotional security for children. Recent evaluations of intensive reunification programs affirm that such approaches, when embedded in trauma-informed and ecological models, are linked to higher rates of successful and sustained restoration (Cunningham et al., 2021; Dunbar et al., 2022).

Another element of parental support that is highly prevalent throughout the literature but is largely absent in Australia in comparison to international counterparts is the support group programs that provide valuable mentorship from fellow birth parents who have lost their children to removal and have worked to have their children reunified back into their care. These are a very common practice in the American states (Enano et al., 2017; Chambers et al., 2019), where partners engage with the State Department of Child Protection and to act as formal supports for parents who are new to navigating the child protection system (Chambers et al., 2019, Bohannan et al., 2016). An important role of these parent partners is not only acting as an intermediary between the State Department personnel, but also holding the parent to account to make the necessary behavioural shifts, often with support from practitioners working with the parents (Chambers et al., 2019). Parent partners who have lived experiences of successful reunification are often able to demonstrate positive coping strategies and discuss how to navigate the complex government and court administrative processes involved with reunification.

Ross et al., (2017) explored the perspectives and experiences of biological parents in the Hunter Valley, New South Wales, Australia, who had experienced removal of their children and were not able to be active participants in the child protection processes relating to reunification. Their study revealed five key areas in which parents needed support and where, without a parent advocate, they felt disempowered, particularly when they were supported only by the caseworker who removed their child in the first instance. The first of these key areas was power and inclusion, with legal and court settings disempowering parents through non-participatory processes when their children were in care. The second was professional relationships with lawyers, child protection workers, and agency workers – knowing what to say and who to trust amid the grief and loss can be overwhelming. The third theme is based on the parent–child relationship and attachment – specifically, the challenges of maintaining a relationship with their children while they are in care, the impact of removal, and the emotions of grief, guilt, loss and shame. Parents discussed the challenges associated with having contact, including not being provided with the details of contact, such as location, times, activities, food and gifts allowed, carer's preferences etc. The fourth theme concerns the immense grief and loss that parents often experienced, having often been in care themselves, and then having their children removed from their care. Parents felt that their normal emotional responses were used against them, to depict them as "unstable" and adduced as a reason they shouldn't have their children in their care. The fifth area focused on parents' identity; parents continue to see themselves as their children's parents despite their children being in care, and they remain focused on their children's health, safety and wellbeing. They felt confronted by being replaced by carers whom their children called 'mum' or 'dad' and felt that they faced considerable barriers to reunification and were unsupported by child protection services.

Reunification Therapy

Reunification therapy serves as a comprehensive, trauma-informed framework aimed at supporting families as they navigate the complex journey of healing and reunification following separation. This therapeutic umbrella encompasses a range of evidence-based modalities tailored to the individual needs of family members, sub-dyads (e.g., parent–child), and the family system as a whole. These modalities are often most effective when implemented concurrently in a coordinated and sequenced manner. Clinical practice and emerging literature suggest that parallel therapeutic engagement, aligned with the distinct developmental and relational needs of each family member, yields optimal outcomes (Cooper & Vetere, 2008; Hughes et al., 2019).

The strategic integration of therapeutic modalities should be grounded in robust assessment processes that identify the biopsychosocial, relational, and developmental needs of each family subsystem. Tailored interventions not only support emotional healing but also promote long-term relational stability and parenting capacity, and the critical factors in the sustainability of reunification (Woods, 2011; Lieberman, Van Horn, & Ippen, 2005).

Case Example: "Family A"

The following vignette illustrates a multi-tiered reunification therapy process grounded in trauma-responsive practice.

Family Context: Joan is a single mother of three children: Cassie (age 7), Lionel (age 2), and James (9 months) at the time of removal. The children were removed eight months prior due to Joan's cohabitation with a partner who was violent and sexually assaulted Cassie. Joan also struggled with alcohol misuse and mental health challenges. Since the removal, Joan has completed a three-month residential rehabilitation program and has sustained sobriety. She has engaged actively with supports and achieved key milestones in the reunification intervention phase, including stable housing, part-time employment, participation in a peer support network, and consistent engagement with parenting education and substance use treatment. Joan still is without a driver's licence and requires furnishings to set up her new home and support to understand the domestic violence cycle.

Joan's Reunification Services Plan (example)

To ensure relational repair and developmental recovery across the family system, the following trauma-informed Reunification Services Plan is recommended.

Reunification Intervention Assessments:

Learner's driver's licence – and then complete her hours with the support service to obtain her Provisional driver's licence. Joan already has her own vehicle. Joan will acquire car seats and learn how to fit the car seats for the respective ages of her children.

Family Contacts – Joan will engage in 3 x weekly visitation with her children in a variety of community-based contexts.

Domestic & Family Violence Program – Joan will engage in the Safe & Together Domestic Violence (David Mandell Program) and in safety planning for herself and her children. Joan will attend her domestic and family violence counselling each week.

Drug & Alcohol Rehabilitation – Joan will continue attending her drug and alcohol rehabilitation classes and counselling appointments each week.

Set up Home – Joan will source resources and set up her baby's nursery and other communal spaces within her home.

Parent Coaching and Psychoeducation: Joan should receive individualised coaching sessions to address parent burnout and blocked care. These sessions should draw on neurodevelopmentally informed parenting models, such as the Neurosequential Model of Therapeutics (Perry, 2009) and the PACE model (Playfulness,

Acceptance, Curiosity, Empathy) (Hughes (2016), to support trauma-sensitive caregiving strategies. This would include Joan coming to understand the neurobiology of trauma (e.g., amygdala hijack, dysregulation), addressing blocked care, which refers to a caregiver's subconscious withdrawal from emotional connection due to chronic stress or trauma triggers (Delaney, 2006) and building strategies to manage parent burnout and emotionally dysregulated behaviours in trauma-impacted children. These elements would then be implemented in the intervention services and the post-reunification services as part of the overall reunification services framework.

Reunification Therapy

Child-Centred Play Therapy: Cassie, Lionel and James should engage in individual play therapy sessions to process trauma, enhance emotional expression, and support psychological resilience. Play therapy is developmentally appropriate and effective in supporting children exposed to complex trauma (Landreth, 2012) and will provide a safe psychological space for Cassie, Lionel and James to symbolically re-enact their traumatic experiences and develop adaptive coping strategies (Landreth, 2012). Research shows that non-directive child-centred play therapy is effective in reducing symptoms of anxiety, aggression, and post-traumatic stress in children exposed to maltreatment and family violence (Bratton et al., 2005). Play supports neurodevelopment by enhancing regulation, strengthening prefrontal cortex functioning, and building pathways for social cognition (Perry, 2009). This will greatly assist the reunification process through the children having an opportunity to process their grief and their trauma with a qualified therapist trained in child mental health.

Theraplay: Joan should participate in Theraplay sessions with each child to rebuild attachment bonds. Theraplay is an evidence-based, attachment-focused play modality designed to promote secure relational patterns through structured, nurturing interactions (Booth & Jernberg, 2010). Theraplay focuses on four dimensions of healthy attachment: structure, engagement, nurture, and challenge (Booth & Jernberg, 2010). These components are critical in repairing disrupted relational patterns, which inevitably occur when children have witnessed domestic violence. Cassie, Lionel and James have lived with a parent with a substance misuse issue and mental health challenges, creating a pattern of relational unavailability for these children and causing disruption in attachment that requires repair. Theraplay is a practitioner-led modality that supports the nurturing and repair of the relationship between the parent and the child. Studies demonstrate that Theraplay improves emotional regulation, increases attachment security, and enhances social responsiveness in children with histories of trauma and disrupted caregiving. Given that Theraplay has also been shown to reduce parenting stress and increase caregiver sensitivity, particularly in high-risk family contexts (Sianko et al., 2016), Theraplay is a strong recommendation for Joan and her children in this reunification intervention.

Filial Therapy: Following initial Theraplay sessions, filial therapy may be introduced to sustain and extend therapeutic gains. Filial therapy will empower Joan to take an active, therapeutic role with Cassie, Lionel and James, reinforcing parental sensitivity and emotional attunement (Guerney, 2000). Filial therapy bridges the therapeutic environment and the home, training caregivers to facilitate therapeutic play sessions to improve attachment and emotional expression (Guerney, 2000). Research indicates that filial therapy leads to statistically significant improvements in child behaviour, parent–child relationships, and parental empathy (Cornett & Bratton, 2014). It is especially effective with parents who have histories of substance use, trauma, or disempowerment, as it builds reflective functioning and emotional attunement. Given Joan has a significant history of disempowerment, following her building attachments with her children it is recommended that she strengthen her engagement with the children through filial therapy.

POST-REUNIFICATION SERVICES

In Australia, the child protection system has long operated under the assumption that reunification represents the successful resolution of child removal and the final point of child protection services involvement. However, emerging evidence both internationally and domestically demonstrates that for families with high and complex support needs, reunification is only the beginning of a longer journey (Rushovich et al., 2021). Without ongoing, structured, and trauma-informed support, these families face a substantial risk of recurrent involvement with child protection, including re-entry into care. The reunification period is a critical time to identify the threats, issues, concerns, and risks that were present when initial removal occurred, and it is essential to be alert to these as re-emergence may occur. When children have been absent from family units and when family contact schedules have been ad hoc, irregular, or not incrementally built up therapeutically over time to repair attachments and resolve the discontinuities in relationships, it can create challenges for family re-integration (Rycus & Hughes, 2008). Given the significant and multifaceted stressors associated with family reunification, families with high and complex needs require intensive, coordinated support both during and following the reunification process. Such sustained intervention is critical to maintaining child and family well-being, preserving family stability, and ensuring fidelity to reunification goals. Ongoing support also reinforces the child's safety, mitigates/reduces the risk of harm or re-entry into care, and safeguards the social and financial investment made in the reunification process.

Throughout the literature there is discussion surrounding the significant number of children re-entering care once reunification breaks down or fails. Such failures arise due to several factors, as outlined above: a lack of supports and services post reunification, insufficient duration of reunification supports, lack of comprehensive assessments, and failure to resolve the issues and risks that led to initial removal of the children in the first instance (Fraser et al., 1996; McDonald et al., 2006). According to Balsells et al. (2013) statistics relating to failed reunification and subsequent re-entry into the child protection system vary by country, with American statistics indicating 19–50% of reunified children returning to the protection system after two or three years (Barth et al., 2008; Biehal, 2006). As noted earlier, in Australia successful reunification is defined as the child not returning to care within twelve months. According to national data, in the 2017–18 year 82% of children who were reunited with their biological families did not return to OOHC, although this did vary across jurisdictions and by Aboriginal status (Cunningham et al., 2021). Longitudinal data is scarce and difficult to access in Australia; however, international data demonstrates that reunification breakdowns continue to occur up to 24 months post-reunification (Chambers et al., 2019). A UK study (Sinclair et al., 2005) found that children who had been placed in foster care and then reunited with their biological families experienced a much higher abuse rates than children who remained in care, with the apparent lack of planning and post-reunification support, guidance and follow-up cited as the reason (McMurtry & Lie, 1992).

Another UK study identified the cumulative impacts of two or more failed reunification attempts for 35% of 180 children who participated in a UK study (Farmer, 2014. The attachment and relational impacts for these children, along with the worsening mental health consequences, are chronic and have lifelong implications for these children. The study noted that 43% of the children and young people were reunified with minimal assessments of the risks of harm and that many of the pre-existing problems were still apparent.

Numerous studies have shown that the 12–24 months following reunification is the highest-risk period for family breakdown and re-entry into care (Malm et al., 2021), with factors such as parental substance use, intergenerational trauma, parental mental illness, housing instability, and the lingering effects of disrupted attachment persisting when children return home. Indeed, the stresses of parenting post-reunification often reactivate or intensify these issues.

In the Australian context, these challenges are magnified by service fragmentation, the short-term nature of reunification support, and limited access to trauma-informed parenting interventions, particularly in rural, regional, and remote areas (Australian Institute of Health and Welfare, 2023c). Where service availability is restricted and cross-sector collaboration is inconsistent, the burden of navigating multiple systems frequently falls on parents who are already experiencing significant psychosocial stress (Australian Institute of Health and Welfare, 2023b; Higgins et al., 2020). The lack of continuity between child protection services and post-reunification therapeutic supports thus creates a gap at precisely the moment families are most vulnerable to relapse, placement disruption, and relational breakdown.

Moreover, families with multiple and intergenerational adversities often require long-term, scaffolded interventions that extend beyond the narrow timelines and compliance-based frameworks of statutory child protection. When intensive needs such as parental mental illness, neurodevelopmental disorders, intergenerational trauma, domestic and family violence, and substance dependency are met with brief, transactional interventions, reunification efforts are not only weakened but rendered unsustainable. Without a system of structured, enduring support, reunification can become a revolving door, contributing to a cycle of repeated removals that exacerbate attachment disruption and compound developmental trauma, causing further cumulative harm and significantly diminishing long-term outcomes for children and families.

Addressing this reality requires the establishment of a specialised, therapeutic post-reunification service system, one that mirrors the principles underpinning the National Disability Insurance Scheme (NDIS). Like the NDIS, such a model would recognise that complex and chronic biopsychosocial conditions require individualised, flexible, and long-term support that is responsive to both the intensity and variability of family needs over time. The NDIS is underpinned by values of equity, person-centred planning, early intervention, and lifelong support for individuals with significant impairments. These same principles are directly applicable to families attempting to rebuild caregiving capacity after statutory removal, where the "impairment" lies not in a singular diagnosis but in a system of relational, environmental, and psychological vulnerability.

A post-reunification scheme modelled on the NDIS could include multidisciplinary care teams, wraparound funding that follows the family rather than the case file, and integrated supports spanning mental health, housing, therapeutic parenting, early childhood services, and cultural healing programs. It would also facilitate continuity across transitions, ensuring that families are not discharged from one service stream without another already in place. This approach would shift the focus from crisis response to developmental repair and relational reunification, enabling practitioners to work proactively rather than reactively.

Crucially, a NDIS-style approach would also permit tiered and scalable support, allowing families to access more intensive interventions during periods of acute stress (e.g., relapse, transitions, court proceedings, family violence matters, unexpected homelessness), and tapering back services during periods of stability, without requiring case closure or full re-assessment. This flexibility is essential in addressing the non-linear and cumulative nature of recovery from complex trauma, especially in families where multiple developmental stages, disabilities, or diagnoses coexist within a single household.

By framing reunification within a structure akin to the NDIS, where long-term investment in functional outcomes is prioritised over short-term procedural closure, the child protection system can finally address the root causes of placement instability and intergenerational involvement with the system. Such a model would not only promote family preservation and reduce re-entry into care but would also represent a fiscally responsible approach, redirecting resources from crisis-driven interventions to preventive capacity-building practices that strengthen family systems over time.

CONCLUSION

This chapter has sought to unpack the multifaceted and often contested terrain of reunification within the Australian child protection system. By critically examining the current landscape, including legislative frameworks, success rates, and systemic limitations, it has illuminated the challenges and inconsistencies in how reunification is understood, assessed, and operationalised across Australian jurisdictions. Despite reunification being an embedded goal within statutory child protection legislation, it remains inconsistently planned for, under-resourced, and frequently approached in a fragmented manner.

Beyond merely identifying the gaps, this chapter has proposed a more comprehensive and therapeutically informed model for reunification, conceptualised as a three-phase service delivery framework: Reunification Intervention, Reunification Therapy, and Post-Reunification Services. These components are not intended to occur in isolation or sequentially, but, rather, as overlapping and interdependent processes that must be initiated early and sustained over time. Each phase responds to a different layer of need – practical, relational, and systemic – recognising that the return of a child to their family does not in itself equate to safety, stability, or healing.

Importantly, the chapter also emphasises the relevance of the cumulative risk and harm framework in understanding reunification outcomes. Children who have experienced repeated disruptions, exposure to chronic neglect or abuse, multiple placements, or failed reunifications are at significantly higher risk of long-term developmental, relational, and psychological harm. These risks do not operate in isolation; rather, they accumulate over time, compounding the vulnerability of children and families. Reunification efforts that fail to account for these layered risks by offering minimal, short-term, or one-size-fits-all interventions risk replicating the very conditions that led to removal in the first place. A lack of sustained support post-reunification not only undermines placement stability but may also exacerbate the cumulative burden of harm experienced by the child.

What has become evident through this discussion is the paucity of robust, longitudinal data within the Australian context that tracks reunification outcomes or evaluates the effectiveness of existing service models. This gap in evidence presents a significant barrier to policy reform, practice improvement, and accountability. It also reinforces the need for a national commitment to developing trauma-informed, family-centred, and evidence-based reunification practices that align with the complexity of the families involved.

Ultimately, this chapter calls for a shift in how reunification is conceptualised, not as a case closure milestone, but as a relational and developmental process that requires investment, clinical skill, and structural support. Just as systems like the NDIS recognise the need for long-term, individualised supports for people with complex needs, so too must the child protection sector begin to view reunified families through a more strategic lens. The alternative is the perpetuation of a system that restores children to families without the resources required to sustain that restoration, an approach that risks traumatisation, cumulative harm, and further systemic failure. Reunification, when done well, holds the potential to be transformative. But this can only be achieved if the system evolves to meet families not just at the point of crisis, but throughout the long journey of repair, reconnection, and resilience-building that follows.

REFERENCES

Australian Broadcasting Corporation. (2024). Foster carers leave the system in droves as cost-of-living pressures bite. *ABC News.* https://www.abc.net.au/news/2024-07-15/foster-carers-leaving-compensation-allowance-cost-of-living/104047836

Australian Housing and Urban Research Institute. (2023). *Crisis accommodation in Australia: Now and for the future* (AHURI Final Report No. 407). AHURI.

Australian Institute of Family Studies. (2022). *Identifying strategies to better support foster, kinship and permanent carers.* Commonwealth of Australia.

Australian Institute of Health and Welfare. (2023a). *Child protection Australia 2021–22* (Cat. no: CWS 92). AIHW. Retrieved from www.aihw.gov.au/reports/child-protection/child-protection-australia-2021-22

Australian Institute of Health and Welfare. (2023b). *Australia's welfare 2023: Data insights – Young people who have experienced child protection.* AIHW.

Australian Institute of Health and Welfare. (2023c). *Child Protection Australia 2021–2022.* Child welfare series no. 75. Cat no. CWS 92. AIHW.

Australian Institute of Health and Welfare. (2025). *Child protection Australia 2023–24.* AIHW.

Balsells, M. A., Pastor, C., Molina, M. C., Fuentes-Pelaez, N., Vaquero, E., & Mundet, A. (2013). Child welfare and successful reunification: Understanding of the family difficulties during the socio-educative process. *Revista de Cercetare si Interventie Sociala*, *42*, 228–247.

Barth, R. P., Weigensberg, E. C., Fisher, P. A., Fetrow, B., & Green, R. L. (2008). Re-entry of elementary aged children following reunification from foster care. *Children and Youth Services Review*, *30*(4), 353–364. DOI: 10.1016/j.childyouth.2007.10.002

Beer, A., Vij, A., Baker, E., Crommelin, L., Dodson, J., Gharaie, E., Li, T., & Horne, S. (2024). *Disruption in regional housing: Policy responses for more resilient markets* (AHURI Final Report No. 424). Australian Housing and Urban Research Institute.

Biehal, N. (2006). *Reuniting looked after children with their families: A research review.* University of York.

Bifulco, A., Moran, P. M., Ball, C., & Bernazzani, O. (2002). Adult attachment style: Its relationship to clinical depression. *Social Psychiatry and Psychiatric Epidemiology*, *37*(2), 50–59. DOI: 10.1007/s127-002-8215-0

Bifulco, A., & Thomas, G. (2013). *Understanding adult attachment in family relationships: Research, assessment and intervention*. Routledge.

Bohannan, T., Gonzalez, C., & Summers, A. (2016). Assessing the relationship between a peer mentoring program and case outcomes in dependency court. *Journal of Public Child Welfare*, *10*(2), 176–196. DOI: 10.1080/15548732.2016.1155523

Booth, P. B., & Jernberg, A. M. (2010). *Theraplay: Helping parents and children build better relationships through attachment-based play* (3rd ed.). Jossey-Bass.

Bratton, S. C., Ray, D., Rhine, T., & Jones, L. (2005). The efficacy of play therapy with children: A meta-analytic review of treatment outcomes. *Professional Psychology, Research and Practice*, *36*(4), 376–390. DOI: 10.1037/0735-7028.36.4.376

Brennan, J., Woolgar, M., & Rutter, M. (2016). *Parenting Role Interview manual*. King's College London.

Bromfield, L., & Higgins, D. (2005). *National comparison of child protection systems*. National Child Protection Clearinghouse, Australian Institute of Family Studies.

Bromfield, L., & Holzer, P. (2008). *A national approach for child protection: Project report*. National Child Protection Clearinghouse, Australian Institute of Family Studies. https://aifs.gov.au/research/research-reports/national-approach-child-protection

Bronson, D. E., Saunders, S., Holt, M. B., & Beck, E. (2008). *Systemic review of strategies to promote successful reunification and to reduce re-entry to care for abused, neglected, and unruly children*. Paper delivered at the Ohio Department of Job and Family Service, Ohio. http://www.ocwtp.net/PDFs/Reun-Reentry%20Final%20Report.pdf

Bryce, I. (2018). A review of cumulative harm: A comparison of international child protection practices. *Children Australia*, *43*(1), 23–31. DOI: 10.1017/cha.2018.3

Bryce, I., & Collier, S. (2022). *Child sexual abuse: Forensic issues in evidence, impact and management*. Routledge.

Bywaters, P., Brady, G., Bunting, L., Daniel, B., Featherstone, B., Jones, C., Morris, K., Scourfield, J., Sparks, T., & Webb, C. (2018). Inequalities in English child protection practices under austerity: A universal challenge? *Child & Family Social Work*, *23*(1), 53–61. DOI: 10.1111/cfs.12383

Cashmore, J., & Parkinson, P. (2008). Children and the law: Do we value our children enough? *The Sydney Law Review*, *30*(1), 1–26.

Chambers, J., Lint, S., Thompson, M., Carlson, M., & Graef, M. (2019). Outcomes of the Iowa partner program evaluation: Stability of reunification and re-entry into foster care. *Children and Youth Services Review, 104*, 1–11. DOI: 10.1016/j.childyouth.2019.05.030

Childhood Foundation. (2022). *Understanding the needs of kinship carers in Australia: Research brief.* Australian Childhood Foundation.

Choate, P. (2009). Parenting capacity assessments in child protection cases. *Forensic Examiner, 18*(1), 52–60.

Cloitre, M., Stolbach, B. C., Herman, J. L., van der Kolk, B., Pynoos, R., Wang, J., & Petkova, E. (2011). A developmental approach to complex PTSD: Childhood and adult cumulative trauma as predictors of symptom complexity. *Journal of Traumatic Stress, 22*(5), 399–408. DOI: 10.1002/jts.20444

Collings, S., McLaine, M., Ciftci, S., & Luu, B. (2024). Working towards reunification in New South Wales: Professional perspectives on navigating complex systems. *Australian Journal of Social Issues, 59*, 752–772. https://doi:org/DOI: 10.1002/ajs4.333

Cooper, J., & Vetere, A. (2008). *Domestic violence and family safety: Systemic approach to working with violence in families.* Wiley-Blackwell.

Coote, G., & Shams, H. (2023, September 24). NSW inquiry to hear from children forced into motels, hotels due to shortage of foster carers. *ABC News.* https://www.abc.net.au/news/2023-09-24/nsw-inquiry-into-kids-in-hotels-motels-due-lack-foster-carers/102895278

Cornett, N., & Bratton, S. C. (2014). The efficacy of filial therapy for parents of children with chronic illness: A pilot study. *International Journal of Play Therapy, 23*(2), 70–82.

Cunningham, M., Shlonsky, A., & Fouché, C. (2021). Reunification in out-of-home care: A rapid evidence review. *Children and Youth Services Review, 128*, 106–120.

Cunningham, T., Bastian, C., Seymour, K., & Wendt, S. (2021). Reunification: Rapid literature review. Flinders University. https://researchnow.flinders.edu.au/en/publications/reunification-rapid-literature-review

Davis, I. P., Landsverk, J., Newton, R., & Ganger, W. (1996). Parental visiting and foster care reunification. *Children and Youth Services Review, 18*(4/5), 363–382. DOI: 10.1016/0190-7409(96)00010-2

Delaney, R. (2006). *Trauma, attachment, and family permanency: Fear can stop you loving*. Wood 'N' Barnes.

Delfabbro, P., Fernandez, E., McCormick, J., & Wilson, S. (2019). *Out-of-home care in Australia: Children and young people's views after five years of the National Standards*. Department of Social Services.

Department of Communities and Justice (DCJ). (2023). *How do relative/kinship carers and foster carers differ? Pathways of Care Longitudinal Study Evidence to Action Note 15*. NSW Government.

Dozier, M., & Bernard, K. (2019). *Coaching parents of vulnerable infants: The Attachment and Biobehavioral Catch-Up approach*. Guilford Press.

Dunbar, A., Savaglio, M., Halfpenny, N., O'Donnell, R., Pileggi, A., & Skouteris, H. (2022). MacKillop Family Services' Family Preservation and Reunification Response for vulnerable families: Protocol for an effectiveness-implementation study. *International Journal of Environmental Research and Public Health, 19*(1), 426.

Edwards, V. J., Holden, G. W., Felitti, V. J., & Anda, R. F. (2003). Relationship between multiple forms of childhood maltreatment and adult mental health in community respondents: Results from the Adverse Childhood Experiences (ACE) study. *The American Journal of Psychiatry, 160*(8), 1453–1460. DOI: 10.1176/appi.ajp.160.8.1453

Enano, S., Freisthler, B., Perez-Johnson, D., & Lovato-Hermann, K. (2017). Evaluating parents in partnership: A preliminary study of a child welfare intervention designed to increase reunification. *Journal of Social Science Research, 43*(2), 236–245.

Farmer, E. (2014). Improving reunification practice: Pathways home, progress and outcomes for children returning from care to their parents. *British Journal of Social Work, 44*(2), 348–366. DOI: 10.1093/bjsw/bcs093

Felitti, V. J., Anda, R. F., Nordenberg, D., Williamson, D. F., Spitz, A. M., Edwards, V., & Marks, J. S. (1998). Relationship of childhood abuse and household dysfunction to many of the leading causes of death in adults: The Adverse Childhood Experiences (ACE) study. *American Journal of Preventive Medicine, 14*(4), 245–258. DOI: 10.1016/S0749-3797(98)00017-8

Fernandez, E., & Lee, J. (2013). Accomplishing family reunification for children in care: An Australian study. *Children and Youth Services Review, 35*(9), 1374–1384. DOI: 10.1016/j.childyouth.2013.05.006

Fish, S., & Hardy, M. (2015). Complex issues, complex solutions: Applying complexity theory in social work practice. *Nordic Social Work Research, 1*(5), 98–114. DOI: 10.1080/2156857X.2015.1065902

Foster Care Association of Victoria. (2024). *Carer snapshot.* FCAV.

Foundation, E. Q. T. (2024, April 12). *More support for foster carers as numbers continue to decline.* EQT Foundation Media Centre. https://www.eqt.com.au/MediaCentre/2024/04/12/More-support-for-foster-carers-as-numbers-continue-to-decline

Fraser, M. W., Walton, E., Lewis, R. E., Pecora, P. J., & Walton, E. K. (1996). An experiment in family reunification: Correlates of outcomes at one year follow-up. *Children and Youth Services Review, 18*(4/5), 335–362. DOI: 10.1016/0190-7409(96)00009-6

Guerney, L. F. (2000). Filial therapy. In Kaduson, H. G., & Schaefer, C. E. (Eds.), *Short-term play therapy for children* (pp. 75–104). The Guilford Press.

Herman, J. (1992). *Trauma and recovery.* Basic Books.

Higgins, D., Bromfield, L., & Richardson, N. (2007). *Child abuse and neglect in Australian families.* Australian Institute of Family Studies.

Hughes, D. A. (2016). *Building the bonds of attachment: Awakening love in deeply troubled children* (3rd ed.). Rowman & Littlefield.

Hughes, D. A., Golding, K. S., & Hudson, J. (2019). *Creating loving attachments: Parenting with PACE to nurture confidence and security in the troubled child.* Jessica Kingsley Publishers.

Jones, L., Malekoff, A., & Bryant, K. (2021). Reunification services and family preservation: A practice-informed review. *Journal of Family Social Work, 24*(2), 157–174.

Kertesz, M., Humphreys, C., & Kiraly, M. (2021). Addressing parental mistrust in child protection contexts: Building relationships to support reunification. *Australian Social Work, 74*(1), 28–40.

Kezelman, C., Hossack, N., Stavropoulos, P., & Burley, P. (2015). *The cost of unresolved childhood trauma and abuse in adults in Australia.* Adults Surviving Child Abuse and Pegasus Economics. Retrieved from https://blueknot.org.au/resources/blue-knot-publications/the-cost-of-unresolved-childhood-trauma-and-abuse-in-adults-in-australia-2/

Kezelman, C., & Stavropoulos, P. (2012). *Practice guidelines for treatment of complex trauma and trauma informed care and service delivery*. Adults Surviving Child Abuse.

Kiraly, M. (2024). Kinship care in the welfare system: The lived experience of Victorian kinship stakeholders. *Children and Youth Services Review*, *157*, 107424.

Kirk, R. (2010). *A comparative study of older-youth families and younger youth families in placement prevention and reunification cases, using traditional case protection services measures and NCFAS and NCFAS-R assessment data*. National Family Preservation Network Project.

Kirk, R. S. (2015a). *Development, intent and use of the North Carolina Family Assessment Scales and their relation to their reliability and their validity of the scales*. National Family Preservation Network.

Kirk, R. S. (2015b). Psychometric properties of the trauma and post trauma well-being assessment domains of the North Carolina Family Assessment Scale for general and reunification services (NCFAS G, R). *Journal of Public Child Welfare*, *9*(5), 444–452. DOI: 10.1080/15548732.2015.1090364

Kirk, R. S., Kim, M., & Griffith, D. P. (2005). *NCFAS-R: North Carolina Family Assessment Scale for Reunification*. University of North Carolina at Chapel Hill.

Landreth, G. L. (2012). *Play therapy: The art of the relationship* (3rd ed.). Routledge. DOI: 10.4324/9780203835159

Lieberman, A. F., Van Horn, P., & Ippen, C. G. (2005). Toward evidence-based treatment: Child–parent psychotherapy with preschoolers exposed to marital violence. *Journal of the American Academy of Child and Adolescent Psychiatry*, *44*(12), 1241–1248. DOI: 10.1097/01.chi.0000181047.59702.58

Macdonald, G., Livingstone, N., Hanratty, J., McCartan, C., Cotmore, R., Cary, M., Glanville, J., & Bywater, T. (2018). The effectiveness, acceptability and cost-effectiveness of psychosocial interventions for maltreated children and adolescents: An evidence synthesis. *Health Technology Assessment*, *22*(52), 1–508.

McDonald, T., Bryson, S., & Poertner, J. (2006). Balancing reunification and re-entry goals. *Children and Youth Services Review*, *28*(1), 47–58. DOI: 10.1016/j.childyouth.2005.02.007

McMurtry, S. L., & Lie, G. Y. (1992). Differential exit rates of minority children in foster care. *Social Work Research & Abstracts*, *28*(1), 42–48. DOI: 10.1093/swra/28.1.42

McWey, L. M., & Cui, M. (2021). Parent–child contact and family reunification in foster care. *Children and Youth Services Review, 128*, 106–152.

Nelson, J., & Landsman, M. (2006). Promoting reunification through evidence-based assessment. *Protecting Children, 21*(1), 36–45.

NSW Department of Communities and Justice. (2023). *How do relative/kinship carers and foster carers differ in their characteristics, wellbeing and support needs? Evidence to Action Note No. 13, Pathways of Care Longitudinal Study (POCLS).* NSW Department of Communities and Justice.

O'Connell, M. (2025). *The cost of late intervention 2024.* The Front Project.

Oosterman, M., & Schuengel, C. (2023). The quality of parent–child contact and its role in family reunification. *Children and Youth Services Review, 149*, 106–783.

Osborn, A., & Bromfield, L. (2007). *Young people leaving care.* National Child Protection Clearinghouse, Australian Institute of Family Studies.

Parnell, S. (2024, December 13). Hundreds of Queensland children living in residential care. *The QLDR*. https://theqldr.com.au/queensland-news/2024/12/13/care-2/

PeakCare & Queensland Family and Child Commission. (2024, June). *Queensland foster carer demographic insights report: The future of foster care*. The Demographics Group. https://www.qfcc.qld.gov.au/queensland-foster-carer-demographic-insights-report-peakcare

Perry, B. D. (2009). Examining child maltreatment through a neurodevelopmental lens: Clinical applications of the neurosequential model of therapeutics. *Journal of Loss and Trauma, 14*(4), 240–255. DOI: 10.1080/15325020903004350

Reed-Ashcraft, K., Kirk, R., & Fraser, M. (2001). The reliability and validity of the North Carolina Family Assessment Scale. *Research on Social Work Practice, 11*(4), 503–520. DOI: 10.1177/104973150101100406

Ross, N., Cocks, J., Johnston, L., & Stoker, L. (2017). *No voice, no opinion, nothing: Parent experiences when children are removed and placed in care.* University of Newcastle.

Rushovich, B., Sepulveda, K., Efetevbia, V., & Malm, K. (2021). A post-reunification service model: Implementation and population served. *Children and Youth Services Review, 122*, 105928. DOI: 10.1016/j.childyouth.2021.105928

Rycus, J. S., & Hughes, R. C. (2008). Assessing risk throughout the life of a child welfare case. In Lindsay, D., & Shlonsky, A. (Eds.), *Child welfare research: Advances for practices and policy* (p. 48). Oxford University Press. DOI: 10.1093/acprof:oso/9780195304961.003.0012

Secretariat of National Aboriginal and Islander Child Care (SNAICC). (2017). *The Family Matters report 2017: Measuring trends to turn the tide on the over-representation of Aboriginal and Torres Strait Islander children in out-of-home care in Australia*. SNAICC.

Sianko, N., Peterson, C. A., Spieker, S. J., & Gillmore, M. R. (2016). Enhancing parent-child relationships through Theraplay in child welfare. *Child & Family Social Work, 21*(1), 83–93.

Sinclair, I., Baker, C., Wilson, K., & Gibbs, I. (2005). *Foster children: Where they go and how they get on*. Jessica Kingsley Publishers.

Teague, R. (2017). *Reunification for children in out-of-home-care-Part 2: Reunification success rates and the consequences of reunification failure*. Queensland Child & Family Commission.

Testa, M. F., & Poertner, J. (2020). *Fostering accountability: Using evidence to guide and improve child welfare policy*. Oxford University Press.

Woods, P. (2011). *Working with parents to support children's learning*. SAGE Publications.

Chapter 5
Nuancing a Validated Tool to Reduce Adversity and Maltreatment for First Nations Children

Simone Collier
https://orcid.org/0009-0008-3658-8535
University of Queensland, Australia

ABSTRACT

This chapter presents the development of the Cumulative Experiences Index – Culturally Responsive (CEI-CR) tool, an assessment tool designed to identify and measure cumulative harm experienced by First Nations children. Building on the validated Cumulative Experiences Index (CEI) tool, the CEI-CR incorporates culturally specific domains, including intergenerational trauma, cultural disconnection, systemic disadvantage, and resilience factors grounded in kinship, culture, and Country. The CEI-CR integrates historical, cultural, and structural considerations to provide a more accurate profile of risk and protective factors. Its purpose is to support early, culturally safe intervention, family preservation, and reunification, rather than justify removal. This chapter outlines the theoretical framework, co-design process with Aboriginal stakeholders, and intended application of the CEI-CR, highlighting its potential to address service gaps and improve outcomes for children experiencing chronic, layered adversity.

DOI: 10.4018/979-8-3373-4064-7.ch005

INTRODUCTION

The ongoing discussion in the literature relating to First Nations persons in Australia centres primarily around their over-representation in the Child Protection and Youth Justice systems. The consequences include over-representation in the adult justice system and poorer health outcomes for adult First Nations persons across their lifespan.

According to the Australian Institute of Health and Welfare (AIHW) (2024), First Nations children are 11 times more likely to be placed in out-of-home care than non-Indigenous children, and this inequality has been steadily increasing over several decades (Yoorrook Justice Commission, 2023; Long & Stephen, 2011).

Evidence from national and international child maltreatment research consistently highlights the profound impact of cumulative harm, where multiple adverse experiences compound over time, impacting on a child's overall safety, development, and lifelong wellbeing (Mathews et al., 2023; Daniel et al., 2011; Felitti et al., 1998). For Aboriginal and Torres Strait Islander children, this accumulation of harm is often intensified by the legacy of intergenerational trauma, systemic disadvantage, cultural disconnection, and the ongoing impacts of colonisation (Royal Commission into the Protection and Detention of Children in the Northern Territory, 2017; SNAICC – Secretariat of National Aboriginal and Islander Child Care).

The AIHW (2023) and the Royal Commission into the Protection and Detention of Children in the Northern Territory (2017) have both identified that Aboriginal children are disproportionately represented in child protection systems, due not to cultural deficits but to the layered and compounding nature of risk factors such as poverty, housing instability, exposure to family violence, and child removal. The Child Maltreatment Study (Mathews et al., 2023) further underscores the need for early identification and intervention in the presence of multiple adversities, linking cumulative exposure to maltreatment with likely elevated risks of mental health disorders, substance misuse, self-harm, suicide, and contact with the justice system.

For Aboriginal children, failing to measure cumulative harm risks overlooking the interconnected and contextual nature of their adversity. Isolated incidents do not reflect the broader systemic and relational impacts these children experience. Without tools and frameworks to measure cumulative adversity, services remain reactive rather than preventative and restorative, often intervening too late, once crisis and statutory thresholds are breached.

Why Is Measuring Harm in First Nations Children Critical for Early and Culturally Responsive Intervention?

Cumulative harm refers to the chronic and compounding impact of multiple adverse experiences over time, and includes factors such as neglect, abuse, family violence, parental mental health and substance misuse, parental criminality and incarceration, and systemic disadvantage. For Aboriginal and Torres Strait Islander children, this harm is often more complex and entrenched due to the intersecting effects of intergenerational trauma, forced removals, loss of culture and language, racism, and ongoing socio-economic marginalisation.

Unlike single-incident harm, cumulative harm builds silently and incrementally over time. Its effects may be subtle in the early stages, but research shows it can lead to profound and enduring disruptions to a child's development, attachment, mental health, and life trajectory outcomes (Mathews et al., 2023; Daniel et al., 2011). Aboriginal children are disproportionately impacted, not because of deficits within families or communities, but due to the compounded weight of unresolved historical injustices (AIHW, 2023; Royal Commission, 2017).

Measuring cumulative harm matters for First Nations children for several reasons (see Infographic 1), including:

Early Detection: It allows practitioners to identify patterns of concern before harm escalates to statutory thresholds, enabling earlier, preventive, and restorative interventions. This is well supported by the Adverse Childhood Experiences (ACE) Study (Felitti et al., 1998), which demonstrated that early identification of multiple adverse experiences reduces the likelihood of poor longer-term health, mental health, and social outcomes. Early detection of cumulative harm is also well supported in the Australian Child Maltreatment Study (Mathews et al., 2023), which confirmed that cumulative exposure to maltreatment is strongly associated with self-harm, suicidality, and contact with the criminal justice system, highlighting the importance of detecting risk early.

Systemic Understanding: It supports a holistic view of the child's lived experience across education, health, justice, and family systems, rather than reducing concerns to isolated events. Daniel et al., (2011) emphasise the need to consider neglect and maltreatment as multi-faceted and persistent over time, not simply isolated incidents. It is argued that recognising patterns across systems improves assessment and intervention accuracy; SNAICC (2023) has also long argued for systems-level perspectives that account for structural drivers of vulnerability, such as poverty, racism, and lack of access to culturally safe services.

Cultural Safety: Measuring cumulative harm recognises the impact of disconnection from kin, culture, and country as a form of harm, which standard risk assessment tools often overlook. The Royal Commission into Aboriginal Deaths in

Custody (RCIADIC) and the Royal Commission into the Protection and Detention of Children in the Northern Territory (2017) both identified disconnection from culture, kin, and country as a core element of harm. Arney et al., (2015) also stress the importance of culturally adapted cumulative harm assessment frameworks that consider historical and systemic trauma for Aboriginal children.

Practice and Policy Alignment: It ensures decisions about removal, reunification, and intervention are informed by a comprehensive picture of risk, resilience, and cultural context. Tilbury (2009) and Scott (2014) highlight that risk assessments lacking a cumulative harm framework often result in fragmented or reactive service responses. Aligning practice with holistic frameworks ensures child-focused, culturally responsive planning. The AIHW (2024) confirms that cumulative risk factors, when unmeasured, can lead to inappropriate removals or missed opportunities for early support.

Restorative Focus: Finally, measuring cumulative harm validates the experience of Aboriginal children and families by acknowledging the social determinants of their vulnerability and linking harm to modifiable systemic causes, not just parental behaviour. This is supported by Bryce (2020) and Atkinson (2013), who both argue for a trauma-informed, restorative model of intervention that considers structural inequalities, not just individual parenting behaviours. This is vital in supporting Aboriginal families with dignity and justice. The Healing Foundation report reinforces that harm cannot be separated from systemic and colonial impacts and that acknowledging this is foundational to healing (The Healing Foundation, 2025).

Figure 1. Representing reasons for measuring cumulative harm in First Nations Children is critical for early and culturally responsive intervention

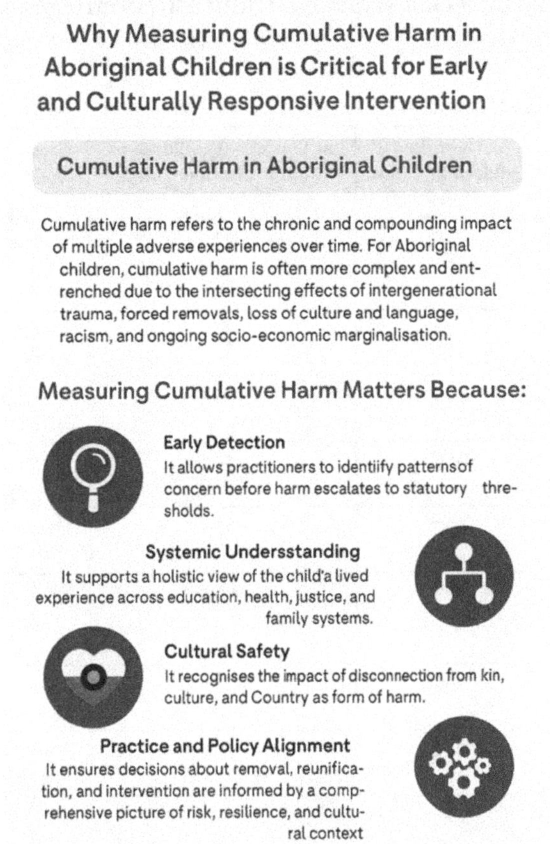
Why Measuring Cumulative Harm in Aboriginal Children is Critical for Early and Culturally Responsive Intervention
Cumulative Harm in Aboriginal Children
Cumulative harm refers to the chronic and compounding impact of multiple adverse experiences over time. For Aboriginal children, cumulative harm is often more complex and entrenched due to the intersecting effects of intergenerational trauma, forced removals, loss of culture and language, racism, and ongoing socio-economic marginalisation.
Measuring Cumulative Harm Matters Because:
Early Detection
It allows practitioners to identiify patternsof concern before harm escalates to statutory thresholds.
Systemic Undersstanding
It supports a holistic view of the child'a lived experience across education, health, justice, and family systems.
Cultural Safety
It recognises the impact of disconnection from kin, culture, and Country as form of harm.
Practice and Policy Alignment
It ensures decisions about removal, reunification, and intervention are informed by a comprehensive picture of risk, resilience, and cultural context

The Crossover Kids – The Accumulated Risks

In Australia, there exists a distinct correlation between children and young people who spend time in out-of-home care and the youth justice system. It is often noted by statutory bodies that the child protection systems are a pipeline into the justice system, and Aboriginal children are significantly over-represented in this population (Crossover Kids: Vulnerable Children in the Youth Justice System, 2020). While Aboriginal children are only 6% of the under-18 Australian population, they make up 40% of children in care and are 11 times more likely to be in out-of-home care than non-Indigenous children (AIHW, 2023). In the Australian youth justice system, Indigenous youth represent over 50% of those in detention on an average day (AIHW, 2023) and are 23 times more likely to be incarcerated than non-Indigenous youth. A study by the Victorian Sentencing Advisory Council (2020) found that two-thirds of children sentenced in the Children's Court in Victoria had prior involvement with child protection, with Indigenous children significantly overrepresented (see Table 1).

Table 1. National patterns across jurisdictions – Crossover kids, (AIHW, 2020)

State/Territory	% Aboriginal Children in Youth Justice	% Aboriginal Children in Child Protection/OOHC	Crossover Kid Risk Factors
Victoria	~17%	~25%	High crossover rates; residential care criminalisation
Queensland	~43%	~40%	OOHC-to-custody pipeline; police involvement in care
New South Wales	~50%	~40%	Inconsistent culturally safe services; care-criminalisation
Western Australia	~75%	~54%	Severe over-policing; systemic removal
South Australia	~60%	~35%	Institutionalisation of trauma responses
Northern Territory	~95%	~85%	Remote dislocation, generational removal, detention default
Tasmania	~20%	~25%	Limited early intervention; small population, same trends
Australian Capital Territory (ACT)	~30%	~25%	Underuse of Aboriginal-led services; kinship care gaps

Across Australia there are some common trends among children and young people in care; equally, there are trends and patterns that are particular when to the individual states and territories. In Victoria, 67% of sentenced children have previous child protection involvement, and Aboriginal children are vastly over-represented in this group. The crossover kids are more likely to be sentenced for more serious offences, be placed into residential care or out-of-home care (OOHC) and be remanded in custody rather than granted bail (AIHW, 2020; AIC, 2022).

In Queensland, research indicates a strong link between OOHC and youth detention, with Aboriginal children making up 43% of youth in detention and a large proportion of children in residential care who have repeated youth justice system contact (AIC, 2022). In New South Wales (NSW), the Child Protection and Youth Justice Systems Review (2021) found Aboriginal children in care were significantly more likely to end up in custody, with a disproportionate number of Aboriginal children enter both systems – protection and justice – due to family disruption, neglect, and lack of culturally appropriate services, while police responses to children and young people in residential care continue to criminalise trauma behaviours. NSW has piloted a Joint Protocol (Child Protection and Youth Justice Systems Review, 2021) to reduce the criminalisation of young people in residential out-of-home care, but uptake has been inconsistent.

Western Australia has one of the highest rates of child removal and youth detention of Aboriginal children per capita, with Aboriginal children being 17 times more likely to be in OOHC and 30 times more likely to be in youth detention. A significant number of children in detention have a prior child protection history, including removal from their families (AIHW, 2020). The Office of the Inspector of Custodial Services has criticised the lack of therapeutic alternatives and over-policing (AIC, 2022). The Northern Territory (NT) likewise has among the highest rates of child protection intervention and youth detention in Australia, with over 90% of children in detention being Aboriginal, many of whom have child protection backgrounds. Many of these young people have experienced remote community dislocation, poverty, and systemic failures, exacerbating crossover risks. A range of youth justice reforms in the NT have rolled back some therapeutic models, increasing the criminalisation of Aboriginal youth (AIC, 2022). The Australian Capital Territory (ACT) has acknowledged the crossover phenomenon, with the Our Booris, Our Way review (2019) highlighting a lack of cultural safety and kinship options in OOHC, and the gaps in early intervention services for Aboriginal families. However, cross-system coordination in the ACT remains limited despite policy attention.

Remond et al. (2023) note studies demonstrating the high risk of intergenerational incarceration in NSW, with children with an incarcerated parent being five times more likely to be imprisoned than a child whose parent/s have no incarceration history.

According to the NSW Bureau of Crime Statistics and Research (2024), there are significant racial disparities in the NSW justice system; Aboriginal children are 12 times more likely to have an incarcerated parent and 61% of Aboriginal people who are in custody also have a parent who is currently or has been imprisoned, in comparison to 30% of non-Aboriginal youth. The cumulative risk factors for a child entering custody increases when parental incarceration is combined with other disadvantages, including:

- early exposure to child protection services
- exposure to pro-criminal thinking and behaviour (role-modelling, normalisation and acceptance of antisocial behaviours) when from families who have a police bias
- housing instability, interpersonal violence and trauma
- problematic gambling, alcohol and drug taking
- bias in policing and statutory responses to crime
- socioeconomic disadvantage

- lower education status, family instability, and poorer health status
- living in out-of-home care
- having a parent incarcerated during their early childhood (0–5 years) (AIHW, 2023).

REASONS FOR THE OVER-REPRESENTATION OF FIRST NATIONS CHILDREN AND THE ACCUMULATION OF HARM IN THEIR LIVES

Historical & Intergenerational Trauma

Factors that have contributed to intergenerational trauma include colonisation, which has resulted in the dispossession of land, culture, language, and identity, and the Stolen Generations, which saw the systemic removal of Aboriginal children and continues to engender mistrust in authorities and fragmented family systems. This has resulted in the widespread and entrenched reluctance among First Nations families to be forthcoming in engaging with statutory authorities, as adverse outcomes of the Australian child removal policies during the Stolen Generations remain vivid (Ralph & Ryan, 2017). Trauma from these events is passed down through the generations, contributing to mental health challenges, substance misuse, criminality, and parenting struggles.

Systemic Racism and Discriminatory Practices

Many Indigenous people continue to feel the weight of biases in mandatory reporting, assessment, and intervention that disproportionately target Aboriginal families, particularly those of lower socio-economic status. Cultural misunderstandings and deficit-based frameworks result in assumptions among those in statutory positions about parenting capacity and differences in how parenting practices are viewed. Police and judicial discretion often result in tougher responses to Aboriginal youth compared to non-Indigenous peers, and this is often reflected in the trends and patterns in state-based data, according to youth advocacy groups.

Poverty and Socioeconomic Disadvantage

Aboriginal families often experience higher rates of unemployment, overcrowded housing, and limited access to healthcare and education, all of which contribute to increased child protection interventions. Within the child protection sector, economic hardship is often interpreted as neglect when evaluating a parent's capacity to care for their children. Many Aboriginal advocacy groups see this as evidence of a need for support, rather than inability to care for their children.

Cumulative Harm and Early System Contact

Aboriginal children often face multiple adversities (family violence, school exclusion, homelessness, disability, health concerns) with limited access to early support services. Once in care, many Aboriginal children are disconnected from kin, Country, and culture, compounding feelings of isolation and trauma.

Poor Care System Outcomes

Children in care are more likely to experience multiple placements, education disruption, and mental health issues. Responses to behavioural issues among children are in residential and foster care placements are often institution-focused, such as calling authorities for behaviour that families would normally manage themselves. When this occurs and police become involved, it results in funnelling Aboriginal children into the justice system. This in turn leads to children entering the 'crossover kids' scenario, with courts and detention becoming part of the child's world – an outcome that could have been avoided if families were able to actively advocate for the child.

Lack of Cultural Safety in Services

Many services lack cultural competency and fail to embed Aboriginal-led frameworks; there is limited use of kinship care placements, culturally appropriate casework, or community-controlled organisations. SNAICC defines cultural safety for First Nations children as 'the child being provided with a safe, nurturing and positive environment where they are comfortable with being themselves, expressing their culture, their spiritual and belief systems, where they are supported by the carer … [who] respects their Aboriginality and therefore encourages their sense of self and identity' (National Office for Child Safety [NOCS] et al., 2021, p 7)

Over-Policing and Criminalisation of Trauma

Aboriginal youth are more likely to be monitored, stopped, searched, and charged for offences that non-Indigenous peers might be cautioned for (Cunneen, 2008; Australian Law Reform Commission, 2018; Snowball, 2009). It is well documented throughout the literature that behaviours stemming from trauma will present as antisocial, and possibly be profoundly impactful, and are criminalised rather than responded to with therapeutic interventions. This includes children with extensive trauma histories who engage in property damage, absconding, and aggression and who are consequently frequently criminalised in residential care settings (Victorian Sentencing Advisory Council 2020). Children in care often report that their emotional responses are misunderstood by carers and the statutory authorities, and this can lead to punitive responses, or being criminalised for emotional distress, particularly in group homes or residential settings (McDowall, 2019).

IDENTIFICATION OF A NEED FOR A TOOL TO MEASURE CUMULATIVE HARM

In 2023, a Cumulative Experiences Index (CEI) tool – a measure of the cumulative harm that is experienced by an individual was developed in Australia by Bryce et al., (2024). This tool can be used to rate a person's adverse childhood experiences as low, medium, or high in severity. The CEI tool assists practitioners in understanding the frequency, duration, and severity of the harm the child or the young person has experienced (Bryce et al., 2024). Before the development of this tool, there was no validated measure to reliably identify and score cumulative harm experienced by a child. A structured decision-making tool combining an actuarial risk assessment and clinical judgment to aid in decision making at the point of intake was therefore developed for child protection workers to use to assist in understanding the cumulative harm experienced by a child. The original CEI tool was formulated by synthesising key components from three foundational frameworks that assess childhood adversity and maltreatment. These were the Adverse Childhood Experiences (ACEs) checklist developed by Felitti et al., (1998), which quantifies exposure to various forms of abuse, neglect, and household dysfunction; Bromfield et al.,'s (2007) conceptual model of cumulative harm, which emphasises the compounding effects of chronic adversity over time; and the Modified Maltreatment Classification System (MMCS) of Barnett et al., (1993), a structured system for coding and categorising different types and severities of maltreatment. By integrating these approaches, the CEI was designed to provide a comprehensive and multidimensional measure of cumulative risk and harm in children's lives, reflecting both the frequency and impact of adverse experiences across developmental stages.

The CEI tool underwent successful testing and evaluation through a structured pilot study, which demonstrated its effectiveness in capturing the complex and layered nature of cumulative harm experienced by children. The pilot confirmed the tool's validity as both a clinical assessment instrument and a practice-informed framework, capable of guiding professionals in identifying patterns of adversity across multiple domains of a child's life. By offering a quantitative scoring system, the CEI enables practitioners to move beyond isolated incidents and instead build a comprehensive picture of risk exposure over time (Bryce et al., 2024). This structured approach supports a continuum of intervention, from assessment and formulation to targeted treatment planning and therapeutic engagement, ensuring that responses are not only trauma-informed but also attuned to the ongoing and compounding effects of adversity on both the child and their family system.

Importantly, the CEI enables practitioners to translate complex trauma histories into a clear, quantifiable profile that informs professional judgement and supports the development of comprehensive case formulations. This process facilitates targeted interventions by integrating assessment with therapeutic treatment planning, while also enhancing engagement with children and families affected by chronic adversity. As such, the CEI serves as a bridge between research, clinical insight, and frontline practice, supporting a coordinated, trauma-informed response to complex child protection concerns.

The initial CEI pilot study involved a small sample of clients engaged with an Intensive Family Support Service. While the pilot demonstrated the CEI's potential utility in identifying and quantifying cumulative adversity and maltreatment, the evaluation did not apply a culturally specific lens. This represents a significant limitation, particularly within the Australian context, where Aboriginal and Torres Strait Islander children remain significantly over-represented in the child protection and youth justice systems.

Given this over-representation, it is imperative that any assessment tool designed to capture cumulative harm be responsive to the cultural, historical, and systemic factors impacting First Nations families. While the pilot findings supported the CEI's viability in informing an assessment, formulation, and intervention planning for families experiencing chronic and layered adversity, the study identified the need for further validation across diverse populations.

To ensure cultural safety and relevance, future implementation and design of the CEI, a key recommendation was that it must include the perspectives of Aboriginal and Torres Strait Islander practitioners, families, and communities. This was needed to support the tool's capacity to guide bespoke, trauma-informed, and culturally responsive interventions, particularly for those families most affected by the intergenerational impacts of colonisation, forced removals, and systemic disadvantage.

While the CEI showed promise in enhancing practice with vulnerable families, its broader efficacy, especially in working with Aboriginal and Torres Strait Islander families, required further development, co-design, and culturally informed validation. Consideration of frameworks such as race-based traumatic stress – which describes the emotional injury caused by hate or fear of a person or group of people as a result of their race (Bryant-Davis, 2007) – has assisted in the development of an expanded and more culturally informed version of the CEI. An understanding of the intergenerational transmission of trauma for Aboriginal peoples – who have been subjected to generations of abuse who continue to live with conditions of disadvantage resulting from colonial polices, to the point of it being considered a form of coercive control – is also highly valued. The CEI framework includes high levels of adverse childhood experiences, including abuse and neglect, household substance misuse, stressful adulthood experiences, including poverty and unemployment, violence, homicide, assaults, domestic violence, criminality, incarceration, witnessing traumatic events, and high levels of discrimination (Bombay et al., 2009).

Further to this, it is argued in the literature that a diagnosis of Post-Traumatic Stress Disorder (PTSD) as described in the Diagnostic and Statistical Manual (DSM) is inadequate in the context of the type of intergenerational trauma experienced by Aboriginal people (Bryant-Davis, 2007; Menzies, 2010; Yellow Horse Brave Heart, 2003, Gone, 2013, Evans-Campbell 2008). Menzies (2010) argues that a diagnosis of PTSD ignores the roles of culture and intergenerational trauma or community trauma and "doesn't connect the person's experiences to broader, systemic conditions that perpetuate and exacerbate the individual's experience" (p.68). Other perspectives likewise state that PTSD is a diagnosis too limited to capture the complex, collective, and vast cumulative trauma that has transpired across generations that Aboriginal people have endured (Gone, 2013; Yellow Horse Brave Heart, 2003). Traditional diagnostic categories such as PTSD often fail to adequately recognise the interconnected nature of historical, intergenerational, and current traumas experienced by Aboriginal people (Evans-Campbell, 2008). These frameworks tend to confine diagnosis to the individual without acknowledging the collective and systemic harms caused by colonisation, forced removals, cultural disconnection, and institutional racism. As a result, trauma is frequently pathologised rather than contextualised, leading to misdiagnosis, inadequate support, and, in many cases, victim-blaming (Bryant-Davis, 2007; Gone, 2013). This deficit-based lens ignores the ongoing impact of structural inequality and erases the resilience, strength, relational and cultural protective factors that are central to Aboriginal and Torres Strait Islander people's healing. A culturally responsive approach must recognise trauma as embedded within a broader socio-political and historical context to avoid further marginalisation and to enable effective, community-led healing pathways.

Herman (1992), in her landmark paper, discussed the framework of Complex Post-Traumatic Stress Disorder (CPTSD) applying to Aboriginal persons who had "prolonged, repeated trauma that can occur only where the victim is in a state of captivity, unable to flee and under the control of the perpetrator" (p.391). Herman argues that in situations of prolonged trauma, the relationship between victim and perpetrator is often underpinned by coercive control. This control can be exerted through direct physical force or a complex interplay of economic dependence, social isolation, psychological manipulation, and structural inequality. When viewed through a cumulative harm lens, Herman's theory resonates deeply with the lived experiences of many Aboriginal and Torres Strait Islander people. For these communities, the impacts of colonisation, such as forced removals, dispossession from land and culture, racialised violence, and systemic marginalisation, have not occurred as isolated events but, rather, as layered and compounding harms over generations (Aguiar & Halseth, 2015).

These experiences of historical trauma are further entrenched by contemporary experiences of poverty, discrimination, child removal, incarceration, and restricted access to culturally safe services. The cumulative effect of these harms establishes conditions that closely align with Herman's definition of coercive control conditions in which individuals and communities are systematically disempowered and denied autonomy. The perpetuation of such control across generations constitutes a form of collective captivity, where freedom, safety, and dignity are persistently undermined by systems that reproduce disadvantage.

This understanding demands a shift away from individualised, deficit-based interpretations of trauma and behaviour, and instead calls for responses that are historically aware, culturally grounded, and trauma-sensitive. Recognising coercive control as a cumulative and systemic phenomenon is essential for developing interventions and policies that address not only the symptoms of trauma, but its deep-rooted structural causes.

As noted above, Herman believes that in these cases the relationship between victim and perpetrator is based on coercive control, whether this state of captivity is based primarily on physical force or on a combination of physical, economic, social and psychological forces. For many Aboriginal people, continuing to live with disadvantage after being subjected to generations of abuses fits the conditions of coercive control (Aguiar & Halseth, 2015).

PTSD and CPTSD are both recognised within clinical literature as trauma-related conditions. However, CPTSD encompasses a broader spectrum of psychological harm that more accurately captures the profound and enduring impacts of chronic, interpersonal, and systemic trauma. For Aboriginal and Torres Strait Islander peoples, whose experiences of trauma are often embedded in colonial history and perpetuated through structural inequality, the CPTSD framework offers a more culturally congruent and clinically appropriate understanding (Atkinson, 2002; Dudgeon et al., 2014). The following sections expand upon the key domains outlined by Herman (1992), as they relate specifically to the lived realities of Aboriginal Australians.

Alterations in Affect Regulation

CPTSD is marked by chronic difficulties in regulating affective states. Emotional responses may become extreme, unpredictable, or flattened. For Aboriginal and

Torres Strait Islander peoples, whose communities have been repeatedly exposed to systemic trauma, affect dysregulation may represent a neurobiological imprint of cumulative harm passed through generations (Atkinson et al., 2010).

Self-harming behaviours, such as cutting, burning, and substance abuse, may emerge as maladaptive coping strategies to manage unresolved grief, cultural disconnection, and being emotionally overwhelmed. These expressions of distress are often misunderstood or criminalised rather than contextualised as survival responses to chronic oppression. Furthermore, sexual behaviours may also become dysregulated, either through extreme inhibition (associated with shame and body dissociation) or risky promiscuity (linked to boundary confusion and poor self-worth stemming from early relational trauma). These patterns are particularly relevant among Aboriginal individuals who have experienced child sexual abuse in institutional or foster care settings, or who have been subjected to punitive policing and child protection systems.

Alterations in Consciousness

Altered states of consciousness, including dissociation, memory fragmentation, and ruminative preoccupation, are central features of CPTSD and reflect the mind's defensive adaptation to overwhelming and prolonged trauma (Herman, 1992; Cloitre et al., 2013). Unlike the more circumscribed re-experiencing symptoms characteristic of PTSD, these alterations in CPTSD are more pervasive and diffuse, often involving a disruption in the continuity of identity and narrative.

For Aboriginal and Torres Strait Islander peoples, these disruptions in consciousness are deeply shaped by intergenerational trauma, forced child removals, and a lack of psychological safety across generations (Atkinson, 2002; Dudgeon et al., 2014). Dissociation may present as emotional numbing, depersonalisation, or blanking out during times of stress, a survival response that enables the individual to psychologically escape when physical escape is not possible (van der Kolk, 2014). Research indicates that children who experience chronic maltreatment or disconnection from attachment figures are particularly vulnerable to developing dissociative responses, which may persist into adulthood without therapeutic intervention (Putnam, 1997; Atkinson et al., 2010).

Furthermore, ruminative preoccupation – characterised by obsessive, repetitive thoughts about past trauma, perceived personal failure, or systemic injustice – is frequently reported by Aboriginal individuals who have experienced prolonged institutional abuse or the disintegration of family and cultural continuity. This mental looping often reflects both unresolved grief and a cognitive attempt to make sense of incoherent and unjust experiences (Zubrick et al., 2010; Dudgeon et al., 2017).

Amnesia or memory gaps surrounding traumatic events are also common in CPTSD. For members of the Stolen Generations and their descendants, these memory disruptions may be compounded by institutional denial, lack of access to family records, and silencing of cultural identity (Human Rights & Equal Opportunity Commission, 1997; Atkinson, 2002). These layers of historical erasure intensify the individual's difficulty in constructing a coherent life narrative, further impairing their sense of continuity and identity.

In these contexts, consciousness is not simply disrupted at the individual level; it is fragmented by systemic and generational forces. The restoration of consciousness and narrative coherence in Aboriginal clients often requires culturally informed therapeutic approaches that integrate storytelling, connection to Country, and recognition of both individual and collective trauma histories (Dudgeon et al., 2014; Gee et al., 2014).

Alterations in Self-Perception

One of the most profound impacts of complex trauma is the erosion of a coherent and positive sense of self. In CPTSD, this often manifests as chronic shame, guilt, and a belief in one's worthlessness or unlovability. For Aboriginal and Torres Strait Islander peoples, such internalised negativity may stem not only from personal trauma but also from systemic devaluation. The effects of colonisation, language loss, removal from kin, and enforced cultural silence have transmitted messages of inferiority and disposability across generations (Dudgeon et al., 2017).

Moreover, the rationalisation of perpetrator behaviour, a coping mechanism seen in many survivors of chronic abuse, further disrupts self-understanding. Aboriginal individuals who have experienced violence or neglect at the hands of authorities, institutions, or carers may internalise the belief that they were somehow responsible or deserving of their treatment. This pathological self-blame entrenches disempowerment and impedes healing unless therapeutic and community-led processes actively work to deconstruct it.

Alterations in Relationships with Others

CPTSD deeply affects the survivor's capacity for trust, intimacy, and boundary-setting. For Aboriginal people, this impact is magnified by the destruction of kinship networks, the criminalisation of cultural practices, and the ongoing removal of children from families. Relationships may be marked by hypervigilance, withdrawal, or a repeated search for a saviour, patterns that reflect deep relational wounds and the absence of safe, reliable attachment figures during childhood (Atkinson, 2002).

Additionally, repeated failures in self-protection are common. This may result from both a learned helplessness developed in environments of chronic threat and from developmental disruptions in learning how to assess and respond to danger.

For those who have cycled through institutional systems such as child welfare, juvenile justice, or incarceration, there may also be a disorganised attachment style that inhibits the formation of stable, healthy relationships. Misunderstanding these behaviours through a deficit lens, rather than viewing them as adaptive survival mechanisms, contributes to ongoing cycles of re-traumatisation and marginalisation.

Alterations in Systems of Meaning

A defining feature of CPTSD is the disruption of spiritual, cultural, and existential beliefs. For Aboriginal and Torres Strait Islander peoples, colonisation forcibly severed ties to ancestral knowledge, sacred sites, language, and dreaming, resulting in a loss not only of external freedoms but of internal frameworks for meaning making. This disconnection is compounded by systemic racism and the delegitimisation of Aboriginal worldviews within mainstream institutions.

The loss of meaning often manifests as nihilism, hopelessness, or a sense of futility. Individuals may feel alienated from cultural practices or uncertain about their identity and place in the world, not knowing where they fit within their family or community. This is especially evident among Stolen Generations survivors and their descendants, who were denied the opportunity to grow up within their cultural systems. Reconnection with cultural identity, Country, and community is therefore not only a protective factor but a necessary condition for healing. Restoring meaning through cultural renewal, storytelling, ceremony, and community leadership is vital in addressing the existential dimensions of complex trauma.

Clinical and Cultural Implications

Herman's model of CPTSD offers a critically important framework for understanding trauma in Aboriginal and Torres Strait Islander communities. While PTSD remains a useful diagnostic construct for certain individuals, its limitations become apparent when applied to trauma that is chronic, relational, collective, and systemically produced. CPTSD enables clinicians and policymakers to engage with the intersections of personal and historical trauma, moving beyond symptom reduction toward holistic, culturally grounded healing.

For Aboriginal Australians, trauma is not an isolated experience; it is embedded in the legacy of colonisation, the ongoing impacts of dispossession, and the intergenerational transmission of grief and harm. Approaching healing through a CPTSD lens facilitates culturally safe practices, encourages strengths-based engagement, and validates the survivor's story within the broader socio-political context. Interventions that embed community-led responses, cultural revitalisation, and trauma-informed care grounded in Aboriginal ways of knowing, being and doing are essential for addressing the full scope of complex trauma.

Resilience as a Collective, Culturally Grounded Response to Cumulative Harm

Exposure to adversity, whether through trauma, poverty, displacement, family violence, or parental incarceration, can leave children vulnerable to cumulative harm, particularly when protective factors are absent or undermined. While adversity may contribute to emotional fragility, it also has the potential to catalyse growth, strength, and resilience, particularly when individuals are embedded within strong social and cultural systems. For Aboriginal and Torres Strait Islander children, resilience is not conceptualised as a solely internal capacity or personality trait. Rather, it is viewed through a culturally grounded and collectivist lens, where the capacity to endure and recover from adversity is nurtured through connections to kin, culture, community, and Country (Young et al., 2017; Dobia et al., 2014).

Aboriginal communities consistently emphasise the significance of Aboriginal ways of knowing, being, and doing in the development and maintenance of resilience among children (Young et al., 2017). This epistemology acknowledges that healing and strength arise from relational connections, cultural identity, and a sense of belonging to one's ancestral land and community. Resilience is therefore deeply relational and situated within a collective cultural identity, rather than an individualised psychological process. Such a view directly challenges Western constructs that frame resilience as a personal trait or behavioural adaptation, instead locating it within interconnected systems of care, spirituality, and intergenerational knowledge.

Protective factors identified across the literature include strong kinship networks, cultural continuity, and community connectedness, particularly in contexts where children experience adversity in their immediate environment, such as the incarceration of a parent, family violence, or state intervention through child protection systems (Kelly et al., 2009; Walker et al., 2014). These protective mechanisms are especially vital when statutory systems remove children from their biological families or when children are exposed to cumulative patterns of harm. Supportive adults, especially elders, extended family members, and respected community figures, play a central role in buffering the impact of adversity by transmitting cultural knowledge, facilitating belonging, and modelling resilience through storytelling, cultural practices, and ceremonies (Gee et al., 2014; Young et al., 2017).

The importance of culturally safe spaces, whether within extended family households, Aboriginal-run community organisations, or inclusive educational environments, cannot be overstated. These settings enable children to remain connected to their identity and community and mitigate the effects of cultural loss and intergenerational trauma. When Aboriginal and Torres Strait Islander children are displaced from such protective networks, their capacity for resilience is significantly compromised (SNAICC, 2019).

Kelly et al. (2009) argue that the emotional well-being and mental health of Aboriginal children and families are most effectively supported through culturally congruent models of care, which may fundamentally diverge from standardised Western practices. Healing is often best facilitated within a context of community, family, and on-Country experiences, where traditional knowledge systems and spiritual connections guide recovery. This challenges dominant paradigms of trauma recovery and mental health intervention, which are frequently grounded in individualistic and clinical models that can inadvertently pathologise or marginalise Aboriginal ways of healing.

Resilience-building for Aboriginal and Torres Strait Islander children exposed to cumulative harm must therefore be underpinned by principles of self-determination, cultural continuity, and relational healing. Government and non-government services that fail to integrate these cultural imperatives risk perpetuating further harm through systems of disconnection and assimilation. Accordingly, efforts to foster resilience must be led by Aboriginal communities themselves and be grounded in culturally safe, trauma-informed, and decolonising frameworks.

Measuring Accumulation: The Cumulative Experiences Index – Culturally Responsive Tool (CEI-CR)

Throughout the development of the CEI, tool the research team remained critically aware of the limitations identified during the pilot phase, particularly the absence of representation from key population groups. Notably, the initial design did not adequately include the perspectives and lived experiences of Aboriginal and Torres Strait Islander children, despite their significant over-representation in both the child protection and youth justice systems. Although this paper presents a theoretical framework for the CEI and proposes its potential application in future pilot studies, deliberate attention has been given to ensuring that the unique vulnerabilities of First Nations children are acknowledged. Equally important is the recognition of the resilience embedded within Aboriginal and Torres Strait Islander communities and the resilience that has been forged through generations of systemic adversity, cultural dislocation, and ongoing marginalisation. The framework aims to be both inclusive and responsive to the cultural, historical, and structural factors that shape cumulative harm and healing within these communities.

An extensive process was undertaken that examined the original CEI, the resilience factors as explained by Young et al., (2017) and the many elements that signify patterns of adversity that have continued to plague Aboriginal and Torress strait Islander families across multiple generations since colonisation. Consultation with individual Indigenous folks, families and family groups occurred during the development and evolution of the Cumulative Experiences Index-Culturally Responsive Tool (CEI-CR) (Collier & Bryce, 2023) has been developed. As with the original CEI, the CEI-CR is designed to complement existing tools rather than being used in isolation or replacing existing tools. It is a tool to be used as part of a toolbox, assisting practitioners to systematically identify contextual information that is frequently missing from a child's profile.

The development of the CEI-CR draws upon established adverse experience scoring systems, notably the MMCS (Barnett et al., 1993) and the ACEs checklist (Felitti et al., 1998). While the MMCS served as a foundational instrument in the original CEI pilot, it was added to in the evolution of the CEI-CR to better reflect the cultural, structural, and intergenerational realities faced by Aboriginal and Torres Strait Islander families. This adaptation was guided by the recognition that standardised trauma measurement tools often fail to capture the contextualised and collective experiences of harm within First Nations communities. As such, the CEI-CR includes additional domains that are highly relevant to Aboriginal and Torres Strait Islander children and parents, including: chronic physical health complaints in both parent and child; welfare dependency; experiences of racism and marginalisation; geographic isolation due to residence in regional, rural, or remote areas; statutory system involvement (e.g., child protection, justice, housing); and the absence or disruption of cultural protocols, practices, spirituality, and kinship connections. Furthermore, it explicitly recognises the enduring impact of intergenerational trauma, including familial ties to the Stolen Generations. These culturally and historically situated domains aim to ensure that the CEI-CR is not only clinically robust but also culturally responsive, providing a more accurate and meaningful tool for understanding cumulative harm within Aboriginal and Torres Strait Islander contexts.

In the development of the CEI-CR, deliberate and culturally respectful consideration was given to the multifaceted elements of resilience that Aboriginal and Torres Strait Islander children have cultivated across generations. These strengths have emerged in response to the profound adversities endured by their ancestors, including colonisation, forced removals, systemic discrimination, and cultural disruption. The resilience observed today reflects intergenerational adaptation, cultural continuity, and collective strength. These elements, summarised in the table below, are intended to assist practitioners in contextualising a child's presentation not only in terms of risk or adversity but also within the framework of normative development. This includes understanding the typical age-related milestones that unfold predictably across developmental domains, including cognitive, emotional, physical, and social, while recognising how cultural and historical contexts shape each child's developmental trajectory.

Table 2. Childhood resilience factors to build resilience in aboriginal children

	Childhood Resilience Factors to build resilience in Aboriginal children (Adapted from Young et al., 2017)										
Resilience Factor	Normative Development (ND) Demonstrate Empathy	ND- Take Pride in Appearance	ND – Demonstrate respect for self & others	ND – Maintain Pro-social Relationships	ND – Attend School, Value Education	ND – Alcohol & Drug Free	Possess Inner Fortitude Strong work ethic, desire to achieve goals	Access to extended family members modelling healthy relationships and behaviours	Awareness of heritage & connection to cultural practices (a strong cultural self-concept)	Access to community Safeguards – camps, mentors, homework centres, sports	Demonstrate Self-regulation
Child's Name											

The use of culturally sensitive assessment tools in child protection practice is critical to ensuring equitable, respectful, and effective engagement with Aboriginal and Torres Strait Islander children and families. Mainstream tools often fail to account for the complex interplay of intergenerational trauma, cultural identity, kinship systems, and community connection that underpin wellbeing in First Nations contexts (Janca et al., 2015). As a result, assessments based solely on Western constructs of harm and parenting risk misinterpret cultural practices, contributing to the ongoing overrepresentation of Aboriginal children in statutory care. Tools such as the Victorian Aboriginal Child and Community Agency (VACCA) Kinship Assessment Guide, the Centre of Best Practice in Aboriginal and Torres Strait Islander Suicide Prevention (CBPATSISP)'s culturally validated screening instruments, and the Children and Family Intensive Support (CaFIS) Cultural Safety Framework provide practitioners with culturally informed approaches to identifying harm, strengths, and healing pathways. Their use enables child protection systems to move beyond deficit-based models toward frameworks grounded in self-determination, cultural continuity, and relational resilience. Embedding these tools into standard practice is essential for upholding the rights of Aboriginal and Torres Strait Islander children to grow up safely, connected to kin, culture, and Country. As with the original CEI, the CEI-CR is not intended to be a holistic assessment to be used in isolation as an assessment of risk, nor is it intended to replace or reduce the value of specific abuse type assessment and scoring tools or the use of structured decision making tools that are used by statutory officers to assess safety and future risk.

The CEI-CR is designed to be an additional information-gathering instrument to support targeted capacity-building for the purpose of family preservation and reunification. It does not function as a predictive risk assessment or a mechanism for justifying child removal from the family of origin. Rather than adopting a deficit-based orientation, the tool seeks to capture contextual factors and relational dynamics that may be impacting family functioning. The data collected is used to inform strengths-based, culturally responsive interventions aimed at enhancing parenting capacity, household stability, and child wellbeing. In particular, the tool is grounded in the principles of resilience in First Nations children, recognising that effective intervention must be informed by cultural identity, kinship structures, and intergenerational healing. It is designed to support a holistic and relational understanding of family strengths and challenges, to empower families to remain safely connected wherever possible.

CONCLUSION

There is extensive literature underscoring the need for practitioners to be guided by trauma-informed frameworks and structured tools that enable the recognition of accumulated risk and its associated harm (Bromfield et al., 2007). Such guidance is vital not only for accurate assessment but also for the development of effective intervention strategies. The CEI-CR reflects this principle by shifting away from an incident-based view of child maltreatment and instead adopting a holistic approach that captures the broader spectrum of adversity a child has experienced over time.

Critically, the CEI-CR incorporates a culturally responsive lens, acknowledging that a child's cultural identity and experiences of connection or disconnection from culture, Country, and community can significantly shape the manifestation and impact of trauma. This approach enables a more nuanced understanding of harm, particularly for Aboriginal and Torres Strait Islander children, who are disproportionately represented in child protection and justice systems. By recognising the role of systemic disadvantage and cultural dislocation as contributing factors, this tool addresses gaps often overlooked by standardised assessment models.

Furthermore, the CEI-CR facilitates the identification of children who may have experienced low to moderate levels of harm across multiple domains, yet who are frequently underserved because their experiences do not meet statutory thresholds for intervention. By making visible the accumulation of risk factors over time, the tool equips clinicians with a structured, evidence-informed process for recognising cumulative harm. The intention is that this tool will enable more accurate formulation of clinical needs and support the planning of timely, targeted, and culturally appropriate interventions, ultimately promoting better outcomes for vulnerable Aboriginal children and their families.

The theoretical foundation of the CEI-CR has been informed by a review of culturally grounded research. This collaborative and culturally responsive development process acknowledges the importance of embedding Indigenous knowledge and perspectives in tools intended to assess and respond to trauma within Aboriginal and Torres Strait Islander communities.

The original evaluation of the CEI tool (Bryce et al., 2024) highlighted its potential to enhance clinical decision-making by offering a structured means to assess not only risk and harm but also protective factors over time. The CEI-CR builds upon this promise by aiming to capture the nuanced and often lower-level but chronic patterns of neglect and abuse that can persist below statutory thresholds yet cause significant cumulative harm. These children frequently present with complex and high-support needs as a result of enduring prolonged adversity. The CEI-CR thus holds considerable potential as a culturally responsive and clinically valid tool to support earlier identification, tailored intervention, and, ultimately, the prevention of ongoing cycles of maltreatment among Aboriginal and Torres Strait Islander children.

Practice Implications and Next Steps

Having developed a tool to measures the cumulative harmful experiences of a target population, the next step is to formulate a pilot study. The aim of the pilot study will be to determine whether the CEI-CR tool accurately and adequately measures cumulative harm, providing a validated measure for Aboriginal and Torres Strait Islander children. This will require involvement from services that work closely with Aboriginal and Torres Strait Islander children, that employ Aboriginal and Torres Strait Islander staff members, and that are invested in using the tool. The construct validity measures need to be carefully considered as comparison tools and need to be deemed culturally appropriate. Research ethics approval will also need to be obtained.

REFERENCES

Aguiar, W., & Halseth, R. (2015). *Aboriginal peoples and historic trauma: The processes of intergenerational transmission*. National Collaborating Centre for Aboriginal Health.

Arney, F., Iannos, M., Chong, A., McDougall, S., & Parkinson, S. (2015). *Enhancing the implementation of the Aboriginal and Torres Strait Islander Child Placement Principle: Policy and practice considerations*. CFCA Paper No. 34. Australian Institute of Family Studies.

Atkinson, J. (2002). *Trauma trails, recreating song lines: The transgenerational effects of trauma in Indigenous Australia*. Spinifex Press.

Atkinson, J. (2013). *Trauma-informed services and trauma-specific care for Indigenous Australian children*. Closing the Gap Clearinghouse.

Atkinson, J., Nelson, J., & Atkinson, C. (2010). Trauma, transgenerational transfer and effects on community wellbeing. In N. Purdie, P. Dudgeon, & R. Walker (Eds.), *Working together: Aboriginal and Torres Strait Islander mental health and wellbeing principles and practice* (pp. 135–144). Commonwealth of Australia.

Australian Institute of Health and Welfare. (2020). *Crossover children: Vulnerabilities in youth justice supervision.* Canberra: AIHW Australian Institute of Criminology (AIC). (2022). *Crossover kids: Youth justice involvement among children known to child protection.* Canberra: AIC. *Research Reports (Montgomery).*

Australian Institute of Health and Welfare. (2023). *The health of people in Australia's prisons 2022*. Australian Government.

Australian Institute of Health and Welfare (AIHW). (2023). *Child Protection Australia 2021–22*. Australian Government. https://www.aihw.gov.au/reports/child-protection/child-protection-australia-2021-22

Australian Institute of Health and Welfare (AIHW). (2024). *Child protection Australia 2021–22 web report* (catalogue number CWS 92). Australian Government. www.aihw.gov.au/getmedia/2cecbc62-8c65-4031-a6df-5fec9422b0cf/child-protection-australia-2021-22.pdf?v=20240516104741&inline=true

Australian Law Reform Commission. (2018). *Pathways to justice – Inquiry into the incarceration rate of Aboriginal and Torres Strait Islander peoples (ALRC Report 133)*. Australian Government. https://www.alrc.gov.au/publication/pathways-to-justice-inquiry-into-the-incarceration-rate-of-aboriginal-and-torres-strait-islander-peoples-alrc-report-133/

Barnett, D., Manly, J. T., & Cicchetti, D. (1993). Defining child maltreatment: The interface between policy and research. In Cicchetti, D., & Toth, S. L. (Eds.), *Child abuse, child development, and social policy* (pp. 7–73). Ablex Publishing.

Bombay, A., Matheson, K., & Anisman, H. (2009). Intergenerational trauma: Convergence of multiple processes among First Nations peoples in Canada. *Journal of Aboriginal Health*, *5*(3), 6–47.

Booris, O., & Way, O. (2019). *Final report*. ACT Government.

Bromfield, L. M., Gillingham, P., & Higgins, D. J. (2007). Cumulative harm: A conceptual framework for child protection. *Australian Social Work*, *60*(2), 258–268. DOI: 10.1080/03124070701323847

Bryant-Davis, T. (2007). Healing requires recognition: The case for race-based traumatic stress. *The Counseling Psychologist*, *35*(1), 135–143. DOI: 10.1177/0011000006295152

Bryce, I. (2020). *Cumulative harm and the need for a restorative framework in child protection*. University of Southern Queensland.

Bryce, I., Collier, S., Harris, L., Higgins, D., & Toohey, J. (2024). Measuring accumulation: Constructing a tool for evaluating cumulative harm in children engaged with an intensive family support service. *Child Abuse Review*, *33*(5), e2897. DOI: 10.1002/car.2897

Centre of Best Practice in Aboriginal and Torres Strait Islander Suicide Prevention. (n.d.). *Best practice screening and assessment tools*. University of Western Australia. https://cbpatsisp.com.au/clearing-house/best-practice-screening-assessment/

Cloitre, M., Shevlin, M., Brewin, C. R., Bisson, J. I., Roberts, N. P., Maercker, A., & Hyland, P. (2013). Evidence for the coherence and integrity of the ICD-11 diagnostic construct of complex post-traumatic stress disorder: A latent profile analysis. *European Journal of Psychotraumatology*, *4*(1), 20706. Advance online publication. DOI: 10.3402/ejpt.v4i0.20706 PMID: 23687563

Commonwealth of Australia. (1991). *Royal Commission into Aboriginal Deaths in Custody: National Report (Vols. 1–5)*. Australian Government Publishing Service. https://www.nla.gov.au/collections/aboriginal-deaths-in-custody

Commonwealth of Australia. (2017). *Royal Commission into the Protection and Detention of Children in the Northern Territory: Final Report (Vols. 1–4)*. Australian Government. https://www.royalcommission.gov.au/child-detention

Cunneen, C. (2008). Understanding restorative justice through the lens of critical criminology. In Shoham, S. G., Knepper, P., & Kett, M. (Eds.), *International handbook of penology and criminal justice* (pp. 1095–1128). CRC Press.

Daniel, B., Taylor, J., & Scott, J. (2011). *Recognizing and helping the neglected child: Evidence-based practice for assessment and intervention.* Jessica Kingsley Publishers Department of Social Services. (2020). *Cultural safety and responsiveness: Child and Family Intensive Support (CaFIS) program guidelines – Annex 3C.* Australian Government. https://www.dss.gov.au/system/files/resources/cafis_3c_-_cultural_safety_and_responsiveness.pdf

Dobia, B., Bodkin-Andrews, G., Parada, R., O'Rourke, V., Gilbert, S., Daley, A., & Roffey, S. (2014). *The Aboriginal Girls Circle: Promoting resilience and cultural connectedness* (Pilot project report). Western Sydney University.

Dudgeon, P., Bray, A., D'Costa, B., & Walker, R. (2017). Decolonising psychology: Validating social and emotional wellbeing. *Australian Psychologist, 52*(4), 316–325. DOI: 10.1111/ap.12294

Dudgeon, P., Milroy, H., & Walker, R. (Eds.). (2014). *Working together: Aboriginal and Torres Strait Islander mental health and wellbeing principles and practice* (2nd ed.). Commonwealth of Australia.

Evans-Campbell, T. (2008). Historical trauma in American Indian/Native Alaskan communities: A multilevel framework for exploring impacts on individuals, families, and communities. *Journal of Interpersonal Violence, 23*, 316. DOI: 10.1177/0886260507312290 PMID: 18245571

Felitti, V. J., Anda, R. F., Nordenberg, D., Williamson, D. F., Spitz, A. M., Edwards, V., Koss, M. P., & Marks, J. S. (1998). Relationship of childhood abuse and household dysfunction to many of the leading causes of death in adults. *American Journal of Preventive Medicine, 14*(4), 245–258. DOI: 10.1016/S0749-3797(98)00017-8 PMID: 9635069

Gee, G., Dudgeon, P., Schultz, C., Hart, A., & Kelly, K. (2014). Aboriginal and Torres Strait Islander social and emotional wellbeing. In Dudgeon, P., Milroy, H., & Walker, R. (Eds.), *Working together: Aboriginal and Torres Strait Islander mental health and wellbeing principles and practice* (2nd ed., pp. 55–68). Department of the Prime Minister and Cabinet.

Gone, J. P. (2013). Redressing First Nations historical trauma: Theorizing mechanisms for indigenous culture as mental health treatment. *Transcultural Psychiatry, 50*(5), 683–706. DOI: 10.1177/1363461513487669 PMID: 23715822

Herman, J. L. (1992). Complex PTSD: A syndrome in survivors of prolonged and repeated trauma. *Journal of Traumatic Stress*, *5*(3), 377–389. DOI: 10.1002/jts.2490050305

Human Rights and Equal Opportunity Commission (HREOC). (1997). *Bringing them home: Report of the National Inquiry into the Separation of Aboriginal and Torres Strait Islander Children from Their Families*. Commonwealth of Australia. https://humanrights.gov.au/our-work/bringing-them-home-report-1997

Janca, A., Lyons, Z., Balaratnasingam, S., Parfitt, D., Davison, S., Laugharne, J., & Winthrop, Z. (2015). Here and Now Aboriginal Assessment (HANAA): Background, development and preliminary evaluation of a culturally appropriate screening tool. *Australasian Psychiatry*, *23*(3), 287–292. DOI: 10.1177/1039856215584514 PMID: 25944764

Kelly, K., Dudgeon, P., Gee, G., & Glaskin, B. (2009). Living on the edge: Social and emotional wellbeing risk and protective factors for serious psychological distress among Aboriginal and Torres Strait Islander people. In N. Purdie, P. Dudgeon, & R. Walker (Eds.), *Working together: Aboriginal and Torres Strait Islander mental health and wellbeing principles and practice* (pp. 87–95). Commonwealth of Australia.

Long, M., & Stephen, R. (2011). Rethinking the 'best interests' of the child: Voices from Aboriginal child and family welfare practitioners. *Australian Social Work*, *64*(1), 96–112. DOI: 10.1080/0312407X.2010.535544

Mathews, B., Pacella, R., Dunne, M. P., Simunovic, M., & Marston, C. (2023). *The Australian Child Maltreatment Study, Final Report*. Queensland University of Technology

McDowall, J. J. (2019). *Out-of-home care in Australia: Children and young people's views after five years of National Standards*. CREATE Foundation. https://create.org.au

Menzies, P. (2010). Intergenerational trauma from a mental health perspective. *Native Social Work Journal*, *7*, 63–85.

National Office for Child Safety. SNAICC, & VACCA. (2021). *Keeping our kids safe: Cultural safety and the national principles for child safe organisations*. National Office for Child Safety. www.childsafety.gov.au/resources/keeping-our-kids-safe

NSW Bureau of Crime Statistics and Research. (2024). *The involvement of young people aged 10 to 13 years in the NSW criminal justice system*. NSW Government.

Ralph, S., & Ryan, K. (2017). Addressing the mental health gap in working with Indigenous youth: Some considerations for non-Indigenous psychologists working with Indigenous youth. *Australian Psychologist, 52*(4), 288–298. DOI: 10.1111/ap.12287

Rémond, M., Zeki, R., Austin, K., Bowman, J., Galouzis, J., Stewart, K.-A., & Sullivan, E. (2023). *Intergenerational incarceration in New South Wales: Characteristics of people in prison experiencing parental imprisonment* (Trends & Issues in Crime and Criminal Justice No. 663). Australian Institute of Criminology.

Royal Commission into the Protection and Detention of Children in the Northern Territory. (2017). *Final report.* Australian Government. https://childdetentionnt.royalcommission.gov.au

Scott, D. (2014). *Intervening to improve life chances for vulnerable children: The importance of culturally appropriate assessment tools.* Child Family Community Australia.

SNAICC – Secretariat of National Aboriginal and Islander Child Care. (2019). *The family matters report 2019: Measuring trends to turn the tide on the over-representation of Aboriginal and Torres Strait Islander children in out-of-home care in Australia.* SNAICC.

SNAICC – Secretariat of National Aboriginal and Islander Child Care. (2023). *Family Matters Report 2023.* SNAICC. https://www.familymatters.org.au

Snowball, L. (2009). *Diversion of Aboriginal youth from juvenile justice system.* NSW Bureau of Crime Statistics and Research. https://www.bocsar.nsw.gov.au/

The Healing Foundation. (2016). *Bringing them home 20 years on.* https://healingfoundation.org.au

The Healing Foundation. (2025). *Are you waiting for us to die? The unfinished business of bringing them home.*

Tilbury, C. (2009). The over-representation of Indigenous children in the Australian child welfare system. *International Journal of Social Welfare, 18*(1), 57–64. DOI: 10.1111/j.1468-2397.2008.00577.x

Victorian Aboriginal Child Care Agency (VACCA). (2010). *Assessing kinship care for Aboriginal children: A practice guide for child protection practitioners.* Victorian Government Department of Human Services. https://www.cpmanual.vic.gov.au/sites/default/files/Asess_kc_aboriginal_chn_cpguide%202304_0.pdf

Victorian Sentencing Advisory Council. (2020). *Crossover kids: Vulnerable children in the youth justice system (Report 1 & 2)*. https://www.sentencingcouncil.vic.gov.au/

Walker, R., Schultz, C., & Sonn, C. (2014). Cultural competence: Transforming policy, services, programs and practice. In Dudgeon, P., Milroy, H., & Walker, R. (Eds.), *Working together: Aboriginal and Torres Strait Islander mental health and wellbeing principles and practice* (2nd ed., pp. 195–220). Department of the Prime Minister and Cabinet.

Yellow Horse Brave Heart, M. (2003). The historical trauma response among natives and its relationship with substance abuse: A Lakota illustration. *Journal of Psychoactive Drugs*, *35*(1), 7–13. DOI: 10.1080/02791072.2003.10399988 PMID: 12733753

Yoorrook Justice Commission. (2023). *Yoorrook for justice: Report into Victoria's child protection and criminal justice systems*. yoorrookforjustice.org.au/wp-content/uploads/2023/08/Yoorrook-for-justice-report.pdf

Young, C., Craig, J. C., Clapham, K., Banks, S., & Williamson, A. (2017). Perspectives on childhood resilience among the Aboriginal community: An interview study. *Australian and New Zealand Journal of Public Health*, *41*(4), 405–410. DOI: 10.1111/1753-6405.12681 PMID: 28712160

Zubrick, S. R., Shepherd, C. C., Dudgeon, P., Gee, G., Paradies, Y., Scrine, C., & Walker, R. (2010). Social determinants of Aboriginal and Torres Strait Islander social and emotional wellbeing. In N. Purdie, P. Dudgeon, & R. Walker (Eds.), *Working together: Aboriginal and Torres Strait Islander mental health and wellbeing principles and practice* (pp. 75–90). Commonwealth of Australia.

Chapter 6
Applying Betrayal Trauma Theory to Addressing Intergenerationally and Systemically Perpetrated Trauma

Maria-Ernestina Christl
https://orcid.org/0000-0003-1718-8583
University of Denver, USA

Adi Rosenthal
University of Denver, USA

Anne P. DePrince
University of Denver, USA

ABSTRACT

Betrayal trauma theory offers an important framework for preventing and responding to cumulative adverse childhood experiences. From its inception, betrayal trauma theory has highlighted the importance of the context in which trauma occurs, with applications ranging from parent-child relationships and romantic relationships to the role of institutions in shaping traumatic experiences. This chapter will address how utilizing betrayal trauma theory can support trauma-informed approaches to protecting children by contextualizing the range of diverse relationships that surround interpersonal trauma and their effects on traumatic experiences and outcomes. Furthermore, we will discuss how researchers and providers at the individual level and at the systemic level can better understand and address the accumulation of

DOI: 10.4018/979-8-3373-4064-7.ch006

betrayals over lifetimes, beginning in childhood and perpetuated via intergenerational transmissions of trauma, through trauma-informed and multidisciplinary approaches to protecting children and their families.

INTRODUCTION

Betrayal trauma theory offers an important framework for preventing and responding to cumulative adverse childhood experiences (ACEs). From its inception, betrayal trauma theory has highlighted the importance of the relational context in which trauma occurs, with applications ranging from parent-child relationships and romantic relationships to the role of institutions and intracultural pressures in shaping human response to traumatic experiences. Betrayal trauma theory can support trauma-informed approaches to protecting children by contextualizing the range of diverse relationships that surround interpersonal trauma and their effects on traumatic experiences and outcomes.

When she introduced betrayal trauma theory, Jennifer Freyd (1996) articulated the importance of the interpersonal nature of trauma, especially when perpetrated by someone close to the victim, drawing from attachment theory (Bowlby, 1982; Bowlby 1988; Ainsworth & Bowlby, 1991; Ainsworth, 1973) and social contracts (Cosmides, 1989). Freyd posited that dependence in the abusive relationship contributed to survival pressures to minimize awareness of abuse to maintain necessary relationships. First applied to the parent-child relationship, children's innate dependence on their caregivers results in a high betrayal when caregivers abuse or neglect their children. In fact, high betrayal traumas have been linked with more severe psychological symptoms, physical health issues (Goldsmith et al., 2012), and distorted expectations of interpersonal relationships (DePrince et al., 2009). Betrayal trauma theory has since been applied to romantic relationships, where financial, emotional, social, and functional dependence increases survivors' seemingly counterintuitive responses to intimate partner violence, such as remaining in abusive relationships. Furthermore, betrayal trauma theory has also been applied to other relationships such as individuals' relationships with institutions and minoritized individuals' relationships to within group members and oppression.

Preventing and responding to adverse childhood experiences requires understanding the social and intergenerational context in which adverse childhood experiences occur to better protect and support children and families – and betrayal trauma theory offers a critical framework for understanding those contexts. Without acknowledging and addressing these factors, critical intervention points are lost, and the perpetuation of adverse childhood experiences is maintained not only by perpetrators but also by providers and systems designed to mitigate risk and harm.

Therefore, this chapter applies a betrayal trauma theory lens to addressing cumulative adverse childhood experiences by contextualizing traumatic experiences through individuals' relationships with perpetrators at the individual and institutional level by first describing the building blocks of betrayal trauma theory within a variety of relationships. Next, we apply betrayal trauma theory to understanding cumulative harm and chronic exposure to adverse childhood experiences. Furthermore, we will discuss the implications of betrayal trauma theory as they relate to trauma-informed prevention and responses. Finally, we will explore how researchers and providers at the individual level and at the systemic level can better understand and address the accumulation of betrayals over lifetimes, beginning in childhood and perpetuated via intergenerational transmissions of trauma, through trauma-informed and multidisciplinary approaches to protecting children and their families.

THE BUILDING BLOCKS OF BETRAYAL TRAUMA THEORY

Betrayal trauma theory draws from attachment theory (Bowlby, 1969, 1980), which posits that infants ensure survival by developing and maintaining attachment to a caregiver. This attachment serves two critical functions. First, the caregiver serves as protection from a variety of threats of harm (e.g., protecting the child from hungry predators, protecting them from abusive perpetrators) and an undeniable source of life-sustaining resources (e.g., shelter from the elements, provision of nourishment). This innate dependence in children forms the foundation of their attachment to their caregivers as children would not survive without the support of their caregivers.

Second, caregivers serve as a "secure base" that provides the child with a safe harbor as the child explores their environment. As children develop, a crucial aspect of their development requires their ability to interact and learn about the world around them. Indeed, children's brains develop synaptic connections during their three years of life at an incredible rate. The following 10 to 12 years, until around age 15, the brain selectively reduces these synapses largely in part due to lived experiences (Haartsen et al., 2016; Huttenlocher, 1984). Regardless of nature of these lived experiences, the child's brain is programmed for survival best suited for its environment. Caregivers play a major role in these formative experiences, ideally, noticing and understanding their child's cue and responding to the child's need with warmth and structure. For example, if a child is at a park with their caregiver and is startled by an unexpected loud sound (i.e., a loud dog barking), the child may run to their secure base, their attuned and responsive caregiver, and/or begin crying as a signal for the parent to come to the child's aid. A well-attuned and responsive caregiver will notice their child's cues and respond in a way that ensures and communicates safety to the child consistently. Of course, it is impossible to notice and respond to every cue; and research has demonstrated that even parent-child relationships with low-risk are often not in synchrony with their child (Tronick & Cohen, 1989). However, when the secure base is in itself the source of fear and harm, the child faces irreconcilable urges: create distance between themselves and the threat and approach their attachment figure for safety and comfort.

Ainsworth and colleagues' work with children identified three styles of attachment (i.e., secure attachment, anxious-avoidant attachment, and anxious-ambivalent attachment). Secure attachment differs from anxious-avoidant and anxious-ambivalent attachment in that securely attached individuals tend to have a positive and healthy emotional bond that is characterized by trust and the ability to express their emotions. Children with secure attachment often become adults who are comfortable and capable of navigating healthy interpersonal relationships as well as regulating their emotions in adaptive ways. In contrast, children with insecure attachment (i.e., anxious-avoidant, anxious-ambivalent), grow up to have more difficulties navigating intimate relationships, whether by fearing abandonment and requiring frequent reassurance or by avoiding emotional intimacy and becoming overly self-reliant. Building on this work, a fourth group of infants emerged demonstrating an approach-avoidance attachment pattern, or disorganized attachment (Main & Solomon, 1990). This pattern of insecure and disorganized attachment is characterized by both anxious and avoidant behaviors that often seem confusing or hard to explain. For example, a child who has disorganized attachment may begin running to their caregiver when fearful and then freeze mid-run and run away from the parent. This style of attachment implies a lack of coherence in the child's behaviors, exhibiting both avoidant and anxious behaviors, and has been found to be present in half to more than three quarters of maltreated children (Cicchetti & Barnett, 1991; Carlson et al., 1989; Barnett et al., 1999; Beeghly & Cicchetti, 1994; Morton & Browne, 1998; Cyr et al., 2010), which has been linked to long-term consequences. Longitudinal studies have found that disorganized attachment at 18 months of age is related to behavioral problems beginning in preschool through high school (Carlson, 1998; Lyons-Ruth et al., 1997; Fearon et al., 2010) as well as psychopathology and dissociative symptoms in adolescence (Carlson, 1998).

Early childhood experiences, especially caregiver behaviors, contribute to individuals' overall ability to relate to others and teaches children how to engage with their environment in such a way to ensure survival. Betrayal trauma theory builds upon attachment theory to understand individuals' responses to trauma and has provided a theoretical framework that helps us understand a variety of responses and outcomes after trauma, especially counterintuitive responses to abuse. Betrayal trauma theory proposes that abuse that occurs within an attachment relationship, such as a parent-child relationship or romantic relationship, is unique to abuse that occurs outside of an attachment relationship, such as abuse perpetrated by a stranger, for example. Betrayal trauma theory recognizes that traumatic experiences vary in the degree to which they involve social betrayal by another person on which the victim depends. For instance, many natural disasters are relatively low in betrayal. Meanwhile, abuse and violence perpetrated by a trusted other, such as a primary caregiver, is relatively high in betrayal. By focusing on the social context of the trauma, betrayal trauma theory offers a unique perspective (for a review, see DePrince & Freyd, 2002). Furthermore, betrayal trauma theory invites survivors, providers, and researchers to emphasize the adaptive quality of a range of responses to trauma, providing opportunities to empower survivors rather than engage in victim-blaming.

Betrayal trauma theory was first proposed to offer an explanation for survivors' experiences of unawareness, minimization, or forgetting of high betrayal traumas via cognitive mechanisms. "Betrayal trauma theory implicates dissociation as a possible mechanism in blocking information about or knowledge of the trauma…Betrayal trauma theory suggests that dissociations or disconnections may occur between normally connected aspects of processing and memory" (DePrince & Freyd, 2008), resulting in unawareness or forgetting of the trauma. In other words, a lack of integration in the processing of threat information may help the victim to maintain the necessary attachment to the perpetrator. Over time, empirical tests of this core assumption of betrayal trauma theory have shown that survivors of high-betrayal traumas are more likely to report dissociation compared to those who experienced low-betrayal traumas or non-interpersonal trauma (Freyd et al., 2005; Goldsmith et al., 2012; Hulette et al., 2008). Furthermore, individuals who have experienced high betrayal trauma have also been shown to have more difficulties detecting betrayals in relationships (e.g., DePrince, 2005).

Typically, detecting betrayals in social relationships is incredibly important to human beings, who rely on coordination and cooperation for survival. Social contracts theory (Cosmides, 1989) suggested that humans have evolved to be able to detect violations of social contracts. It is adaptive to notice when another individual has violated a social contract because it allows one to withdraw from the relationship or confront the offender. Betrayal trauma theory, however, pointed out that detecting betrayal may not be adaptive in the short-run for those experiencing abuse at the hands of someone they depend on for survival. Instead, noticing violations of the social contract and responding to them by withdrawing or fighting back could be counterproductive or even dangerous when maintaining the relationship is necessary for survival. Freyd coined the term "betrayal blindness" to refer to minimizing awareness, knowledge, or memory of abuse in necessary-but-abusive relationships. As she and others would go on to discover, betrayal blindness can be broadened beyond the original abusive relationship to other betrayals with implications for revictimization risk, for instance (DePrince, 2005).

Extending Betrayal Trauma Theory

Betrayal trauma theory was initially developed and studied in the context of understanding abuse in parent-child relationships. Over time, the theory has also been applied and examined in the context of a variety of other social contexts as researchers and clinicians explored social dependence and violations in other kinds of relationships, including romantic. Although the parent-child relationship is heavily influential and sets the stage for other relationships, research has demonstrated that the presence of a safe, stable, and nurturing relationship can help buffer the effects of childhood maltreatment (Afifi & MacMillan, 2011; Meng et al., 2018), underscoring the importance of social relationships and dependence.

Romantic Relationships

Like attachment theory, betrayal trauma theory was initially applied to parent-child relationships and then was extended to romantic relationships. Betrayal trauma theory provides explanations for counterintuitive responses to abuse or violence from romantic partners, such as staying with an abusive partner. While dependence in adult relationships may seem less obvious compared to parent-child relationships, researchers studying intimate partner violence have identified several forms of dependence in adulthood, including economic, structural, emotional, and functional dependence (Bornstein, 2006; Gelles, 1976; Kalmuss & Straus, 1982; Strube & Barbour, 1983; Strube & Barbour, 1984).

Economic dependence refers to the degree to which an individual relies on the offender's income and has been linked with risk for IPV and remaining in an abusive relationship (Anderson & Saunders, 2003; Kim & Gray, 2008; Gelles, 1976; Woffordt et al., 1994). Similarly, increased economic dependence has been found to be associated with increased likelihood of returning to an abusive relationship (Rusbult & Martz, 1995). Another study found that both subjective and objective ratings of economic dependence were linked to victimization (Kalmuss & Strauss, 1982; Strube & Barbour, 1983; Strube & Barbour, 1984). Furthermore, Bornstein (2006) found a bidirectional relationship between financial dependence and abuse such that a more financially dependent woman is more likely to continue in an abusive relationship than a more economically independent woman, and abuse in a relationship is positively associated with financial dependence. In addition to economic disparity between partners leading to economic dependence, economic dependence can also occur if the perpetrator uses threats or intimidation to take control over finances (Scott et al., 2002)

Structural dependence refers to logistical restrictions that create obstacles to ending the relationship such as marriage, children, or living together. Women who reported that they have nowhere else to go if they leave the abuser, have been found to be more likely to remain in the abusive relationship (Strube & Barbour, 1983, 1984). Strube and Barbour (1983, 1984) also found that women were less likely to have left the abuser at follow-up if she had reported being married to the abuser and having children to consider at the initial intake. Stahly (2000) identified that victims of abuse "may fear loss of the children, either through custody proceedings or through kidnapping by the abuser," which may lead the victim to maintain the relationship (pg. 244). Another form of structural dependence is immigration status. If an individual's authorized immigration status is determined by their relationship with a perpetrator, this dependence can also impact decisions to exit a relationship. Similarly, this can be used as a threat against the individual (Erez & Gregory, 2009).

Emotional dependence refers to reliance on a partner for support and emotional care regardless of if an individual is able to meet these needs independently (Bornstein 1992, 1993). Emotional dependence is measured through social dependence as well as reported feelings of love and commitment. Strube and Barbour (1983, 1984) found that women who reported staying in an abusive relationship at first because of love were more likely to be in the relationship at follow-up compared to women who did not report initially staying with the perpetrator out of love. Women were also more likely to have left the relationship by follow-up if they had been in the relationship for a shorter amount of time, signaling lower levels of commitment (Strube & Barbour, 1984). Women have been found to be more emotionally dependent than men, which increases their risk for experiencing intimate partner violence (Castillo-Gonzáles et al., 2024).

Functional dependence refers to an individual's reliance on another person due to physical or mental disabilities. Women with mental or physical disabilities have increased dependence on abusive partners and suffer longer periods of abuse when compared to women without disabilities due to mental and physical constraints (Young et al., 1997). These constraints not only limit their ability to leave an abusive relationship but also weaken their ability to defend themselves. Furthermore, women with disabilities are perceived as more vulnerable to abuse by others (Young et al., 1997). Functional dependence can be determined by assessing physical or mental disabilities which the victim relies on the offender for help.

Institutions

Almost two decades after Freyd introduced Betrayal trauma theory, Smith and Freyd (2014) extended the theory to incorporate individuals' dependence on larger systems that shape our society. In the *American Psychologist*, they argued that we are dependent on institutions that surround our daily lives, whether we trust the institution or not. They acknowledge the different relationships individuals may have with institutions. Smith and Freyd utilize examples to illustrate this point. For example, after experiencing sexual assault on a college campus, a victim may seek help from the institution itself, the police, and/or medical services, demonstrating a level of "trust" in the institution to respond to their help seeking. In contrast, an individual who is distrustful that the court system will take their reports of domestic violence seriously is still dependent on the judicial institutions. Other institutions that are intertwined with society that can perpetrate institutional betrayal against their constituents include schools, which provide education and childcare; religious institutions, which provide moral and spiritual guidance and community; and workplaces, which are necessary to subsist in our capitalist society.

Institutional betrayal describes institutions' acts of commission or omission that harm their members. Specifically, institutional betrayal refers to ways institutions actively or passively fail to prevent a trauma from occurring and/or respond appropriately after a trauma occurs. For example, an institution perpetrates institutional betrayal against its members by creating an environment where trauma is common or normal (e.g., hazing practices) and/or inadequately responding to reports of trauma (e.g., dismissing claims that an institutionally sanctioned individual is sexually abusing members). Research has demonstrated that institutional betrayal is linked to a host of negative outcomes, such as poorer mental and physical health outcomes and loss of trust.

Although this area of research is newer compared to that the literature examining the impact of betrayal trauma in the context of interpersonal relationships, researchers have begun to examine the extent and impact of betrayal on individuals perpetrated or perpetuated by larger institutions. In fact, empirical studies investigating the prevalence and consequences of institutional betrayal have been conducted in relation to a variety of institutions, including higher education, the military, healthcare systems, religious institutions, and judicial systems (see Christl et al., 2024 for review). For example, investigations into the Catholic Church revealed institutional patterns in which priests previously accused of child abuse continued to have contact with other children (e.g., Böhm et al., 2014; Dale & Alpert, 2007). Here, abusive individuals with institutionally sanctioned power, who were trusted by faith practitioners to morally and spiritually guide them, actively harmed those who were entrusted to their care, constituting an act of commission. Moreover, in response to complaints, religious leaders' responses allowed for continued abuse by accused church leaders, further betraying the institution's members (act of omission). In higher education, concerning patterns of institutional betrayal have also been identified. Investigative reporting revealed that institutions of higher education have also been failing students through action and inaction. For example, some universities have supported campus subcultures, such as athletics and Greek life, where abuse is normalized (commission) or minimized and dismissed their institutional responsibility to protect their students (omission) by permitting student athletes to continue competing despite accusations of sexual assault.

The consequences of institutional betrayal have been shown to negatively impact both psychological and physical well-being. Experiences of institutional betrayal have been found to be related to symptoms of posttraumatic stress disorder, depression, and anxiety (Lee et al., 2021; Lett et al., 2020; Smith et al., 2016; Hannann et al., 2021; Wright et al., 2017). Furthermore, institutional betrayal has been associated with dissociation (Smith & Freyd, 2017; Smith, 2017), suicidal ideation (Monteith et al., 2019a), and increased odds of attempting suicide (Monteith et al., 2016). In terms of physical health, institutional betrayal has been associated with higher overall number of physical illness symptoms and poorer physical functioning and lower energy levels (Smith and Freyd, 2017; Smith, 2017).

The social damage inflicted by institutional betrayal cannot be ignored. Studies examining individuals' engagement with the systems that have betrayed them demonstrate reductions in engagement in the institution. For example, military veterans who had experienced institutional betrayal perpetrated by the military reported lower levels of willingness to engage in veteran-related services, preferring to seek care elsewhere or giving up on veteran resources (Bloeser et al., 2021; Monteith et al., 2021). Although disengaging with institutions that have betrayed you may serve as protective, other research suggests that doing so comes with grave consequences, such as losing one's military career (Monteith et al., 2019) or non-compliance with healthcare behaviors (Smith, 2017).

Given the complex and interconnected nature of individuals' relationships to larger systems, disengagement from harmful institutions may be impossible, especially when systems causing harm are embedded into the fabric of society. Researchers examining institutional betrayal have indeed found that institutional betrayal is also perpetrated and perpetuated by United States governing institutions. For example, Gutowski & Goodman (2020) found that experiences of institutional betrayal occur within the United States court systems, documenting the experiences of mothers seeking legal custody of their children in the context of intimate partner violence. Rosenthal et al. (2025) found that caregivers involved in a child protective services investigation, despite whether they were the individual being investigated for abuse, also described experiences of institutional betrayal in child protective services. Straus (2016) documented evidence that the U.S. government has perpetrated institutional betrayal against its constituents by surveying more than 200 adult U.S. citizens' experiences of institutional betrayal related to ten controversial events in which U.S. political or public institutions were involved (e.g., government's response to Hurricane Katrina, police shootings of unarmed African Americans, police corruption). Cromer et al., (2018) surveyed a sample of Native Americans located in Oregon regarding institutional betrayal related to historical trauma. These studies demonstrate that entities central to individuals' lives, such as government institutions, can also perpetrate institutional betrayal.

Cultural Betrayal

Betrayal trauma theory has also been applied to larger sociocultural contexts to further contextualize interpersonal abuse. Jennifer Gómez coined the term cultural betrayal trauma to describe the unique vulnerability experienced by a victim of minoritized race and ethnicities (Gómez, 2012; 2017; 2019). Gómez further contextualizes interpersonal trauma by calling to the forefront the impact of societal trauma, such as discrimination, genocide, slavery, and police brutality, on minoritized groups and protective forces such as intracultural trust. As a response to systemic societal trauma, members of cultural groups pool defense resources as a protective measure. This intracultural trust refers to the relationships between cultural group members based on loyalty and responsibility, conferring a form of dependence between in-group members.

Cultural betrayal draws on both betrayal trauma and institutional betrayal. Like betrayal trauma, cultural betrayal occurs in the context of within-groups where a social contract exists between perpetrator and victim. By nature of within-group identification, an intracultural trust exists, which is then violated by the in-group perpetrator. At a more macro level, like institutional betrayal, the perpetrator's group membership represents the larger minoritized cultural group due to historical oppression that assumes minorities represent their entire group rather than operate as individuals (Platt et al., 2009). Furthermore, intracultural pressure to protect the minoritized perpetrator at the expense of the victim for the sake of the minoritized group exacerbates the effects of trauma.

In essence, oppressed groups form within-group dependence based in connection and loyalty to buffer the effects of societal trauma conferred by oppressors, which then leads to intracultural pressure from other in-group members that require the victim to remain silent. For example, if a minoritized person is assaulted by an individual from the same minoritized group, other members of that within group may pressure the victim to remain silent or punish the individual for speaking out "against" their fellow marginalized counterpart to protect the reputation of the group as a form of guarding against societal oppression.

Research on cultural betrayal trauma has revealed evidence that within-group interpersonal trauma symptoms, such as depression and sleep issues, were stronger for minoritized individuals when compared to those in the majority (Gómez & Freyd, 2018). Studies examining the relationship between cultural betrayal trauma and trauma outcomes in a variety of minoritized groups have also been published. For example, cultural betrayal has been found to have an indirect effect on hallucinations through dissociation (Gómez, 2018) in male Latinos (Gómez, 2017b) and Asian American/Pacific Islanders (Gómez, 2017a).

BETRAYAL TRAUMA AND ADVERSE CHILDHOOD EXPERIENCES

Researchers at the Centers for Disease Control and Prevention and Kaiser Permanente found evidence that childhood trauma had negative impacts on long term health (Felitti et al., 1998). Adults who had experienced four or more adverse childhood experiences (ACEs) were at significantly higher risk for a multitude of negative health outcomes (e.g., depression, alcoholism, suicide attempt, heart disease, cancer) compared to those who did not report experiencing ACEs. Cumulative and graded effects have been identified, where those who report more ACEs also are at increased risk for a variety of negative consequences (Boullier & Blair, 2018). The impact of the ACEs Study has led to an increased interest in understanding the impact of adverse experiences in childhood as well as in preventing childhood adversity.

Examining the ACEs items with a Betrayal trauma lens can help those working on preventing and responding to ACEs understand how to better understand the impact of ACEs and mechanisms for prevention. Notably, both the physical and emotional abuse items anchor the respondent to reflect on whether a parent or stepparent perpetrated any physical or emotional abuse. In line with betrayal trauma theory, the impact of direct or indirect harm caused by a parent or parental figure is especially potent given the child's dependence on the adult.

Furthermore, an individual may endorse emotional or physical abuse that was perpetrated by an adult that lived in the child's home, regardless of whether they were the parent or stepparent. Although not at the hands of a parent or stepparent, traumatic experiences perpetrated at home, ostensibly a place of security, violate a social contract between individuals. Additional contextualizing of the relationship between the abuser and child can help elucidate additional levels of betrayal in this situation, and it is critical to think through this adult's relationship to the child and to the child's caregivers. For example, if the adult is an abusive relative, the child may or may not disclose the abuse due to direct or indirect messages from a parent or primary caregiver. If the adult is a nonrelative but is financially critical to the home, for example, this may lead to a lack of disclosure due to direct or indirect messages from the child's caregivers who are dependent on the perpetrator. This may be additionally harmful in the context of cultural betrayal, for example, if the child is taught to protect their abuser to protect the family name or reputation.

Experiencing neglect was not included as part of ACEs until the second wave of the ACEs Study. Neglect in itself implies a violation of the social contract between child and caregiver. The child's dependence on the caregiver requires the child to trust that the caregiver will provide necessary life-sustaining resources, such as food and a clean and safe environment. Emotional neglect implies the absence of necessary socioemotional care that the child requires from their caregiver. Given the basis of attachment includes responsiveness to the child's needs, emotional neglect can result in insecure attachment and subsequent cognitive or behavioral mechanisms that maintain the dysfunctional relationship.

The application of Betrayal trauma theory to ACEs related to household challenges can be better understood by examining the contextual nature of the household stressors. Respondents to the ACEs questionnaire indicate whether their mother was treated violently by their father or mother's partner. Although not directly perpetrated against the child, witnessing violence perpetrated by a close other against one's mother, or other caregiver, can also be considered betrayal trauma. Indeed, multiple instances of betrayal trauma are co-occurring. First, the victim of the intimate partner violence is experiencing betrayal trauma, which may vary depending on the level of dependence on the perpetrator. The victim's dependence on the perpetrator is related to their ability to notice and respond to the violence in a way that protects themselves and their child(ren). The child's dependence on both adults results in experiences of betrayal trauma. Indeed, so-called failure-to-protect laws, which are active across the United States at varying degrees, often fail to contextualize the role of dependence when domestic violence occurs in a home with children.

Similarly, applying betrayal trauma theory to ACEs items related to household substance abuse, household mental illness, parental separation, and incarceration of a household member requires providers, researchers, and policymakers to contextualize the adverse experiences. Household substance abuse, household mental illness, parental separation, and household member incarceration imply negative consequences on caregivers' ability to care for their dependents. Addiction, serious mental illness, and absence/inconsistency all negatively impact a caregivers' ability to notice and respond to their child's needs, ultimately violating the social contract between caregiver and child. Furthermore, substance abuse and mental illness are associated with increased risk for abusive parenting, further conferring betrayal trauma. The absence of a caregiver, whether due to parental separation or incarceration, increases stress at home for a variety of reasons, which may reduce present caregivers' ability to notice and respond to their dependents' needs. This reduction in ability to notice and respond to their child's needs increases risk for additional aversive experiences, such as sibling abuse or sexual abuse by a relative, resulting in cumulative betrayal trauma. Furthermore, families where ACEs are present are more likely to require support from systems, which may also result in institutional betrayal. The domino effect of betrayal trauma seems endless.

CUMULATIVE HARM: REVICTIMIZATION AND INTERGENERATIONAL CYCLES OF TRAUMA AND ABUSE

Betrayal trauma may contribute to repeated exposure to traumatic events, referred to as revictimization. Researchers have found that experiences of betrayal trauma may impact cognitive mechanisms that allow individuals to accurately gauge other's trustworthiness, which may increase risk for further violation. Specifically, experiencing high betrayal trauma early in life may lead to suppression of individuals' innate adeptness at identifying dishonesty and unfairness (Zurbriggen & Freyd, 2004). Researchers have also found that those who had experienced high betrayal trauma were more likely to remain in a relationship after a betrayal of trust (Gobin & Freyd, 2009), putting them at risk for revictimization by another perpetrator. DePrince (2005) found that individuals who had been revictimized performed more poorly on tasks requiring them to detect social violations. Evidence shows higher dissociation and amnesia rates in those abused by parents versus non-parents (Freyd et al., 2001). Thus, experiencing betrayal trauma and using cognitive strategies like self-blame, idealization, and minimizing abuse, known as "betrayal blindness," can hinder recognizing abuse in relationships (Babcock et al., 2016; DePrince et al., 2009; DePrince, 2005) and thus increase risk of revictimization.

Similarly, betrayal trauma theory can also be used to explain intergenerational transmission of trauma exposure (Freyd, 1996). Approximately one-third of those who are physically or sexually abused or extremely neglected will perpetrate one of these forms of abuse with their own children (Kaufman & Zigler, 1987; Newcomb et al., 2001; Pears et al., 2001; Kim, 2009). Further, even if caregivers who were abused in childhood don't perpetrate abuse against their own children themselves, their children at still at risk for abuse from others. For example, child victims of sexual abuse are more likely to have a non-offending mother who also experienced childhood sexual abuse (Avery et al., 2002; McCloskey et al., 2000; Font et al., 2020). Children who were abused are also more likely to enter into abusive relationships in adulthood (McMahon et al., 2015), thus increasing the likelihood that their children will witness interpersonal violence or be exposed to abuse themselves and continuing the cycle of victimization (Avery et al., 2002). In the same way that betrayal blindness may impede an individual's ability to detect abuse in their own future interpersonal relationships (DePrince et al., 2009; DePrince, 2005), betrayal blindness also reducing caregivers' capacity to detect abusive behaviors in those who may pose a risk to their child or recognize their own parenting behaviors as abusive (Egeland et al., 1996). Further evidence for the role of betrayal trauma in intergenerational continuity comes from findings that mothers who had been revictimized were more likely to have children with experiences of interpersonal trauma, suggesting that dissociation from childhood betrayal may involve a persistent unawareness of future threats to themselves and their children (Hulette et al., 2011). In fact, Fenerci and Allen (2018) found that rates of intergenerational continuity of child maltreatment are higher when caregivers experienced abuse by their caregiver compared to caregivers who experienced abuse by someone else. Similarly, maternal betrayal trauma has been found to be related to higher levels of dissociation in their own children (Chu & DePrince, 2006), and mothers that experienced betrayal trauma and engaged in high levels of dissociation were more likely to have children that were also abused by someone they were close to and engage in dissociation (Hulette et al., 2011).

IMPLICATIONS FOR TRAUMA-INFORMED PREVENTION, RESPONSE, AND INTERVENTION

As highlighted by betrayal trauma theory and its various applications, the contextualization of ACEs via attachment and dependence and the violation of social contracts is imperative to adequately prevent and address ACEs and their long-term negative and self-perpetuating outcomes. The complexity of these issues requires a multilevel approach from primary prevention to therapeutic interventions that disrupt the intergenerational transmission of abuse to institutional action and commitment to avoid perpetration of betrayal to its constituents. Given the role of betrayal trauma in revictimization and intergenerational transmission of trauma, prevention and intervention are inextricably linked. Providing caregivers, educators, providers, researchers, policymakers, and other professionals with education related to the role of relational context between victims and perpetrators and the larger socioecological and systemic pressures allow those involved in prevention to recognize the histories of betrayal trauma perpetrated by individuals in power against those who do not hold the power. Therefore, providing education related to institutional and cultural betrayal requires an intersectional approach (Crenshaw, 1989). Increasing all stakeholders' awareness, however, is not enough, and a radical reform (or revolution) is warranted across systems so that the relational context of trauma and abuse can be fully addressed.

Institutional Response

Given the central role of institutions in the continuation of betrayal trauma, it is critical that institutional actors make an effort to avoid acting in ways that may be experienced as betraying. In their study of institutional betrayal in child maltreatment investigations, Rosenthal et al. (2025) heard from caregivers about what actions are associated with experiences of betrayal. Caregivers identified that betrayal experiences were largely tied to the manner by which institutional actors communicated with them. Positive experiences with the quality and quantity of communication between institutional actors and constituents led caregivers to feel respected, supported, and protected. Conversely, the manner of communication could also convey blame, lack of investment, and discriminatory beliefs consistent with experiences of institutional betrayal. In this same study, participants also indicated that institutions perpetrated betrayal when they excluded constituents from processes, invalidate their traumatic or distressing experiences, fail to follow through on promises, and make discriminatory decisions based on the identities of constituents.

Institutions can thus interrupt the continuation of betrayal trauma by taking concrete steps to help constituents feel included and respected. For example, given the importance of communication and inclusion in preventing betrayal, institutions are urged to make their data, policies, and processes publicly available and to prioritize ongoing communication with and solicitation of feedback from constituents. Freyd (2018) provides recommendations to address discrimination-related experiences of institutional betrayal that urge institutions to shift from focusing on basic compliance with civil rights laws to more preventative approaches to mitigate risk of discrimination. To do so, Freyd (2018) suggests training staff on biases, ensuring staff reflect the identities and values of the communities served, and decreasing subjective and individual-level decision-making through a system of checks and balances.

Therapeutic Intervention

Therapeutic intervention can serve as a critical avenue for reducing both revictimization and the intergenerational transmission of betrayal trauma. Betrayal trauma theory posits that "betrayal blindness"—a lack of awareness or memory of betrayal perpetrated by a trusted other—can be an adaptive response that allows individuals, particularly children, to preserve essential attachment relationships in the face of interpersonal trauma (Freyd, 1996). However, this adaptive mechanism may come with consequences that impact risk for revictimization. When betrayal remains unacknowledged, learning and memory integration processes may be disrupted, thereby increasing the risk of future victimization (DePrince, 2005; Freyd et al., 2007).

Re-engaging with interpersonally traumatic experiences in the context of a therapeutic relationship may offer a reparative opportunity. Specifically, therapy can facilitate increased awareness of past betrayals, counteracting minimization or betrayal blindness, and enabling survivors to re-integrate their experiences and construct new meanings. In theory, this process may improve survivors' ability to detect risk and engage in more effective safety behaviors in future relationships (Freyd & Birrell, 2013).

Several evidence-based trauma therapies already incorporate mechanisms that support this form of cognitive and emotional integration. For instance, Trauma-Focused Cognitive Behavioral Therapy (TF-CBT) includes the development of a trauma narrative, which assists clients in confronting and processing previously suppressed or minimized traumatic experiences (Cohen et al., 2017). Similarly, Child-Parent Psychotherapy (CPP) emphasizes the principle of "speaking the unspeakable," encouraging both survivors and clinicians to name and process traumatic events that may have been silenced within the family system (Lieberman et al. 2020). By bringing suppressed trauma into conscious awareness, survivors may become better equipped to use these memories adaptively, particularly in assessing and responding to interpersonal risk.

As clinical psychologists that study and work with children, parents, and families impacted by interpersonal trauma, we propose an approach to intervening on the intergenerational transmission of abuse through a community-based group therapy approach. Parenting interventions are the gold standard for reducing maltreatment risk and have proven effective (Desai et al., 2017; Altafim et al., 2016), yet their implementation is limited. Many focus on a single generation, overlooking intergenerational influences. For instance, child-focused programs like *The Incredible Years* (Webster-Stratton, 2005, 2015) prioritize social-emotional development but do not address caregivers' own traumatic experiences of adverse childhood experiences. Effective interventions should integrate caregivers' own histories of ACEs, as addressing their own experiences enhances engagement and behavior change (Butler et al., 2020). Addressing their own childhood trauma and providing explicit psychoeducation about the impact of betrayal trauma allows individuals to bring past experiences to awareness in order to guide their current decision-making.

Lewis (2025) interviewed survivors of maternal abuse who are now raising their own children and found that recognizing and naming the abuse was central to their healing. Women reported that "motherhood acted as both a mirror and a magnifier serving to bring long-buried memories to the surface and prompt participants to reflect more critically on the emotional environment in which they were raised" (pg. 123). For these women, returning to the childhood memories that were previously minimized in the context of parenthood and therapy served as a catalyst for change.

In addition to integrating the caregivers' own childhood experiences, intergenerationally focused interventions must also highlight the experiences and needs of the child. Interventions that focus solely on the caregiver's behaviors, such as the *Triple P- Positive Parenting Program* (Sanders, 1999), are also limiting. Caregivers benefit from education about children's needs, maintaining child safety, and strengthening parent-child relationships, especially when they lack modeling of these skills from their own caregivers. Integrating caregiver's own childhood experiences and traumas, their adult caregiving experiences, and their child's experiences, is optimal for targeting intergenerational continuity.

Another key limitation of widely used parenting interventions is their focus on individual families or parent-child dyads (e.g., Parent-Child Interaction Therapy). Group therapy offers unique benefits for breaking intergenerational abuse cycles. Caregivers with childhood trauma often experience isolation, distrust, shame, and disempowerment (Reddan, 2023). Group therapy helps normalize trauma-related experiences, reducing shame, and fostering connection. Altruism, a key component of group therapy, allows participants to support others, strengthening self-efficacy (Yalom & Leszcz, 2020). Additionally, witnessing change in others fosters hope for personal transformation. A meta-analysis by Mew and colleagues found that maternal social support is an important mediator in the intergenerational transmission of trauma (2025). By enhancing self-efficacy, hope, and social support, group therapy may improve well-being and reduce trauma-related risks for intergenerational abuse.

SUMMARY

In sum, interpersonal violence is a pervasive and detrimental phenomenon that negatively impacts individuals, families, communities, and generations beyond the physical harm transmitted. Violence perpetrated by close others, like parents and romantic partners, as well as by social groups and institutions is especially harmful given the attachment and dependence intrinsic to these relationships. This chapter applies betrayal trauma theory to understanding and addressing ACEs across interpersonal, institutional, and cultural contexts. Building on attachment theory, betrayal trauma theory emphasizes that trauma within dependent relationships, such as between child and caregiver, romantic partners, or between individuals and social institutions, carries unique and often more severe consequences than trauma occurring outside of these contexts. Survivors may suppress or remain unaware of abuse (i.e., betrayal blindness) to preserve essential attachments, leaving them vulnerable to a host of long-term psychological and physical consequences that increase risk for revictimization and perpetuating cycles of harm.

We have discussed betrayal trauma theory's extension from parent-child dynamics to romantic partnerships, institutional systems (e.g., schools, religious institutions, the military), and cultural contexts where societal trauma intersects with intracultural trust. These frameworks reveal how betrayal operates not only interpersonally but also structurally, with consequences that can include psychological distress, physical illness, social disengagement, and intergenerational trauma transmission. Applying betrayal trauma theory to the ACEs framework underscores that adverse experiences are not isolated events but occur within webs of dependence and betrayal that amplify their impact.

Finally, the chapter highlights implications for trauma-informed prevention and intervention. Effective strategies require multilevel, cross-disciplinary efforts that both acknowledge contextual dependence and interrupt intergenerational cycles of trauma. Group-based, community-focused interventions that integrate caregivers' own trauma histories alongside parenting supports are particularly promising, offering opportunities to reduce isolation, foster resilience, and strengthen protective family relationships.

CONCLUSION

Betrayal trauma theory offers a powerful framework for contextualizing and responding to cumulative and intergenerational trauma. By understanding the influence of dependence, attachment, and the violation of social contracts, betrayal trauma theory reframes survivors' responses as adaptive, challenges victim-blaming narratives, and illuminates the pathways through which harm is perpetuated across relationships, systems, and generations. Recognizing the role of betrayal at interpersonal, institutional, and cultural levels reveals critical intervention points for both prevention and treatment.

To break cycles of harm, practitioners, researchers, and policymakers must adopt trauma-informed, multigenerational approaches that address both individual experiences and systemic failures. Supporting caregivers in processing their own trauma, strengthening parent-child relationships, and fostering community connections are vital to disrupting intergenerational transmission. Likewise, holding institutions accountable for betrayal is essential for restoring trust and preventing future harm.

Ultimately, applying betrayal trauma theory to ACEs demonstrates that healing and prevention are inseparable from context. Protecting children and families requires not only individual interventions but also systemic change that prioritizes safety, trust, and equity across all levels of society.

REFERENCES

Afifi, T. O., & MacMillan, H. L. (2011). Resilience following child maltreatment: A review of protective factors. *Canadian Journal of Psychiatry, 56*(5), 266–272. DOI: 10.1177/070674371105600505 PMID: 21586192

Ainsworth, M. D. (1973). The development of infant mother attachment. In Caldwell, B. M., & Ricciuti, H. N. (Eds.), *Review of child development research* (Vol. 3). University of Chicago Press.

Ainsworth, M. S., & Bowlby, J. (1991). An ethological approach to personality development. *The American Psychologist, 46*(4), 333–341. DOI: 10.1037/0003-066X.46.4.333

Altafim, E. R. P., Pedro, M. E. A., & Linhares, M. B. M. (2016). Effectiveness of ACT raising safe kids parenting program in a developing country. *Children and Youth Services Review, 70*, 315–323. DOI: 10.1016/j.childyouth.2016.09.038

Anderson, D. K., & Saunders, D. G. (2003). Leaving an abusive partner: An empirical review of predictors, the process of leaving, and psychological well-being. *Trauma, Violence & Abuse, 4*(2), 163–191. DOI: 10.1177/1524838002250769 PMID: 14697121

Avery, L., Hutchinson, K. D., & Whitaker, K. (2002). Domestic Violence and Intergenerational Rates of Child Sexual Abuse: A Case Record Analysis. *Child & Adolescent Social Work Journal, 19*(1), 77–90. DOI: 10.1023/A:1014007507349

Babcock, R., Fenerci, R. L., Chu, A. T., & DePrince, A. P. (2016). Intergenerational transmission of trauma-related distress: Maternal betrayal trauma, parenting attitudes, and behaviors. *Journal of Aggression, Maltreatment & Trauma, 25*(4), 382–399. DOI: 10.1080/10926771.2015.1129655

Barnett, D., Ganiban, J., & Cicchetti, D. (1999). Maltreatment, negative expressivity, and the development of type D attachments from 12- to 24-months of age. *Monographs of the Society for Research in Child Development, 64*(3), 97–118. DOI: 10.1111/1540-5834.00035 PMID: 10597544

Beeghly, M., & Cicchetti, D. (1994). Child maltreatment, attachment, and the self system: Emergence of an internal state lexicon in toddlers at high social risk. *Development and Psychopathology, 6*(1), 5–30. DOI: 10.1017/S095457940000585X

Bloeser, K., McCarron, K. K., Merker, V. L., Hyde, J., Bolton, R. E., Anastasides, N., Petrakis, B. A., Helmer, D. A., Santos, S., Litke, D., Pigeon, W. R., & McAndrew, L. M. (2021). "Because the country, it seems though, has turned their back on me": Experiences of institutional betrayal among veterans living with Gulf War Illness. *Social Science & Medicine*, *284*, 114–211. DOI: 10.1016/j.socscimed.2021.114211 PMID: 34271400

Böhm, B., Zollner, H., Fegert, J. M., & Liebhardt, H. (2014). Child sexual abuse in the context of the Roman Catholic Church: A review of literature from 1981–2013. *Journal of Child Sexual Abuse*, *23*(6), 635–656. DOI: 10.1080/10538712.2014.929607 PMID: 24911986

Bornstein, R. F. (1993). *The dependent personality*. Guilford Press.

Bornstein, R. F. (2006). The complex relationship between dependency and domestic violence: Converging psychological factors and social forces. *The American Psychologist*, *61*(6), 595–606. DOI: 10.1037/0003-066X.61.6.595 PMID: 16953747

Boullier, M., & Blair, M. (2018). Adverse childhood experiences. *Paediatrics and Child Health (Oxford)*, *28*(3), 132–137. DOI: 10.1016/j.paed.2017.12.008

Bowlby, J. (1969). Attachment and Loss. Vol. 1, Attachment. New York: Basic Books, 1982. Bowlby, J. (1980). Attachment and Loss. Vol. 3, Loss. New York: Basic Books.

Bowlby, J. (1982). Attachment and loss: Retrospect and prospect. *The American Journal of Orthopsychiatry*, *52*(4), 664–678. DOI: 10.1111/j.1939-0025.1982.tb01456.x PMID: 7148988

Bowlby, J. (1988). *A secure base: Parent-child attachment and healthy human development*. Basic books.

Butler, J., Gregg, L., Calam, R., & Wittkowski, A. (2020). Parents' perceptions and experiences of parenting programmes: A systematic review and metasynthesis of the qualitative literature. *Clinical Child and Family Psychology Review*, *23*(2), 176–204. DOI: 10.1007/s10567-019-00307-y PMID: 31820298

Carlson, E. A. (1998). A prospective longitudinal study of attachment disorganization/disorientation. *Child Development*, *69*(4), 1107–1128. DOI: 10.1111/j.1467-8624.1998.tb06163.x PMID: 9768489

Carlson, V., Cicchetti, D., Barnett, D., & Braunwald, K. (1989). Disorganized/disoriented attachment relationships in maltreated infants. *Developmental Psychology*, *25*(4), 525–531. DOI: 10.1037/0012-1649.25.4.525

Castillo-Gonzáles, M., Mendo-Lázaro, S., León-del-Barco, B., Terán-Andrade, E., & López-Ramos, V. M. (2024). Dating violence and emotional dependence in university students. *Behavioral Sciences (Basel, Switzerland)*, *14*(3), 176. DOI: 10.3390/bs14030176 PMID: 38540479

Chu, A., & DePrince, A. P. (2006). Development of dissociation: Examining the relationship between parenting, maternal trauma and child dissociation. *Journal of Trauma & Dissociation*, *7*(4), 75–89. DOI: 10.1300/J229v07n04_05 PMID: 17182494

Cicchetti, D., & Barnett, D. (1991). Attachment organization in pre-school-aged maltreated children. *Development and Psychopathology*, *3*, 397–411. DOI: 10.1017/S0954579400007598

Cohen, J. A., Mannarino, A. P., & Deblinger, E. (2017). *Trauma-Focused CBT for Children and Adolescents: Treatment Applications*. Guilford Press.

Cosmides, L. (1989). The logic of social exchange: Has natural selection shaped how humans reason? Studies with the Wason selection task. *Cognition*, *31*(3), 187–276. DOI: 10.1016/0010-0277(89)90023-1 PMID: 2743748

Crenshaw, K. (1989). Demarginalizing the intersection of race and sex: A black feminist critique of antidiscrimination doctrine, feminist theory and antiracist politics. *University of Chicago Legal Forum*, (1), 8, 139–167.

Cromer, L. D., Gray, M. E., Vasquez, L., & Freyd, J. J. (2018). The relationship of acculturation to historical loss awareness, institutional betrayal, and the intergenerational transmission of trauma in the American Indian experience. *Journal of Cross-Cultural Psychology*, *49*(1), 99–114. DOI: 10.1177/0022022117738749

Cyr, C., Euser, E. M., Bakermans-Kranenburg, M. J., & Van Ijzendoorn, M. H. (2010). Attachment security and disorganization in maltreating and high-risk families: A series of meta-analyses. *Development and Psychopathology*, *22*(1), 87–108. DOI: 10.1017/S0954579409990289 PMID: 20102649

Dale, K. A., & Alpert, J. L. (2007). Hiding behind the cloth: Child sexual abuse and the Catholic Church. *Journal of Child Sexual Abuse*, *16*(3), 59–74. DOI: 10.1300/J070v16n03_04 PMID: 18032240

DePrince, A. P. (2005). Social cognition and revictimization risk. *Journal of Trauma & Dissociation*, *6*(1), 125–141. DOI: 10.1300/J229v06n01_08 PMID: 16150689

DePrince, A. P., Combs, M. D., & Shanahan, M. (2009). Automatic relationship-harm associations and interpersonal trauma involving close others. *Psychology of Women Quarterly*, *33*(2), 163–171. DOI: 10.1111/j.1471-6402.2009.01486.x

DePrince, A. P., & Freyd, J. J. (2002). The intersection of gender and betrayal in trauma. In Kimerling, R., Oumette, P. C., & Wolfe, J. (Eds.), *Gender and PTSD* (pp. 98–113). Guilford Press.

Desai, C. D., Reece, J. A., & Shakespeare-Pellington, S. (2017). The prevention of violence in childhood through parenting programmes: A global review. *Psychology Health and Medicine*, *22*(1), 166–186. DOI: 10.1080/13548506.2016.1271952 PMID: 28133982

Egeland, B., & Susman-Stillman, A. (1996). Dissociation as a mediator of child abuse across generations. *Child Abuse & Neglect*, *20*(11), 1123–1132. DOI: 10.1016/0145-2134(96)00102-0 PMID: 8958463

Erez, E., Adelman, M., & Gregory, C. (2009). Intersections of immigration and domestic violence: Voices of battered immigrant women. *Feminist Criminology*, *4*(1), 32–56. DOI: 10.1177/1557085108325413

Fearon, R. P., Bakermans-Kranenburg, M. J., van IJzendoorn, M. H., Lapsley, A. M., & Roisman, G. I. (2010). The significance of insecure attachment and disorganization in the development of children's externalizing behavior: A meta-analytic study. *Child Development*, *81*(2), 435–456. DOI: 10.1111/j.1467-8624.2009.01405.x PMID: 20438450

Felitti, V. J., Anda, R. F., Nordenberg, D., Williamson, D. F., Spitz, A. M., Edwards, V., & Marks, J. S. (1998). Relationship of childhood abuse and household dysfunction to many of the leading causes of death in adults: The Adverse Childhood Experiences (ACE) Study. *American Journal of Preventive Medicine*, *14*(4), 245–258. DOI: 10.1016/S0749-3797(98)00017-8 PMID: 9635069

Fenerci, R. L. B., & Allen, B. (2018). From mother to child: Maternal betrayal trauma and risk for maltreatment and psychopathology in the next generation. *Child Abuse & Neglect*, *82*, 1–11. DOI: 10.1016/j.chiabu.2018.05.014 PMID: 29842995

Font, S., Cancian, M., Berger, L. M., & DiGiovanni, A. (2020). Patterns of intergenerational child protective services involvement. *Child Abuse & Neglect*, *99*, 104247. DOI: 10.1016/j.chiabu.2019.104247 PMID: 31715518

Freyd, J. J. (1996). *Betrayal trauma: The logic of forgetting childhood abuse*. Harvard University Press.

Freyd, J. J. (1996). *Betrayal trauma: The logic of forgetting childhood abuse*. Harvard University Press.

Freyd, J. J., & Birrell, P. J. (2013). *Blind to betrayal: Why we fool ourselves we aren't being fooled*. Wiley.

Freyd, J. J., DePrince, A. P., & Gleaves, D. H. (2007). The state of betrayal trauma theory: The need for more research. *Journal of Trauma & Dissociation*, *8*(3), 1–8. DOI: 10.1300/J229v08n03_01 PMID: 18032341

Freyd, J. J., Klest, B., & Allard, C. B. (2005). Betrayal trauma: Relationship to physical health, psychological distress, and a written disclosure intervention. *Journal of Trauma & Dissociation*, *6*(3), 83–104. DOI: 10.1300/J229v06n03_04 PMID: 16172083

Gelles, R. J. (1976). Abused wives: Why do they stay? *Journal of Marriage and Family*, *38*(4), 659–668. DOI: 10.2307/350685

Gobin, R. L., & Freyd, J. J. (2009). Betrayal and revictimization: Preliminary findings. *Psychological Trauma: Theory, Research, Practice, and Policy*, *1*(3), 242–257. DOI: 10.1037/a0017469

Goldsmith, R. E., Freyd, J. J., & DePrince, A. P. (2012). Betrayal trauma: Associations with psychological and physical symptoms in young adults. *Journal of Interpersonal Violence*, *27*(3), 547–567. DOI: 10.1177/0886260511421672 PMID: 21987504

Gómez, J. M. (2012). Cultural Betrayal trauma theory: The impact of culture on the effects of trauma. In Blind to Betrayal. Retrieved from https://sites.google.com/site/betrayalbook/betrayal-research-news/ cultural-betrayal

Gómez, J. M. (2017). *Cultural Betrayal trauma theory*. University of Oregon.

Gómez, J. M. (2017a). Does ethno-cultural betrayal in trauma affect Asian American/Pacific islander college students' mental health outcomes? An exploratory study. *Journal of American College Health*, *65*(6), 432–436. DOI: 10.1080/07448481.2017.1341896 PMID: 28617143

Gómez, J. M. (2017b). Does gender matter? An exploratory study of cultural betrayal trauma and hallucinations in Latino undergraduates at a predominantly White university. Advanced online publication. *Journal of Interpersonal Violence*, 088626051774694.

Gómez, J. M. (2018). What's in a Betrayal? Trauma, Dissociation, and Hallucinations Among High-Functioning Ethnic Minority Emerging Adults. *Journal of Aggression, Maltreatment & Trauma*, *28*(10), 1181–1198. DOI: 10.1080/10926771.2018.1494653

Gómez, J. M. (2019). Group dynamics as a predictor of dissociation for Black victims of violence: An exploratory study of cultural Betrayal trauma theory. *Transcultural Psychiatry*, *56*(5), 878–894. DOI: 10.1177/1363461519847300 PMID: 31046633

Gómez, J. M., & Freyd, J. J. (2018). Psychological outcomes of within group sexual violence: Evidence of cultural betrayal. *Journal of Immigrant and Minority Health*, *20*(6), 1458–1467. DOI: 10.1007/s10903-017-0687-0 PMID: 29288343

Gutowski, E., & Goodman, L. A. (2020). "Like I'm invisible": IPV survivor-mothers' perceptions of seeking child custody through the family court system. *Journal of Family Violence*, *35*(5), 441–457. DOI: 10.1007/s10896-019-00063-1

Haartsen, R., Jones, E. J., & Johnson, M. H. (2016). Human brain development over the early years. *Current Opinion in Behavioral Sciences*, *10*, 149–154. DOI: 10.1016/j.cobeha.2016.05.015

Hannan, S. M., Zimnick, J., & Park, C. (2021). Consequences of sexual violence among college students: Investigating the role of PTSD symptoms, rumination, and institutional betrayal. *Journal of Aggression, Maltreatment & Trauma*, *30*(5), 586–604. DOI: 10.1080/10926771.2020.1796871

Hulette, A. C., Freyd, J. J., Pears, K. C., Kim, H. K., Fisher, P. A., & Becker-Blease, K. A. (2008). Dissociation and posttraumatic symptoms in maltreated preschool children. *Journal of Child & Adolescent Trauma*, *1*(2), 93–108. DOI: 10.1080/19361520802083980 PMID: 28255424

Hulette, A. C., Kaehler, L. A., & Freyd, J. J. (2011). Intergenerational associations between trauma and dissociation. *Journal of Family Violence*, *26*(3), 217–225. DOI: 10.1007/s10896-011-9357-5

Huttenlocher, P. R. (1984). Synapse elimination and plasticity in developing human cerebral cortex. *American Journal of Mental Deficiency*, *88*(5), 488–496. PMID: 6731486

Kalmuss, D. S., & Straus, M. A. (1982). Wife's marital dependency and wife abuse. *Journal of Marriage and Family*, *44*(2), 277–286. DOI: 10.2307/351538

Kaufman, J., & Zigler, E. (1987). Do abused children become abusive parents? *The American Journal of Orthopsychiatry*, *57*(2), 186–192. DOI: 10.1111/j.1939-0025.1987.tb03528.x PMID: 3296775

Kim, J. (2009). Type-specific intergenerational transmission of neglectful and physically abusive parenting behaviors among young parents. *Children and Youth Services Review*, *31*(7), 761–767. DOI: 10.1016/j.childyouth.2009.02.002

Kim, J., & Gray, K. A. (2008). Leave or stay? Battered women's decision after intimate partner violence. *Journal of Interpersonal Violence*, *23*(10), 1465–1482. DOI: 10.1177/0886260508314307 PMID: 18309037

Lee, J. Y., Micol, R. L., & Davis, J. L. (2021). Intimate partner violence and psychological maladjustment: Examining the role of institutional betrayal among survivors. *Journal of Interpersonal Violence, 36*(15-16), 7505–7522. DOI: 10.1177/0886260519836783 PMID: 30879384

Lett, K., Tamaian, A., & Klest, B. (2020). Impact of ableist microaggressions on university students with self-identified disabilities. *Disability & Society, 35*(9), 1441–1456. DOI: 10.1080/09687599.2019.1680344

Lewis, A. J. (2025). *Interrupting the Cycle of Psychological Betrayal Trauma in Mother-Daughter Relationships* (Doctoral dissertation, Alliant International University).

Lieberman, A. F., Ghosh Ippen, C., & Van Horn, P. (2020). *Don't hit my mommy! A manual for child-parent psychotherapy with young witnesses of family violence* (3rd ed.). Zero to Three Press.

Lyons-Ruth, K., Easterbrooks, M. A., & Cibelli, C. D. (1997). Infant attachment strategies, infant mental lag, and maternal depressive symptoms: Predictors of internalizing and externalizing problems at age 7. *Developmental Psychology, 33*(4), 681–692. DOI: 10.1037/0012-1649.33.4.681 PMID: 9232383

Main, M., & Solomon, J. (1990). Procedures for identifying infants as disorganized/disoriented during the Ainsworth strange situation. In Greenberg, M. T., Cichetti, D., & Cummings, E. M. (Eds.), *Attachment in the Preschool Years: Theory, Research and Intervention* (pp. 121–160). University of Chicago Press.

McCloskey, L. A., & Bailey, J. A. (2000). The intergenerational transmission of risk for child sexual abuse. *Journal of Interpersonal Violence, 15*(10), 1019–1035. DOI: 10.1177/088626000015010001

McMahon, K., Hoertel, N., Wall, M. M., Okuda, M., Limosin, F., & Blanco, C. (2015). Childhood maltreatment and risk of intimate partner violence: A national study. *Journal of Psychiatric Research, 69*, 42–49. DOI: 10.1016/j.jpsychires.2015.07.026 PMID: 26343593

Meng, X., Fleury, M. J., Xiang, Y. T., Li, M., & D'arcy, C. (2018). Resilience and protective factors among people with a history of child maltreatment: A systematic review. *Social Psychiatry and Psychiatric Epidemiology, 53*(5), 453–475. DOI: 10.1007/s00127-018-1485-2 PMID: 29349479

Mew, E., Bonumwezi, J., & Lowe, S. (2025). *Family-level mediators in the intergenerational transmission of maternal childhood trauma: Systematic review and meta-analysis of pooled effect measures* [Poster]. *American Psychological Association Conference*, Denver, CO.

Monteith, L. L., Bahraini, N. H., Matarazzo, B. B., Soberay, K. A., & Smith, C. P. (2016). Perceptions of institutional betrayal predict suicidal self-directed violence among veterans exposed to military sexual trauma. *Journal of Clinical Psychology*, *72*(7), 743–755. DOI: 10.1002/jclp.22292 PMID: 27007795

Monteith, L. L., Gerber, H. R., Brownstone, L. M., Soberay, K. A., & Bahraini, N. H. (2019). The phenomenology of military sexual trauma among male veterans. *Psychology of Men & Masculinity*, *20*(1), 115–127. DOI: 10.1037/men0000153

Monteith, L. L., Holliday, R., Schneider, A. L., Miller, C. N., Bahraini, N. H., & Forster, J. E. (2021). Institutional betrayal and help-seeking among women survivors of military sexual trauma. *Psychological Trauma: Theory, Research, Practice, and Policy*, *13*(7), 814–823. DOI: 10.1037/tra0001027 PMID: 33764096

Morton, N., & Browne, K. D. (1998). Theory and observation of attachment and its relation to child maltreatment: A review. *Child Abuse & Neglect*, *22*(11), 1093–1104. DOI: 10.1016/S0145-2134(98)00088-X PMID: 9827314

Newcomb, M. D., & Locke, T. F. (2001). Intergenerational cycle of maltreatment: A popular concept obscured by methodological limitations. *Child Abuse & Neglect*, *25*(9), 1219–1240. DOI: 10.1016/S0145-2134(01)00267-8 PMID: 11700694

Pears, K. C., & Capaldi, D. M. (2001). Intergenerational transmission of abuse: A two-generational prospective study of an at-risk sample. *Child Abuse & Neglect*, *25*(11), 1439–1461. DOI: 10.1016/S0145-2134(01)00286-1 PMID: 11766010

Platt, M., Barton, J., & Freyd, J. J. (2009). A betrayal trauma perspective on domestic violence. *Violence against women in families and relationships*, 185-207.

Reddan, F. (2023). *How do adult survivors of childhood abuse, experience and understand their capacity to trust in relationships?* (Doctoral dissertation, Dublin City University).

Rosenthal, A., Christl, M. E., Wright, N., Olomi, J., Dmitrieva, J., & DePrince, A. P. (2025). Applying an institutional betrayal lens to caregiver perceptions of child maltreatment investigations. *Journal of Trauma & Dissociation*, *26*(3), 314–330. DOI: 10.1080/15299732.2025.2481029 PMID: 40107839

Rusbult, C. E., & Martz, J. M. (1995). Remaining in an abusive relationship: An investment model analysis of nonvoluntary dependence. *Personality and Social Psychology Bulletin, 21*(6), 558–571. DOI: 10.1177/0146167295216002

Sanders, M. R. (1999). Triple P-Positive Parenting Program: Towards an empirically validated multilevel parenting and family support strategy for the prevention of behavior and emotional problems in children. *Clinical Child and Family Psychology Review*, *2*(2), 71–90. DOI: 10.1023/A:1021843613840 PMID: 11225933

Scott, E. K., London, A. S., & Myers, N. A. (2002). Dangerous dependencies: The intersection of welfare reform and domestic violence. *Gender & Society*, *16*(6), 878–897. DOI: 10.1177/089124302237893

Smith, C. P. (2017). First, do no harm: Institutional betrayal and trust in health care organizations. *Journal of Multidisciplinary Healthcare*, *10*, 133–144. DOI: 10.2147/JMDH.S125885 PMID: 28435281

Smith, C. P., & Freyd, J. J. (2014). Institutional betrayal. *The American Psychologist*, *69*(6), 575–587. DOI: 10.1037/a0037564 PMID: 25197837

Smith, C. P., & Freyd, J. J. (2017). Insult, then injury: Interpersonal and institutional betrayal linked to health and dissociation. *Journal of Aggression, Maltreatment & Trauma*, *26*(10), 1117–1131. DOI: 10.1080/10926771.2017.1322654

Stahly, G. B. (2000). Women with children in violent relationships: The choice of leaving may bring the consequence of custodial challenge. *Journal of Aggression, Maltreatment & Trauma*, *2*(2), 239–251. DOI: 10.1300/J146v02n02_11

Straus, E. (2016). *Political Scandal: The effects of government betrayal on American citizens*. [Doctoral dissertation, California School of Professional Psychology].

Strube, M. J., & Barbour, L. S. (1983). The decision to leave an abusive relationship: Economic dependence and psychological commitment. *Journal of Marriage and Family*, *45*(4), 785–793. DOI: 10.2307/351791

Strube, M. J., & Barbour, L. S. (1984). Factors related to the decision to leave an abusive relationship. *Journal of Marriage and Family*, *46*(4), 837–844. DOI: 10.2307/352531

Tronick, E. Z., & Cohn, J. F. (1989). Infant-Mother Face-to-Face Interaction: Age and Gender Differences in Coordination and the Occurrence of Miscoordination. *Child Development*, *60*(1), 85–92. DOI: 10.2307/1131074 PMID: 2702877

Webster-Stratton, C. (2005). The Incredible Years: A training series for the prevention and treatment of conduct problems in young children.

Webster-Stratton, C. (2015). The Incredible Years® series: A developmental approach. In *Family-Based Prevention Programs for Children and Adolescents* (pp. 54-79). Psychology Press. wife abuse. *Journal of Marriage and Family*, *44*, 277–286.

Woffordt, S., Mihalic, D. E., & Menard, S. (1994). Continuities in marital violence. *Journal of Family Violence*, *9*(3), 195–225. DOI: 10.1007/BF01531948

Wright, N. M., Smith, C. P., & Freyd, J. J. (2017). Experience of a lifetime: Study abroad, trauma, and institutional betrayal. *Journal of Aggression, Maltreatment & Trauma*, *26*(1), 50–68. DOI: 10.1080/10926771.2016.1170088

Yalom, I., & Leszcz, M. (2020). *The Theory and Practice of Group Psychotherapy*. Basic Books.

Young, M. E., Nosek, M. A., Howland, C. A., Chanpong, G., & Rintala, D. H. (1997). Prevalence of abuse of women with disabilities. *Archives of Physical Medicine and Rehabilitation*, *78*(12), S34–S38. DOI: 10.1016/S0003-9993(97)90219-7 PMID: 9422005

Zurbriggen, E. L., & Freyd, J. J. (2004). The link between child sexual abuse and risky sexual behavior: The role of dissociative tendencies, information-processing effects, and consensual sex decision mechanisms.

Chapter 7
Childhood Maltreatment Over Generations:
A Scoping Review on the Theoretical Frameworks and Proposed Interventions in the Literature

Crysta Bowe
https://orcid.org/0009-0008-6935-6327
Charles Sturt University, Australia

Cate Thomas
https://orcid.org/0000-0001-9386-0269
Charles Sturt University, Australia

Patricia Mackey
https://orcid.org/0000-0003-3978-0115
Charles Sturt University, Australia

ABSTRACT

Intergenerational child maltreatment, in which abuse or neglect in childhood reoccurs over generations within the same family, is a consequential yet poorly understood challenge in child protection policy and practice. Using systemic methodology, this scoping review reveals the explanatory theoretical frameworks on intergenerational child maltreatment in the literature, explores diverse intervention approaches, and finds correlations between different facets of the data. A variety of theoretical frameworks and suggested interventions are articulated in the literature, with attachment theory being most prominent and practices focusing more strongly on various ap-

DOI: 10.4018/979-8-3373-4064-7.ch007

proaches to direct service provision and future research than to reflective practice and intervention at a systemic or structural level. This data, alongside correlations between different aspects of the data, holds implications for policy, practice, and research, including broadening intervention options to cater for the diversity of people seeking support and critiquing existing paradigms driving research and practice.

INTRODUCTION

Child maltreatment that reoccurs over generations presents a considerable challenge in child protection systems and contexts worldwide, with a notable body of evidence finding correlations between a parent's childhood experiences of abuse and neglect and child protection interventions in their own subsequent parenting (Armfield et al., 2021; Bartlett et al., 2017; Madigan et al., 2019; Thornberry et al., 2012). Much of the current literature has concentrated on identifying mediating and moderating factors (individual, social, and contextual influences) for intergenerational continuity or discontinuity of child maltreatment (Dixon et al., 2009; Langevin et al., 2021). This, while an essential contribution to the field, is not equivalent to a conceptualisation of *why* child maltreatment may re-occur over generations (Geiger et al., 2015).

This gap is addressed by an exploration of the explanatory theories surrounding intergenerational child abuse and neglect. Theoretical frameworks are foundational to the experiences of families engaging with child protection systems. They inform child protection practice, policy, regulation, and legislation; assist in the organisation of knowledge; underpin training and professional accreditation requirements; and guide further research (Schelbe & Geiger, 2017; Young et al., 2014). Perhaps most importantly, theoretical standpoints predicate clinical and statutory practice interventions with families (Schelbe & Geiger, 2017), a process that may largely operate on an unconscious level on the part of the practitioner but has potentially profound and long-term impacts for families involved with child protection systems.

This chapter describes the process, results, and implications of a scoping review of the literature on the theories applied to intergenerational child maltreatment alongside the proposed intervention approaches. It begins with a brief review of similar literature before going on to outline the methodology. The findings, including the explanatory theories and hypotheses the literature applies to explain why parents who have experienced child maltreatment are more likely to have children who are subjected to harm, the intervention approaches and considerations indicated in the literature, and an exploration of the correlations and trends relating to various features in the selected papers, are then discussed. This piece also provides a dialogue on the implications of the results for child protection practice, policy, and research, as well as a discussion on the strengths and limitations of the review.

BACKGROUND

Scoping reviews involve systematically investigating the literature on a topic to map the knowledge; identify thematic concepts and literature gaps; and inform policy, practice, and future research (Colquhoun et al., 2014; Peters et al., 2021). This thorough and replicable process of exploration and analysis is a fitting approach to gaining a deeper understanding of the theoretical frameworks and recommended interventions in the literature on intergenerational continuity of child maltreatment.

Scoping and other systematic-type reviews of this type are not entirely absent in the literature on intergenerational child maltreatment. Marshall et al., (2022) conducted a review of the theoretical frameworks applied to victim-to-victim cycles of maltreatment (in which the parent who experienced childhood maltreatment is not the perpetrator of the abuse or neglect experienced by their child), finding that attachment theory followed by traumatic stress models (involving the sequalae of trauma and its impacts on psychological functioning) were most frequently applied. Chamberlain, Gee, et al., (2019) completed a review of theoretical constructs in their exploration of the impact of parental childhood maltreatment during the perinatal period (pre-natal to 2 years post-partum), identifying attachment theory as the most commonly applied, followed by social learning theory. This review also mapped the strategies and interventions evaluated or described in the literature, finding a diversity of professional approaches (Chamberlain, Gee, et al., 2019). Other reviews (scoping, systematic and meta-analyses) have summarised or included causation theories as an element of their review, while primarily focusing on mapping the evidence correlating parental maltreatment in childhood to outcomes for children or mediating and moderating factors (Assink et al., 2018; Langevin et al., 2021; Zhang et al., 2023). Still others have focused on the evidence for a particular theoretical framework in the intergenerational childhood maltreatment literature (e.g. attachment theory or epigenetic transmission) (Chamberlain, Ralph, et al., 2019; Langevin et al., 2023; Zhou & Ryan, 2023).

METHODOLOGY

This scoping review draws upon the five-stage framework proposed by Arksey and O'Malley (2005) and elements of its enhancement by Levac et al., (2010). The stages involve clarifying the research question, identifying relevant studies, selecting studies, charting the data, and collating and reporting the results. The optional sixth stage of Arksey and O'Malley's framework, the consultation exercise, was not conducted as part of this review.

Identifying the Research Question

The initial stage in the methodology involves clarifying the research questions (Arksey & O'Malley, 2005) and linking them to the goals, purpose, and rationale for the study (Levac et al., 2010). The review seeks to answer the following questions:

1. Which theoretical frameworks does the literature apply to explain intergenerational recurrence of child maltreatment?
2. What intervention strategies does the literature propose in work with families who have experienced or are at risk of intergenerational child maltreatment?
3. Are there any trends, patterns, and correlations apparent in the literature on explanatory theories and proposed interventions on intergenerational continuity of child maltreatment?

Identifying Relevant Studies

Stage two involves decisions about the design and conduct of the search strategy, including selection of databases, search terms, and search strategies outside of the usage of electronic databases (Arksey & O'Malley, 2005). In accord with Levac et al., (2010)'s recognition of the need to balance comprehensiveness with feasibility in situations where searches result in vast amounts of literature, searches of a limited number of relevant databases (Academic Search Complete [EBSCO Host], PubMed, Scopus, and ProQuest) were conducted. These searches took place in December 2023 and January 2024.

In order to limit the scope of results, the combination of the three key factors (child maltreatment, intergenerational considerations, and theoretical conceptualisations) was entered over three lines of the advanced search function, linked by the joining term 'AND' (see Table 1). Truncation was used to collect relevant results (e.g., "generational" to locate results covering "intergenerational", "transgenerational", "multigenerational", and others, including their hyphenated variations) and wildcards were applied to collect key words containing both American and British/Australian spellings (e.g., "conceptuali?ations"). Title, keywords, and abstract, or "everywhere except full text" were searched where there was the option to apply these limiters. Where facilitated by the database, the limiter of "peer-reviewed" was also selected. No date limiters were applied as this review recognises the historical value of dated papers and, as one aspect of the review, seeks to explore whether (and if so how) theoretical conceptualisations and recommended interventions have changed over time.

Table 1. Search terms

*intergenerational OR multigenerational OR transgenerational OR cross-generational OR generational OR *generational OR generations OR cycle OR cycles*	AND
"child abuse" OR "child neglect" OR "child maltreatment" OR "childhood maltreatment" OR "child victimi?ation" OR "adverse childhood experiences" OR "child protection" OR "child protect" OR "child welfare" OR "looked after" OR "out-of-home care"*	AND
"transmission theories" OR "theories of transmission" OR "theoretical understandings" OR "theoretical constructs" OR "theoretical frameworks" OR "conceptual frameworks" OR "mechanisms of transmission" OR conceptuali?ations OR explanation OR explanations OR perspective OR perspectives	

A total of 1567 potentially relevant studies were identified in this initial search. Four hundred and thirty-two duplicates were identified and removed, leaving 1135 results for the initial screening.

To identify relevant results that may be published in sources outside of peer-reviewed journals, or not accessible or retrievable through the identified search terms, supplementary searching is a useful approach (Arksey & O'Malley, 2005; Cooper et al., 2017; Richards, 2008). As the review progressed, hand searching of key journals (particularly special issues), scanning reference lists and citations of sources during the full text review, and identifying sources from existing knowledge and professional networks revealed 57 additional results, for a total of 1192 records for initial screening.

Selection of Studies

Stage three involves clarifying the inclusion and exclusion criteria to determine which studies are included in the final analysis and review (Arksey & O'Malley, 2005). These decisions are collaboratively refined and revisited during iterative searches and reviews of sources so as to facilitate familiarity with the literature before arriving at a final decision (Arksey & O'Malley, 2005; Rumrill et al., 2010). Through this process, it was established that this review sought to include all papers written in English on intergenerational child maltreatment which articulated at least one clear explanatory theoretical framework. The selected studies could, but were not required to, propose or describe at least one intervention approach.

Covidence was used to select relevant studies. In the initial wave of review, the title and abstract of each result were scanned. Results which did not obviously pertain to intergenerational continuity of child maltreatment (e.g. dating violence, elder abuse, health and education outcomes of children, criminology, and parental separation) were excluded. Also excluded were papers written in languages other than English, papers that did not mention or allude to theories or explanations, papers that contributed to the knowledge on intergenerational child maltreatment without offering a theoretical framework, and papers on parenting styles and childhood experiences that did not meet the threshold for maltreatment (e.g. non-abusive parenting approaches such as corporal punishment and harsh parenting, domestic violence where children or parenting were not mentioned). Following this process, 146 results remained.

As titles and abstracts cannot always be relied upon as representative of the full scope of the article (Badger et al., 2000), a full text review was conducted to identify the papers which met the inclusion criteria and to remove those that did not. This review identified and excluded studies into the longitudinal impacts of abuse and neglect on the child without concentrating on parenting or maltreatment to subsequent generations. It also excluded those which mention one or more theory briefly without providing explanation or contextualisation of these theoretical frameworks.

Further clarification of inclusion and exclusion criteria were collaboratively ascertained to limit the scope of results to a manageable number and to ensure results were pertinent to the research questions (Levac et al., 2010). Results that did not offer a clear *explanatory* theoretical framework (for instance, human rights or person-centred frameworks which do not seek to explain the mechanisms behind intergenerational transmission) were excluded. Papers exploring the aetiology of intergenerational child maltreatment from a position of mediators and moderators (e.g., parental age, mental health diagnoses, social networks, types of abuse, levels of empathy, neurological defects, or intellectual disabilities), while potentially relevant from a systems or developmental theoretical perspective, were also excluded if they did not articulate a clear theoretical framework.

Other decisions required a more nuanced approach. Papers which concentrated on intergenerational continuity of Adverse Childhood Experiences (ACEs), a ten-item childhood trauma checklist correlated to adverse outcomes in later life (Felitti, 2002; Felitti et al., 1998), were considered and included only if the paper's focus was on intergenerational child maltreatment. This was in recognition of the fact that, while many of the ACEs relate directly to child abuse or neglect, others (parental loss due to separation or death, and the incarceration of or mental health diagnosis for a household member) do not necessarily or inevitably correlate with or denote child maltreatment. Similarly, intergenerational studies focusing on Early Maladaptive Schemas (EMSs), deleterious core beliefs about the self, others, and the world which develop due to unmet emotional needs in childhood (Young, 1999; Young et al., 2003), were not automatically included. Instead, it was acknowledged that a variety of parental behaviours, which may or may not meet the threshold for maltreatment, can result in unmet emotional needs and resulting EMSs. Therefore, only results which concentrated on child maltreatment in conjunction with EMSs were included. A third group of studies, those focused on historical or collective trauma related to colonisation, also underwent a process of consideration. This was in recognition of the fact that child removals were often an element of the colonisation process, as seen in the Stolen Generations and the Canadian residential school system (Atkinson, 2002; McCallum, 2022), and that subsequent maltreatment of Stolen or removed children reverberated over the generations. Results pertaining to colonisation trauma were included if a primary focus of the paper was on child maltreatment (as opposed to other elements of intergenerational oppression and disadvantage for Indigenous people).

Disagreements between authors were identified through Covidence, in which each of the authors of this review recommended papers be included or excluded from the review, and resolved through discussion between the three authors. Following the full text review 72 results remained, as demonstrated at Figure 1 below.

Figure 1. PRISMA diagram

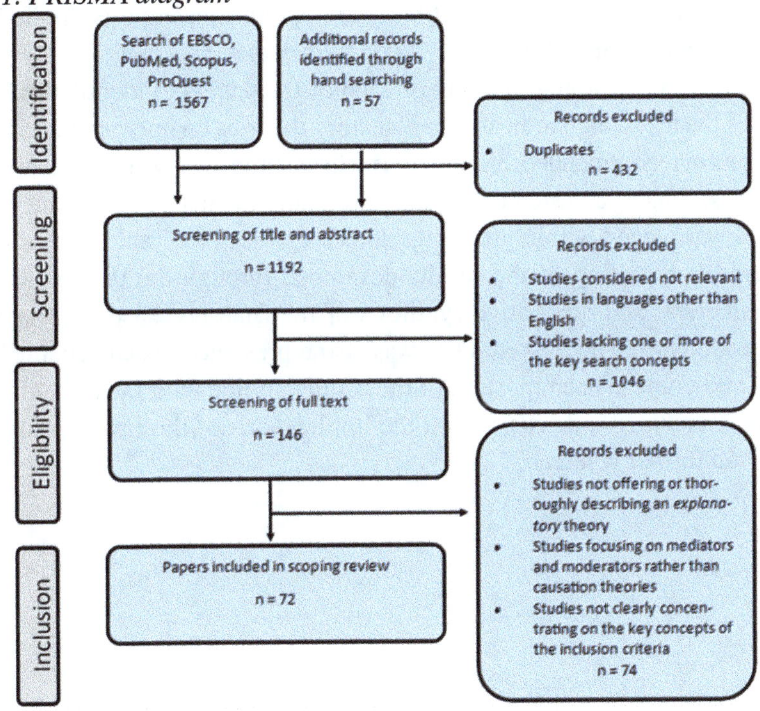

Charting the Data

The fourth stage in Arksey and O'Malley (2005) process for conducting scoping reviews involves charting the data within the included studies for synthesis and thematic interpretation. In accord with Levac et al.'s (2010) recommendations, the data charting form was developed collaboratively and was revised and updated continuously as the data was extracted and new themes became apparent. The key elements supporting an exploration of the research questions, including type of paper, date of publication, location of study, cohort of research participants, maltreatment type studied, were identified and data extracted. A data charting form was developed using Microsoft Excel, allowing data to be sorted and analysed under the different components.

Collating, Summarising, and Reporting the Results

Levac et al.,'s (2010) three step process of analysis (numerical summary and qualitative thematic analysis), reporting, and applying meaning is applied to the final stage of Arksey and O'Malley's (2005) framework. The qualitative analysis of the data involved a thorough reading of each of the papers to identify and extract elements of the text which indicated explanatory theories on intergenerational child maltreatment or recommended interventions. These summaries were then thematically analysed, resulting in a nested organisation of data in which specific interventions or theories was placed within groupings and categories (see Table 2, below).

A narrative reporting of the results developed through the themes that arose from a numerical and qualitative synthesis of the findings, ensuring that the research questions were addressed. Data was also represented visually, using Sankey diagrams and graphs. The reporting of the results, in line with Levac et al., (2010) suggestions, included a discussion on the implications of the findings for policy, practice, and further research.

Table 2. Included papers

Citation	Type of paper	Data sources	Focus/cohort	Type of maltreatment	Location of study	Theoretical framework/s articulated	Theoretical framework/s (coding)	Proposed intervention/s articulated	Proposed intervention/s (coding)
Abbassi & Aslinia (2010)	Review *(narrative)*	•Existing literature		•Domestic and family violence		•Social learning theory and social cognitive theory	•LEARNING: social learning, legitimisation	•Exploration of how children view their roles and the modelling in the family •Emphasis on healthy adaptive behaviour and discouragement of maladaptive behaviour	•DIRECT INTERVENTION: develop parenting skills, emotional and behavioural regulation skills
Aguiar & Halseth (2015)	Grey literature *(organisational publication)*	•Existing literature	•Indigenous *(Canadian Aboriginal residential school survivors)*		Canada	•Psychological processes *(brain development and psychological processes, attachment with caregiver, emotional self-regulation, reading and adapting to social cues)* •Physiological processes *(biological and epigenetic)* •Social processes *(learned coping strategies and impaired parenting/attachment, suppression of Aboriginal culture, interruption of healthy Indigenous child-rearing practices)*	•RELATIONAL: attachment •DEVELOPMENTAL: physiological, mental health •SYSTEMS: ecological, current adversity •HERITABILITY: epigenetic •CULTURAL: cultural, Indigenous	•transcend Western conceptualisations of trauma, including collective and cumulative trauma Aboriginal people have experienced over generations •Re-establish pride and identity through "culture as treatment" (Gone 2013)	•TARGET COHORT: community work •DIRECT INTERVENTION: cultural healing •SYSTEMIC APPROACH: attend to ideologies

continued on following page

Table 2. Continued

Citation	Type of paper	Data sources	Focus/cohort	Type of maltreatment	Location of study	Theoretical framework/s articulated	Theoretical framework/s (coding)	Proposed intervention/s articulated	Proposed intervention/s (coding)
Alexander (2015)	Book	•Existing literature				•Attachment theory •Family systems theory •Developmental evolutionary-based perspective	•RELATIONAL: attachment, family systems •DEVELOPMENTAL: physiological •HERITABILITY: genetic, epigenetic •CULTURAL: culture	•Parent-child interventions to increase mother's sensitivity, e.g., video feedback interventions •Address mother's childhood trauma and link to parenting and increase reflective functioning, e.g., Mothers and Toddlers Program (MTP) •Awareness of therapists' countertransference reactions •Supporting involvement of fathers •Couples therapy (emotionally focused, reflective functioning) •Family therapy •Differential susceptibility - identifying and treating children most at risk based on genetic assessment •Parenting interventions pre-birth for epigenetic changes	•TARGET COHORT: individual parent, family system, parent-child dyad, parent couple/ caregivers •TIMING: perinatal •ASSESSMENT: biological/genetic •DIRECT INTERVENTION: acknowledge and integrate trauma, enhance parental attunement, develop parenting skills, specific models •REFLECTIVE PRACTICE: manage countertransference •RESEARCH: gender pathways

continued on following page

Table 2. Continued

Citation	Type of paper	Data sources	Focus/cohort	Type of maltreatment	Location of study	Theoretical framework/s articulated	Theoretical framework/s (coding)	Proposed intervention/s articulated	Proposed intervention/s (coding)
Alink et al. (2019)	Review *(introduction to special issue)*	•Existing literature	•Parents			•Social learning theory •Social information processing •Attachment theory •Neurophysiological models •Developmental psychopathology models •Heritability models	•RELATIONAL: attachment •DEVELOPMENTAL: physiological, mental health •HERITABILITY: genetic •CORE BELIEFS: social information processing •LEARNING: social learning	•Group Attachment-Based Intervention (GABI) (Steele et al. 2019) •Notes paucity in research on fathers and seeks to address this	•TARGET COHORT: family system, group work •DIRECT INTERVENTION: specific models •RESEARCH: fathers/ other carers
Amos & Segal (2018)	Conceptual paper *(proposes therapeutic model)*	•Existing literature	•Childhood •Mother			•Bio-behavioural explanation of personality development •Attachment theory •Defences against threat *(anti-predator and group living defences)* •Structural dissociation	•RELATIONAL: attachment, family systems •DEVELOPMENTAL: physiological •UNPROCESSED TRAUMA: dissociation	•Parallel Parent and Child Therapy (P-PACT). Incorporates Parallel Parent and Child Narrative (PPCN), Adult Exploration of Attachment Interview (AEAI), and self-other differentiation	•TARGET COHORT: individual parent, individual child, parent-child dyad •TIMING: childhood •DIRECT INTERVENTION: acknowledge and integrate trauma, enhance parental attunement, self-other differentiation, specific
Amos et al. (2011)	Conceptual paper *(proposes therapeutic model) (includes*	•Existing literature	•Childhood •Mother			•Motivational systems perspective of personality development •Relational trauma *(attachment disorganisation)* •Structural dissociation and experiential avoidance	•RELATIONAL: attachment •DEVELOPMENTAL: physiological •UNPROCESSED TRAUMA: dissociation	•Parallel Parent Child Narrative/Parent and Child Therapy (PPCN/PACT). Involves detoxifying and integrating the dissociated parts of the personality (activation, exposure, counter-conditioning) that are triggered by parent-child relationship	•TARGET COHORT: individual parent, individual child, parent-child dyad •TIMING: childhood •DIRECT INTERVENTION: acknowledge and integrate trauma, enhance parental attunement, specific models

continued on following page

Table 2. Continued

Citation	Type of paper	Data sources	Focus/cohort	Type of maltreatment	Location of study	Theoretical framework/s articulated	Theoretical framework/s (coding)	Proposed intervention/s articulated	Proposed intervention/s (coding)
Arons (2005)	Case study	•Case study material	•Mother •Perinatal *(mother and infant son)*		North America	•Attachment •Psychodynamic	•RELATIONAL: attachment •UNPROCESSED TRAUMA: psychodynamic	•"Name, metabolise, and flexibly respond to painful, dissociated or frightening experiences" (p 102) •mother-infant psychotherapy	•TARGET COHORT: parent-child dyad •TIMING: long term •DIRECT INTERVENTION: acknowledge and integrate trauma, use of therapeutic relationship, strengths-based
Babcock Fenerci & DePrince (2018)	Research study	•Self-report *(questionnaires, e.g., traumatic event screening inventory, trauma appraisal questionnaire, trauma symptom*	•Mother •Childhood *(children aged 2-5)*		North America	•Dissociated trauma related cognitions *(post-trauma appraisals and disorganised memory)*	•UNPROCESSED TRAUMA: dissociation	•Re-organising, reframing, restructuring parents' memories and appraisals of their trauma •Future studies incorporating fathers and using multimethod, multireporter, longitudinal, randomised control approaches	•DIRECT INTERVENTION: acknowledge and integrate trauma, enhance parental attunement •RESEARCH: fathers/ other carers, longitudinal prospective studies
Belsky (1993)	Review *(narrative)*	•Existing literature		•Physical abuse •Neglect		•Developmental-ecological context, immediate interactional context, and broader context •Learning •Parents' philosophies of discipline •Internal working model •Personality •Societal-cultural context	•RELATIONAL: attachment •DEVELOPMENTAL: psychosocial •SYSTEMS: ecological, current adversity •LEARNING: social learning, legitimacy •CULTURAL: culture, Afr-Amer	•Addressing poverty, young parenting, lack of education •Providing pre- and post- natal emotional support and guidance. •Attention to the level of support provided by the spouse and to stepparents	•DIRECT INTERVENTION: develop parenting skills, home visiting programs •SYSTEMIC APPROACH: alleviate disadvantage, attend to ideologies •RESEARCH: fathers/ other carers

continued on following page

Table 2. Continued

Citation	Type of paper	Data sources	Focus/cohort	Type of maltreatment	Location of study	Theoretical framework/s articulated	Theoretical framework/s (coding)	Proposed intervention/s articulated	Proposed intervention/s (coding)
Bennett (2021)	Book section	•Existing literature				•Attachment •Emotional, behavioural, cognitive and developmental sequelae •Neurocognitive defects •Cognitive schema	•RELATIONAL: attachment •DEVELOPMENTAL: physiological, mental health •CORE BELIEFS: schema	•Early intervention and treatment •An always available adult •Interventions with child for self-esteem, coping, behaviours •Parental interventions addressing factors such as poverty, mental health, substance use •Research into the efficacy of treatments for evidence-based and evidence-informed intervention	•TARGET COHORT: individual parent, individual child •TIMING: early intervention •DIRECT INTERVENTION: build informal networks, strengths-based •SYSTEMIC APPROACH: alleviate disadvantage •RESEARCH: evaluation
Berthelot et al. (2015)	Research study	•Self-report *(questionnaires, semi structured interviews)* •Observation *(strange situation procedure)*	•Mother •Perinatal *(mothers in third trimester of pregnancy and post-natal)*		Canada	•Attachment •Deficits in mentalisation and reflective functioning regarding trauma	•RELATIONAL: attachment •UNPROCESSED TRAUMA: dissociation	•Helping parents comprehend the impacts of trauma on their self as an individual and a parent. •Reflective functioning regarding trauma	•DIRECT INTERVENTION: acknowledge and integrate trauma, enhance parental attunement
Borelli et al. (2019)	Research study	•Self-report *(checklists completed by parent, semi-structured interview)*	•Mother	•Child sexual abuse	Canada	•"Traumatic shrapnel" affecting the entire family system •Maternal trauma-reflective functioning	•RELATIONAL: family systems •UNPROCESSED TRAUMA: dissociation	•Support mothers' mentalisation of own trauma •Family-based approaches •Treat mental health	•TARGET COHORT: family system •DIRECT INTERVENTION: acknowledge and integrate trauma, enhance parental attunement, emotional and behavioural regulation skills

continued on following page

Table 2. Continued

Citation	Type of paper	Data sources	Focus/cohort	Type of maltreatment	Location of study	Theoretical framework/s articulated	Theoretical framework/s (coding)	Proposed intervention/s articulated	Proposed intervention/s (coding)
Buchheim et al. (2022)	Research study	•Self-report *(questionnaires e.g., childhood trauma questionnaire, adult attachment projective picture system)* •Observation *(strange situation procedure)* •Biological *(laboratory procedures exploring HPA functioning and genetics related to oxytocin)*	•Mother •Perinatal *(birth to 12 months)*		Germany	•Attachment •Genetic and biological stress susceptibility •Social support	•RELATIONAL: attachment •SYSTEMS: ecological •HERITABILITY: genetic	•Social support reduced maternal stress and psychopathology •Personalised and tailored treatment based on genetic risk •Possible pharmacological treatments •Future research into the oxytocinergic system in mother-child dyads	•DIRECT INTERVENTION: build informal networks, oxytocin •RESEARCH: biological
Buss et al. (2017)	Review *(narrative)*	•Existing literature	•Perinatal *(prenatal)*			•Gestational biological *(epigenetic and physical alterations in gestational biological environment)*	•DEVELOPMENTAL: physiological •HERITABILITY: epigenetic	•Screening women for child maltreatment in pre-conception and early pregnancy •Future research involving neurodevelopmental assessments at birth •Studies into intergenerational effects in the gender of offspring	•TIMING: perinatal •ASSESSMENT: screening •RESEARCH: biological, gender pathways

continued on following page

Table 2. Continued

Citation	Type of paper	Data sources	Focus/cohort	Type of maltreatment	Location of study	Theoretical framework/s articulated	Theoretical framework/s (coding)	Proposed intervention/s articulated	Proposed intervention/s (coding)
Chamberlain et al. (2019)	Review *(scoping)*	•Existing literature	•Perinatal *(prenatal to 2 years)*			•Attachment •Belsky's sociological model •"Ghosts/Angels in the Nursery" •Relational developmental •Object relations theory •Resilience theories •Social learning •Family systems •Child sexual assault theoretical healing model •Anger theories	•RELATIONAL: attachment, family systems •SYSTEMS: ecological •UNPROCESSED TRAUMA: psychodynamic •LEARNING: social learning, legitimacy •CULTURAL: Indigenous	•Perinatal period as an opportunity for effective intervention •Care services to be trauma-informed •Research into fathers and other carers & Indigenous people •Flexible, short-term evaluations strategies designed in collaboration with families/communities	•TIMING: perinatal •SYSTEMIC APPROACH: trauma-informed services •RESEARCH: fathers/ other carers, evaluation
Cicchetti & Rizley (1981)	Research study	•Self-report *(structured interview)*			England	•Developmental theories •Transactional	•DEVELOPMENTAL: physiological, psychosocial •SYSTEMS: ecological		
Cordero et al. (2012)	Research study	•Biological *(measurement of plasma corticosterone, post- mortem brain analysis)*	•Animal			•Biological factors	•DEVELOPMENTAL: physiological •HERITABILITY: epigenetic	•Research into biological mechanisms	•RESEARCH: biological

continued on following page

Table 2. Continued

Citation	Type of paper	Data sources	Focus/cohort	Type of maltreatment	Location of study	Theoretical framework/s articulated	Theoretical framework/s (coding)	Proposed intervention/s articulated	Proposed intervention/s (coding)
Cornett (1985)	Review *(narrative)*	•Existing literature		•Physical abuse		•Psychanalytic self-psychology	•UNPROCESSED TRAUMA: psychodynamic	•Treating the individual abuser, entire family, and in groups •A treatment emphasis on empathy and reparenting	•TARGET COHORT: individual parent, family system, parent couple/ caregivers, group work •TIMING: childhood •DIRECT INTERVENTION: acknowledge and integrate trauma, use of therapeutic relationship, enhance parental attunement, flexible approach
DeGregorio (2013)	Conceptual paper *(proposes conceptual model)*	•Existing literature				•Neuropsychological methods *(the "social brain" [p.160])*	•RELATIONAL: attachment •DEVELOPMENTAL: physiological, psychosocial	•Parenting interventions aware of and tailored to the potential neurological deficits in the social brain and subsequent insecure attachment (e.g., Parenting with Feeling, Neurosequential Model of Therapeutics) •Evaluation and dissemination of neuropsychological approaches	•ASSESSMENT: biological/genetic •DIRECT INTERVENTION: specific models •RESEARCH: evaluation
Delsol & Margolin (2004)	Review *(systemic-like)*	•Existing literature		•Domestic and family violence		•Social learning •Legitimacy of violence •Attachment disruption •Family disruption •Continuity of anti-social behaviour •Genetics and heritability	•RELATIONAL: attachment, family systems •HERITABILITY: genetics •LEARNING: social learning, legitimacy •CULTURAL: culture		

continued on following page

Table 2. Continued

Citation	Type of paper	Data sources	Focus/cohort	Type of maltreatment	Location of study	Theoretical framework/s articulated	Theoretical framework/s (coding)	Proposed intervention/s articulated	Proposed intervention/s (coding)
Duthie et al. (2019)	Book section	•Existing literature	•Indigenous *(Indigenous Australians and Canadians)*			•Colonisation •Social inequity/ inequality	•SYSTEMS: ecological, current adversity •CULTURAL: cultural, Indigenous	•Incorporate Indigenous worldviews •Indigenous representation & community organisation •Public health approaches, delivered early, to support families and communities •Practitioner reflection, including personal and societal assumptions and practitioners' own culture as well as that of 'others', and power •More robust data and evaluations	•TIMING: early intervention •DIRECT INTERVENTION: specific models, flexible approach •SYSTEMIC APPROACH: attend to ideologies, trauma-informed services •SELF-REFLECTION: recognise/challenge assumptions •RESEARCH: evaluation
Finzi-Dottan & Harel (2014)	Research study	•Self-report *(questionnaires - e.g., emotional control questionnaire, child abuse potential inventory, childhood trauma questionnaire, perceived stress scale)*	•Perinatal •Childhood *(aged up to 6)* •Parents		Israel	•Belsky's developmental-ecological model *(social information processing, parenting and attachment, contextual factors)*	•RELATIONAL: attachment •SYSTEMS: ecological, current adversity •CORE BELIEFS: social information processing •CULTURAL: culture	•Parental interventions, provided over a longer term, to enhance emotional control, behaviour management strategies, attunement/ sensitivity to children •Provide support to reduce parental stress	•TARGET COHORT: individual parent •TIMING: long term •DIRECT INTERVENTION: enhance parental attunement, develop parenting skills, emotional and behavioural regulation skills •SYSTEMIC APPROACH: alleviate disadvantage

continued on following page

Table 2. Continued

Citation	Type of paper	Data sources	Focus/cohort	Type of maltreatment	Location of study	Theoretical framework/s articulated	Theoretical framework/s (coding)	Proposed intervention/s articulated	Proposed intervention/s (coding)
Geiger et al. (2015)	Book section	•Existing literature				•Social learning •Attachment •Ecological frameworks •Resilience and protective factors •Trauma and epigenetics	•RELATIONAL: attachment •SYSTEMS: ecological •HERITABILITY: epigenetic •LEARNING: social learning	•Aging-out of care process presents unique opportunities for intervention •Develop interventions that consider parents' histories and include teaching parental skills and treat mental health •Researchers and practitioners to understanding effects of multigenerational child maltreatment •Build understanding on social imitation of violence based on gender and longitudinal studies enrolling children before birth	•TIMING: adolescence •DIRECT INTERVENTION: develop parenting skills, pharmacological •SYSTEMIC APPROACH: trauma-informed services •RESEARCH: fathers/ other carers, longitudinal prospective studies, gender pathways
Green (1976)	Research study *(includes case studies)*	•Self-report *(structured interviews)* •Case study material	•Mother *(mothers under supervision of child protection agencies)*	•Child protection involvement	North America	•Environmental stress •Personality characteristics of parent •Contributions of child	•DEVELOPMENTAL: psychosocial •SYSTEMS: ecological, current adversity •UNPROCESSED TRAUMA: psychodynamic	•Non-critical, need-satisfying therapy with parent with focus on increasing self-esteem •Encourage friendships - consider group therapy •Once trust and rapport built, work on connections between childhood experiences and parenting •Address feelings elicited by therapist	•TARGET COHORT: individual parent, group work •TIMING: childhood, long term •DIRECT INTERVENTION: use of therapeutic relationship, develop parenting skills, build informal networks, home visiting programs •REFLECTIVE PRACTICE: manage countertransference

continued on following page

Table 2. Continued

Citation	Type of paper	Data sources	Focus/cohort	Type of maltreatment	Location of study	Theoretical framework/s articulated	Theoretical framework/s (coding)	Proposed intervention/s articulated	Proposed intervention/s (coding)
Hall (2011)	Research study	•Self-report *(semi-structured interviews)*	•Mother *(mothers who had experienced child abuse and did not repeat abuse*		North America	•Attachment *(customised)* •Social learning •Biological developmental *(reveal gaps)* •Strengths-based	•RELATIONAL: attachment •DEVELOPMENTAL: physiological •SYSTEMS: ecological •LEARNING: social learning	•Non-dominant cultural views of "healthy parenting" •Customised view of attachment •Building on strengths •Diverse/eclectic parenting role models •Strengths-based focus to research	•DIRECT INTERVENTION: flexible approach, build informal networks, strengths-based •SYSTEMIC APPROACH: attend to ideologies •REFLECTIVE PRACTICE: recognise/ challenge assumptions •RESEARCH: intergenerational discontinuity
Herzberger (1983)	Book section	•Existing literature				•Social-cognitive perspective *(involves "teaching children that aggressive behaviour is appropriate, failing to teach children an internalised morality, transferring a particular self or interpersonal perspective from adult to child" [p. 326])*	•CORE BELIEFS: social information processing •LEARNING: social learning, legitimacy		

continued on following page

Table 2. Continued

Citation	Type of paper	Data sources	Focus/cohort	Type of maltreatment	Location of study	Theoretical framework/s articulated	Theoretical framework/s (coding)	Proposed intervention/s articulated	Proposed intervention/s (coding)
Howell et al. (2021)	Review *(narrative)*	•Existing literature				•Biological factors •Caregiver mental health and parenting •Social ecological viewpoint •Resilience	•DEVELOPMENTAL: physiological, psychosocial, mental health •SYSTEMS: ecological, current adversity •HERITABILITY: epigenetic •CULTURAL: culture	•Interventions that focus on the "interconnected systems that perpetuate adversity across time" (p. 9) •Interventions in pregnancy, other developmental junctures •Interventions and research with all caregivers, not just biological mothers •Sibling studies to explore differing outcomes in children from the same families	•TARGET COHORT: parent couple/caregivers •TIMING: perinatal •DIRECT INTERVENTION: specific models, develop parenting skills, build informal networks, strengths-based, cultural healing •SYSTEMIC APPROACH: alleviate disadvantage, attend to ideologies •RESEARCH: fathers/ other carers, intergenerational discontinuity
Hurst & Sawatzky (1996)	Research study	•Self-report *(questionnaire - personal authority in the family system, semi-structured interview with genogram providing framework for discussion)*	•Parents *(parents of families involved with child protection and referred to counselling)*	•Child protection involvement	Canada	•Bowenian family systems theory	•RELATIONAL: family systems	•Clarifying context through family assessment	•ASSESSMENT: multigenerational

continued on following page

Table 2. Continued

Citation	Type of paper	Data sources	Focus/cohort	Type of maltreatment	Location of study	Theoretical framework/s articulated	Theoretical framework/s (coding)	Proposed intervention/s articulated	Proposed intervention/s (coding)
Huth-Bocks et al. (2013)	Research study	•Self-report *(questionnaires, e.g. childhood trauma questionnaire, conflict tactics Scale-2, PTSD checklist, interviews)*	•Mother •Perinatal *(pregnant mothers who had experienced relational trauma in childhood and/or*		North America	•Attachment theory *(transformation in pregnancy from being protected/cared for to protecting/caring)* •Relational trauma and PTSD	•RELATIONAL: attachment •DEVELOPMENTAL: psychosocial, mental health	•Assessment and treatment of pregnant womens' past and current relational trauma, including emotional and psychological	•TIMING: perinatal •ASSESSMENT: screening, different forms of maltreatment
Iyengar et al. (2019)	Review *(narrative)*	•Existing literature	•Mother			•Attachment perspectives •Neuroscience perspectives	•RELATIONAL: attachment •DEVELOPMENTAL: physiological	•Mentalisation, reflective functioning, and attachment reorganisation	•DIRECT INTERVENTION: acknowledge and integrate trauma, enhance parental attunement
Juul et al. (2016)	Research study	•Biological *(maternal cortisol samples)* •Self-report *(interviews for maternal trauma exposure, Inventory for mental health)* •Observation *(videotaped mother- child interactions following stressor to infant)*	•Mother •Perinatal *(mothers in post-partum period)*		North America	•HPA axis dysregulation •Affective quality of mother-infant interactions	•RELATIONAL: attachment •DEVELOPMENTAL: physiological	•Consider trauma history in assessment and treatment of postpartum psychiatric illness	•ASSESSMENT: screening

continued on following page

Table 2. Continued

Citation	Type of paper	Data sources	Focus/cohort	Type of maltreatment	Location of study	Theoretical framework/s articulated	Theoretical framework/s (coding)	Proposed intervention/s articulated	Proposed intervention/s (coding)
Kim & Strathearn (2017)	Review *(narrative)*	•Existing literature	•Mother •Perinatal *(mothers and infants aged 12 months)*			•Attachment research •Oxytocin research	•RELATIONAL: attachment •DEVELOPMENTAL: physiological	•Support reorganising attachment for mothers who experienced early maltreatment •Artificially introducing oxytocin through pharmacological treatments (with caution) •Further studies on oxytocin dysregulation depending on the characteristics, timing, duration, re-occurrence of trauma	•DIRECT INTERVENTION: acknowledge and integrate trauma, oxytocin •RESEARCH: biological
Kim (2012)	Review *(narrative)*	•Existing literature				•Dodge's social information processing •Nesbert's cultural cognitive theory •Turiel's social-cognitive domain theory *(considers each theory through a cultural value system lens)*	•SYSTEMS: ecological •LEARNING: legitimacy •CORE BELIEFS: social information processing •CULTURAL: culture		
Kim et al. (2011)	Research study	•Self-report *(structured interview, questionnaires -e.g., inventory of parent and peer attachment, adult attachment*	•Mother *(non-offending mothers)*	•Child sexual abuse	North America	•Attachment representations	•RELATIONAL: attachment	•Learn about mothers' attachment relationship experiences/patterns when working with families of sexually abused children	•ASSESSMENT: attachment

continued on following page

Table 2. Continued

Citation	Type of paper	Data sources	Focus/cohort	Type of maltreatment	Location of study	Theoretical framework/s articulated	Theoretical framework/s (coding)	Proposed intervention/s articulated	Proposed intervention/s (coding)
Köhler-Dauner et al. (2019)	Research study	•Self-report *(questionnaires e.g., atypical maternal behaviour instrument for assessment and classification childhood trauma questionnaire)* •Observation *(strange situation protocol)* •Biological *(salivary cortisol measurement)*	•Mother •Perinatal *(mothers and infants)*		Germany	•Mother-child interaction •HPA response	•DEVELOPMENTAL: physiological, psychosocial	•Interventions improving maternal behaviour and parent-infant relationships	•DIRECT INTERVENTION: enhance parental attunement
Lecic-Tosovski et al. (2014)	Review *(narrative)*	•Existing literature		•Domestic and family violence		•Personality development •Vulnerability to mental health disorders •Family systems communication dysfunction	•RELATIONAL: family systems •DEVELOPMENTAL: psychosocial, mental health •CORE BELIEFS: social information processing	•Psychoeducation of healthy parenting •Early detection and treatment of trauma	•TIMING: early intervention •DIRECT INTERVENTION: develop parenting skills

continued on following page

Table 2. Continued

Citation	Type of paper	Data sources	Focus/cohort	Type of maltreatment	Location of study	Theoretical framework/s articulated	Theoretical framework/s (coding)	Proposed intervention/s articulated	Proposed intervention/s (coding)
Levendosky (2013)	Review *(concluding remarks on special issue)*	•Existing literature		•Domestic and family violence		•Psychodynamically informed framework •Disruptions to attachment *(internal working models)* and parenting •Social information processing •Defences - *projection* •Social learning •Social-cognitive schema	•RELATIONAL: attachment •UNPROCESSED TRAUMA: psychodynamic, dissociation •CORE BELIEFS: social information processing •LEARNING: social learning	•Mom's Empowerment Program (MEP) - a group therapy influenced by interpersonal therapy (Graham-Bermann & Miller, 2013) •Kernberg's transference-focused psychotherapy (Bogat et. al, 2013) •Ongoing assessment of past abuse to account for limited disclosure at onset, safety planning,	•TARGET COHORT: group work •ASSESSMENT: continuous •DIRECT INTERVENTION: acknowledge and integrate trauma, use of therapeutic relationship, specific models
Levendosky et al. (2012)	Review *(narrative) (includes case study)*	•Existing literature •Case study material		•Domestic and family violence		•Attachment *(internal working model)*	•RELATIONAL: attachment	•Acknowledge diversity in situations and interventions •Treatment encouraging exploration of trauma history and the meaning made of it, within the support of a safe therapeutic relationship •Studies into the father-infant attachment, and prospective longitudinal studies from infancy into adulthood	•DIRECT INTERVENTION: acknowledge and integrate trauma, use of therapeutic relationship, flexible approach •RESEARCH: fathers/ other carers, longitudinal prospective studies

continued on following page

Table 2. Continued

Citation	Type of paper	Data sources	Focus/cohort	Type of maltreatment	Location of study	Theoretical framework/s articulated	Theoretical framework/s (coding)	Proposed intervention/s articulated	Proposed intervention/s (coding)
Lomanowska et al. (2017)	Review *(narrative)*	•Existing literature	•Animal *(animal and human research subjects)*			•Psychological mediators of parenting •Physiological mediators of parenting •Genes •Epigenetics	•DEVELOPMENTAL: psychosocial, physiological •HERITABILITY: genetic, epigenetic	•Systemic policies aimed at reducing stressors •Interventions in the perinatal period building parents' emotional regulation, attention/ response to child's signals, ability to manage stress •Further biological research, including longitudinal studies and those incorporating fathers	•TIMING: perinatal •DIRECT INTERVENTION: emotional and behavioural regulation skills, enhance parental attunement •SYSTEMIC APPROACH: alleviate disadvantage •RESEARCH: fathers/ other carers, longitudinal prospective studies, biological
Markward et al. (2000)	Review *(narrative)*	•Existing literature		•Domestic and family violence *(substance abuse, women abuse, and child abuse)*		•Diathesis stress model *(social learning and adverse conditions)* •Biochemical •Genetic •PsychosOcial factors •External factors	•DEVELOPMENTAL: physiological, psychosocial •SYSTEMS: ecological, current adversity •HERITABILITY: genetic •LEARNING: social learning, legitimacy •CULTURAL: culture	•Focus on assessments that include social history, genograms, eco-maps	•ASSESSMENT: multigenerational

continued on following page

Table 2. Continued

Citation	Type of paper	Data sources	Focus/cohort	Type of maltreatment	Location of study	Theoretical framework/s articulated	Theoretical framework/s (coding)	Proposed intervention/s articulated	Proposed intervention/s (coding)
Marshall et al. (2022)	Review *(systematic scoping)*	•Existing literature				•Attachment •Traumatic stress models •Family systems •Ecological framework •Developmental •Biological *(neurophysiological and heritability)*	•RELATIONAL: attachment, family systems •DEVELOPMENTAL: mental health, physiological •HERITABILITY: genetic •SYSTEMS: ecological	•Family and attachment-based treatment involving search for resilience such as child-parent psychotherapy (Cicchetti et al., 2006), Minding the Baby (Sadler et al., 2013) •Treatment of parents' mental health problems •Psychoeducation and therapy to foster more positive parenting practices •Examining the role of fathers in research	•TIMING: perinatal •DIRECT INTERVENTION: enhance parental attunement, specific models, strengths-based, pharmacological •RESEARCH: fathers/ other carers
McCollum (2015)	Conceptual paper *(proposes conceptual model) (includes*	•Existing literature •Case study material			North America	•Multigenerational dissociation	•UNPROCESSED TRAUMA: dissociation	•Support clients to build coherent narratives, expand their life stories, consider their multigenerational context	•DIRECT INTERVENTION: acknowledge and integrate trauma
McMillen & Rideout (1996)	Review *(narrative)*	•Existing literature				•It's in the genes: heritability •It's learned: socialisation theories •It's affect regulation: Bowen and others •It's cognitive: attachment theory •It's unmet needs: self-psychology •It's multiply determined: risk and protection	•RELATIONAL: family systems, attachment •DEVELOPMENTAL: psychosocial •SYSTEMS: ecological •UNPROCESSED TRAUMA: psychodynamic •HERITABILITY: genetic •LEARNING: social learning, legitimacy	•Multiple interventions based around different theories of transmission	•TARGET COHORT: individual parent, individual child •DIRECT INTERVENTION: acknowledge and integrate trauma, use of therapeutic relationship, enhance parental attunement, self- other differentiation, develop parenting skills, build informal networks, strengths-based

continued on following page

Table 2. Continued

Citation	Type of paper	Data sources	Focus/cohort	Type of maltreatment	Location of study	Theoretical framework/s articulated	Theoretical framework/s (coding)	Proposed intervention/s articulated	Proposed intervention/s (coding)
Merrill et al. (2021)	Research study	•Self-report *(questionnaires, e.g., adverse childhood experiences, brief infant sleep questionnaire, child behaviour checklist)* •Biological *(blood DNA and DNA methylation collection and analysis)*	•Father •Perinatal *(paternal ACEs and infants aged 3 months)*			• Biological •Epigenetic	•DEVELOPMENTAL: physiological •HERITABILITY: epigenetic	•Research topic of paternal ACES and infant DNAm prospectively as well as retrospectively	•RESEARCH: longitudinal prospective studies
Meulewaeter et al. (2019)	Research study	•Self-report *(interviews*	•Mother *(mothers with substance use disorders)*		Belgium	•Attachment	•RELATIONAL: attachment	•Healing early trauma, coping strategies, supporting parent-infant attachment, parenting support in treating substance abusing mothers •Attachment, self-regulation and competency model (ARC) •Evaluate the use of parenting interventions on substance using mothers •Future studies that discover protective factors and post-traumatic growth	•TIMING: long term •DIRECT INTERVENTION: acknowledge and integrate trauma, enhance parental attunement, specific models •RESEARCH: intergenerational discontinuity, evaluation

continued on following page

Table 2. Continued

Citation	Type of paper	Data sources	Focus/cohort	Type of maltreatment	Location of study	Theoretical framework/s articulated	Theoretical framework/s (coding)	Proposed intervention/s articulated	Proposed intervention/s (coding)
Mielke et al. (2016)	Research study	•Self-report *(semi-structured interview)* •Observation *(standardised mother- child interaction task)* •Biological *(brain MRI*		•Physical abuse •Child sexual abuse	Germany	•Biological-cognitive development *(maternal sensitivity brain region reduced – compensated for by cognitive empathic brain region)*	•DEVELOPMENTAL: physiological, psychosocial	•Further research on the "neuronal basis of maternal sensitivity" (p. 65)	•RESEARCH: biological
Mitkovic Voncina et al. (2017)	Review *(narrative)*	•Existing literature				•Psychodynamic, attachment and mentalisation frameworks •Cognitive behaviour frameworks •Personality and psychiatric disorders •Neurodevelopment, stress sensitivity and oxytocin •Brain and parenting •Genetic and epigenetic	•RELATIONAL: attachment •DEVELOPMENTAL: psychosocial, physiological •UNPROCESSED TRAUMA: psychodynamic •HERITABILITY: genetic, epigenetic •CORE BELIEFS: schema, social information processing •LEARNING: social learning	•Psychological interventions focused on parenting schemata or attachment patterns •Interventions during pregnancy and the post-natal period •Longitudinal prospective studies concentrating on interaction between biological and other factors	•TIMING: perinatal •DIRECT INTERVENTION: enhance parental attunement, oxytocin •RESEARCH: longitudinal prospective studies, biological
Moog et al. (2022)	Review *(narrative)*	•Existing literature	•Perinatal			•Maternal sequalae •Gestational biology •Maternal biology	•DEVELOPMENTAL: physiological •HERITABILITY: epigenetic	•Focus on interventions during the perinatal period •Research on paternal impacts on gestational biology	•TIMING: perinatal •RESEARCH: fathers/ other carers, biological

continued on following page

Table 2. Continued

Citation	Type of paper	Data sources	Focus/cohort	Type of maltreatment	Location of study	Theoretical framework/s articulated	Theoretical framework/s (coding)	Proposed intervention/s articulated	Proposed intervention/s (coding)
Morton & Brown (1998)	Review *(systemic-like)*	•Existing literature				•Attachment	•RELATIONAL: attachment	•Attachment based interventions aimed at increasing parental sensitivity through education, modelling and support or working through internal working models of attachment •Assess infant attachment	•DIRECT INTERVENTION: enhance parental attunement, develop parenting skills •ASSESSMENT: screening, attachment
Narang & Contreras (2000)	Research study	•Self-report *(questionnaires, e.g., modified child history questionnaire, dissociation experiences scale II, physical child abuse potential inventory)*	•Adolescence/ youth	•Physical abuse (college students' physical child abuse potential)	North America	•Dissociation	•UNPROCESSED TRAUMA: dissociation	•Target dissociative tendencies - helping family members accept the reality of their abuse history and its effects	•DIRECT INTERVENTION: acknowledge and integrate trauma

continued on following page

Table 2. Continued

Citation	Type of paper	Data sources	Focus/cohort	Type of maltreatment	Location of study	Theoretical framework/s articulated	Theoretical framework/s (coding)	Proposed intervention/s articulated	Proposed intervention/s (coding)
Narang & Contreras (2005)	Research study	•Self-report *(questionnaires, e.g., modified child history questionnaire, family environment scale, dissociation experiences scale II, physical child abuse potential inventory)*	•Mother •Childhood *(mothers and elementary school-aged children)*	•Physical abuse	North America	•Dissociation	•UNPROCESSED TRAUMA: dissociation	•Targeting the dissociation in the parent through recalling and integrating •Prevent dissociation in children through building cohesiveness, expressiveness, and conflict-resolution skills into the family system •Affect regulation and emotional regulation skills •Research including fathers and longitudinal studies to test findings in this study	•TARGET COHORT: family system •DIRECT INTERVENTION: acknowledge and integrate trauma, use of therapeutic relationship, emotional and behavioural regulation skills •RESEARCH: fathers/ other carers, longitudinal prospective studies
Negriff at al. (2020)	Research study	•Self-report *(longitudinal study involving the comprehensive trauma Interview and inventories measuring adolescents' self-report of mental health symptoms)*	•Adolescence/ youth •Childhood *(children/ adolescents aged 9-13 and their caregivers - maltreatment group involved in Children and Family Services, comparison group from school lists)*	•Child protection involvement	North American	•Re-victimisation and violence exposure in adulthood •Other adversities in adulthood	•DEVELOPMENTAL: mental health •SYSTEMS: current adversity	•Assessment of parental adversities may be more important that assessing offspring risk of maltreatment •Intervening to meet basic needs, reduce stressors, build emotional regulation •Larger sample sizes of fathers	•ASSESSMENT: adversities •DIRECT INTERVENTION: emotional and behavioural regulation skills •SYSTEMIC APPROCH: alleviate disadvantage •RESEARCH: fathers/ other carers

continued on following page

Table 2. Continued

Citation	Type of paper	Data sources	Focus/cohort	Type of maltreatment	Location of study	Theoretical framework/s articulated	Theoretical framework/s (coding)	Proposed intervention/s articulated	Proposed intervention/s (coding)
Newton (2019)	Review *(narrative)*	•Existing literature	•Indigenous *(Indigenous Australians and child neglect)*	•Neglect	Australia	•Ecological systems theory *(parenting deficits and inadequacies in social structures/environment)* •Loss of passing on of child-rearing practices and culture	•SYSTEMS: ecological, current adversity •CULTURAL: Indigenous	•Working within an ecological framework •Deliver services to communities rather than purely individuals or families •Trauma informed approaches informed by Indigenous understandings	•TARGET COHORT: community work •DIRECT INTERVENTION: cultural healing •SYSTEMIC APPROACH: alleviate disadvantage, attend to ideologies, trauma-informed services
Ney (1989)	Review *(narrative)*	•Existing literature				•Triquetra *(perpetrator, victim and observer each have a role)* • Re petition compulsion as individual tries to understand and resolve early experiences	•UNPROCESSED TRAUMA: psychodynamic	•Treating all parties (victim, perpetrator, observer) •Re-enacting old problems in the therapeutic relationship for resolution	•TARGET COHORT: individual parent, family system, parent couple/ caregivers •DIRECT INTERVENTION: use of therapeutic relationship
Özcan et al. (2016)	Research study	•Self-report *(questionnaires, e.g., sociodemographic data form, adult attachments style scale, childhood trauma questionnaire)*	•Mother •Adolescence/ youth *(mothers with psychiatric disorders and their children aged over 16)*		Turkey	•Attachment	•RELATIONAL: attachment •DEVELOPMENTAL: mental health		

continued on following page

Table 2. Continued

Citation	Type of paper	Data sources	Focus/cohort	Type of maltreatment	Location of study	Theoretical framework/s articulated	Theoretical framework/s (coding)	Proposed intervention/s articulated	Proposed intervention/s (coding)
Putallaz et al. (1998)	Review *(narrative)*	•Existing literature	•Mothers •Animals *(includes human and non-human primate*			•Cognitive schema of relationships/attachment •Modelling •Socioeconomic status	•RELATIONAL: attachment •SYSTEMS: current adversity •UNPROCESSED TRAUMA: dissociation •CORE BELIEFS: schema •LEARNING: social learning	•Influences of gender of both parent and child	•RESEARCH: fathers/ other carers, gender pathways
Quinton & Rutter (1984)	Research study	•Self-report *(interview)*	•Parents *(parents of children in care)*	•Child protection involvement	England	•Effects on personality and coping •Transmission of material disadvantage	•DEVELOPMENTAL: psychosocial •SYSTEMS: ecological, current adversity		
Ramo-Fernández et al. (2015)	Review *(narrative)*	•Existing literature				•Epigenetic alterations	•HERITABILITY: epigenetic	•Epigenetic research on sperm cells, studies into biological and epigenetic functions following trauma, epigenetic changes following recovery from trauma,	•RESEARCH: fathers/other carers, intergenerational discontinuity, biological, gender pathways
Renner & Slack (2006)	Research study	•Self-report *(annual surveys completed by families)* •Organisational/ governmental data		•Domestic and family violence	North America	•Social learning theory *(learned helplessness)*	•LEARNING: social learning	•Children who have experienced one form of maltreatment be assessed for other forms of maltreatment	•ASSESSMENT: multigenerational, different forms of maltreatment •RESEARCH: longitudinal prospective studies

continued on following page

Table 2. Continued

Citation	Type of paper	Data sources	Focus/cohort	Type of maltreatment	Location of study	Theoretical framework/s articulated	Theoretical framework/s (coding)	Proposed intervention/s articulated	Proposed intervention/s (coding)
Rodriguez & Tucker (2011)	Research study	•Self-report *(questionnaires, e.g., child abuse potential inventory, parenting scale, parental attachment questionnaire, abuse history index)*	•Mother •Adolescence/ youth *(mothers of children aged 12-17 who were receiving therapy for behavioural issues)*		North America	•Attachment	•RELATIONAL: attachment	•Research with fathers	•RESEARCH: fathers/ other carers
Rosso (2022)	Review *(narrative)*	•Existing literature		•Physical abuse		•Psychoanalytic	•UNPROCESSED TRAUMA: psychodynamic	•Long term intensive treatment •Parent-child psychotherapy •Individual psychoanalytic treatment of parent •Mentalisation-based treatment •Evaluations of psychoanalytic treatments •Awareness and management of negative countertransference	•TARGET COHORT: individual parent, parent-child dyad •TIMING: childhood, early intervention, long term •DIRECT INTERVENTION: acknowledge and integrate trauma, use of therapeutic relationship, enhance parental attunement, emotional and behavioural regulation skills •REFLECTIVE PRACTICE: manage countertransference, supervision and support •RESEARCH: evaluation

continued on following page

Table 2. Continued

Citation	Type of paper	Data sources	Focus/cohort	Type of maltreatment	Location of study	Theoretical framework/s articulated	Theoretical framework/s (coding)	Proposed intervention/s articulated	Proposed intervention/s (coding)
Seng et al. (2013)	Research study	•Self-report *(questionnaires, e.g., traumatic events questionnaire, trauma symptoms checklist, parental bonding instrument, maternal antenatal attachment*	•Mother •Perinatal *(pregnant mothers in second or third trimester)*		North America	•Prenatal attachment •"Ghosts in the nursery"	•RELATIONAL: attachment •UNPROCESSED: psychodynamic		
Shelbe & Geiger (2017)	Book	•Existing literature				•Psychodynamic models (parental psychopathology) •Social learning theory •Social information processing theory •Attachment theory •Ecological models	•RELATIONAL: attachment •DEVELOPMENTAL: mental health •SYSTEMS: ecological •CORE BELIEFS: social information processing •LEARNING: social learning •CULTURAL: culture, African American	•Earlier the intervention, the better •Screening tools and targeting specific populations •Home visiting programs •Parent training using promising models •Improve parents' ability to develop and maintain adult relationships •Consider cultural context •Longitudinal prospective studies, with participants enrolled before birth	•TIMING: early intervention •ASSESSMENT: screening, adversities •DIRECT INTERVENTION: specific models, develop parenting skills, emotional and behavioural regulation skills, build informal networks, home visiting programs •SYSTEMIC APPROACH: alleviate disadvantage, attend to ideologies •RESEARCH: fathers/ other carers, longitudinal prospectives studies, evaluation

continued on following page

Table 2. Continued

Citation	Type of paper	Data sources	Focus/cohort	Type of maltreatment	Location of study	Theoretical framework/s articulated	Theoretical framework/s (coding)	Proposed intervention/s articulated	Proposed intervention/s (coding)
Sheppard (2003)	Research study	•Self-report *(interviews with social workers and mothers of children subject to child protection intervention, questionnaires - Beck depression inventory, depression social assessment scale)*	•Parents *(parents with depression involved in child protection systems)*	•Child protection involvement	England	•Attachment and bonding •Depression	•RELATIONAL: attachment •DEVELOPMENTAL: mental health	•Needs assessment •Families' needs to be considered within a longitudinal lens and theoretical understanding	•ASSESSMENT: multigenerational, adversities •RESEARCH: longitudinal prospective studies
Sperlich et al. (2017)	Conceptual paper *(proposes conceptual framework)*	•Existing literature	•Perinatal			•Unresolved trauma and PTSD and depression •Trauma theory •Attachment theory	•RELATIONAL: attachment •DEVELOPMENTAL: mental health	•Interventions at certain points in the childbearing year •Screening and identifying women with maltreatment history •Specialised support to manage triggers during labour and parenting support	•TARGET COHORT: parent-child dyad, parent couple/caregivers •TIMING: perinatal •ASSESSMENT: screening

continued on following page

Table 2. Continued

Citation	Type of paper	Data sources	Focus/cohort	Type of maltreatment	Location of study	Theoretical framework/s articulated	Theoretical framework/s (coding)	Proposed intervention/s articulated	Proposed intervention/s (coding)
Steele (1970)	Book section	•Existing literature •Case study material				•Misconception of the infant (as a need satisfying object or as "bad") •Lack of motherliness (lack of confidence in the world, lack of empathy and attunement) •Ego and superego development •Narcissism and masochism •Parental psychopathology	•RELATIONAL: attachment •DEVELOPMENTAL: mental health •UNPROCESSED TRAUMA: psychodynamic •CORE BELIEFS: social information processing, Schema	•Dynamic psychotherapy with parents with an emphasis on the therapist dealing with own emotional responses and the therapeutic relationship •Support parent to look towards other adults for support rather than the child	•DIRECT INTERVENTION: acknowledge and integrate trauma, build informal networks •TIMING: long term •REFLECTIVE PRACTICE: manage countertransference
Stob et al. (2020)	Case study	•Case study material	•Mother *(mother and son-age not specified)*			•Attachment and mentalisation	•RELATIONAL: attachment	•Enhance mentalisation abilities through The Family Cycle activity	•DIRECT INTERVENTION: acknowledge and integrate trauma, enhance parental attunement, specific models,

continued on following page

Table 2. Continued

Citation	Type of paper	Data sources	Focus/cohort	Type of maltreatment	Location of study	Theoretical framework/s articulated	Theoretical framework/s (coding)	Proposed intervention/s articulated	Proposed intervention/s (coding)
Tomison (1996)	Grey literature *(organisational publication)*	•Existing literature				•Social learning theory •Biological or genetic components •Interaction of gene and environment •multi-factor approach	•SYSTEMS: ecological •HERITABILITY: genetic •LEARNING: social learning	•Promotion of beliefs running counter to the use of physical punishment •Explicit training in parenting and conflict management •Early intervention strategies •Future research on caregivers other than the mother, trigenerational studies, adult sibling studies to explore discontinuity, gender pathways exploration	•TARGET COHORT: individual parent •TIMING: early intervention •ASSESSMENT: different forms of maltreatment •DIRECT INTERVENTION: develop parenting skills, specific models •SYSTEMIC: attend to ideologies •RESEARCH: fathers/ other carers, longitudinal prospective studies, intergenerational discontinuity, gender pathways
Wilson & Scarpa (2011)	Book section	•Existing literature				•HPA axis vulnerabilities •Ecological framework	•DEVELOPMENTAL: physiological •SYSTEMS: ecological	•Interventions in the HPA axis and stress management (e.g., relaxation activities) •Parental training to increase confidence •Future research into gender differences in intergenerational child maltreatment	•TARGET COHORT: individual parent •DIRECT INTERVENTION: develop parenting skills, emotional and behavioural regulation skills •RESEARCH: gender pathways

continued on following page

Table 2. Continued

Citation	Type of paper	Data sources	Focus/cohort	Type of maltreatment	Location of study	Theoretical framework/s articulated	Theoretical framework/s (coding)	Proposed intervention/s articulated	Proposed intervention/s (coding)
Zajac et al. (2019)	Research study	•Self-report *(questionnaires, e.g., childhood trauma questionnaire, adult attachment interview)* •Observation *(controlled study introducing parenting intervention, observations of parent-*	•Parents *(parents involved with child protective services)*	•Child protection involvement	North America	•Attachment states of mind	•RELATIONAL: attachment	•Assessing for attachment states of mind •Prospective, longitudinal study to explore effects of different types of maltreatment	•ASSESSMENT: attachment •RESEARCH: longitudinal prospective studies
Zeanah & Zeanah (1989)	Book section	•Existing literature				•Attachment and internal working models	•RELATIONAL: attachment	•Research into the processes of overcoming early trauma	•RESEARCH: intergenerational discontinuity
Zonnevijlle & Hildebrand (2019)	Research study	•Self-report *(questionnaires, e.g., Young schema questionnaire, Egna Minnen Betraffande Uppfostran for children, experiences in close relationships scale-revised)*	•Adolescence/ youth *(youth under 18 in care facility)*	•Child protection involvement	Netherlands	•Schema	•CORE BELIEFS: schema	•Screening for early maladaptive schemas among youth and parents	•ASSESSMENT: schema

RESULTS

Overview of Results

The 72 results were published between 1970 to 2022. Two of the results were published between 1970-1979, six between both 1980-1989 and 1990-1999, seven between 2000-2009, 42 between 2010 and 2019, and nine between 2020- 2022. Of the 30 papers which specify a location (26 of them research studies) all are from the global north, with 15 conducted in North America, four in Canada, three in Germany, three in England, and one each in Australia, Belgium, Israel, the Netherlands, and Turkey.

There are 26 reviews (20 narrative reviews, four scoping or otherwise systemic-like, and two other), 28 research studies, nine books or book sections, three case studies, five conceptual papers, and two instances of grey literature. The majority of papers (mostly reviews) uses existing literature as their source of knowledge (42), with self-report measures (27), observation (seven), case study material (six), biological samples (six), and organisational or governmental data (one) also comprising data sources.

A range of cohorts or areas of focus are targeted in the selected papers. The majority of research studies focus on human participants, with only three exploring animal subjects. Twenty-two of the papers study mothers, with only one concentrating on fathers and six on parents (often parents of children in care or otherwise involved with child protection systems) more generally. The perinatal period is well represented in the literature, with 14 papers focusing their research on this timeframe. In contrast, five of the results concentrate on adolescence or youth, and six on childhood. Three of the papers cover intergenerational child maltreatment for Indigenous families and communities. A diversity of abuse types is investigated, with seven papers applying their discussions to domestic and family violence, six to physical abuse, three to child sexual abuse, and two to neglect. Seven results explore experiences of families involved in child protection systems. Twenty of the papers do not specify a cohort or maltreatment type, covering the concept broadly.

Theoretical Frameworks

The results articulate a variety of theoretical frameworks to explain the concept of intergenerational child maltreatment. Importantly, the vast majority of results refer to more than one theory and/or theoretical framework, either successively exploring them or blending theories to generate original outlooks. Figure 2 (below) visually represents the quantity of results referring to each of the theoretical perspective and theory.

Figure 2. Theoretical frameworks in the reviewed literature

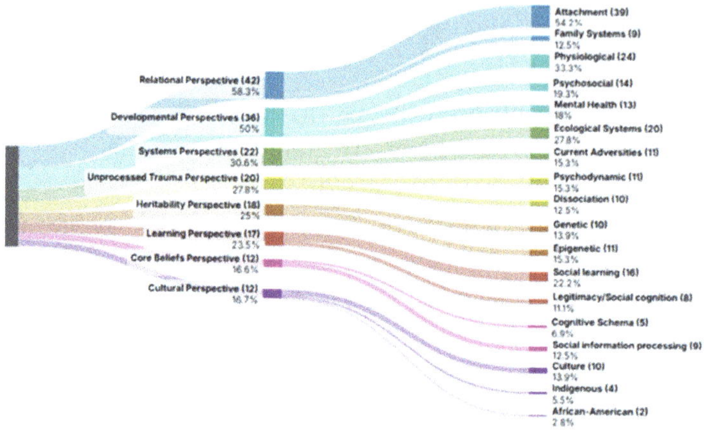

Relational Perspectives

Relational perspectives, holding that the intergenerational continuity of childhood maltreatment occurs due to disruptions to the relational patterning between parent and child, is dominant in the reviewed literature. Forty-two (58.3%) of the reviewed papers apply this theoretical perspective.

Attachment

Attachment theory concerns the physical proximity and emotional attunement between child and caregiver, positioning the nature and quality of parent-child relationship as central to an individual's capacity to form and maintain healthy relationships throughout life, including with their own children (Ainsworth, 1978; Bowlby, 1979). Mirroring other comparable reviews (Chamberlain, Gee, et al., 2019; Marshall et al., 2022), this theoretical construct was most prevalent in the reviewed literature, with 39 papers (54.2%) referring to attachment theory as an explanation for intergenerational child maltreatment.

Several of the results focus on specific facets of attachment theory. Internal working models, or the mental views one holds about oneself and others as a result of early attachment experiences, is frequently referred to (Amos et al., 2011; Levendosky et al., 2012; Marshall et al., 2022; Özcan et al., 2016; Zeanah & Zeanah, 1989). This concept is described by Kim et al., (2011) as "an unconscious interpretive filter through which social experiences are understood" (p. 500), with several papers emphasising the link between a parent's interpretation of their child's communication and the potential for insensitive or maltreating parenting practices (Amos & Segal, 2018; Meulewaeter et al., 2019; Morton & Browne, 1998; Steele, 1970). Other results refer to the internal dilemma of a child innately drawn both towards their abusive parent for survival and away from this parent for their safety (Amos et al., 2011; Arons, 2005; Kim & Strathearn, 2017), a concept originally referred to as "fright without solution" (Main & Hesse, 1990, p. 484). Amos and Segal (2018) expanded this concept into "terrified shame without solution" (p. 2), including the child's predicament of both pursuing the attuned mirroring from a parent that is essential for the development of self and avoiding the experience of shame that occurs when attempts to engage are met with non-responsiveness. Other papers explore attachment as a prenatal, as well as postnatal, phenomenon (Seng et al., 2013; Sperlich et al., 2017), make note of the wider and more holistic view of attachment (beyond the parent-child dyad and incorporating attachment to extended family and kinship groups) held by many Indigenous communities (Aguiar & Halseth, 2015), and refer to the differing and sometimes hierarchal attachments to primary carer, secondary carers, and peers (Kim et al., 2011; Morton & Browne, 1998). Additionally, Hall (2011) suggests that an alternate view of attachment "timetables" (p. 46) for mothers who had experienced abuse or neglect in childhood may be necessary, describing findings in her study relating to a research subject requiring additional time to develop the sense of emotional safety needed to securely attach to her baby.

Family Systems

Family systems theories are also represented in the reviewed literature with nine results (12.5%) making some mention of this theoretical construct or a concept deriving from it. Family systems theories focus on the roles and energies between family members, amplifying that stress, trauma, and adversity affecting one family member reverberates throughout the entire family system over generations (Alexander, 2015; Delsol & Margolin, 2004; Marshall et al., 2022), remaining as "traumatic shrapnel … long after the immediate threat is gone" (Borelli et al., 2019, p. 8). Hurst and Sawatzky (1996) applies Bowen's family systems theory (Bowen, 1966), which has a particular emphasis on intergenerational patterns. Additionally, several papers describe the Bowenian concept of "differentiation of self" (Bowen, 1972), which holds that healthy development is attained through balancing individual autonomy and relational connection, and hindered by emotional fusion (over-identification and enmeshment with family of origin) or emotional cut-off (distance from and animosity towards family of origin) (Chamberlain, Gee, et al., 2019; Hurst & Sawatzky, 1996; Marshall et al., 2022; McMillen & Rideout, 1996). Further, the Bowenian notion of "multigenerational transmission" (Bowen, 1978), referring to the way levels of differentiation of self may continue and compound over generations, partly due to the propensity towards partnering (and having children) with others who have similar levels of emotional fusion or cut-off, is referenced in the literature (Hurst & Sawatzky, 1996; Marshall et al., 2022).

Developmental Perspectives

Developmental perspectives suggest that maltreatment, particularly if sustained in sensitive developmental periods, can alter an individual's ability to navigate life's challenges, thereby impacting their parenting instincts and potentially resulting in maltreatment to their offspring. Within the reviewed literature, 36 (50%) of the results apply a developmental perspective.

Physiological Developmental Theories

Twenty-four results (33.3%) describe the physiological impairments of early adversity, including to the hypothalamic-pituitary-adrenal axis (stress response system) (Cordero et al., 2012; Howell et al., 2021; Juul et al., 2016; Köhler-Dauner et al., 2019), to neurological development (Buss et al., 2017; DeGregorio, 2013; Iyengar et al., 2019; Mielke et al., 2016), and to the hormones and chemicals necessary for functions of parenting (lyengar et al., 2019; Kim & Strathearn, 2017). Papers consider the interdependence between each of these biological systems (Lomanowska et al., 2017), with Moog et al. (2022, p. 2) noting that brain regions involved in "neuroendocrine control, autonomic regulation vigilance, emotional regulation, and fear conditioning" (p. 2) were altered and affected by childhood maltreatment, and Mitkovic Voncina et al. (2017) introducing the concept of the "mind-brain-body interplay" (p. 1), or the interconnected alterations in psychological, neurological, and somatic domains that may influence intergenerational continuity of child maltreatment.

Psychosocial Developmental Theories

Other results focus on psychosocial impacts, with 14 papers (19.3%) describing the lasting difficulties in emotional and relational wellbeing following a history of child maltreatment and the impacts of these challenges on parenting. These studies often examine characteristics of the parental personality and coping strategies affected by early trauma, including difficulties with emotional regulation and stress management (Lomanowska et al., 2017; Mitkovic Voncina et al., 2017; Wilson & Scarpa, 2011), skewed perceptions and interpretations of situational and relational data (Green, 1976; Lomanowska et al., 2017), and perceptions of problems in interpersonal relationships (Green, 1976; Lecic-Tosevski et al., 2014). Further, the data implies parents' experiences of early maltreatment is correlated to lower levels of empathy (Mielke et al., 2016) and self-esteem (McMillen & Rideout, 1996), and increased levels of hostility (Belsky, 1993; Howell et al., 2021), deviance (Quinton & Rutter, 1984), and neuroticism (Mitkovic Voncina et al., 2017).

Mental Health

The sequalae of early abuse and its correlation with mental health disorders in adulthood is also positioned as a causation factor for intergenerational child maltreatment. This theory as a possible explanation for intergenerational child maltreatment is proposed in 13 (18%) of the reviewed papers. Recognising the increased susceptibility to mental health disorders following childhood abuse and neglect, these papers explore the prevalence of mental health issues among parents who had experienced early maltreatment and the impact on the next generation (Bennett, 2021; Howell et al., 2021; Özcan et al., 2016). Several studies refer to the influences of different psychological disorders, such as depression (Sheppard, 2003; Sperlich et al., 2017), post-traumatic stress disorder (PTSD) and complex post-traumatic stress disorder (C-PTSD) (Aguiar & Halseth, 2015; Sperlich et al., 2017), and personality disorders (Huth-Bocks et al., 2013) on the risk of intergenerational child maltreatment. Alink et al., (2019) notes that some symptoms of psychological disorders, such as passivity and withdrawal (which are more likely in depression and some manifestations of PTSD) may result in parental neglect rather than abuse, while Bennett (2021), referring to a study by Lyons-Ruth et al., (2005), reports that parental characteristics associated with many mental health disorders often result in disorganised attachment in their children, even in the absence of the child experiencing maltreatment.

Systems Perspectives

Theoretical perspectives concentrating on the interaction between external (systemic and societal) and individual or familial factors are discussed in 22 results (30.6%). These papers make note of the mutual and reciprocal influences, or "transactive risk factors" (Cicchetti & Rizley, 1981, p. 44) between individual, family, culture, community, and society and emphasise the importance of looking beyond the individual and the family system when considering the aetiology of intergenerational child maltreatment.

Ecological Systems

Brofenbrenner's (1979) ecological systems theory, which concentrates on the layers of influence between individuals and their family (micro), community (meso), societal (exo), and cultural or ideological (macro) environments, is indicated in 20 (27.8%) of the reviewed papers. These discussions hold that it is the combination of a multiplicity of risk factors across "multiple, interacting layers" (Geiger et al., 2015, p. 70), rather than any sole or dominant causation factor, that may result in intergenerational child maltreatment.

Some studies focus on particular elements of the ecological system. Many explore the macro level, describing an overrepresentation of some cultural or social groups in child protection systems due to societal bias and overreporting (Hall, 2011) and the Western worldviews and ideologies on which policies and laws are based (Duthie et al., 2019; Kim, 2012; Newton, 2019). Others explore the impact of trauma on the micro level, focusing on the ontogenic system (characteristics of individuals), including physical health, hypothalamic-pituitary-adrenal axis, methylation of DNA, and neurological development (for both parents who have experienced maltreatment and their offspring), and the reverberations of these ontogenic forces into other wider levels of the system (Belsky, 1993; Mitkovic Voncina et al., 2017; Wilson & Scarpa, 2011). Still others concentrate on the meso level, commenting on the role and quality of social and community resources the family is able to access (Buchheim et al., 2022; Hall, 2011; Howell et al., 2021). A number of papers refer to Belsky's sociological or process model of parenting (Belsky, 1993), which is based in Brofenbrenner's theory and considers the integrated role of parental characteristics, child characteristics, cultural and social values regarding child-rearing, and stressors deriving from social or political influences in child rearing behaviours (Chamberlain, Gee, et al., 2019; Cicchetti & Rizley, 1981; Finzi-Dottan & Harel, 2014; Geiger et al., 2015; Schelbe & Geiger, 2017; Tomison, 1996).

Current Adversities

The impact of current environmental stressors is central to 11 (15.3%) of the reviewed papers. Markward et al. (2000) propose a "diathesis-stress perspective" (p. 237), which views families' current adversities as potential triggers for existing vulnerabilities, thereby constructing conditions in which child maltreatment may be more likely to occur. Several others echo this view, some suggesting that an equally pertinent consideration when examining intergenerational child maltreatment is the intergenerational transmission of poverty, oppression, and disadvantage (Duthie et al., 2019; Howell et al., 2021; Negriff et al., 2020; Putallaz et al., 1998; Quinton & Rutter, 1984). Quinton and Rutter (1984), for instance, wonder whether childhood abuse and neglect may "predispose (an individual) to social and environmental disadvantages which then impede or interfere with parenting" (p. 231).

Unprocessed Trauma Perspectives

Twenty of the reviewed papers (27.8%) apply the perspective that unacknowledged and unprocessed trauma presents symptomatically. These perspectives theorise that the risk of intergenerational continuity of child maltreatment is perpetuated by the triggering of unresolved or dissociated trauma that occurs in the parent-child dynamic.

Psychodynamic

Eleven results (15.3%) apply psychodynamic theories to the concepts of intergenerational continuity of child maltreatment, focusing on unconscious and subliminal process through which parents project their experience onto their child. Fraiberg et al.'s (1975) concept of "ghosts in the nursery", an analogy for the re-enactment of childhood experiences (of which parents are often unaware) in the relationships with their children is referenced in several of the discussions (Arons, 2005; Chamberlain, Gee, et al., 2019; Rosso, 2022; Seng et al., 2013), with Chamberlain, Gee, et al., (2019) adding Lieberman et al.'s (2005) positive reframe of "angels in the nursery", which focuses on the unconscious intergenerational transmission of nurturing parenting experiences. Several papers refer to "self-psychology" (Kohut, 1971, 1977), positioning the psychological injury to the development of self that is experienced by many parents who were harmed as children as central to the risk of intergenerational maltreatment (Cornett, 1985; McMillen & Rideout, 1996; Rosso, 2022; Steele, 1970). These papers suggest that these parents may experience intense and predominant needs for the love, acceptance, and admiration that they were unable to consistently attain as children and may attempt to meet these needs in their interactions with their children. Thus, authors submit, identical unmet needs develop in these children as they put aside their own developmental needs to meet those of their parent (Cornett, 1985; McMillen & Rideout, 1996). Alternatively, Steele (1970) notes that parents may respond with abusive or neglectful behaviours when the children fail to satisfy these needs

Various specific psychodynamic concepts are applied in the reviewed papers to the concepts of intergenerational child maltreatment. Ney (1989), for instance, refers to Freud's (1936) concept of the "repetition compulsion" (p. 595), in which traumatic situations similar to those the individual experienced in childhood are unconsciously sought out or recreated throughout life in an attempt to resolve them. Other authors discuss the role of the psychoanalytic ego, superego and id (Cornett, 1985; Steele, 1970). The notion of "projective identification" (Klein, 1946), in which people may project disavowed thoughts, feelings, and qualities about the self onto another, is also mentioned (Levendosky, 2013; Mitkovic Voncina et al., 2017), with Levendosky (2013) suggesting that a parent who has experienced violence may unconsciously view their child as helpless and vulnerable like the self (or, equally, through projection, as aggressive and hostile like their abuser).

Dissociation

Dissociation, or some form of disconnect from memories, thoughts, emotions, embodied self, is also positioned in the reviewed literature as an explanation for intergenerational child maltreatment, with nine results (12.5%) applying this theory. The reviewed literature positions dissociation as an adaptive, survival-orientated response to trauma and abuse which provides children with the option to endure, rather than avoid, violence (Levendosky, 2013; McCollum, 2015). However, it can result in unintegrated memory or knowledge, thus impeding the logical placement of the maltreatment experience within a coherent contextual framework (Narang & Contreras, 2000) and resulting in skewed memories, perceptions, and senses of self that interfere with parenting sensitivity (Babcock Fenerci & DePrince, 2018; Levendosky, 2013; Narang & Contreras, 2005).

The reviewed literature finds that deficits in parents' memories, cognitions and reflections on their own past trauma predicted maltreatment towards or emotional and relational difficulties for offspring (Babcock Fenerci & DePrince, 2018; Berthelot et al., 2015; Borelli et al., 2019). Putallaz et al., (1998) referred to the concept of "splitting" (p. 393), whereby the trauma memory is psychologically separated from the self and spoken about without emotion or integration. Similarly, Amos et al., (2011), citing Van der Hart et al., (2006) describes "structural dissociation of the personality" (p. 495), in which the personality becomes divided in an attempt to avoid the overwhelming traumatic experience. The authors go on to explain that the attachment experiences of parenthood may retrigger these dissociated parts, thus perpetuating the risk of intergenerational child maltreatment. McCollum (2015) introduced the concept of "multigenerational dissociation" (p. 563), in which child abuse is both re-enacted and denied over generations and with family members appearing unaware that maltreatment occurred or that the experience was harmful or distressing.

Heritability Perspectives

A theoretical perspective based in heritability is also present in the reviewed literature. Eighteen papers (25%) refer to potential genetic or epigenetic influences contributing to the risk of intergenerational child maltreatment.

Genetics

Ten papers (13.9%) reference the genetic heritability of biological systems influencing parenting practices and the trauma response to maltreatment. Some refer to "behavioural genetics" (Alink et al., 2019, p. 3), emphasising the potential heritability of genes implicated in stress responses and temperament (Alink et al., 2019; Buchheim et al., 2022) or the endocrine systems influencing hormones associated with maternal behaviours, such as oxytocin, serotonin, and dopamine (Lomanowska et al., 2017). Others apply a "differential susceptibility" (Alexander, 2015, p. 112) perspective, suggesting that the presence or absence of certain genes may influence resilience and the ability to overcome early experiences of abuse and neglect (Buchheim et al., 2022; Lomanowska et al., 2017; Markward et al., 2000). The question of what specific genetic material is being transmitted in intergenerational continuity of child maltreatment, such as low intellectual capacity or mental illness, is raised (McMillen & Rideout, 1996), with authors noting the dearth of research on this theory in human subjects (Alink et al., 2019), the compounding variables of co-occurring environmental factors (Alink et al., 2019; Delsol & Margolin, 2004; Lomanowska et al., 2017; Marshall et al., 2022), and the challenges translating this theory into change-orientated practice (McMillen & Rideout, 1996). Indeed, McMillen and Rideout (1996) describe genetic explanations as "a poor model for social intervention" (p. 381), noting that practitioners holding a purely genetic theoretical viewpoint can, at best, hope to assist second generation family members predict and prepare for the challenges they may be predisposed to.

Epigenetic

An alternate, and perhaps more useful, heritability perspective in the reviewed literature refers to epigenetic alterations, the changes to how the gene is expressed or silenced based on the conditions in which an organism exists. The epigenetic, or gene by environment, theory is proposed in 11 (15.3%) of the reviewed papers. Authors note that "epigenetic plasticity" (Mitkovic Voncina et al., 2017, p. 50; Ramo-Fernández et al., 2015, p. 714) can be stimulated within the germ cell (sperm or oocyte [pre-ova]) resulting in the child being conceived with certain epigenetic markers (Buss et al., 2017; Mitkovic Voncina et al., 2017; Moog et al., 2022; Ramo-Fernández et al., 2015). They also express that the gestational biological environment (Aguiar & Halseth, 2015; Alexander, 2015; Buss et al., 2017; Ramo-Fernández et al., 2015), and the postnatal environment (Alexander, 2015; Buss et al., 2017; Merrill et al., 2021) can epigenetically alter gene expression. Several papers refer to rodent studies which demonstrate that different maternal behaviours result in changes to the way DNA, often associated with the stress response, manifests, both in the animal subjects and up to two generations of offspring (Lomanowska et al., 2017; Merrill et al., 2021; Mitkovic Voncina et al., 2017; Ramo-Fernández et al., 2015). Other discussions reference similar research in human subjects (Lomanowska et al., 2017; Moog et al., 2022). Importantly, the reviewed literature emphasises that epigenetic effects resulting from introduced stressors and adversities are reversable when nurturing environments are introduced (Mitkovic Voncina et al., 2017), with Alexander (2015) suggesting that positive relational experiences may help an individual to epigenetically overcome biological and genetic challenges and Howell et al., (2021) noting the potential for positive epigenetic changes to individual children following the delivery of programs and supports to their parent/s.

Learning Perspectives

Learning perspectives, which hold that parenting behaviours are learnt and repeated, are represented in 17 (23.5%) of the results. These refer to both the reproduction of parenting behaviours implicitly learnt in childhood (Abbassi & Aslinia, 2010; Renner & Slack, 2006) and the role of individual appraisal of these modelled behaviours within a cultural and societal context (Belsky, 1993; Chamberlain, Gee, et al., 2019).

Social Learning

Social learning theory (Bandura, 1977), which holds that the modelling and reinforcement of behaviours results in their imitation, is anecdotally positioned in the literature as one of the two primary theories espoused to explain intergenerational child maltreatment (the other being attachment theory) (Cordero et al., 2012; McMillen & Rideout, 1996; Mitkovic Voncina et al., 2017; Renner & Slack, 2006). However, its occurrence within the reviewed literature is less prevalent than might be expected. This may be partially due to the inclusion and exclusion criteria applied to the review. Certainly, much of the literature on "cycles of violence", which refers to the repetition of violence experienced as children in subsequent adult relationships, draws upon social learning theory (Mitkovic Voncina et al., 2017). "Cycles of violence" literature was excluded from this review unless there was a specific focus on maltreatment to the following generation. Nevertheless, social learning theory is mentioned in 16 (22.2%) papers. Abbassi and Aslinia (2010) refer to "vicarious learning" (p. 19), asserting that simply witnessing family violence may result in its reproduction over generations, while Herzberger (1983), citing Feshbach (1974, 1980), suggests that children of abusive parents "learn 'retaliatory norms' or social rules for the expression of aggression" (p. 319). Renner and Slack (2006) offer the concept of "learned helplessness" (p. 603) as a socially learned behaviour. The authors express that people who have witnessed or experienced violence in childhood may be vulnerable to disempowerment, helplessness, and perceptions of the self as unable to escape the violence or exhibit influence over their situation. Hence, they may be more susceptible to re-victimisation in adult relationships, to which their children may also be exposed.

Legitimacy and Social Cognition

Eight (11.1%) of the reviewed papers note that a purely modelling application (observation and repetition of behaviours) of social learning theory does not satisfactorily explain "cross-typal" (McMillen & Rideout, 1996, p. 382) child maltreatment (where, for instance, a parent experienced childhood neglect while the child was physically abused) or the intergenerational *dis*continuity of maltreatment (Chamberlain, Gee, et al., 2019; McMillen & Rideout, 1996). Some authors suggest that social cognition theory (Bandura, 1978), which considers how behaviours are not only learnt, but how they are triggered and maintained, may be a more appropriate theoretical construct (Abbassi & Aslinia, 2010; Chamberlain, Gee, et al., 2019). Others refer to the perceived legitimacy of the behaviour (Belsky, 1993; Delsol & Margolin, 2004) based on factors such as the child's levels of identification with or differentiation from their perpetrators (Delsol & Margolin, 2004), their views on whether the self or other is to blame (Herzberger, 1983), their experiences of multiple versus singular forms and instances of violence within the home (Delsol & Margolin, 2004), and the role of reinforcement through societal and cultural modelling of behaviours similar to those observed in the family home (Kim, 2012; Markward et al., 2000). Thereby, a simultaneous consideration of children's agency in the meaning-making process about the acceptability or unacceptability of behaviours and the contextual and environmental factors which may reinforce the learnt behaviour are integrated (Delsol & Margolin, 2004; Herzberger, 1983; McMillen & Rideout, 1996).

Core Beliefs Perspectives

A further theoretical perspective outlined in the reviewed literature concerns the core beliefs an individual holds about their own worth and the reliability of their social environment. Discussions contend that these core beliefs, which often derive from early experiences of abuse and neglect, affect parenting behaviours as well as the implicit messages passed on to offspring. Twelve papers (16.6%) suggest this perspective to explain intergenerational child maltreatment.

Cognitive Schema

Cognitive schema theory (and schema therapy) believes that people develop cognitive appraisals of themselves and their environment, often referred to early maladaptive schemas (EMSs) (Young, 1999; Young et al., 2003) or "mental models" (Putallaz et al., 1998, p. 401) as a result of their experiences of being parented. These schemas become generalised, "operat(ing) outside of conscious awareness" (Putallaz et al., 1998, p. 394) and affect a person's conduct in all social and relational situations (Mitkovic Voncina et al., 2017). Five (6.9%) of the reviewed papers refer to this theory, noting that individuals who experienced early maltreatment may develop expectations that their needs for safety, stability, and connection will not be met, resulting in maladaptive behaviour and, potentially, maltreatment of their own children (Bennett, 2021; Mitkovic Voncina et al., 2017; Steele, 1970).

Zonnevijlle and Hildebrand (2019) explore the correlations between EMSs of parents and their adolescent children in a youth care facility, finding both correlating and compensatory EMSs in parents and children. Both parents and children in the studied cohort scored in the clinical range for self-sacrifice (belief that others' needs take precedence over one's own) and unrelenting standards/hyper-criticalness (self-imposition of unattainable standards). A correlation between a parent's impaired limits schema category (entitlement and insufficient self-control) and a child's disconnection/rejection schema category (abandonment, mistrust/abuse, and emotional deprivation) was noted, suggesting that children may develop "schemas that 'answer' or respond to parents' schemas rather than just replicate them" (Zonnevijlle & Hildebrand, 2019, p. 197)

Social Information Processing

Social information processing theory, which concerns cognitive schemas specifically related to the interpretation and response to social interactions, often in relation to aggression, (Dodge, 1986; Milner, 1993) is represented in nine (12.5%) results. Authors consider the hypothesis that parents who have experienced early maltreatment may perceive their child's behaviour as hostile and blameworthy, thereby responding with aggression or withdrawal (Alink et al., 2019; Finzi-Dottan & Harel, 2014; Lecic-Tosevski et al., 2014; Steele, 1970). Mitkovic Voncina et al., (2017), for instance, propose that a parent's "aggression-related schemata" (p. 50) is stored in the long-term memory and can be activated by contextual factors such as the child's behaviours and life stressors.

Cultural experiences and perspectives

Twelve (16.7%) of the results emphasise the role of culture in the conceptualisation and experience of intergenerational child maltreatment. These discussions note the collective experiences and values of cultural groups and their interactions with state systems, which are generally designed and conducted from a dominant cultural perspective.

Cultural Perspectives

Ten (13.9%) of the reviewed papers refer to the influence of culture on perceptions of intergenerational child maltreatment. Some examine the cross-cultural differences in definitions of child maltreatment, parenting roles played by different gendered parents, expectations of children, beliefs about violence in general, and attitudes towards disclosure of abuse and neglect (Alexander, 2015; Belsky, 1993; Delsol & Margolin, 2004; Finzi-Dottan & Harel, 2014; Markward et al., 2000). Kim (2012), citing studies by Lansford et al., (2004) and Deater-Deckard et al., (1996) which found that physical discipline was correlated with child aggression among Caucasian American children but not among Black American children, suggests that the cultural meanings ascribed to violence may influence its sequalae and intergenerational continuity. Other discussions refer to experiences of racism and discrimination resulting in systemic inequities and stressors which both increase the risk of child maltreatment and result in the over-representation of some cultural groups in child protection systems (Duthie et al., 2019; Howell et al., 2021; Newton, 2019).

Indigenous

Four (5.5%) of the reviewed papers explore Indigenous perspectives, focusing on Australian and Canadian contexts. These papers note that child removals are a function of colonisation, resulting in a legacy of intergenerational child maltreatment and intergenerational involvement in child protection systems (Aguiar & Halseth, 2015; Chamberlain, Gee, et al., 2019; Duthie et al., 2019; Newton, 2019). These discussions focus on the role of historic trauma in degrading traditional Indigenous healing and child rearing practices and replacing them with dominant Western models which fail to incorporate a wider cultural understanding of Indigenous parenting practices (Aguiar & Halseth, 2015; Duthie et al., 2019; Newton, 2019). Newton (2019), for instance, refers to an example of Aboriginal children being taken into care as there was no food in the home, when the cultural norms for the family involved eating as a community at an Auntie's house, where the food was stored.

African American

A similar observation is made for African American families in two (2.8%) of the reviewed papers. Schelbe and Geiger (2017) note that the more authoritarian parenting attitudes that studies identify in African American parents may be due to the valid need for parental authority to protect children from dangers that are present within their environment as a result of systemic racism and disadvantage. Belsky (1993) places these same parenting approaches into a historic context, noting that the legacy of slavery instilled in African American families a "'submit or die'" (p. 423, citing Wright, 1982, p. 241) mentality, which is passed on to children over the generations through an emphasis on obedience and respect for authority.

Integrated Perspectives

The review reveals that it is rare for any one theoretical construct to be applied in isolation. Indeed, only 21 of the results (29.2%) relied on only one theoretical framework to explain the reasons for intergenerational child maltreatment. These studies often acknowledged other theories concerning transmission mechanisms while expressing that their discussion was targeting a specific area of knowledge or theoretical perspective (e.g., Herzberger, 1983; Narang & Contreras, 2000; Ramo-Fernández et al., 2015; Renner & Slack, 2006). The vast majority of the results take an integrated approach (Kim, 2012), holding that intergenerational continuity of child maltreatment is "multiply determined" (McMillen & Rideout, 1996, p. 387) and positioning singular theories as "contributing rather than determining agents" (Belsky, 1993, p. 418) in the intergenerational recurrence of child maltreatment.

Several papers, particularly the reviews, describe and consider each of their selected theories in isolation before moving on to the next (Alink et al., 2019; Chamberlain, Gee, et al., 2019; Geiger et al., 2015; Marshall et al., 2022; Tomison, 1996), sometimes with a section focused on the integration of theories (McMillen & Rideout, 1996; Schelbe & Geiger, 2017). Others consider the influence of one theorised aetiology of intergenerational child maltreatment on another, suggesting, for instance, that the mental health diagnoses of a parent due to their trauma history may lead to insecure attachment with their child (mental health and attachment theories) (Sheppard, 2003), that violence-related dysfunction within family systems is entrenched in receptive communication difficulties when benign social cues are interpreted as threatening (family systems and social information processing theories) (Lecic-Tosevski et al., 2014), or that oxytocin and vasopressin deficits are evident in mothers who experienced child maltreatment, thus biologically impacting on her ability to bond with and attune to her baby (physiological development and attachment) (Aguiar & Halseth, 2015; Kim & Strathearn, 2017).

Intervention Frameworks

A number of intervention approaches or strategies are promoted in the reviewed literature, with 65 of the 72 papers including some discussion on the implications of their findings for practice, policy or research. These include recommendations for *who* the practical or therapeutic intervention should be aimed towards, *when* the intervention is best delivered, and *what* the approach (to assessment, treatment, and reflective work on the part of the practitioner) should comprise. Papers also make recommendations about policy and legislative amendments and future research directions that may affect the way that services are designed and delivered. The recommended intervention approaches and a comparison of the number of results are outlined in Figure 3 below.

Figure 3. Proposed interventions in the reviewed literature

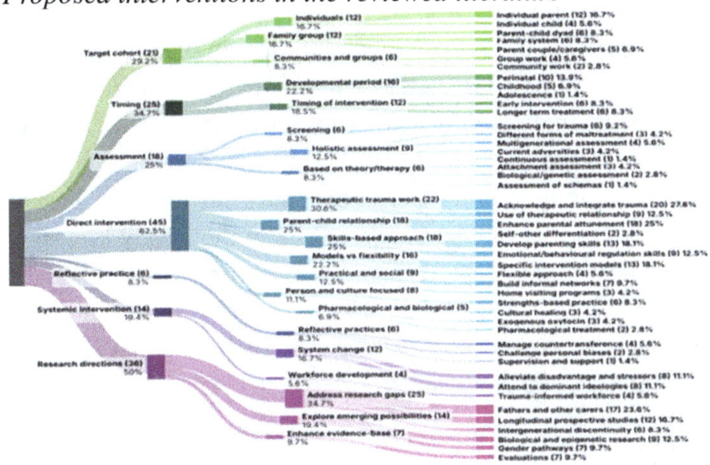

Target Cohort

Twenty-one of the reviewed papers (29.1%) make recommendations about the individuals or groups to target for engagement. Noteworthy, the majority of these do not limit their recommendations to only one individual or cohort, sometimes suggesting staggered or adjunctive therapeutic responses (Alexander, 2015; Amos & Segal, 2018; Green, 1976) or a simultaneous focus on a range of family members and groups when planning and delivering supports (Cornett, 1985; Levendosky, 2013; Rosso, 2022).

Individual Parent

Twelve results (16.7%) recommend individual work with the parent as an effective intervention. Many such papers frame unresolved parental trauma as the precursor of the child's experiences of abuse or neglect, advocating for parents to have the opportunity for trauma processing, mourning, healing, and meaning-making of their own trauma (Bennett, 2021; McMillen & Rideout, 1996; Ney, 1989). Some discussions reflect that the experience of parenthood and the child itself may trigger the parent's early trauma memories and experiences, resulting in frightening and attachment-disrupting parental responses (Alexander, 2015; Amos et al., 2011; Bennett, 2021; Ney, 1989). Papers note that any therapeutic focus on the child may provoke resentment and competitiveness in the parent, who may perceive such attention as a threat to their parental role and interrupt or cease treatment (Green, 1976; Rosso, 2022). These authors, therefore, caution against simultaneous work with both parent and child.

Many papers focusing on individual parent therapy place an emphasis on non-critical and "need satisfying" (Green, 1976, p. 427) treatment with parents to provide a corrective and empathic relational experience (Alexander, 2015; Cornett, 1985; Green, 1976; McMillen & Rideout, 1996). Others focus on interventions with individual parents to counteract and compensate for the insufficient or flawed modelling of parenting and behaviour that parents received in their early life, suggesting the need to provide interventions that offer alternate parenting paradigms and approaches (Finzi-Dottan & Harel, 2014; Tomison, 1996) and skills to recognise and regulate emotional and behavioural responses when encountering triggers and stressors (Bennett, 2021; Rosso, 2022; Wilson & Scarpa, 2011).

Individual Child

Individual therapy with the child as part of the intervention is proposed in four (5.6%) of the reviewed papers. Amos and Segal (2018), citing Beebe et al. (2010), note that traumatised children have internalised the experience of not being "sensed, known or recognized (sic) by their mothers" (p. 2) resulting in the development of internal working models that require deliberate re-working in therapy. Other authors focus on interrupting the ramifications of trauma in individual work with children through building resilience and esteem as well as increasing opportunities and skills for safety-seeking (Bennett, 2021; McMillen & Rideout, 1996).

Parent-Child Dyad

Dyadic work with a parent (usually a mother) and child is recommended in six (8.3%) of the results. These discussions centralise the necessity of relational repair in healing from relational trauma and interrupting its intergenerational progression. Alexander (2015) makes note of the efficacy of supports that increase the mother's sensitivity to the child as among the more useful interventions. Amos and co-authors' (2011; 2018) propose, as part of their model, a shared (mother and child equally involved) relational history taking and opportunities for connection in play-based therapy. Parent-child psychotherapy is mentioned in two papers (Arons, 2005; Rosso, 2022), with the case study presented by Arons (2005) involving attention to the connections and emotions between mother, infant, and therapist to metabolise trauma and increase affective proficiency. Sperlich et al., (2017) proposes a dyadic approach during the pre-natal and perinatal period, recognising that the mother-child relationship commences prior to birth and positioning this timeframe as opportune for the resolution of relational disruptions resulting from childhood maltreatment.

Family System

Six (8.3%) of the reviewed papers advocate for a family-based approach in addressing intergenerational trauma. Authors note that positive family interactions can buffer against the progression of trauma into mental health challenges such as PTSD or dissociation and thereby interrupt the intergenerational continuity of child abuse and neglect (Alink et al., 2019; Borelli et al., 2019; Narang & Contreras, 2005). Ney's (1989) discussion on the "triquetra of abuse" (p. 597) places emphasis on the role of perpetrator, victim, and observer within family systems (among other systems) in maintaining the maltreatment dynamic and promotes interventions with individuals in all three of these roles. Alexander (2015) positions family work as a critical step in the process but proposes a staged approach to the target group for therapy where abuse has been perpetrated by a family member, suggesting the introduction of family therapy later in the process and after individual and dyadic approaches and when safety can be ensured.

Parent Couple/Caregivers

Five (6.9%) of the results note the criticality of including fathers or secondary caregivers in the assessment and intervention process, often noting the narrow focus on the mother in traditional interventions addressing intergenerational child maltreatment (Howell et al., 2021; Sperlich et al., 2017). The knowledge in the reviewed papers also infers that the selection of partner is often based on the individual's attachment style and their own family-of-origin history, perhaps, some authors assert, as a subconscious attempt to re-enact and resolve past traumas (Cornett, 1985; Ney, 1989), thus calling for interventions involving both parents. Authors point out that two adults with insecure attachment and interpersonal trauma experiences may be more likely to experience conflict and instability, sometimes to the point of domestic violence, thus noting the need to focus on the relational dynamics between the caregivers (Alexander, 2015; Cornett, 1985; Ney, 1989). Alexander (2015) explores the impacts of interparental conflict or cooperative co-parenting in interrupting or facilitating intergenerational child maltreatment, suggesting that supporting father involvement in children's lives and providing couples therapy to parents as effective points of intervention to ensure children receive consistent parenting messages and relational modelling.

Group Work

Group work is recommended in four (5.6%) of the papers. These discussions make note of the positive influence of social supports, positioning group work as an opportunity to form informal networks and develop empathetic communication skills in a peer context (Cornett, 1985; Green, 1976; Levendosky, 2013). Authors note some limitations to the benefits of group work, including a decreased efficacy for those with higher levels of childhood maltreatment (Alink et al., 2019) and the need for accompanying and longer-term therapeutic supports to overcome and integrate the experiences of interpersonal violence (Levendosky, 2013).

Community Work

Two papers (2.8%) argue for a focus on work with communities, rather than solely with individuals or families, specifically when working with Indigenous people (Aguiar & Halseth, 2015; Newton, 2019). Newton (2019) asserts that such an approach is more likely to resolve the underlying issues that contribute to intergenerational child maltreatment and achieve more sustainable change due to the community experiences of colonisation trauma and the adaptive but often harmful coping mechanisms that are sometimes widely utilised within communities.

Timing

Of the reviewed papers, 25 (34.7%) make recommendations on the timing of interventions. Some encourage intervening at particular developmental stages as either optimal times for change or times when there may be a higher risk of child maltreatment (Amos & Segal, 2018; Moog et al., 2022). Others endorse interventions that are delivered early, when experiences of maltreatment and disadvantage are less severe (Duthie et al., 2019; Schelbe & Geiger, 2017), or interventions with the capacity for longer term work to more thoroughly address the complexities of intergenerational child maltreatment (Meulewaeter et al., 2019; Rosso, 2022).

Perinatal

Ten papers (13.9%) identified the perinatal period as an ideal period for intervention. Several of these papers refer to this time period as more critical for safe and nurturing parenting experiences, noting the profound sensitivity to maltreatment during embryonical and foetal development and infancy (when development is most rapid and dependant on environmental influence) in comparison to other developmental periods (Alexander, 2015; Buss et al., 2017; Howell et al., 2021; Lomanowska et al., 2017; Moog et al., 2022; Sperlich et al., 2017). Others refer to the increased risk of specific mental health challenges and behavioural reactions for mothers with a history of child maltreatment in the prenatal and postnatal periods which may increase the risk of intergenerational child maltreatment (Marshall et al., 2022; Mitkovic Voncina et al., 2017). Some papers, for instance, note that a mother's trauma can be triggered in the perinatal period by experiences of perinatal health care, birth and breastfeeding, or by the crying infant (Chamberlain, Gee, et al., 2019; Sperlich et al., 2017). Mitkovic Voncina et al., (2017) describes the correlations between a mother's depression or dissociation and reduced bonding behaviours of the mother-baby dyad.

Other results take a more strengths-focused approach to this time period, with Chamberlain, Gee, et al., (2019) suggesting that the perinatal period "offers a window of opportunity to transform the 'vicious cycle of trauma' into a 'virtuous cycle of healing'" (p. 28). Authors note that the often-universal provision of professional and health support during pregnancy and early childhood offers enhanced prospects for engagement and intervention with mothers who had experienced child maltreatment (Moog et al., 2022; Sperlich et al., 2017). Additionally, the hormonal, neurobiological and psychological changes occurring within the mother during pregnancy and the post-partum period are positioned as a potential accelerator of attachment and "relational reorganisation" (Huth-Bocks et al., 2013, p. 281) making this an ideal time to offer support (Chamberlain, Gee, et al., 2019; Huth-Bocks et al., 2013; Lomanowska et al., 2017; Mitkovic Voncina et al., 2017). Huth-Bocks et al., (2013), for example, expresses that "mothers" mental representations of self and others are reactivated and reworked throughout pregnancy" (p. 282), referring to the psychological shift mothers often make during pregnancy from being protected and cared for to providing protection and care. The authors go on to note that a history of childhood maltreatment can impede this psychological transition, further emphasising the importance of intervention during this timeframe.

Childhood

Five papers (6.9%) refer to childhood as a particularly challenging period for the parent-child relationship. Authors note that the traumatised parent's need for recognition and connection can be sated by an infant's unconditional dependency, suggesting that when the child asserts a need for differentiation (as they inevitably do as they grow from infancy into toddlerhood and childhood) strong reactions are triggered in the parents, often underpinned by the further erosion of self-esteem as they perceive themselves as unwanted or un-needed (Cornett, 1985; Green, 1976; Rosso, 2022). Discussions also refer to the development of aggressive and controlling or submitting and appeasing behaviours (agonic mode) in both parents and children when early attachment experiences have been paired with fear or danger, thus resulting in an enmeshed, other-focused, and combative parent-child relationships (Amos et al., 2011; Amos & Segal, 2018).

Adolescence

One paper (Geiger et al., 2015) (1.4%) positions adolescence as a critical period for intervention with children aging out of formal out-of-home care. The authors accentuate the vulnerability of adolescents in care, and the importance of interventions customised to their unique histories, strengths, and needs to prepare them for adulthood and possible parenthood.

Early Intervention

Early intervention to address intergenerational child maltreatment is advised in six (8.3%) of the reviewed papers. Many of these discussions note the criticality of identifying the early signs of maltreatment and ensuring timely treatment and support (Bennett, 2021; Lecic-Tosevski et al., 2014; Rosso, 2022; Tomison, 1996). Duthie et al., (2019) advocates for a public health approach, providing "society wide early interventions that provide timely, accessible supports and resources" (p. 336) to address the over-representation of Indigenous children in child protection systems, emphasising the importance of cultural grounding in the provision of such services. Similarly, Schelbe and Geiger (2017), citing Widom and Wilson (2015), note that the more effective supports are early interventions that take a "multidimensional approach" (p. 78), with access to resources such as health care and parenting support.

Longer Term Treatment

Six results (8.3%) promote longer term service provision to address intergenerational child maltreatment. Papers refer to the evidence suggesting that shorter term parenting or therapeutic interventions are less likely to be effective with parents who have experienced childhood maltreatment (Finzi-Dottan & Harel, 2014; Rosso, 2022). The literature comments on the challenges and time required to establish a sense of psychological safety, a foundational and critical need, with people who have experienced child maltreatment (Arons, 2005; Steele, 1970). Meulewaeter et al., (2019) describe mothers with early trauma experiences as "fighting against distrust, nonetheless searching for a safe caregiving environment" (p. 12) while Green (1976) points out that many maltreated and potentially maltreating parents experience suspicion and mistrust of authority following a history of disempowerment and tension in their relationships with people in authority (including their own parents) which needs to be recognised and overcome before any meaningful therapeutic work can take place.

Assessment

The reviewed literature also contains recommendations on how to identify families in need of services and their specific support needs, with 18 results (25%) making some comment on the type or approach to assessment. These include recommendations for screening for parental trauma (Morton & Browne, 1998; Sperlich et al., 2017), more holistic or thorough trauma-focused assessment processes (Hurst & Sawatzky, 1996; Levendosky, 2013), and assessments focused on or derived from a particular theory surrounding intergenerational child maltreatment or modality of treatment (DeGregorio, 2013; Zonnevijlle & Hildebrand, 2019).

Screening for Trauma

Six of the reviewed papers (9.2%) encourage screening for maternal trauma or maltreatment. A number of these advise such screening at intake to prenatal care (Buss et al., 2017; Huth-Bocks et al., 2013; Sperlich et al., 2017), with Sperlich et al., (2017) suggesting that pre-pregnancy mental health disorders may be likely to lead to the continuation or reappearance of such disorders during pregnancy. Some authors propose the use of a screening tool for identified risk factors, including parental history of maltreatment (Morton & Browne, 1998; Schelbe & Geiger, 2017); however, note the potential for inaccuracies in the use of such tools (Morton & Browne, 1998) and caution against positioning parental child maltreatment as overly deterministic (Schelbe & Geiger, 2017). Schelbe and Geiger (2017) also promote screening for strengths and protective factors alongside risks.

Multigenerational Assessment

Four papers (5.6%) advise an intergenerational lens to the assessment process, in which experiences over several generations are considered and brought to awareness. A thematic commonality in these papers is the suggestion of a longitudinal lens to assessment, the use of genograms, and the exploration of intergenerational histories (Hurst & Sawatzky, 1996; Markward et al., 2000; Sheppard, 2003). Renner and Slack (2006) indicate the need to explore parental experiences of early abuse and their link to victimisation in adult relationships, which also put offspring at risk. Hurst and Sawatzky (1996) express that "crisis-plagued families" (p. 707) may be representing a "'normal'" (p. 707) pattern of interactions in the context of their intergenerational history, thus centralising the importance of multigenerational assessment in understanding a family's presentation and historic context. Markward et al., (2000) notes the need for further investigation into the interplay between internal (biogenetic and psychosocial) factors and external (cultural and societal) context in which families live, promoting practice that incorporates ecomaps, genograms and social histories.

Different Forms of Maltreatment

Three of the results (4.2%) contend that a focus on multiple types of childhood maltreatment is necessary for a holistic assessment, arguing that maltreatment types rarely occur in isolation. Renner and Slack (2006), for instance, point out that type-to-type maltreatment (in which the parent and child experiences the same type of childhood maltreatment) may not be the only intergenerational pathway of child maltreatment, urging an assessment that involves asking parents about all forms of violence and maltreatment during their childhood. Huth-Bocks et al., (2013) centralises the relevance of exploring the often overlooked emotional and psychological maltreatment, arguing that this form of trauma is more prevalent than physical or sexual violence and has equally deleterious consequences to mothering. Tomison (1996) makes a similar argument for the overlooked and harmful effects of child neglect.

Current Adversities

Three papers (4.2%) articulate the view that an understanding of a family's current challenges and needs is a vital element of the assessment, noting the correlations between early maltreatment experiences and structural or systemic disadvantage in adult life. Negriff et al., (2020), for instance, found that family stressors, such as poverty, health problems, social isolation, and the death of family members may be more prevalent for parents who had experienced child maltreatment and, in turn, may affect their ability to provide safe and nurturing parenting. Others indicate the need for assessments which identify the specific resources and supports a family may need, such as mental health or addiction supports, housing, and education (Schelbe & Geiger, 2017; Sheppard, 2003) within a theoretical framework that facilitates a thorough and contextual case conceptualisation (Sheppard, 2003).

Continuous Assessment

One paper (Levendosky, 2013), citing Bogat et al., (2005) (1.4%), notes that assessment is not necessarily a point in time process. The authors point out that the full extent of the maltreatment is often not disclosed at the commencement of treatment, resulting in the need to normalise omission of information and provide several opportunities over the course of the intervention for individuals to provide further information about their maltreatment experiences.

Attachment Assessment

Three results (4.2%) propose assessing the attachment between parent and child. Morton and Browne (1998) wonders whether traditional attachment assessments, such as the Strange Situation, which observes the child's reactions when an unknown adult enters the room and their parent leaves the room then returns, may be too lengthy and not suitable, proposing the development of a new and simplified attachment assessment procedure. Kim et al., (2011) notes the central role of familial attachments in helping children overcome sexual abuse, suggesting that an understanding of parents' and intergenerational relatives' attachment experiences and styles may assist in case formulation to help children heal from abuse. Zajac et al., (2019) proposes that assessing family members' attachment states of mind (the internal representation of attachment figures and ways of managing thoughts and feelings about others) may help to identify families at highest risk for intergenerational child maltreatment.

Biological and Genetic Assessment

Assessments focused on human biology are considered in two papers (2.8%). Alexander (2015) reports that various interventions have been found to be more effective with children with certain genes and epigenetic markers associated with neural plasticity and dopamine transporter genotype, implying that an understanding of the presences or absence of these alleles and markers may help to select interventions most helpful for the individual. DeGregorio (2013) explores the neurodevelopmental impacts of childhood trauma, suggesting a "comprehensive neuropsychological profiling of parents who have experienced childhood trauma" (p. 163) to identify the areas of the brain that have been impacted and to recommend interventions based on the individual's neurological strengths and limitations.

Assessment of Schemas

One study (Zonnevijlle & Hildebrand, 2019) (1.4%) recommends assessing the early maladaptive schemas of parents and youths involved with child protective services. The authors note that such an assessment may help family members to better understand themselves and their coping mechanisms in the context of their early experiences and inform intervention strategies.

Direct Intervention

A considerable number of the reviewed results (45 papers or 62.5%) make recommendations on direct practice approaches that may be helpful in addressing intergenerational child maltreatment. These include therapeutic work to reframe and resolve the trauma (Cornett, 1985; Iyengar et al., 2019; Narang & Contreras, 2000), skill-building in parenting and affect management (Howell et al., 2021; Rosso, 2022), and strengthening the parent-child relationship (Alexander, 2015). Suggestions about the use of specific models of treatment versus flexibility of approach (DeGregorio, 2013; Hall, 2011) and practical support to individuals and families (McMillen & Rideout, 1996; Schelbe & Geiger, 2017) are made. These results also recommend direct intervention with an emphasis on cultural healing (Aguiar & Halseth, 2015), strengths (Hall, 2011), and biological or pharmacological treatment (Geiger et al., 2015; Kim & Strathearn, 2017).

Acknowledge and Integrate Trauma

Twenty of the reviewed papers (27.8%) advocate for approaches that place the emphasis on therapeutically exploring and detoxifying the early maltreatment experiences, the meanings ascribed to it, and the relation of these experiences to current functioning and parenting. These discussions imply that early life traumas which remain unacknowledged, unprocessed, and unresolved emerge behaviourally and with a specific propensity for intergenerational manifestation, therefore necessitating trauma resolution work (Amos et al., 2011; Arons, 2005; Iyengar et al., 2019; McCollum, 2015; Narang & Contreras, 2000).

Authors frequently suggest that making visible the trauma and its impacts, or some form of exposure, is a necessary element to treating intergenerational abuse or neglect. Narang and Contreras (2000), for instance, position a therapeutic goal as helping family members to "reclaim dissociated thoughts and affect as parts of the self" (p.662) and "fully accept(ing) the reality of their abuse history, as well as accepting that the abuse affected them negatively" (p. 662), while McMillen and Rideout (1996) refer to studies finding that the parent survivors of childhood maltreatment who were able to place a coherent narrative around their trauma experiences were more likely to have securely attached children. Some papers note that the attachment experiences of parenthood may activate early trauma memories, unsettling the experiential avoidance that has been relied on throughout life and incidentally creating an exposure event that brings trauma memories to consciousness (Alexander, 2015; Amos et al., 2011; Amos & Segal, 2018; Iyengar et al., 2019). The trigger of parenthood is considered to offer both opportunities (for healing within the parent through the new relationship with the child) and dangers (of destabilising the parent's existing, albeit often maladaptive, coping mechanisms and disrupting the provision of safe nurturing care the child) (Amos et al., 2011; Iyengar et al., 2019).

Supporting parents to examine and alter the cognitions and meanings they ascribe to the trauma is also centralised. Babcock Fenerci and DePrince (2018) note that "negative post trauma appraisals" (p. 132) and disorganisation in trauma memories is associated with more dysfunctional mother-child relationships, suggesting that targeting these facets is a critical aspect of treatment. Recognising that trauma experiences often result in low self-worth and the development of shame, the reviewed literature refers to the need for a reappraisal of self-concept within the therapeutic space. Steele (1970) reflects on parental attritions of a child's behaviour as potential manifestations of their own negative self-perception, viewing "the offspring as another edition of his own bad childhood self" (p. 457) and thus parenting through this skewed perspective. Amos and Segal (2018) introduce, as part of the therapeutic history taking process, the reframing of existing interpretations of behaviours as "understandable mistakes" (p. 623) and seeking the positive intentions behind actions. Other authors similarly suggest that a service user's sense of self-worth may increase through the acceptance and unconditional positive regard inherent in the therapeutic relationship (Green, 1976; Levendosky et al., 2012; McMillen & Rideout, 1996).

Other discussions examine the belief systems specific to relationships that people with unresolved trauma may hold (such as the conviction that attempts to connect will be met with undesired outcomes), advocating for interventions that support a re-evaluation of these expectations in mothers who have experienced childhood maltreatment (Iyengar et al., 2019). Several papers prioritising this approach refer to terms such as "earned security" and "attachment reorganisation" (Iyengar et al., 2019; Kim & Strathearn, 2017), in which the traumatised parent is able to update their internal working models and attachment styles later in life (Alexander, 2015; Iyengar et al., 2019), thereby attaining a default relational expectation of safety and connection that is enacted in the parent-child relationship.

Use of the Therapeutic Relationship

Nine of the reviewed papers (12.5%) place the emphasis on the therapeutic connection as a representation of other relational experiences and an opportunity for relational change. Arons (2005), for instance, describes a case vignette in which the mother and therapist attended closely to communication in therapy and linked this to patterns of emotional connection between mother and child. Some of the reviewed authors refer to the narcissistic vulnerability (Cornett, 1985; Rosso, 2022), or fragile sense of self (Amos & Segal, 2018), of parents with a childhood history of maltreatment, presenting as a negative self-concept and damaged self-esteem. Indeed, a number of papers suggests that this narcissistic fragility may, at times, have unconsciously led to parenthood itself, with the adult creating a child to meet their need for recognition and connection. This culminates in parent-child role-reversal in which the child, to some degree, satisfies and comforts their parent (Green, 1976; McMillen & Rideout, 1996; Rosso, 2022) rather than receiving adequate comfort and satisfaction themself. Cornett (1985) points out that parents who have not experienced empathy will struggle to provide it to their children, promoting the goal of providing an empathic environment in individual and family therapy. Green (1976) notes that the delicate self-esteem of a traumatised parent means they may perceive advice as criticism, and therefore their dependency needs must be met before introducing explicit behavioural change. Thus, the literature places an emphasis on empathetic, non-critical, and "need satisfying" (Green, 1976, p. 427) therapy with parents to provide a corrective and empathic relational experience (Alexander, 2015; Cornett, 1985; Green, 1976; McMillen & Rideout, 1996).

The tendency of relational trauma to repeat and echo throughout subsequent relationships the person may encounter is also referenced in these papers, with authors positioning the therapeutic relationship as an opportunity for the purposeful and skilful use of transference to re-enact and potentially resolve the trauma (Levendosky, 2013; Narang & Contreras, 2005; Ney, 1989) or to "reparent" the adult who has experienced early maltreatment (Cornett, 1985; Green, 1976). Many of these papers refer to Kohut's (1971) "self-psychology" and "self-object" theory, suggesting that the clinician or helping professional can act as a self-object (person who helps someone to meet their foundational and necessary psychological needs) for the service-user, therefore mitigating against the manifestation of these unmet needs in the parent-child relationship (Cornett, 1985; McMillen & Rideout, 1996; Rosso, 2022). McMillen and Rideout (1996) notes the therapist as self-object "build(s) compensatory structures or inner resources" (p.387), so that the service user is able to gradually develop the skills to praise and soothe themselves.

Enhance Parental Attunement

Eighteen papers (25%) propose interventions that focus on developing parental attentiveness and sensitivity to their child's needs to interrupt intergenerational child maltreatment. Köhler-Dauner et al. (2019), for instance, found that the levels of cortisol stress reactivity in infants are mediated by the emotional caregiving they receive, rather than their parents' experiences of child maltreatment, suggesting that supporting parents to develop more attuned and sensitive parenting styles may mitigate intergenerational child maltreatment. Lomanowska et al. (2017) proposes interventions aimed towards "in the context of parent-child interaction, attention to infant signals, contingent responding and positive regard" (p.132).

Parental "mentalisation", or the ability to recognise behaviours (one's own and others) as manifestations of internal beliefs, emotions and cognitions which exist in the context of current and past experience, is referred to in these papers as key to promoting parent-child attachment (Borelli et al., 2019; Iyengar et al., 2019; Stob et al., 2020). Other authors use the term "reflective functioning", a closely related concept of mentalising specific to attachment (Alexander, 2015; Babcock Fenerci & DePrince, 2018; Iyengar et al., 2019). Still others refer to "trauma specific" mentalisation and reflective functioning, involving deliberate attention to the correlations between trauma experiences and internal psychological states (Berthelot et al., 2015; Borelli et al., 2019; Stob et al., 2020). Such papers hold that it is not the trauma itself, but the deficits in parental mentalisation or reflective functioning regarding their own and their child's mental states that prevent the formation of a secure and safe parent-child relationship (Berthelot et al., 2015; Mitkovic Voncina et al., 2017). Such papers promote mentalisation-based therapy, which spans the individual self-explorative trauma therapy with parents (described in detail above, under "acknowledge and integrate trauma") in conjunction with fostering parental curiosity and interest in the child's unique internal experiences within context as an explanation for behaviour (Alexander, 2015; Rosso, 2022; Stob et al., 2020).

Self-Other Differentiation

Two of the reviewed papers (2.8%) promote "self-other differentiation", or the development of independent yet connected sense of self, in interventions for intergenerational child maltreatment. McMillen and Rideout (1996) make note of Bowen's (1972) approach towards therapy with families who are excessively enmeshed or distant and advise helping individual family members to "establish an 'I' position" (p. 384) as well as providing psychoeducation on how family systems can operate. Similarly, Amos and Segal (2018) focus on self-other differentiation in treatment through exploring both the parent's and child's inner world and the interactions between these two connected, yet disparate, beings. The authors note that this process can present significant challenges for the mother's sense of worth and identity but often result in profound empathic development in her perception of and response to her child.

Develop Parenting Skills

Thirteen papers (18.1%) recommend explicit teaching approaches for parents through coaching, providing psychoeducation and feedback, and modelling safe parenting practices. Some authors encourage training in discipline and behaviour management strategies to increase parent's confidence and skill, thereby interrupting intergenerational child maltreatment (Belsky, 1993; Finzi-Dottan & Harel, 2014; McMillen & Rideout, 1996; Schelbe & Geiger, 2017; Tomison, 1996; Wilson & Scarpa, 2011). Others recommend enhancing parental knowledge of child development and theoretical concepts such as attachment theory, resulting in parents developing appropriate expectations of their child and, consequently, interpreting and responding to their child's communication with increased sensitivity and empathy (Alexander, 2015; Howell et al., 2021; Morton & Browne, 1998; Schelbe & Geiger, 2017). Alexander (2015) contends that video feedback interventions which facilitate reflection on both the positive and less sensitive parent-child interactions are particularly helpful, while Howell et al., (2021) makes note of the evidence base suggesting parenting programs have attained positive results in improving outcomes for children experiencing mental health challenges, including the evidence on epigenetic changes following the provision of such programs.

Emotional and Behavioural Regulation Skills

Teaching the skills to manage stress and associated emotional and behavioural reactions is recommended in nine (12.5%) of the reviewed papers. Several of these support interventions aimed towards cultivating the capacity to recognise and understand emotional states (Abbassi & Aslinia, 2010; Borelli et al., 2019; Rosso, 2022) and enhancing the ability to manage emotions and choose behaviours rather than acting on impulse (Abbassi & Aslinia, 2010; Finzi-Dottan & Harel, 2014; Lomanowska et al., 2017). Wilson and Scarpa (2011) refer to trauma's tendency to disrupt the functioning of the hyper-pituitary-adrenal (stress regulation) system, proposing interventions that provide stress management skills such as relaxation techniques, with an ultimate goal of altering the biological stress response through gene-environment interaction (Lomanowska et al., 2017; Wilson & Scarpa, 2011). Narang and Contreras' (2005) discussion on dissociation recommends supporting families to develop "cohesion, expressiveness, and conflict resolution skills" (p. 676).

Specific Intervention Models

Thirteen of the reviewed papers (18.1%) refer to, briefly evaluate, or recommend specific intervention models or approaches to treat intergenerational child maltreatment. Some centre their discussion around the theoretical basis and practical application of a specific treatment approach that the authors have developed, modified, or applied to the child protection context. Amos et al (2011; 2018), for instance, propose a dyadic psychotherapeutic approach, titled variously Parallel Parent Child Narrative and Parent and Child Therapy (PPCN/PACT) and Parallel Parent and Child Therapy (P-PACT), which uses specific approaches at different phases of treatment to reframe negative appraisals of the parent-child relationship and make links between early experiences of being parented and current parenting. Stob et al.,'s (2020) Family Cycle Activity involves promoting the aforementioned mentalisation through reflection on trauma experiences and their sequalae, both for the parent and the child, with the goal of shifting attention from behaviour to holistic experience.

Papers also refer to established and often evidence-based models of treatment that may be useful in addressing intergenerational child maltreatment. These include trauma-informed approaches such as the Attachment, Self-Regulation and Competency (ARC) Model which recognises and addresses the effects of trauma on relationships, emotional regulation, and self-esteem (Meulewaeter et al., 2019); Neurosequential Model of Therapeutics (and specifically one branch, the Neurosequential Model of Caregiving), which identifies and enhances key areas of the brain affected by trauma (DeGregorio, 2013); and Mom's Empowerment Program, a group therapy approach aimed at reducing of the traumatic impact of past abuse (Howell et al., 2021; Levendosky, 2013). Models specifically aimed at increasing parenting capacity and parent-child attachment are also mentioned, including the Parent Aide Program (Tomison, 1996), Minding the Baby (Marshall et al., 2022), the Incredible Years Programme (DeGregorio, 2013; Schelbe & Geiger, 2017), Parenting with Feeling (DeGregorio, 2013), Group Attachment-Based Intervention (Alink et al., 2019), and the Mothers and Toddlers Programme (Alexander, 2015). Duthie et al., (2019) mentions Signs of Safety, an assessment and intervention approach specifically developed for statutory child protection in collaboration with Indigenous Australians.

Flexible Approach

On the other hand, four papers (5.6%) promote malleability and responsiveness to families' diverse needs when providing interventions. Levendosky et al. (2012) note that people who have experienced violence and maltreatment display a heterogeneity and often pattern-less sequalae of vulnerabilities, requiring person-centred and adaptable intervention approaches. Hall (2011) notes that parents reported more success when they felt able to "be flexible with parenting approaches in response to feedback from their child(ren)" (p. 46-47), incorporating elements of their learnings from different sources or parenting role models in response to the situation rather than applying a parenting model with fidelity. Cornett (1985) suggests flexible parenting education groups, involving parents who have experienced childhood maltreatment alongside those who have not for shared learning and co-regulation, while Duthie et al., (2019) promotes the needs for less rigidity around timeframes in the implementation and delivery of programs and services.

Build Informal Networks

The benefits of supportive personal relationships are noted in the reviewed literature, with the enhancement of social and interpersonal networks proffered as an intervention in seven papers (9.7%). Papers recommend that support be provided to parents to develop and maintain healthy relationships with other adults (Schelbe & Geiger, 2017) and to increase access to relational or community resources (Howell et al., 2021; McMillen & Rideout, 1996). Green (1976) indicated that as parents strengthen their adult relationships, they will be less reliant on their children to meet their emotional and dependency needs. In one study (Hall, 2011), parents (study subjects) reported that the lack of social support was a source of stress and suggested support groups led by parents with similar experiences to address this risk factor.

Authors also propose increasing the range of safe and nurturing adults that children are able to access as an intervention in intergenerational child maltreatment. Schelbe and Geiger (2017), for example, identify a "strong prosocial relationship with at least one caring adult" (p.52) as a key protective factor. Bennett (2021) focuses on building resilience in vulnerable children through an "always available adult" (p.1241), while McMillen and Rideout (1996) recommends providing children with or teaching them the skills to access other environmental contexts or safe adults in times of danger.

Home Visiting Programs

Three papers in the reviewed literature (4.2%) make note of the value of home visiting supports to provide practical assistance to families. The discussions included advocacy for specially trained visitors to provide emotional support to parents alongside parenting and health information and guidance (Belsky, 1993; Green, 1976), with some focus on home visiting programs during the perinatal period (Belsky, 1993; Schelbe & Geiger, 2017)

Strengths-Based Practice

A strengths-focused approach is emphasised in six (8.3%) of the reviewed papers. Bennett (2021), citing Leitch (2017), notes that an unintended consequence of the trauma informed care model was a deficit lens, expressing that a "strengths-based and action orientated" (p. 1241) approach is more likely to foster resilience. Hall (2011) likewise points out that research into intergenerational child maltreatment has been focused on pathology and the high rates of intergenerational continuity, focusing her research on the voices and strategies of mothers who experienced early maltreatment and had children who did not experience abuse or neglect. McMillen and Rideout (1996) encourage providing family members with opportunities to recognise and develop their unique skills and talents, thus facilitating a sense of task accomplishment, mastery, and a more positive sense of self. Marshall et al., (2022) note that "even the most discouraged families have been successful at times…" (p. 110), emphasising the need to identify and call attention to the positive aspects that are observed in the professional/family relationship. The case study described by Arons (2005) demonstrates such an approach, describing the articulation of parental strengths by the therapist, with words such as "'you let him know that you could feel he was angry… you had some good ideas about how to calm him…'" (p.117).

Cultural Healing

Three of the results (4.2%) note the importance of considering culture in the interventions with families at risk of intergenerational child maltreatment. Aguiar and Halseth (2015), citing Gone (2013), suggests "culture as treatment" (p. 23). The authors note that healing through reconnection to culture may rebuild the sense of self-worth and identity that was degraded during the colonisation process. Newton (2019) notes that the child removal in Aboriginal communities has inhibited the passing on of cultural child-rearing practices to the next generation, while Howell et al., (2021) advocates for "culturally sensitive treatment paradigms" (p. 7) which recognise and respond to historic colonisation traumas.

Exogenous Oxytocin

Three of the reviewed papers (4.2%) discuss the possibilities of the administration of oxytocin, a hormone found to be reduced in people who have experienced early life maltreatment, and which is crucial for bonding and parenting (Kim & Strathearn, 2017). Authors explore the potential for pharmacological treatments targeting the oxytocinergic systems to improve stress management and facilitate secure parent-child attachment (Buchheim et al., 2022; Kim & Strathearn, 2017). The controversies of this approach are noted, with Mitkovic Voncina et al. (2017) emphasising the need for future biological research on the efficacy and associated risks, and Kim and Strathearn (2017) acknowledging that additional and externally administered oxytocin may disrupt the adaptive internal mechanisms that the individual has developed to maintain a level of stability and coping skills, thus increasing risk.

Pharmacological Treatment

Two papers (2.8%) make note of the use of pharmaceutical interventions, alongside counselling and other approaches. Geiger et al. (2015) notes that such an approach has the potential to reverse the trauma related neurological adaptions in offspring, while Marshall et al. (2022) accentuates the importance of mental health treatment, which may include pharmacological interventions, for mothers in the critical perinatal period.

Reflective Practice

Six papers (8.3%) note the importance of reflective practice on the part of the practitioner to identify the emotions and personal biases that may emerge when working with families who have experienced intergenerational child maltreatment (Duthie et al., 2019). Authors promote such practices to ensure that personal views and reactions do not negatively affect the families and children with whom they are working with (Duthie et al., 2019; Green, 1976; Rosso, 2022) and to mitigate against burn out (Rosso, 2022).

Manage Countertransference

Four papers within the reviewed literature (5.6%) acknowledge that engaging and interacting with themes of child maltreatment can evoke strong emotions and reactions on the part of the practitioner. Authors outline the potential for therapists to instinctively "dislike or condemn" (Green, 1976, p. 426) parents who have caused harm to vulnerable children, to identify as a rescuer of children, to feel challenged or ineffectual when working with parents who present as dismissing, ambivalent, confronting or unappreciative, or to deny the abuse or attribute it to accidental forces (Alexander, 2015; Green, 1976; Rosso, 2022; Steele, 1970). Hence, it is argued, attending to these emotional experiences and, thereby, managing negative countertransference in the therapeutic space are positioned as central and ongoing tasks when working with families who have experienced intergenerational child maltreatment (Alexander, 2015; Rosso, 2022; Steele, 1970).

Challenge Personal Biases

Two results (2.8%) urge thoughtful examination of the self to make visible and scrutinise any biases and assumptions that may influence practice. Duthie et al., (2019), discussing cultural safety, notes the need for practitioners to reflect on their own culture rather than only the "cultures of 'others'" (p. 339), to recognise and question any stereotypes or assumptions, and to hold awareness of the personal power and privilege. Hall (2011) suggests questioning an automatic and often subconscious application of attachment theory when working with parents who have experienced early abuse, noting that the model may not adequately explain or support this cohort and that openness to other, client-led, ways of thinking may be more useful.

Supervision and Support

One paper (1.4%) makes note of the high potential for burn out among professionals working with families who are at risk of intergenerational child maltreatment, advising supports to mitigate against this. Rosso (2022), citing Tuohy (1987) endorses supervision and peer support, shared decision making through case reviews, and the option of engaging in additional workplace activities such as professional development, research, and teaching.

Systemic Interventions

Macro level interventions are proposed in 14 (19.4%) of the reviewed papers. These discussions amplify the benefits; indeed, the criticality of change to the systems and processes that guide and inform direct practice. Recommendations include whole of population interventions that reduce the stressors and systemic disadvantage experienced by some families (Bennett, 2021; Howell et al., 2021), addressing the reliance on dominant ideologies and values that inform systems (Aguiar & Halseth, 2015; Duthie et al., 2019; Newton, 2019), and increasing the skill of the workforce (Chamberlain, Gee, et al., 2019; Geiger et al., 2015).

Alleviate Disadvantage and Stressors

Alleviating poverty and disadvantage are proposed as interventions in eight (11.1%) of the results, which propose a combination of providing financial or material support and increasing access to supports and services that may mitigate the risk of intergenerational child maltreatment. Key themes of access to an adequate income, education, and community supports emerge (Belsky, 1993; Bennett, 2021; Howell et al., 2021; Negriff et al., 2020; Schelbe & Geiger, 2017). Schelbe and Geiger (2017), for instance, note that the translation of knowledge about risk factors for intergenerational child maltreatment into systemic practice indicates the need for programs providing tangible support, such as housing, financial benefits, health and food provision services, as well as ensuring access to education, therapy, and social support. Howell et al. (2021) advocates for a "multisectoral response" (p. 7), involving addressing the systemic issues that inhibit families from accessing services and increasing opportunities for income, employment, community spaces, education, and other services. Newton (2019) emphasises the need for culturally suitable service delivery with Indigenous Australians, noting the historical context of child removals has resulted in fear and reluctance to seek help and engage with services, and for systemic supports that address the underlying disadvantage experienced by Indigenous communities as a whole.

Attend to Dominant Ideologies

Eight (11.1%) of the results emphasise that the underlying basis of the legislative and political structures, and the practice that occurs within them, is entrenched in the dominant ideologies, values, and beliefs which shape societies. These papers call for attention to these societal ideologies and a reform of systems to ensure than non-dominant ontologies and values are incorporated in legislation and policy. Hall (2011) points out that conceptualisations of "healthy" (p. 45) parenting is defined by the dominant culture, suggesting the re-evaluation and re-appraisal of paradigms that guide practice with attention to the views of parents with a history of abuse. The author notes that these parents may identify alternate approaches and solutions to be more helpful than interventions imposed upon them by contemporary societal standards and values. Some papers propound the promotion of alternate beliefs and ideologies about the discipline of children through legislative change and public education so as to proclaim the unacceptability of certain behaviours, such as domestic violence and child abuse and neglect, to the population at large (Belsky, 1993; Schelbe & Geiger, 2017; Tomison, 1996).

Others, taking a cultural lens, note the "structural racism" (Howell et al., 2021, p. 7) inherent in the institutions and systems. These discussions suggest that dominant Western conceptualisation of trauma and subsequent intervention approaches are inadequate and unsuited for Indigenous and culturally diverse peoples. Papers refer to the mismatch of Western policies with both the compounding and collective traumas experienced by Indigenous people and other cultural minorities (Aguiar & Halseth, 2015; Duthie et al., 2019) and the worldviews and approaches to parenting within non-dominant populations, which are not understood by or incorporated into the policies and procedures that drive child protection systems (Newton, 2019; Schelbe & Geiger, 2017). Hence, these dialogues prescribe a scrutiny of the values driving systems and the incorporation of alternate cultural beliefs and ontologies.

Trauma-Informed Services

Four papers (5.6%) encourage the development of a more trauma-informed workforce (comprising all professionals engaging with families and children, not just specialised therapists or child protection workers). Authors assert that such a measure may avoid the triggering of trauma responses in service users and promote sensitive and insightful professional interpretations and case formulations (Chamberlain, Gee, et al., 2019; Duthie et al., 2019; Newton, 2019). Geiger et al., (2015) notes that children born into families who have experienced intergenerational trauma may be "primed to respond to stress much differently than their peers" (p. 80), thus requiring different understandings and interventions by professionals. The authors also counsel that all service users should be initially treated as though they have experienced trauma (Geiger et al., 2015).

Research Directions

Mapping recommendations for future research is not an explicit goal of this scoping review and is not explored comprehensively in this discussion. However, the indivisibility of research and practice, alongside the capacity for research to make meaningful contributions to intervention approaches, mean that recommendations for future research directions cannot be entirely omitted from this discussion. Several noteworthy themes, explored within 35 (48.6%) of the results, are deserving of some discussion due to thematic commonality and the potential to inform intervention approaches. These comprise addressing identified literature gaps (Howell et al., 2021; Zajac et al., 2019), exploring new and emerging possibilities (Alexander, 2015; Hall, 2011), and building the evidence base for interventions (Bennett, 2021; Schelbe & Geiger, 2017).

Fathers and Other Carers

The overemphasis in the research on mothers' caregiving characteristics and early experiences of maltreatment is expressed in the reviewed literature, with 17 results (23.6%) calling for future research into the role of other carers. The majority of these note the need to include fathers, but some note the diversity of family compositions and suggest research that incorporates same-sex parents, stepparents, and other supplementary carers such as grandparents (Geiger et al., 2015; Howell et al., 2021). As Lomanowska et al., (2017) notes, parents "exist within a family context, affect one another's parenting, and participate in a dynamic that also contributes to children's development" (p. 122).

Negriff et al., (2020) notes that the pathways and mechanisms of intergenerational transmission may operate differently for mothers compared to fathers, advocating for future studies that observe the mechanisms separately. Other discussions hold that the level of practical and emotional support provided to the mother by a secure partner relationship may be a relevant variable in the study of intergenerational child maltreatment that is deserving of further study (Moog et al., 2022; Putallaz et al., 1998). Levendosky et al., (2012) refers to the dearth of studies into the attachment relationship between children and carers who perpetrate domestic and family violence (more frequently fathers or male caregivers), suggesting that children could develop self-conceptualisations that align with either the aggressor or the victim. The authors point out, however, the safety risks of involving fathers who perpetrate violence in such research. Research into the genetic or epigenetic contributions of the biological father is also proposed (Lomanowska et al., 2017; Moog et al., 2022), with Ramo-Fernández et al., (2015), for instance, encouraging future epigenetic research on the germ cells of fathers exposed to adversity to help understand the intergenerational continuity of child maltreatment.

Longitudinal Prospective Studies

Twelve of the reviewed papers (16.7%) call for research that takes a prospective and longitudinal lens. Many authors reflect on the limitations of retrospective studies (the more commonly utilised in research into intergenerational child maltreatment), which look backwards in time through exploring whether maltreating parents experienced abuse or neglect in their own childhood. Authors note that such studies risk both the over-reporting of child maltreatment (as parents may falsely report childhood harm, be affected by recall bias, or have diverse interpretations of what constitutes maltreatment [Merrill et al., 2021; Sheppard, 2003; Tomison, 1996; Zajac et al., 2019]) and the under-reporting of childhood maltreatment (as parents may idealise their childhood and their relationship with their parents as a coping mechanism, have varied beliefs about the definitions of abuse and neglect, or choose not to disclose so as to avoid the retriggering of painful memories [Sheppard, 2003; Tomison, 1996]). Further, authors argue that retrospective approaches are almost universally conducted in high-risk groups (where maltreatment is confirmed or suspected), potentially leading to skewed estimations of the rates of intergenerational child maltreatment (Renner & Slack, 2006; Tomison, 1996) and the omission of insight into intergenerational *dis*continuity of child maltreatment (Tomison, 1996).

These discussions call for longitudinal prospective studies, (following families forward in time to measure childhood maltreatment experiences). Several authors suggest the enrolment of participants in early childhood, or even before the child's birth (Schelbe & Geiger, 2017), and studying these families over generations. Studies also emphasise that participants should be representative of the general population (Schelbe & Geiger, 2017) and propose studying two groups of children (one in which parents were maltreated in childhood, the other a control group) into adulthood and parenthood (Tomison, 1996). Several papers surmise that such a methodological approach is required to better understand the variables involved in intergenerational child maltreatment, such as the intergenerational effects of different types of abuse and neglect (Zajac et al., 2019), the psychological and biological considerations (Lomanowska et al., 2017; Mitkovic Voncina et al., 2017), the timing of the adversity (Widom, 2015, in Geiger et al., 2015), and the influence of various risk factors such as dissociation (Narang & Contreras, 2005) and attachment representations (Zajac et al., 2019). The logistic and practical difficulties conducting such research, due to the expense and time commitment required, is noted in the reviewed literature (Widom, 2015, in Geiger et al., 2015,; Tomison, 1996).

Intergenerational Discontinuity

Six (8.3%) of the reviewed papers propose a strengths and resilience lens in future research, pointing out that that the continuation of child maltreatment over generations is far from deterministic and may be the exception rather than the norm (Tomison, 1996) and urging research into protective and recovery-orientated factors present for survivors of childhood maltreatment (Hall, 2011; Meulewaeter et al., 2019; Zeanah & Zeanah, 1989). Some papers suggested sibling studies to explore the phenomenon of intergenerational discontinuity of child maltreatment, noting that children in the same household frequently experience similar abuse yet often have differing trajectories in terms of their own adult functioning and parenting (Howell et al., 2021; Tomison, 1996). Ramo-Fernández et al. (2015), for example, note that survivors of child maltreatment differ in terms of responsiveness to therapy, encouraging research into the epigenetic processes that predict or correlate with effective recovery, while Zeanah and Zeanah (1989) proposes further research that explores Belsky and Pensky's (1988) concept of "lawful discontinuity" (p. 191), or the capacity to form and maintain successful relationships in adulthood as a mediator of intergenerational child maltreatment.

Biological and Epigenetic Factors

Recognising that much of the research into biological and epigenetic processes involved in intergenerational child maltreatment is in its infancy, nine studies (12.5%) recommend further research into this field of enquiry. Papers call for additional studies on the gene-environment interactions, or the capacity for epigenetic change over the lifespan (Lomanowska et al., 2017; Ramo-Fernández et al., 2015), neurological structures and functions associated with experiencing and perpetrating child maltreatment (Mielke et al., 2016), correlations between early maltreatment experiences and the functioning of genes associated with hormones implicated in mothering, such as the dopamine, serotonin, vasopressin and oxytocin systems (Kim & Strathearn, 2017; Lomanowska et al., 2017), and the impacts of gestational biology (Buss et al., 2017; Moog et al., 2022).

Gender Pathways

Seven (9.7%) of the reviewed papers suggest further research into the ways that intergenerational continuity of child maltreatment may follow different trajectories depending on gender. Geiger et al., (2015), for instance, makes note of research finding that males may display aggression and impulsiveness as trauma responses while women tend towards relational and communication difficulties. Similarly, Ramo-Fernández et al., (2015) indicates that females are at increased risk of internalising behaviours, sometimes resulting in PTSD or depression, while males may exhibit violent and antisocial behaviours. Alexander (2015) expresses that boys may be more likely to respond to a mother's maltreatment with the more classical symptoms of disorganised attachment, such as punitive controlling and internalising and externalising behaviours, whereas girls may be more inclined to an "approach, affiliation, and compliance" (p. 213), or "tend and befriend" (p. 213) trauma response. Authors find indications that these gender differences may be due to number of factors, such as differences in hormonal functioning and brain development in different genders (Alexander, 2015; Geiger et al., 2015), socialisation practices positioning women as "'kin keepers'" (Putallaz et al., 1998, p. 416) with elevated relational and interpersonal responsibilities (Alexander, 2015), and decreased cortisol levels in females who have experienced maltreatment compared to increased levels in males (Alexander, 2015; Wilson & Scarpa, 2011).

Evaluations

Seven (9.7%) of the reviewed papers suggest that programs and frameworks addressing intergenerational child maltreatment receive regular and rigorous evaluation. Some discussions call for evaluation and the establishment of an evidence-based on specific intervention approaches in intergenerational child maltreatment, such as parenting programs (Schelbe & Geiger, 2017), psychoanalytic treatment approaches (Rosso, 2022), and neuropsychological therapeutic approaches (DeGregorio, 2013). Duthie et al., (2019) proposes evaluations which assess the effectiveness of interventions for different groups or cohorts of service users, rather than the whole-of-population evaluations, in order to tailor treatments to the needs of particular groups or communities. Bennett (2021) refers to the societal emphasis on funding and delivering evidence-based treatments for consumer and agency partner confidence as driving the need for evaluations. Chamberlain, Gee, et al., (2019), on the other hand, emphasises the value of frequent evaluation in delivering practice that is responsive to the needs of families and for early identification of unforeseen conditions or outcomes.

Trends, Patterns, and Correlations

Analysis of the relationships between different aspects of the data deepens insight into the ways in which various focuses or nuances within the literature may explain and respond to intergenerational child maltreatment uniquely. This discussion explores correlations based on the publication date of the paper, the cohort it studies, and the type of maltreatment it concentrates upon. Further, and perhaps more crucially, this section of the review finds and describes themes in the co-occurrences of theoretical frameworks and proposed interventions, as well as the interconnections between theoretical perspective and interventions recommendation in the 72 results explored in this discussion.

Publication Date

The data reveals changes to the leading theories applied to intergenerational child maltreatment over time. Relational perspectives (particularly attachment theory over family systems theory), developmental perspectives (with physiological outlooks increasing and psychosocial outlooks decreasing), and systems perspectives have remained dominant, albeit fluctuating, in the reviewed literature over time. In contrast, the heritability perspective has seen a gradual increase since the 1980s, with genetic theories influencing studies in the 1990s and 2000s and epigenetic theories more prominent in the subsequent time periods, likely reflecting the development of the collective knowledge in the field of genetics and epigenetics. Unprocessed trauma theories have declined somewhat since the 1970s, also gradually shifting in focus from psychodynamic theories towards dissociation theories. Learning theories increased, reaching their peak in the 1990s before declining again. Figure 4, Figure 5, Figure 6 and Figure 7 (below) show the changes in a selection of the aforementioned theories and theoretical perspectives over time.

Figure 4. Relational theories over time

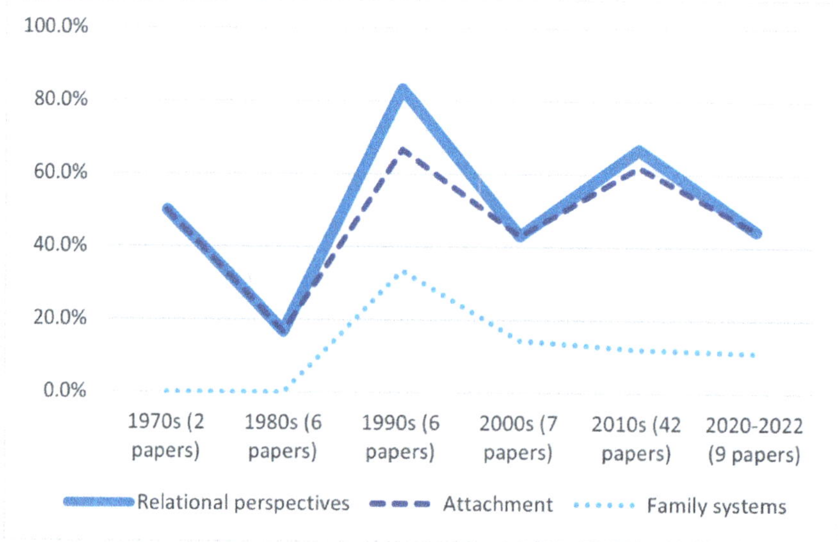

Figure 5. Developmental theories over time

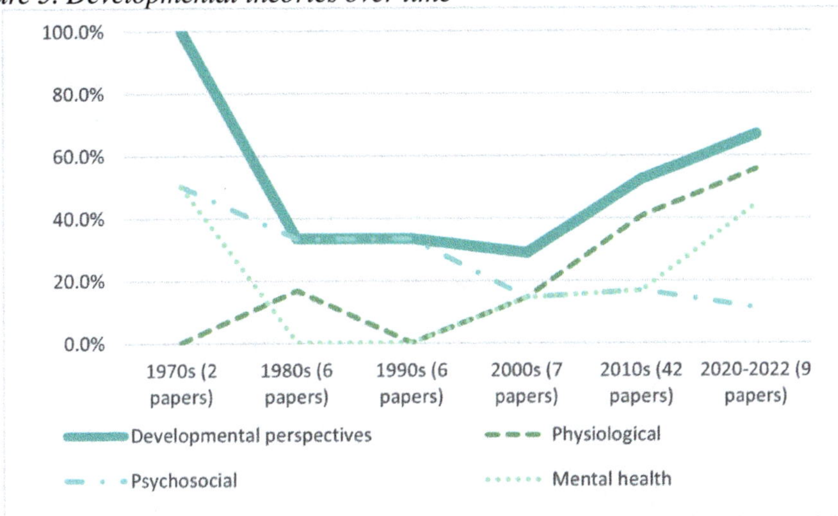

Figure 6. Unprocessed trauma theories over time

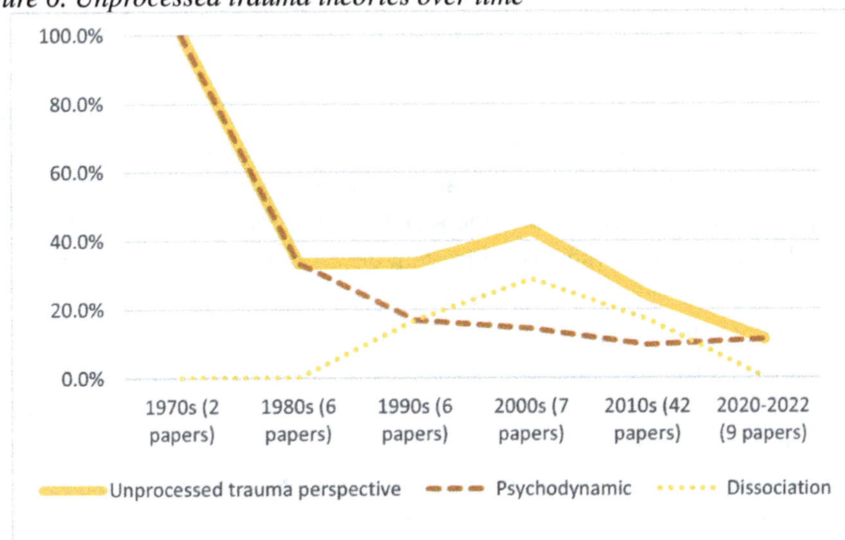

Figure 7. Heritability theories over time

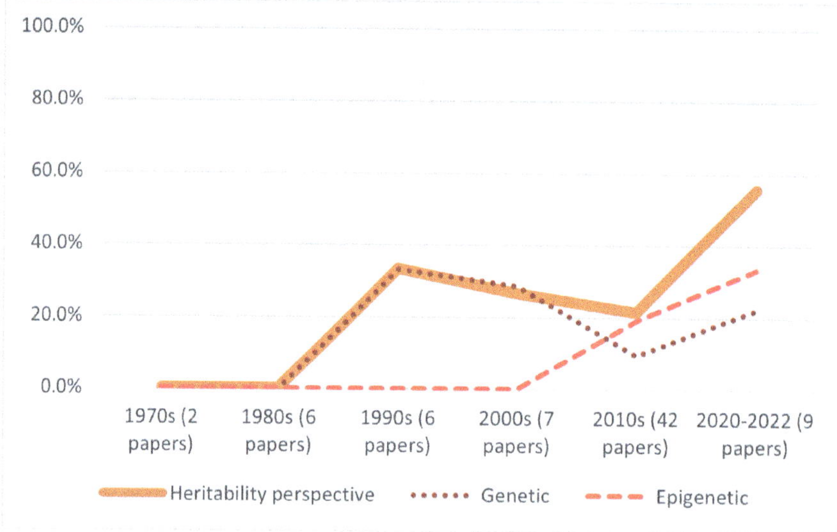

Similarly, the recommended intervention approaches differ according to the decade in which the paper was published, as noted in Figure 8, Figure 9, Figure 10, and Figure 11, below. Results published in the 1980s were least likely to offer a proposed intervention, with only 3 of the 6 papers (50%) making suggestions relating to direct practice, the target group, and future research, while 100% of those published in the 1970s, 1990s and 2020s make some recommendations.

Advocacy for future research increased over time (see Figure 9, below). The rise in promotion of research on fathers and other carers, gender pathways, and biological and epigenetic functions in recent decades may reflect our burgeoning bioscientific knowledge of the mechanisms of intergenerational trauma, while the growing attention to evaluations in the past two and half decades may be a product of neoliberalism ideals, with its attention to measurability and evidence-based practice (Healy, 2022). In contrast, reflective practices were by far most prominent in the 1970s (with a focus on the psychoanalytic attention to transference and countertransference), before decreasing to nil and then rearising slightly in the 2010s and 2020s.

Suggestions relating to direct practice (the largest of the intervention categories) remain consistently notable over time, although differences in the focus of these proposed interventions are observable. While some approaches, such as acknowledging and integrating trauma, enhancing parental attunement, developing parenting skills, and building informal networks have fluctuated but remained prominent over time, other intervention approaches have increased or decreased. Cultural healing and pharmaceutical approaches or exogenous oxytocin have only been recognised in the reviewed literature since 2010, perhaps representing bioscientific developments and increasing attention to alternative healing approaches. Strengths-based practice and emotional and behavioural regulation skills also increased over time, as did the use of specific models (again, potentially a product of a neoliberal focus on measurable and manualised treatment models). On the other hand, the use of the therapeutic relationship to re-enact and resolve trauma became less frequently recommended over time in the reviewed literature, while practical and social interventions declined before rearising in recent decades.

Figure 8. Proposed intervention categories over time

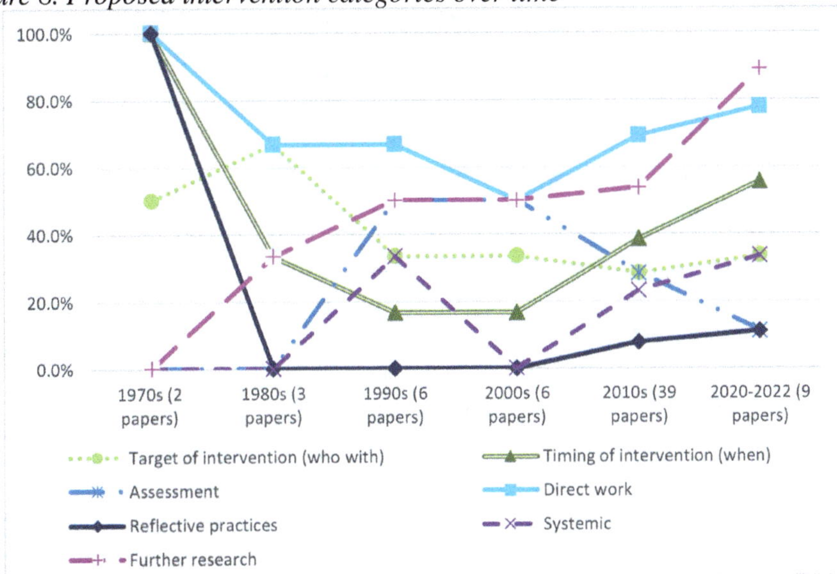

Figure 9. Proposed research directions over time

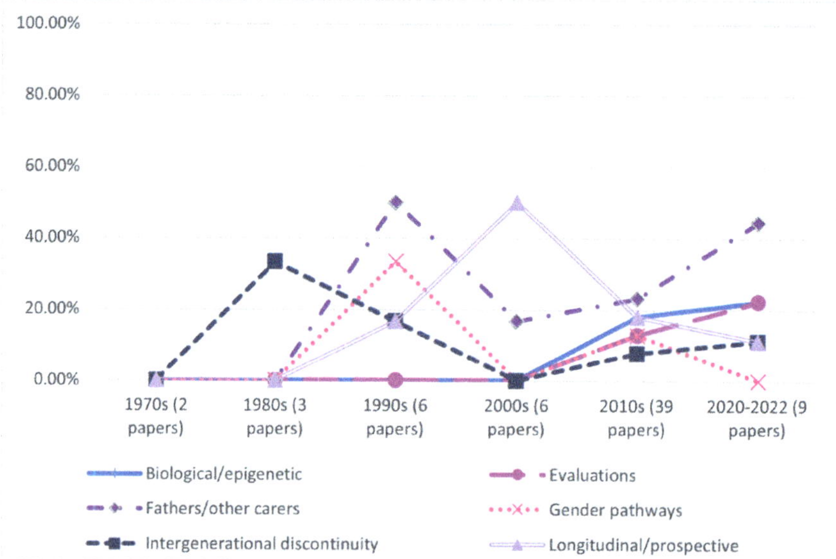

Figure 10. Proposed therapeutic trauma work over time

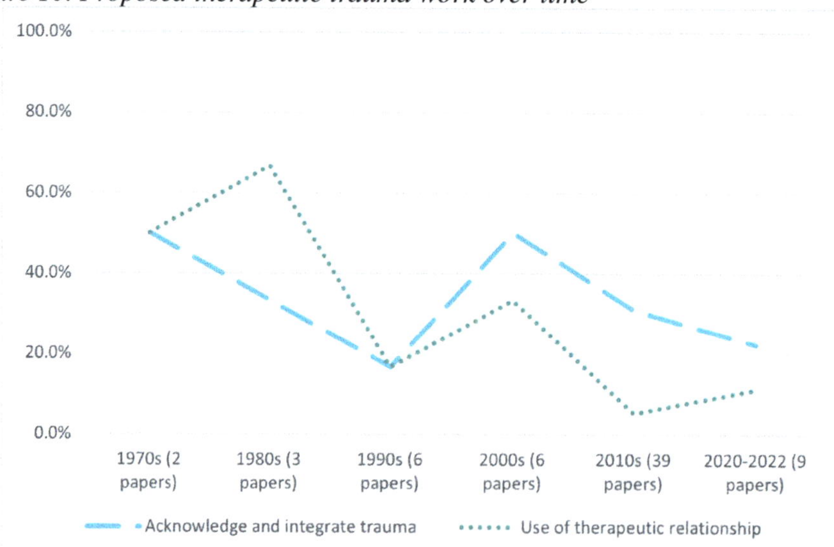

Figure 11. Proposed use of models vs flexibility over time

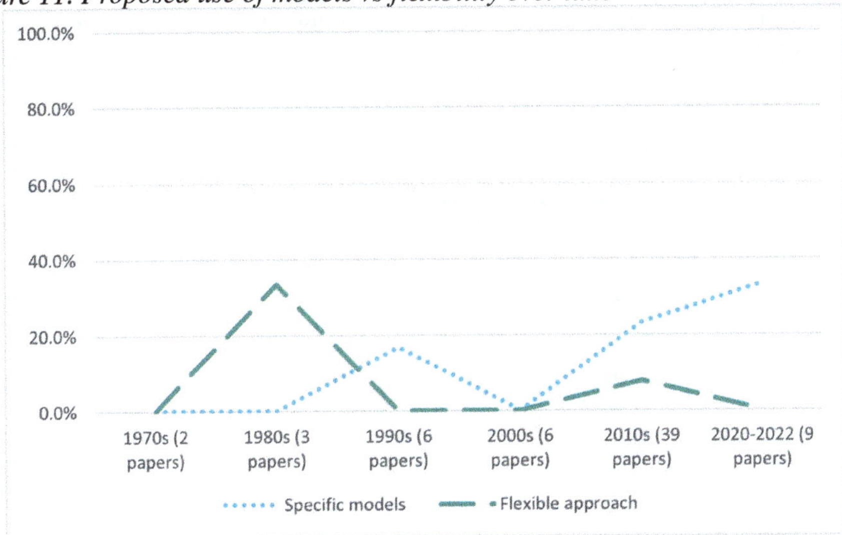

Cohort studied

An analysis of the 41 results which targeted their study towards a particular cohort (such as mothers, both parents, or families involved in child protection systems) or developmental period (such as childhood or the perinatal period) also reveals theoretical and interventional trends and themes (see Figure 12 and Figure 13 below). Unsurprisingly, the literature studying Indigenous people strongly expresses cultural theoretical perspectives (100%) and cultural healing interventions (50%) as well as the systemic theoretical perspective (100%) and systemic interventions (100%). This dominance in systems perspectives and interventions in Indigenous papers significantly outweighs that articulated in studies on other cohorts or developmental periods.

Relational perspectives, particularly attachment theory, are robustly apparent in many of the studied cohorts, particularly the perinatal period (100%), parents (83.3%), and mothers (77.3%). The developmental and heritability perspectives are noted most frequently in literature studying fathers (100% each) and animal studies (100% for developmental and 66.6% for heritability). The developmental theoretical perspective is also the most pronounced in studies focusing on the perinatal period (57.1%), while papers studying fathers and animal studies are most likely to suggest further research as an intervention (100% each), although future research is well represented in results exploring all the identified cohorts. More attention to assessment considerations is expressed as suitable interventions with both parents

(50%) and with adolescents (40%), while studies focused on the perinatal period are, unsurprisingly, more likely to recommend interventions during the perinatal period (35.7%).

Figure 12. Cohort studied: Theoretical perspective

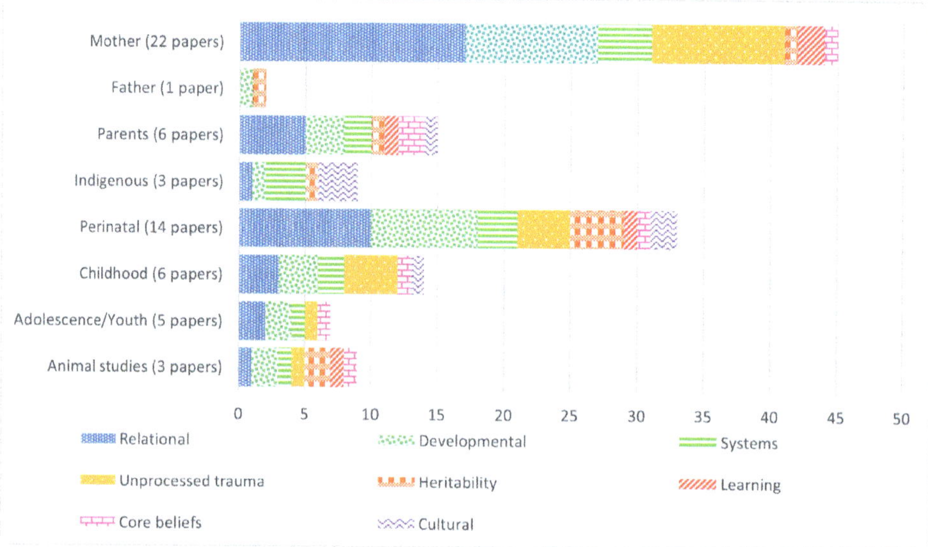

Figure 13. Cohort studied: Proposed intervention category

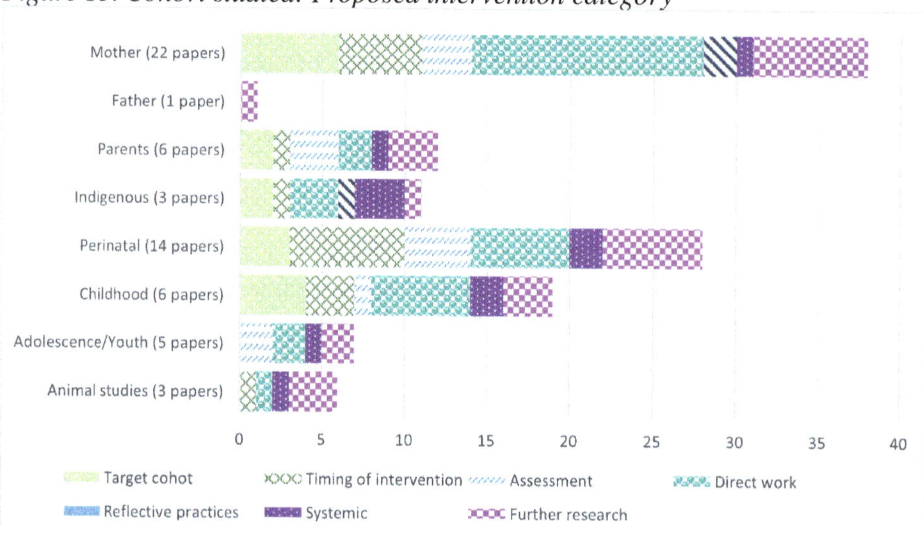

Maltreatment Type

The type of maltreatment (such as physical abuse or domestic violence) specifically studied in 23 of the reviewed papers also reveal trends in theoretical perspective and intervention preferences. Papers focused on domestic and family violence, for example, are most likely to articulate the learning perspective (71.4%) and to recommend direct service-user to practitioner interventions (57.1%) (specifically developing parenting skills, acknowledging and integrating trauma, and the use of the therapeutic relationship [28.6% each]). Results exploring involvement with child protection systems are correlated most prominently with the developmental theoretical perspective (57.1%) and practices that involve assessment (71.4%).

Physical abuse is strongly linked to the unprocessed trauma perspective (66.6%) and likely to correlate with proposed direct interventions involving acknowledging and integrating the trauma (66.6%) and the use of the therapeutic relationship (50%) as well as interventions attending to specific target individuals or groups (individual parent, family system, group work, couples, and the parent-child dyad) (50%). Papers focused on child sexual abuse included the most diversity in theories and suggested approaches, aligning slightly more towards the relational perspective (66.6%) and towards direct interventions involving emotional and behavioural regulation, enhancing parental attunement to their child, and integration of trauma (33.3% each). The small sample on neglect is most strongly correlated with cultural theoretical perspectives and systems perspectives (100% each) and in systemic interventions and direct work with service users (100% each). Figure 14 and Figure 15 (below) visually depict a number of the trends described.

Figure 14. Maltreatment type: Theoretical perspective

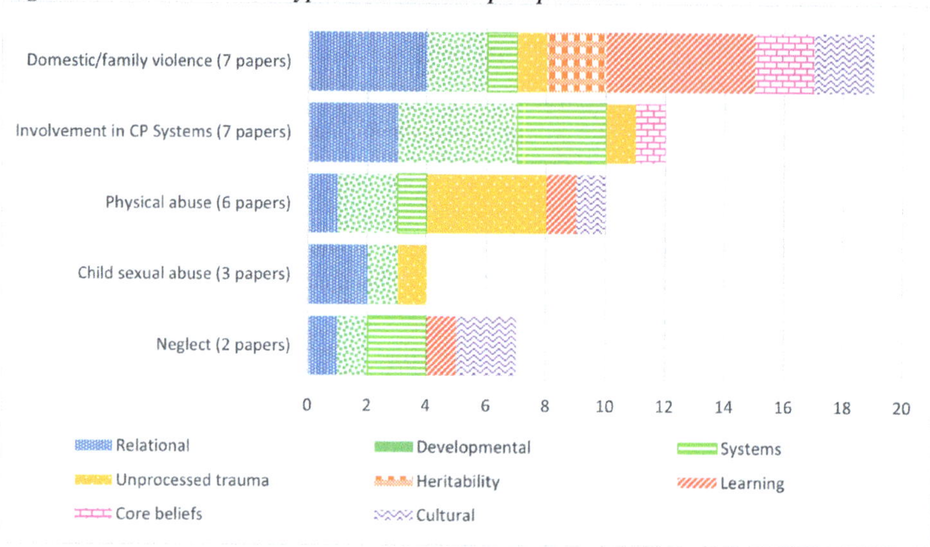

Figure 15. Maltreatment type: Intervention category

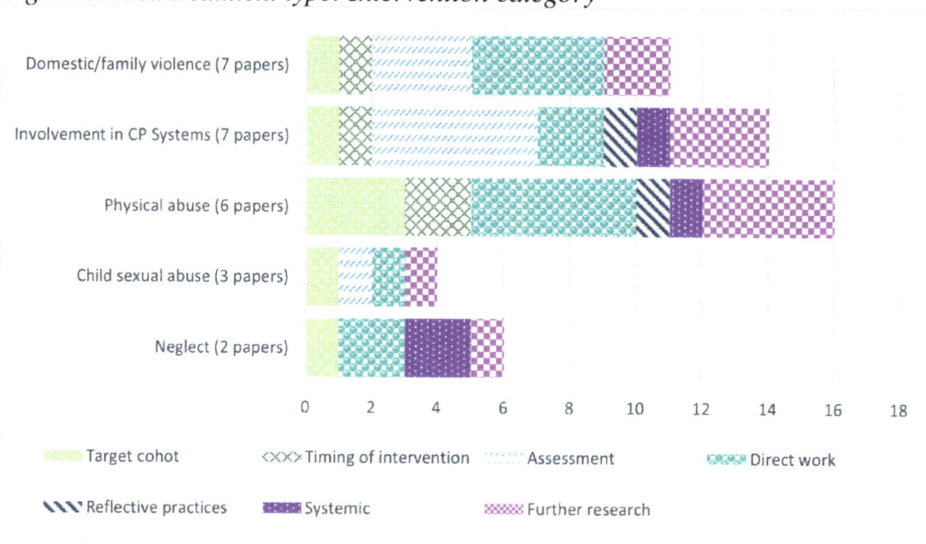

Co-occurrence of Theoretical Perspectives and Proposed Interventions

An analysis of theoretical perspectives which commonly co-occur in the reviewed literature provides some indication of the ways in which theoretical perspectives are likely to be blended or integrated, sometimes resulting in fresh insights explaining intergenerational child maltreatment. The unprocessed trauma perspective is most likely to occur in isolation (i.e., papers with no other theory concurrently articulated) (35.5%). On the other hand, results expressing cultural and systemic perspectives are least likely to express a sole perspective (0% each). Relational perspectives and, to a slightly lessor degree, developmental theories co-occur alongside the broadest range of other theories, potentially relating to the higher numbers of results expressing these theoretical frameworks.

Patterns emerge regarding the types of theoretical perspectives most likely to co-occur. Papers expressing heritability perspectives often tend to concurrently articulate developmental theories (72.2%). Those referring to cultural perspectives are most likely to also include systems perspectives (83.3%) and, reciprocally, the systems perspective has a higher proportion of results that also named cultural theories (45.5%) than other theoretical frameworks. Learning perspectives and core beliefs perspectives also align with one another in this review (41.2% of learning perspectives also naming core beliefs perspectives, and 58.3% of core beliefs concurrently identifying learning theories). Core belief theories are also likely to simultaneously name relational theories (75%). Figure 16, below, visually represents the co-occurrence of theoretical perspectives,

Figure 16. Co-occurrence of theoretical perspectives

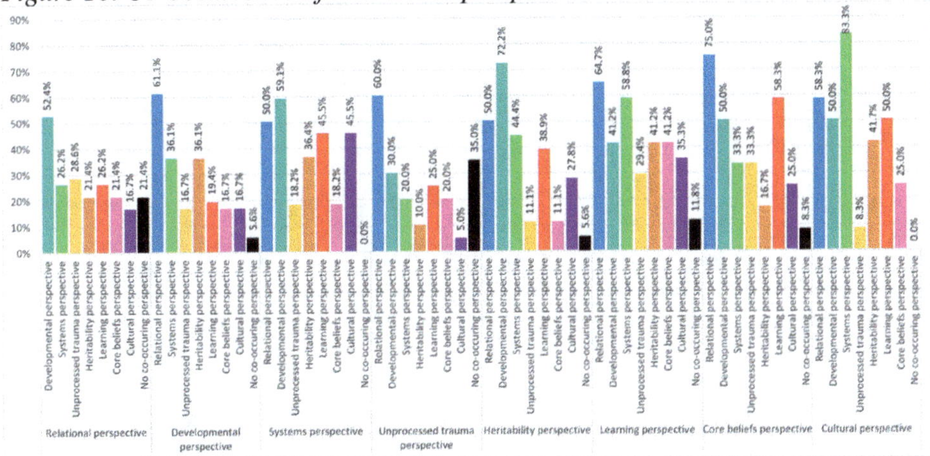

An examination of the co-occurrence of proposed interventions also offers valuable insight into the ways in which approaches to address the issue are likely to merge and coalesce, potentially resulting in unique and tailored practice approaches. Figure 17, Figure 18, and Figure 19, below, provides a visual representation of recommended interventions that coincide in the reviewed literature.

Interventions involving direct practice are endorsed alongside a range of other recommendations in the reviewed literature, most strongly in systemic change, reflective practices, working with individuals, and working with communities or groups (100% each). Encouragement of future research also frequently co-occurs alongside other proposed interventions, with 100% of the direct practices involving biological or pharmacological interventions and 75% of systemic interventions concurrently proposing further research.

Considerations on the timing of service delivery are most likely to occur alongside recommendations for building the evidence base through further research (85.7%) and reflective practices (83.3%). Advice regarding the target cohort is most strongly represented in papers which also propose person and culture focused direct intervention (75%).

Systemic interventions display a varied correlation with other intervention approaches, including direct practice (person and culture focused work [62.5%] and practical and social interventions [55.6%]) while the two largest subcategories of direct practice in the reviewed literature, therapeutic trauma work and intervening in the parent-child relationship, were least likely to concurrently suggest systemic work (0% and 11.1% respectively). Research aimed towards building an evidence base for practice was also correlated with systemic interventions (57.1%).

Figure 17. Co-occurrence of proposed interventions (target cohort, timing, and assessment)

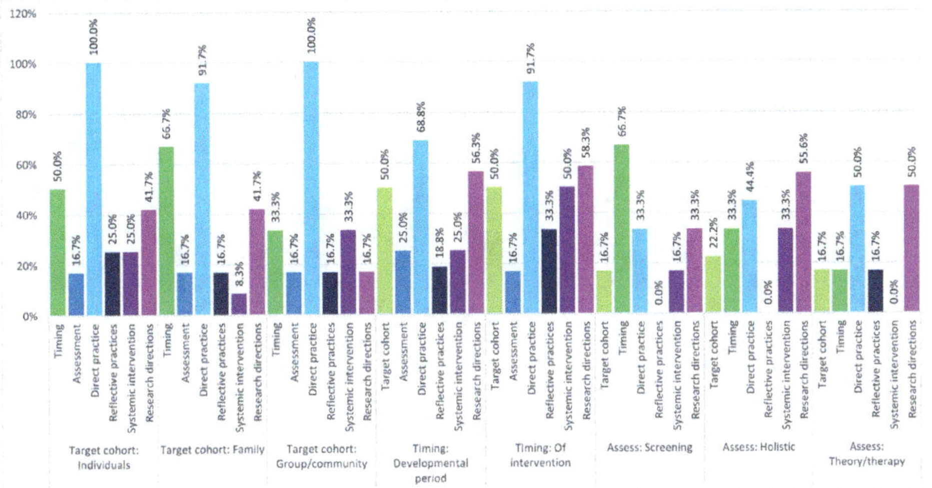

Figure 18. Co-occurrence of proposed interventions (direct practice)

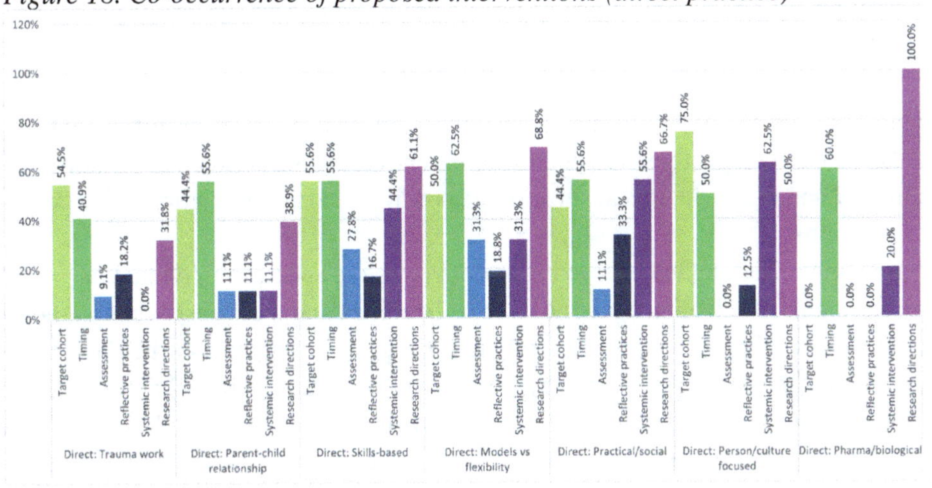

Figure 19. Co-occurrence of proposed interventions (reflective practices, systemic intervention, and research directions)

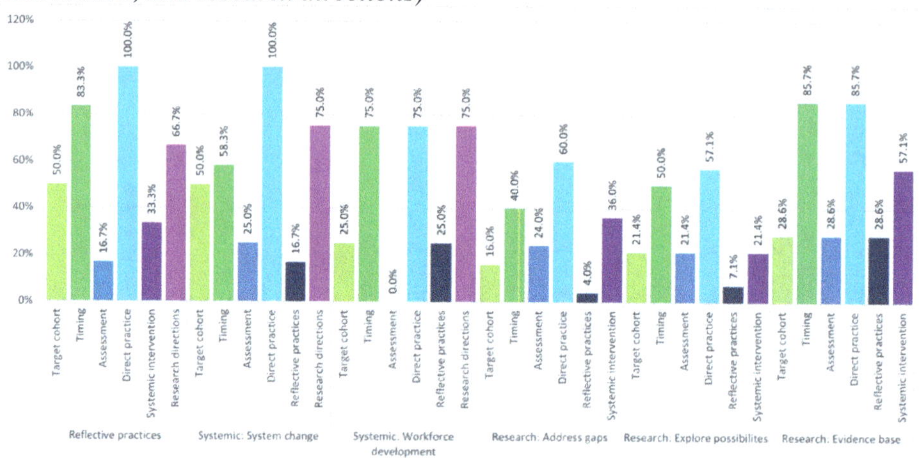

Theoretical Alignment and Proposed Interventions

Patterns are also located when exploring connections between the papers' theoretical alignment and the interventions they propose. Figure 20 (below) illustrates correlations between theoretical perspective and intervention category. Figure 21, Figure 22, Figure 23, and Figure 24 visually represent a selection of the analysis of theoretical perspectives to specific interventions, while Figure 25, Figure 26, Figure 27 and Figure 28 reveal some of the specific theories in relation to proposed interventions.

Recommendations for interventions delivered to a specific individual or group are reasonably evenly distributed across the theoretical perspectives, although those delivered to individuals are most likely to be suggested by papers articulating the unprocessed trauma perspective (35% for individual parents and 15% for individual children). Community interventions are most likely to be advised by cultural (16.7%) and systems perspectives (9.1%), and endorsement for group work most prominent in core beliefs perspectives (16.7%).

Views on the timing of the intervention reveals a preference for work during the perinatal period, particularly in heritability perspectives (38.9%), developmental perspectives (25%), and cultural perspectives (25%). Advice for early intervention is most common in core beliefs perspectives (25%), cultural perspectives (16.7%), and systems perspectives (13.6%), while that for long term engagement with professionals is foremost in unprocessed trauma perspectives (20%), reflective of the longer time frames of therapy common in such depth therapy.

Approaches to the assessment of individuals and families are recommended across the range of theoretical perspectives, although absent in Indigenous theories and comparatively low in unprocessed trauma perspectives (5%). The relational perspective (11.9%) and the developmental perspective (13.9%) are most likely to recommend screening for trauma, and the systems perspective displays increased attention to assessments of current adversities (9.1%). The learning perspective, particularly social learning, is most likely to recommend holistic assessments including multigenerational assessment (11.8%), assessment of different forms of maltreatment (11.8%), ongoing assessment (5.9%), and assessing for current adversities (5.9%).

Some form of direct practice is endorsed by results within all theoretical perspectives. Practices based in therapeutic trauma work are most notable in the unprocessed trauma perspective (70% for acknowledge and integrate trauma and 40% for the use of the therapeutic relationship), while those stemming from a goal of improving the parent child relationship, particularly enhancing parental attunement, are strongest in the unprocessed trauma perspective (45%) and relational perspective (31%). Endorsed interventions aimed towards developing parenting skills are prominent in cultural perspectives (41.7%), systems perspectives (40.9%), and the learning perspective (35.3%), and those proposing the development of informal social networks are strongest in the systems perspective (27.3%). Working in fidelity to specific models is somewhat prominent throughout the theoretical perspectives. Flexibility in approach is far less so, but higher in cultural (8.3%) and systems (9.1%) perspectives. Unsurprisingly, culturally healing is highly endorsed in the cultural perspective (25%) and pharmacological interventions are most notable in the heritability perspective (11.1% for exogenous oxytocin and 11.1% for pharmaceuticals).

Reflective practices are most evident in the unprocessed trauma perspectives (15% for management of countertransference and 5% for accessing supervision and support). Papers based in systems and cultural perspectives also encourage reflection upon personal biases (9.1% and 8.3% respectively).

A systemic approach to intervention is most strongly represented in cultural perspectives and systems perspectives, in particular, attending to and challenging the dominant societal ideologies and their translation to policy and practice (50% for cultural and 36.4% for systemic), followed by alleviating disadvantage (41.7% for cultural and 27.3% for systemic). The unprocessed trauma perspective is least likely to propose any type of systemic intervention.

Recommendations for future research in general are more prominent in the heritability perspective (77.8%) and least apparent in the unprocessed trauma perspective (30%, with 18.2% recommending evaluations for a more rigorous evidence-based of psychodynamic theories). Papers aligned with the cultural perspective are also likely to propose evaluations for a more robust evidence-based on alternative healing approaches (25%). The heritability, systems, and developmental perspectives are most inclined towards future research exploring biological and epigenetic functions of intergenerational child maltreatment (38.9%, 31.8% and 19.4% respectively), while research on fathers and other carers is propounded more significantly in papers expressing heritability, learning, and systems perspectives (44.4%, 41.2%, and 40.9% respectively). Future research exploring intergenerational influences based on gender of the offspring are strongest in heritability theories (27.8%), followed by systems theories (18.2%) and learning theories (17.6%).

Figure 20. Theoretical perspectives: Proposed intervention category

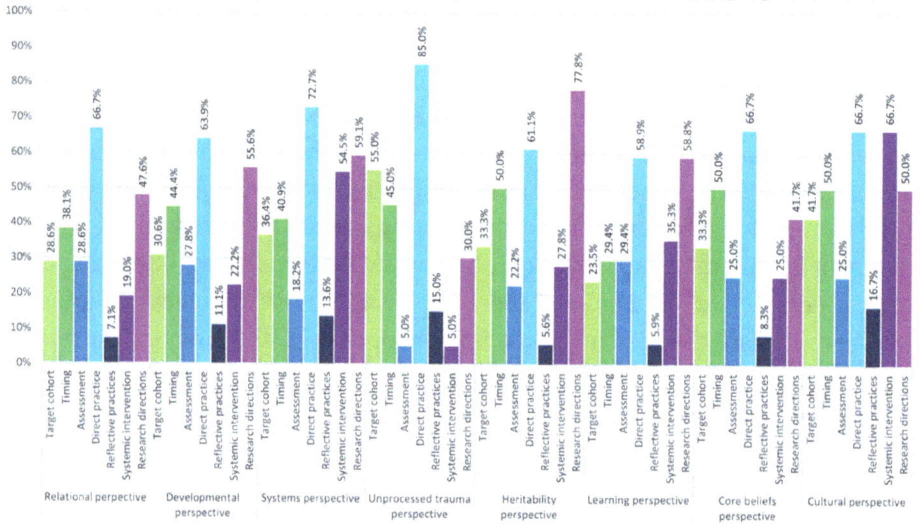

Figure 21. Theoretical perspective: Target cohort

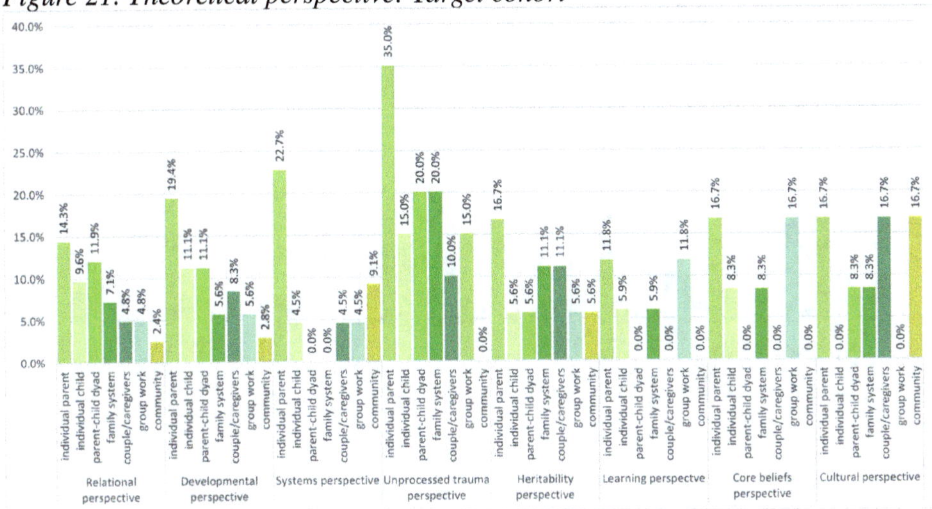

Figure 22. Theoretical perspective: Direct practice (part a)

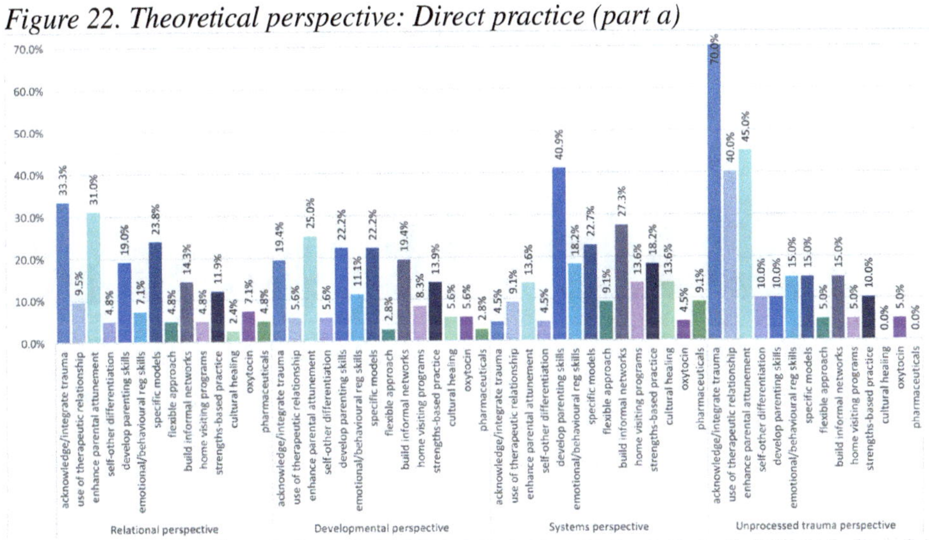

Figure 23. Theoretical perspective: Direct practice (part b)

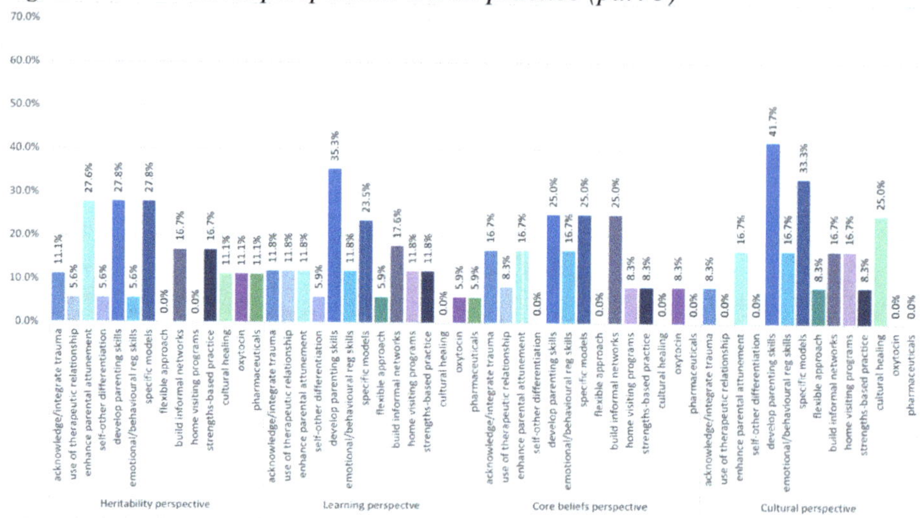

Figure 24. Theoretical perspective: Research directions

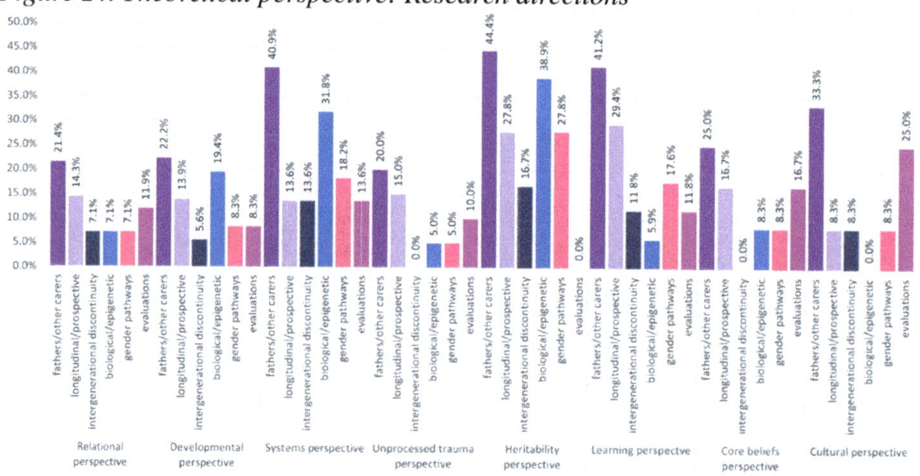

Figure 25. Attachment theory: Proposed interventions

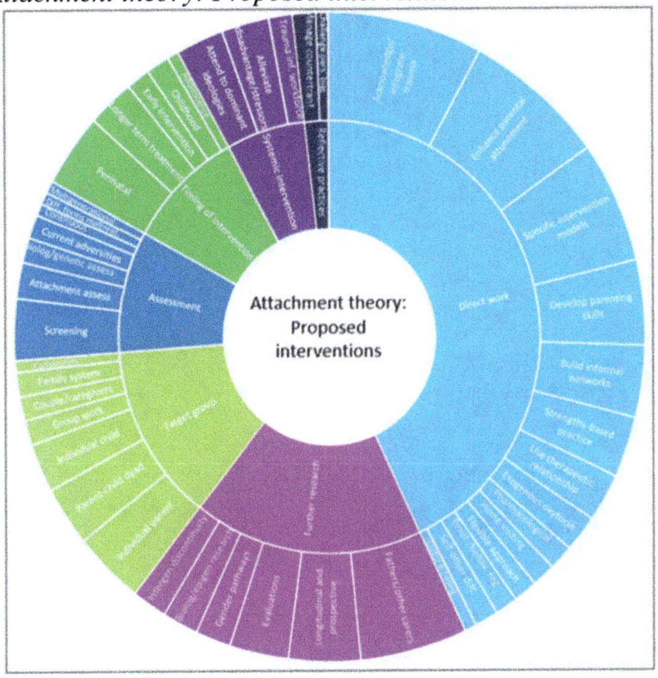

Figure 26. Ecological systems theory: Proposed interventions

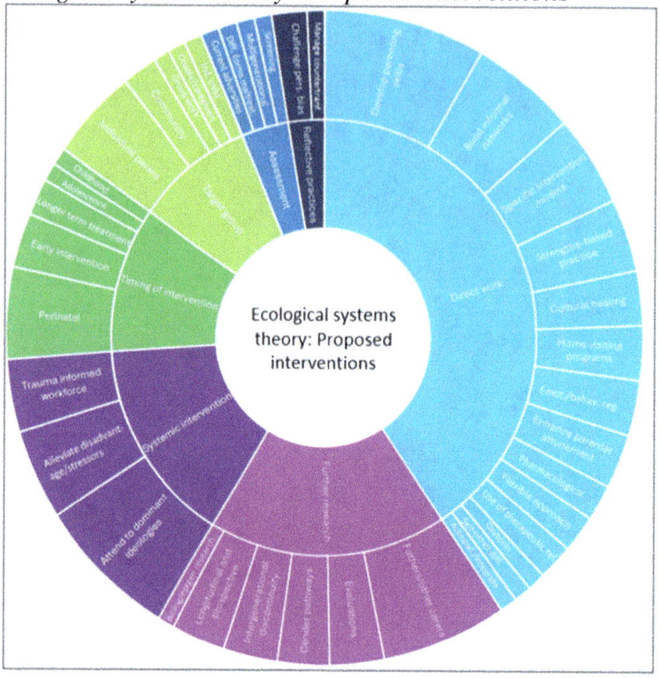

Figure 27. Social learning theory: Proposed interventions

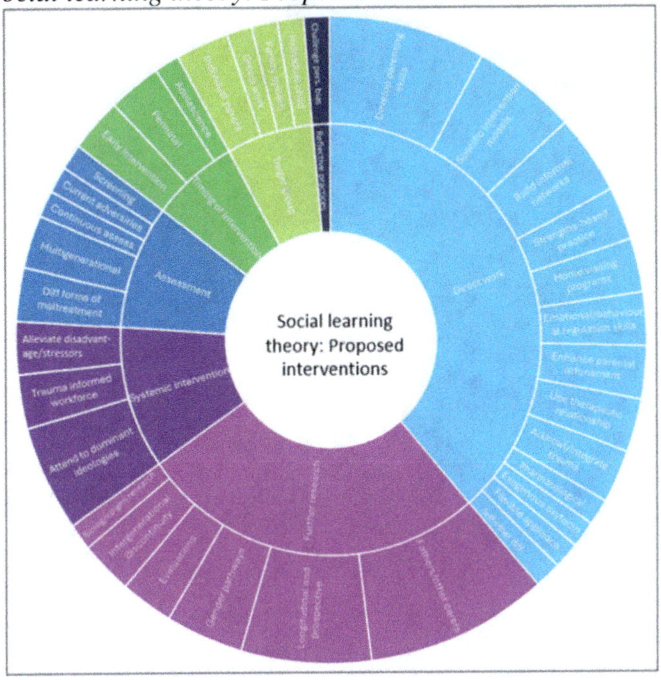

Figure 28. Indigenous theories: Proposed interventions

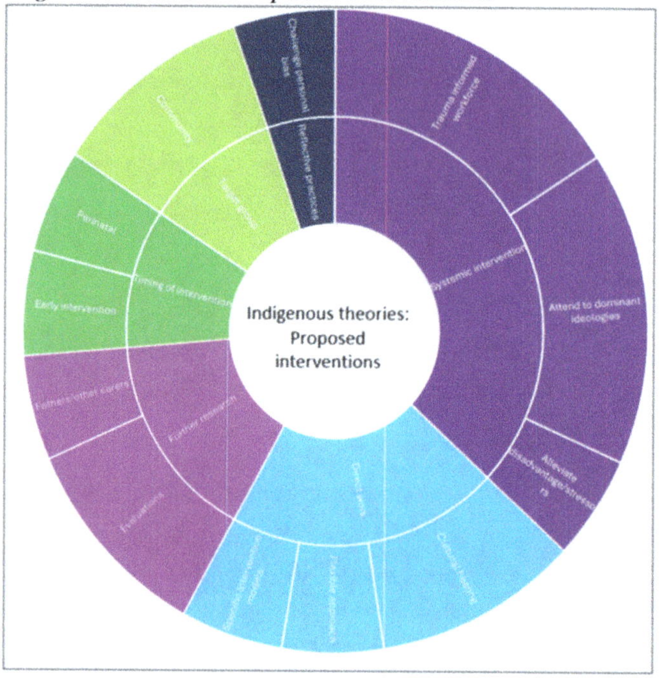

DISCUSSION

This scoping review aimed to develop insight into the theoretical frameworks applied in the literature to explain intergenerational child abuse and neglect; to map the interventions endorsed or propounded in the literature on the topic; and to reveal patterns and trends in relation to the expressed theories, the proposed interventions and the correlations between the two. The findings emphasise the diversity of explanatory theories and recommended interventions as well as reveal the more dominant theories and treatments within the reviewed literature, including those which are predisposed to co-occur. Findings also illuminate the pathways from theoretical framework to recommended intervention, as well as the influences of different facets of the research, such as time period, cohort studied, and maltreatment type.

Implications for Policy and Practice

For some decades, practitioners and policymakers working in the field of child protection have noticed the prevalence of intergenerational child maltreatment, expressed concern about the phenomenon, and emphasised the importance of designing interventions to address this public health challenge (Geiger et al., 2015; Islam et al., 2023; Jaffee et al., 2013). The insights provided by this review reveal a number of useful themes and trends within the research that are translatable to child protection policy and practice.

With some anomalies, the reviewed literature reveals links between theoretical perspectives and the proposed interventions they may be naturally inclined towards. Results articulating unprocessed trauma theories, for example, are most likely to coincide with recommendations for long term direct therapy with individual parent survivors of childhood maltreatment. Attachment theory is correlated strongly with interventions aimed towards enhancing a parent's attunement to their child (albeit slightly less significantly than with interventions aimed at acknowledging and integrating trauma), while those involving the learning perspective include preferred interventions based on building parental skills in parenting and managing emotions. Further, papers expressing systems theories and cultural theories frequently correspond with systemic theories and proposed interventions at a structural or macro level, and the heritability perspective is most likely to recommend further research, particularly that exploring fathers and biological and epigenetic inquiry. Thus, the relevance of theory to practice is demonstrated. In comparison to practice frameworks, theoretical frameworks are less well articulated by practitioners and organisations; yet, they have inextricable links to the type of intervention delivered. Making overt these theories, which motivate and drive practice, allows for greater insight, transparency and cognisance and is, therefore, a vital reflective practice for both individual professionals and for organisations or structures.

Variations in the prominence of different theories and interventions are apparent when sorted according to decade of publication, often mirroring the dominant ideologies of the era. Psychodynamic theories and interventions are most common in papers published in the 1970s, when, despite the emergence of behaviouralism and cognitive therapies, psychoanalysis and the "talking cure" remained a more established and orthodox therapeutic approach (Sharma, 2023; Woolfolk, 2015) before declining over subsequent decades. Heritability theories, physiological developmental theories, and pharmaceutical interventions have gradually increased over the past two to three decades as the knowledge on the role of epigenetics and biology in trauma responses emerged and expanded (DeGregorio, 2013; Yehuda & Bierer, 2009). Papers advocating for interventions based in specific treatment models, as opposed to a flexible and nimble approach to therapy, increased from the 1990s onwards, perhaps as a response to the rise of neoliberalism and New Public Management (with their values of privatisation, economic rationalism, free market competition, and the measurement of performance to ensure accountability), resulting in funding packages and delivery of services based upon "proven" effectiveness and a robust evidence-base (Healy, 2022; Jacobsson & Meeuwisse, 2020). In policy and practice, a deep awareness of the political, economic, and social factors influencing the era in which we live and practice, alongside a mindfulness of the mutable nature of these factors, results in a more holistic appreciation for the pertinence of the macro system on the interaction between practitioner and service-user.

Further, the data reveals theoretical and intervention preferences according to specific area of enquiry. Studies on domestic and family violence is correlated with the learning perspective in the reviewed literature, reflecting broader trends in which social learning theory is applied to explain why children exposed to violence may grow into adults who experience or perpetrate violence (Copp et al., 2019). The reviewed papers focusing on parents with involvement in child protection systems are often related to assessment interventions, an unsurprising connection as assessment of safety and risk is a central task in child protection work. Relational perspectives are most prominent in the perinatal period, a critical timeframe for attachment and relational reliance. Direct interventions are most likely to be recommended in studies concentrating on mothers, perhaps mirroring a broader observation (and concern) that the female caregiver is often more likely to be expected and compelled to engage with systems following concerns for the safety of children (Nygren et al., 2021; Zanoni et al., 2013). Cultural perspectives and interventions are most common in papers focused on neglect, a reflection of the critique of Western child protection systems for misinterpreting and making assumptions about cultural parenting practices, thus ascribing neglect to healthy cultural practices (Newton, 2019; Nietz, 2019). Knowledge of such inclination towards certain theories and approaches within specific fields of research is critical for the acknowledgement of bias in these specific fields of practice and, potentially, could result in the broadening of frameworks applied to each area of enquiry for deeper comprehension and interpretation.

Indigenous families are frequently overrepresented in the child protection systems and addressing this disproportionality is a priority for child protection policy in many jurisdictions worldwide (Australian Institute of Health and Welfare, 2025; Quinn et al., 2022). The findings in this review hold significant implications for this topic. In comparison to papers exploring other cohorts and theories in this review (even surpassing papers expressing systemic perspectives), results focused on Indigenous people and articulating Indigenous or cultural theoretical perspectives are strongly correlated with systemic theories and argue persuasively for systemic change. This illustrates the concept of the more disenfranchised (Indigenous families experience more oppression, systemic racism, poverty and the reverberations of colonisation [Duthie et al., 2019; Menzies, 2019]) or those who feel a sense of solidarity with these groups being more likely to initiate structural change, while the issue may be overlooked or left unattended by groups benefitting from this inequal power distribution (Curtin et al., 2016; Strolovitch, 2006). Arguably, professionals involved with families who experience intergenerational child maltreatment have an intrinsic responsibility to acknowledge and address disadvantage and oppression as part of the treatment model (Bennett et al., 2020) rather than simply make change at a micro level. Thus, advocacy and potentially activism alongside Indigenous peoples and groups affected by other forms of oppression and disadvantage are positioned as a core aspect of engagement with families who experience intergenerational child maltreatment.

Papers on Indigenous experience and theory are also more likely to recommend the inclusion of cultural healing as a recognised method of intervention, community work, and the reflective practice of acknowledging personal bias. There are many diverse approaches to interventions and healing, often deriving from cultural practices that Western child protection contexts are unaware, or only minimally aware, of. These may, therefore, be absent in the training of practitioners, funding decisions, and in practice itself. Practitioners, policymakers, and education providers are therefore challenged to expand their understanding of the therapeutic needs and preferences of Indigenous people (and, indeed, all people) and to customise their approach accordingly.

Further, interventions involving evaluations are frequent in papers articulating Indigenous theories (50%) and cultural perspectives (25%) as a pathway towards building an evidence base and for the inclusion of cultural approaches and understandings in the accepted (and funded) interventions (Chamberlain, Gee, et al., 2019; Duthie et al., 2019). However, a significant body of work notes that this neoliberal public management approach conflicts with Indigenous ontologies (Luke et al., 2022; Poirier et al., 2022; Sullivan, 2018), expressing that evidence-based practice is individualistic and competitive, thus ignoring the Indigenous attention to collaboration and interconnection between community and land; that it overlooks Indigenous research methodologies in favour of scientific rigour; and that it focuses on economic rationalism, resulting in an "audit society" (Power, 1997) which undermines Indigenous self-determination and the autonomy of Aboriginal community controlled organisations. Decolonisation involves a recognition that colonisation is more than "…invasions, occupation and taking of resources…" (Green, 2023, p. 109), simultaneously involving an imposition of value driven practices and structures (Green, 2023). Therefore, perhaps a more decolonialising approach involves a critical examination, and perhaps a deconstruction, of the emphasis on evidence-based practice as it is conceptualised and enacted in contemporary child protection policy.

The reviewed literature reveals a notable dominance in attachment theory (named in 54.2% of the results, in comparison to between 35% and 2.8% for the remainder of the individual theories expressed). This prevalence of attachment theory is consistent with other systemic-like reviews on intergenerational child maltreatment (Chamberlain, Gee, et al., 2019; Marshall et al., 2022), revealing a penchant for this theory within the child protection literature. Direct intervention approaches focusing on the parent-child relationship are among the most significant in this review (although not foremost; this position is held by therapeutic trauma work). Further, specific treatment models proposed in the reviewed papers are often attachment based, such as Minding the Baby (Marshall et al., 2022), the Incredible Years Program (DeGregorio, 2013; Schelbe & Geiger, 2017), and Group Attachment-Based Intervention (Alink et al., 2019). The dominance of attachment theory, therefore, appears to exude quite profoundly into the interventions that are delivered and experienced by families who have experienced intergenerational harm, challenging practitioners to reflect on the often broad and uncritical application of attachment theory and to consider its fit for specific groups and situations. Attachment theory, for instance, has been critiqued as a theory reflecting a primarily Western dyadic view of caregiving bonds, overlooking the wider and more holistic views of connection with extended family and country held by many other, often Indigenous, cultures (Choate et al., 2020; Ryan, 2011), while a sole, uncritical, and misrepresented application of attachment theory in family and child protection courts has resulted in mistaken assumptions about the experiences and needs of children (Forslund et al., 2022).

Theoretical frameworks and interventions that are marginally represented in the review are equally consequential to those which are prominent. Reflective practices, involving management of countertransference, supervision, and building awareness of personal biases, are recommended in only six (8.3%) of the 72 reviewed papers. Reflective practices are often positioned as vital activities in social work, psychology, psychotherapy and other professions which are likely to provide support to families experiencing intergenerational child maltreatment (Chard & Hansel, 2006; Ferguson, 2018; Fook, 2015). Further, working with child abuse and neglect is certainly recognised as a demanding role, in which professionals are confronted with vicarious trauma, highly emotional service-users, elevated workloads, and substantial rates of burnout (McFadden et al., 2015; Rosso, 2022). Reflective practices in child protection unveil subconscious emotions and biases, provide space for emotional debrief and processing, explore possibilities of alternate perspectives, and advance learning (Chard & Hansel, 2006; McKeown & Yeung, 2023). It is perhaps surprising, therefore, that such limited attention is paid to the role of reflective practices in the reviewed literature. This vital component of professional practice may require further promotion and centralisation in child protection research, policy and practice.

Implications for Research

Papers explored in the review itself identify a number of areas for further research, most prominently research focusing on fathers to balance the field's unequal attention to mothers. This is certainly a valid proposition, particularly given that the research in the area of intergenerational transmission of trauma has found differences in the ways in which fathers' trauma affects children, in comparison to trauma through the maternal line (Franklin et al., 2010; Gapp et al., 2014). Equally, the incitement in the reviewed papers towards future research into longitudinal studies, gender pathways, epigenetic and biological research, and determining the efficacy of certain programs or approaches is supported and encouraged to advance collective understanding.

This review also identifies additional opportunities for further research. Firstly, all of the 30 papers specifying a location were conducted in the global north, most frequently North America (15, or 50%). Increased attention to research in a more diverse range of nations and communities, including those in the global south, is encouraged, which may involve increased attention to translating services to ensure papers from different countries and cultures are accessible to one another. Such studies may reveal further theoretical frameworks explaining intergenerational child maltreatment and unique interventions on a global level, providing pathways towards practice that may cater more efficiently for the diverse range of families affected by intergenerational child maltreatment.

Secondly, this review provides an overview of the ways in which intergenerational child maltreatment is conceptualised and responded to in the *literature*, which may or may not reflect the theories and interventions preferred by practitioners and policy makers with direct involvement with individuals and families who have experienced childhood maltreatment. Future research with professionals working with families who have experienced intergenerational child abuse and neglect will provide additional insights into the ways in which theories and interventions are actualised and translated into practice and, ultimately, the experiences of service provision received by service-users.

Strengths and Limitations

This review covers a broad range of timeframes, forms of abuse, focuses of studies, and types of publication. This can be viewed as both a strength and a limitation. There is some controversy, for instance, about whether to study different child abuse types separately, with many authors holding the view that abuse types are not comparable, each having a differing etiology and sequalae (Berzenski & Yates, 2022; Rosso, 2022). Others recognise the frequent comorbidity in abuse types and recommend that multiple forms of maltreatment be studied concurrently (Belsky, 1993; Berzenski & Yates, 2011; Finzi-Dottan & Harel, 2014; Geiger et al., 2015). Similarly, many scoping reviews include limits on the publication dates of included papers (Tricco et al., 2016), a practice that ensures the results are relevant for contemporary discourse as well as limiting results to a more manageable number, but may exclude potentially relevant papers depending on the research question

(Alexander et al., 2024). The focus of this review (particularly the third research question on trends, patterns, and correlations in the literature on explanatory theories and proposed interventions on intergenerational continuity of child maltreatment) involved locating themes in the literature on intergenerational child maltreatment base, initiating the separate consideration and analysis of papers based on, not only date of publication, but other identifiers within the literature such as maltreatment type and cohort studied. This approach provides a deeper and more nuanced understanding of the ways in which theoretical frameworks and intervention approaches correlate differently to one another and other factors, however resulted in a more complex and lengthy process of review, analysis, and written description.

The small sample sizes for some of these independently analysed groups of papers is a further limitation of the review. There were two papers published between 1970 and 1979, for instance, two studying child neglect specifically, and only one focused on fathers. This raises queries about the generalisability of the findings in this review and whether the included papers are representative of the general views within these more specific areas of study.

CONCLUSION

Addressing and treating child abuse or neglect that re-occurs over generations is a prominent area of focus within the field of child protection (policy, research, and practice), with interventions and understandings applied uniquely to this specific experience of childhood maltreatment. This scoping review of the literature locates a vast range of theoretical perspectives and applied interventions in intergenerational child maltreatment, often integrated with one another. It also finds correlations between theories, interventions, and other components of the selected papers, offering additional insights and implications. Overall, this review reveals that explanatory theories and chosen interventions with families and children who have experienced maltreatment over generations are not simply based on personal or professional preference or style, nor are they purely based on the perceived or expressed needs of service-users. Instead, they are a culmination of the dominant ideologies within the individual, the practice or research topic, and the culture and society in which they are researched, disseminated, and enacted. Hence, it is imperative for professionals, policymakers, and academics working in this field to identify and reflect on the theoretical frameworks driving practice, to recognise these as products of wider ideologies, and to critically examine child protection policy and practice through this enhanced lens.

REFERENCES

Abbassi, A., & Aslinia, S. D. (2010). Family violence, trauma and social learning theory. *Journal of Professional Counseling, Practice, Theory, & Research, 38*(1), 16–27. DOI: 10.1080/15566382.2010.12033863

Aguiar, W., & Halseth, R. (2015). *Aboriginal peoples and historic trauma: The processes of intergenerational transmission*. National Collaborating Centre for Aboriginal Health Centre.

Ainsworth, M. D. S. (1978). The Bowlby-Ainsworth attachment theory. *Behavioral and Brain Sciences, 1*(3), 436–438. DOI: 10.1017/S0140525X00075828

Alexander, L., Cooper, K., Peters, M. D. J., Tricco, A. C., Khalil, H., Evans, C., Munn, Z., Pieper, D., Godfrey, C. M., McInerney, P., & Pollock, D. (2024). Large scoping reviews: Managing volume and potential chaos in a pool of evidence sources. *Journal of Clinical Epidemiology, 170*, 111343. Advance online publication. DOI: 10.1016/j.jclinepi.2024.111343 PMID: 38582403

Alexander, P. C. (2015). *Intergenerational cycles of trauma and violence: An attachment and family systems perspective*. WW Norton & Company.

Alink, L. R. A., Cyr, C., & Madigan, S. (2019). The effect of maltreatment experiences on maltreating and dysfunctional parenting: A search for mechanisms. *Development and Psychopathology, 31*(1), 1–7. DOI: 10.1017/S0954579418001517

Amos, J., Furber, G., & Segal, L. (2011). Understanding maltreating mothers: A synthesis of relational trauma, attachment disorganization, structural dissociation of the personality, and experiential avoidance. *Journal of Trauma & Dissociation, 12*(5), 495–509. DOI: 10.1080/15299732.2011.593259 PMID: 21967177

Amos, J., & Segal, L. (2018). Disrupting intergenerational maternal maltreatment in middle childhood: Therapeutic objectives and clinical translation. *Frontiers in Psychiatry, 9*, 623. DOI: 10.3389/fpsyt.2018.00623 PMID: 30538646

Arksey, H., & O'Malley, L. (2005). Scoping studies: Towards a methodological framework. *International Journal of Social Research Methodology, 8*(1), 19–32. DOI: 10.1080/1364557032000119616

Armfield, J. M., Gnanamanickam, E. S., Johnston, D. W., Preen, D. B., Brown, D. S., Nguyen, H., & Segal, L. (2021). Intergenerational transmission of child maltreatment in South Australia, 1986–2017: A retrospective cohort study. *The Lancet. Public Health, 6*(7), 450–461. DOI: 10.1016/S2468-2667(21)00024-4 PMID: 33939966

Arons, J. (2005). "In a black hole": The (negative) space between longing and dread: Home-based psychotherapy with a traumatized mother and her infant son. *The Psychoanalytic Study of the Child, 60*(1), 101–127. DOI: 10.1080/00797308.2005.11800748 PMID: 16649677

Assink, M., Spruit, A., Schuts, M., Lindauer, R., van der Put, C. E., & Stams, G.-J. J. M. (2018). The intergenerational transmission of child maltreatment: A three-level meta-analysis. *Child Abuse & Neglect, 84*, 131–145. DOI: 10.1016/j.chiabu.2018.07.037 PMID: 30086419

Atkinson, J. (2002). *Trauma trails: Recreating song lines: The transgenerational effect of trauma in Indigenous Australia*. Spinifex Press.

Australian Institute of Health and Welfare. (2025). *Closing the Gap targets: Key findings and implications*. https://www.aihw.gov.au/reports/indigenous-australians/closing-the-gap-targets-key-findings-implications/contents/child-protection

Babcock Fenerci, R. L., & DePrince, A. P. (2018). Intergenerational transmission of trauma: Maternal trauma–related cognitions and toddler symptoms. *Child Maltreatment, 23*(2), 126–136. DOI: 10.1177/1077559517737376 PMID: 29092624

Badger, D., Nursten, J., Williams, P., & Woodward, M. (2000). Should all literature reviews be systematic? *Evaluation and Research in Education, 14*(3-4), 220–230. DOI: 10.1080/09500790008666974

Bandura, A. (1977). *Social learning theory*. Prentice Hall.

Bandura, A. (1978). Social learning theory of aggression. *Journal of Communication, 28*(3), 12–29. DOI: 10.1111/j.1460-2466.1978.tb01621.x PMID: 690254

Bartlett, J. D., Kotake, C., Fauth, R., & Easterbrooks, M. A. (2017). Intergenerational transmission of child abuse and neglect: Do maltreatment type, perpetrator, and substantiation status matter? *Child Abuse & Neglect, 63*, 84–94. DOI: 10.1016/j.chiabu.2016.11.021 PMID: 27914238

Beebe, B., Jaffe, J., Markese, S., Buck, K., Chen, H., Cohen, P., Bahrick, L., Andrews, H., & Feldstein, S. (2010). The origins of 12-month attachment: A microanalysis of 4-month mother-infant interaction. *Attachment & Human Development, 12*(1/2), 3–141. DOI: 10.1080/14616730903338985 PMID: 20390524

Belsky, J. (1993). Etiology of child maltreatment: A developmental-ecological analysis. *Psychological Bulletin, 114*(3), 413–434. DOI: 10.1037/0033-2909.114.3.413 PMID: 8272464

Belsky, J., & Pensky, E. (1988). Developmental history, personality, and family relationships: Towards an emergent family system. In Hinde, R. A., & Stevenson-Hinde, J. (Eds.), *Relationships within families: Mutual influences.* Claredon Press.

Bennett, D. B. (2021). Implications of maltreatment for young children. In Geffner, R., & White, J. W. (Eds.), *Handbook of interpersonal violence and abuse across the lifespan: A project of the National Partnership to End Interpersonal Violence Across the Lifespan (NPEIV)* (pp. 1225–1248). Springer International Publishing.

Bennett, K., Booth, A., Gair, S., Kibet, R., & Thorpe, R. (2020). Poverty is the problem – not parents: So tell me, child protection worker, how can you help? *Children Australia, 45*(4), 207–214. DOI: 10.1017/cha.2020.39

Berthelot, N., Ensink, K., Bernazzani, O., Normandin, L., Luyten, P., & Fonagy, P. (2015). Intergenerational transmission of attachment in abused and neglected mothers: The role of trauma-specific reflective functioning. *Infant Mental Health Journal, 36*(2), 200–212. DOI: 10.1002/imhj.21499 PMID: 25694333

Berzenski, S. R., & Yates, T. M. (2011). Classes and consequences of multiple maltreatment: A person-centered analysis. *Child Maltreatment, 16*(4), 250–261. DOI: 10.1177/1077559511428353 PMID: 22146858

Berzenski, S. R., & Yates, T. M. (2022). Revisiting a multidimensional model of intergenerational transmission of child maltreatment. In Krugman, R. D., & Korbin, J. E. (Eds.), *Handbook of child maltreatment* (2nd ed., pp. 351–370). Springer. DOI: 10.1007/978-3-030-82479-2_17

Bogat, G. A., Levendosky, A. A., & Eye, A. (2005). The future of research on intimate partner violence: Person-oriented and variable-oriented perspectives. *American Journal of Community Psychology, 36*(1/2), 49–70. DOI: 10.1007/s10464-005-6232-7 PMID: 16134044

Borelli, J. L., Cohen, C., Pettit, C., Normandin, L., Target, M., Fonagy, P., & Ensink, K. (2019). Maternal and child sexual abuse history: An intergenerational exploration of children's adjustment and maternal trauma-reflective functioning. *Frontiers in Psychology, 10*, 1062. DOI: 10.3389/fpsyg.2019.01062 PMID: 31156503

Bowen, M. (1966). The use of family theory in clinical practice. *Comprehensive Psychiatry, 7*(5), 345–374. DOI: 10.1016/S0010-440X(66)80065-2 PMID: 5922263

Bowen, M. (1972). On the differentiation of self. In Framo, J. (Ed.), *Family Interaction: A Dialogue Between Family Researchers and Family Therapists.* Springer Books.

Bowen, M. (1978). *Family therapy in clinical practice.* Aronson.

Bowlby, J. (1979). The Bowlby-Ainsworth attachment theory. *Behavioral and Brain Sciences, 2*(4), 637–638. DOI: 10.1017/S0140525X00064955

Brofenbrenner, U. (1979). *The ecology of human development.* Harvard University Press. DOI: 10.4159/9780674028845

Buchheim, A., Ziegenhain, U., Kindler, H., Waller, C., Gündel, H., Karabatsiakis, A., & Fegert, J. (2022). Identifying risk and resilience factors in the intergenerational cycle of maltreatment: Results from the trans-gen study investigating the effects of maternal attachment and social support on child attachment and cardiovascular stress physiology. *Frontiers in Human Neuroscience, 16*, 890262–890262. DOI: 10.3389/fnhum.2022.890262 PMID: 35923749

Buss, C., Entringer, S., Moog, N. K., Toepfer, P., Fair, D. A., Simhan, H. N., Heim, C. M., & Wadhwa, P. D. (2017). Intergenerational transmission of maternal childhood maltreatment exposure: Implications for fetal brain development. *Journal of the American Academy of Child and Adolescent Psychiatry, 56*(5), 373–382. DOI: 10.1016/j.jaac.2017.03.001 PMID: 28433086

Chamberlain, C., Gee, G., Harfield, S., Campbell, S., Brennan, S., Clark, Y., Mensah, F., Arabena, K., Herrman, H., & Brown, S. (2019). Parenting after a history of childhood maltreatment: A scoping review and map of evidence in the perinatal period. *PLoS One, 14*(3), 1–41. DOI: 10.1371/journal.pone.0213460 PMID: 30865679

Chamberlain, C., Ralph, N., Hokke, S., Clark, Y., Gee, G., Stansfield, C., Sutcliffe, K., Brown, S. J., & Brennan, S. (2019). Healing the past by nurturing the future: A qualitative systematic review and meta-synthesis of pregnancy, birth and early postpartum experiences and views of parents with a history of childhood maltreatment. *PLoS One, 14*(12), 1. DOI: 10.1371/journal.pone.0225441 PMID: 31834894

Chard, K. M., & Hansel, J. E. (2006). Supervising therapists working with traumatised children. In K. T, Neill (Ed.), *Helping others help children: Clinical supervision of child psychotherapy* (pp. 193-207). American Psychological Association. DOI: 10.1037/11467-011

Choate, P. W., CrazyBull, B., Lindstrom, D., & Lindstrom, G. (2020). Where do we go from here? Ongoing colonialism from attachment theory. *Aotearoa New Zealand Social Work, 32*(1), 32–44. DOI: 10.11157/anzswj-vol32iss1id702

Cicchetti, D., & Rizley, R. (1981). Developmental perspectives on the etiology, intergenerational transmission, and sequelae of child maltreatment. *New Directions for Child and Adolescent Development, 1981*(11), 31–55. DOI: 10.1002/cd.23219811104

Colquhoun, H. L., Levac, D., O'Brien, K. K., Straus, S., Tricco, A. C., Perrier, L., Kastner, M., & Moher, D. (2014). Scoping reviews: Time for clarity in definition, methods, and reporting. *Journal of Clinical Epidemiology*, *67*(12), 1291–1294. DOI: 10.1016/j.jclinepi.2014.03.013 PMID: 25034198

Cooper, C., Booth, A., Britten, N., & Garside, R. (2017). A comparison of results of empirical studies of supplementary search techniques and recommendations in review methodology handbooks: A methodological review. *Systematic Reviews*, *6*(1), 234. DOI: 10.1186/s13643-017-0625-1 PMID: 29179733

Copp, J. E., Giordano, P. C., Longmore, M. A., & Manning, W. D. (2019). The development of attitudes toward intimate partner violence: An examination of key correlates among a sample of young adults. *Journal of Interpersonal Violence*, *34*(7), 1357–1387. DOI: 10.1177/0886260516651311 PMID: 27229921

Cordero, M. I., Poirier, G. L., Marquez, C., Veenit, V., Fontana, X., Salehi, B., Ansermet, F., & Sandi, C. (2012). Evidence for biological roots in the transgenerational transmission of intimate partner violence. *Translational Psychiatry*, *2*(4), 10. DOI: 10.1038/tp.2012.32 PMID: 22832906

Cornett, C. (1985). The cyclical pattern of child physical abuse from a psychoanalytic self-psychology perspective. *Child & Adolescent Social Work Journal*, *2*(2), 83–92. DOI: 10.1007/BF00757474

Curtin, N., Kende, A., & Kende, J. (2016). Navigating multiple identities: The simultaneous influence of advantaged and disadvantaged identities on politicization and activism. *The Journal of Social Issues*, *72*(2), 264–285. DOI: 10.1111/josi.12166

Deater-Deckard, K., Dodge, K. A., Bates, J. E., & Pettit, G. S. (1996). Physical discipline among African American and European American mothers: Links to children's externalizing behaviors. *Developmental Psychology*, *32*(6), 1065–1072. DOI: 10.1037/0012-1649.32.6.1065

DeGregorio, L. J. (2013). Intergenerational transmission of abuse: Implications for parenting interventions from a neuropsychological perspective. *Traumatology*, *19*(2), 158–166. Advance online publication. DOI: 10.1177/1534765612457219

Delsol, C., & Margolin, G. (2004). The role of family-of-origin violence in men's marital violence perpetration. *Clinical Psychology Review*, *24*(1), 99–122. https://doi.org/https://doi.org/10.1016/j.cpr.2003.12.001. DOI: 10.1016/j.cpr.2003.12.001 PMID: 14992808

Dixon, L., Browne, K., & Hamilton-Giachritsis, C. (2009). Patterns of risk and protective factors in the intergenerational cycle of maltreatment. *Journal of Family Violence*, *24*(2), 111–122. DOI: 10.1007/s10896-008-9215-2

Dodge, K. A. (1986). A social information processing model of social competence in children. In Perlmutter, M. (Ed.), *The Minnesota symposium on child psychology: Cognitive perspectives of children's social and behavioural development* (pp. 77–125). Lawrence Erlbaum Associates.

Duthie, D., Steinhauer, S., Twinn, C., Steinhauer, V., & Lonne, B. (2019). Understanding trauma and child maltreatment experienced in Indigenous communities. In Lonne, B., Scott, D., Higgins, D. J., & Herrenkohl, T. I. (Eds.), *Re-visioning public health approaches for protecting children* (Vol. 9, pp. 327–347). Springer International Publishing. DOI: 10.1007/978-3-030-05858-6_20

Felitti, V. J. (2002). The relation between adverse childhood experiences and adult health: Turning gold into lead. *The Permanente Journal*, *6*(1), 44–47. DOI: 10.7812/TPP/02.994 PMID: 30313011

Felitti, V. J., Anda, R. F., Nordenberg, D., Williamson, D. F., Spitz, A. M., Edwards, V., Koss, M. P., & Marks, J. S. (1998). Relationship of childhood abuse and household dysfunction to many of the leading causes of death in adults: The adverse childhood experiences (ACE) study. *American Journal of Preventive Medicine*, *14*(4), 245–258. DOI: 10.1016/S0749-3797(98)00017-8 PMID: 9635069

Ferguson, H. (2018). How social workers reflect in action and when and why they don't: The possibilities and limits to reflective practice in social work. *Social Work Education*, *37*(4), 415–427. DOI: 10.1080/02615479.2017.1413083

Feshbach, S. (1974). The development and regulation of aggression: Some research gaps and a proposed cognitive analysis. In Wit, J. D., & Hartup, W. W. (Eds.), *Determinants and origins of aggressive behavior*. Mouton.

Feshbach, S. (1980). Child abuse and the dynamics of human aggression and violence. *Child abuse: An agenda for action*, 48-60.

Finzi-Dottan, R., & Harel, G. (2014). Parents' potential for child abuse: An intergenerational perspective. *Journal of Family Violence*, *29*(4), 397–408. DOI: 10.1007/s10896-014-9592-7

Fook, J. (2015). Reflective practice and critical reflection. In Lishman, J. (Ed.), *Handbook for practice learning in social work and social care: Knowledge and theory* (3rd ed., pp. 440–454). Jessica Kingsley Publishers.

Forslund, T., Granqvist, P., van Ijzendoorn, M. H., Sagi-Schwartz, A., Glaser, D., Steele, M., Hammarlund, M., Schuengel, C., Bakermans-Kranenburg, M. J., Steele, H., Shaver, P. R., Lux, U., Simmonds, J., Jacobvitz, D., Groh, A. M., Bernard, K., Cyr, C., Hazen, N. L., Foster, S., & Duschinsky, R. (2022). Attachment goes to court: Child protection and custody issues. *Attachment & Human Development, 24*(1), 1–52. DOI: 10.1080/14616734.2020.1840762 PMID: 33427578

Fraiberg, S., Adelson, E., & Sharpiro, V. (1975). Ghosts in the nursery: A psychodynamic approach to the problems of impaired infant-mother relationships. *Journal of the American Academy of Child and Adolescent Psychiatry, 14*(3), 387–421. PMID: 1141566

Franklin, T. B., Russig, H., Weiss, I. C., Gräff, J., Linder, N., Michalon, A., Vizi, S., & Mansuy, I. M. (2010). Epigenetic transmission of the impact of early stress across generations. *Biological Psychiatry, 68*(5), 408–415. DOI: 10.1016/j.biopsych.2010.05.036 PMID: 20673872

Freud, S. (1936). *Inhibitions, symptoms and anxiety*. Hogarth.

Gapp, K., Jawaid, A., Sarkies, P., Bohacek, J., Pelczar, P., Prados, J., Farinelli, L., Miska, E., & Mansuy, I. M. (2014). Implication of sperm RNAs in transgenerational inheritance of the effects of early trauma in mice. *Nature Neuroscience, 17*(5), 667–669. DOI: 10.1038/nn.3695 PMID: 24728267

Geiger, J. M., Schelbe, L., Hayes, M. J., Kawam, E., Katz, C. C., & Klika, J. B. (2015). Intergenerational transmission of maltreatment: Ending a family tradition. In Daro, D., Cohn Donnelly, A., Huang, L., & Powell, B. (Eds.), *Advances in Child Abuse Prevention Knowledge* (pp. 67–91). Springer., DOI: 10.1007/978-3-319-16327-7_4

Gone, J. P. (2013). Redressing First Nations historical trauma: Theorizing mechanisms for Indigenous culture as mental health treatment. *Transcultural Psychiatry, 50*(5), 683–706. DOI: 10.1177/1363461513487669 PMID: 23715822

Green, A. H. (1976). A psychodynamic approach to the study and treatment of child-abusing parents. *Journal of the American Academy of Child Psychiatry, 15*(3), 414–429. DOI: 10.1016/S0002-7138(09)61617-4 PMID: 965619

Green, S. (2023). Colonisation, post-colonisation and decolonisation. In Holscher, D., Hugman, R., & McAuliffe, D. (Eds.), *Social work theory and ethics: Ideas in practice* (pp. 101–120). Springer. DOI: 10.1007/978-981-19-1015-9_7

Hall, S. (2011). "It's going to stop in this generation": Women with a history of child abuse resolving to raise their children without abuse. *Harvard Educational Review, 81*(1), 24–49,150. DOI: 10.17763/haer.81.1.m8202r3804uvmv68

Healy, K. (2022). *Social work theories in context: Creating frameworks for practice* (3rd ed.). Bloomsbury Publishing.

Herzberger, S. D. (1983). Social cognition and the transmission of abuse. In Finkelhor, D., Gelles, R. J., Hotaling, G. T., & Straus, M. A. (Eds.), *The dark side of families: Current family violence research* (pp. 317–329). SAGE Publications.

Howell, K. H., Miller-Graff, L. E., Martinez-Torteya, C., Napier, T. R., & Carney, J. R. (2021). Charting a course towards resilience following adverse childhood experiences: Addressing intergenerational trauma via strengths-based intervention. *Children (Basel, Switzerland), 8*(10), 844. DOI: 10.3390/children8100844 PMID: 34682109

Hurst, N. C., & Sawatzky, D. D. (1996). Families with multiple problems through a Bowenian lens. *Child Welfare, 75*(6), 693–693. PMID: 8936483

Huth-Bocks, A. C., Krause, K., Ahlfs-Dunn, S., Gallagher, E., & Scott, S. (2013). Relational trauma and posttraumatic stress symptoms among pregnant women. *Psychodynamic Psychiatry, 41*(2), 277–301. DOI: 10.1521/pdps.2013.41.2.277 PMID: 23713621

Islam, S., Jaffee, S. R., & Widom, C. S. (2023). Breaking the cycle of intergenerational childhood maltreatment: Effects on offspring mental health. *Child Maltreatment, 28*(1), 119–129. DOI: 10.1177/10775595211067205 PMID: 35073784

Iyengar, U., Rajhans, P., Fonagy, P., Strathearn, L., & Kim, S. (2019). Unresolved trauma and reorganization in mothers: Attachment and neuroscience perspectives. *Frontiers in Psychology, 10*, 110. DOI: 10.3389/fpsyg.2019.00110 PMID: 30761051

Jacobsson, K., & Meeuwisse, A. (2020). 'State governing of knowledge' - constraining social work research and practice. *European Journal of Social Work, 23*(2), 277–289. DOI: 10.1080/13691457.2018.1530642

Jaffee, S. R., Bowes, L., Ouellet-Morin, I., Fisher, H. L., Moffitt, T. E., Merrick, M. T., & Arseneault, L. (2013). Safe, stable, nurturing relationships break the intergenerational cycle of abuse: A prospective nationally representative cohort of children in the United Kingdom. *The Journal of Adolescent Health, 53*(4), 4–10. DOI: 10.1016/j.jadohealth.2013.04.007 PMID: 24059939

Juul, S. H., Hendrix, C., Robinson, B., Stowe, Z. N., Newport, D. J., Brennan, P. A., & Johnson, K. C. (2016). Maternal early-life trauma and affective parenting style: The mediating role of HPA-axis function. *Archives of Women's Mental Health, 19*(1), 17–23. DOI: 10.1007/s00737-015-0528-x PMID: 25956587

Kim, K. (2012). The role of culture in theories of the intergenerational transmission of violence. *Child & Family Social Work*, *17*(4), 395–405. DOI: 10.1111/j.1365-2206.2011.00793.x

Kim, K., Trickett, P. K., & Putnam, F. W. (2011). Attachment representations and anxiety: Differential relationships among mothers of sexually abused and comparison girls. *Journal of Interpersonal Violence*, *26*(3), 498–521. DOI: 10.1177/0886260510363416 PMID: 20442447

Kim, S., & Strathearn, L. (2017). Trauma, mothering, and intergenerational transmission: A synthesis of behavioral and oxytocin research. *The Psychoanalytic Study of the Child*, *70*(1), 200–223. DOI: 10.1080/00797308.2016.1277897

Klein, M. (1946). Notes on some schizoid mechanisms. In *The writings of Melanie Klein* (pp. 1–24). Free Press.

Köhler-Dauner, F., Fegert, J. M., Anna, B., Krause, S., Gündel, H., Waller, C., & Ziegenhain, U. (2019). Maternal behavior affects child's attachment-related cortisol stress response. *Journal of Child and Adolescent Psychiatry*, *1*(1), 46–60. DOI: 10.14302/issn.2643-6655.jcap-19-2737

Kohut, H. (1971). *The analysis of the self: A systematic approach to the psychoanalytic treatment of narcissistic personality disorders*. International Universities Press.

Kohut, H. (1977). *The restoration of the self.* International Universities Press.

Langevin, R., Gagné, M., Brassard, A., & Fernet, M. (2023). Intergenerational continuity of child maltreatment: The role of maternal emotional dysregulation and mother–child attachment. *Psychology of Violence*, *13*(1), 1–12. Advance online publication. DOI: 10.1037/vio0000409

Langevin, R., Marshall, C., & Kingsland, E. (2021). Intergenerational cycles of maltreatment: A scoping review of psychosocial risk and protective factors. *Trauma, Violence & Abuse*, *22*(4), 672–688. DOI: 10.1177/1524838019870917 PMID: 31455161

Lansford, J. E., Deater-Deckard, K., Dodge, K. A., Bates, J. E., & Pettit, G. S. (2004). Ethnic differences in the link between physical discipline and later adolescent externalizing behaviors. *Journal of Child Psychology and Psychiatry, and Allied Disciplines*, *45*(4), 801–812. DOI: 10.1111/j.1469-7610.2004.00273.x PMID: 15056311

Lecic-Tosevski, D., Draganic-Gajic, S., Pejovic-Milovancevic, M., Popovic-Deusic, S., Christodoulou, N., & Botbol, M. (2014). Child is father of the man: Child abuse and development of future psychopathology. *Psychiatriki*, *25*(3), 185–191. PMID: 25367662

Leitch, L. (2017). Action steps using ACEs and trauma-informed care: A resilience model. *Health & Justice*, *5*(1), 1–10. DOI: 10.1186/s40352-017-0050-5 PMID: 28455574

Levac, D., Colquhoun, H., & O'Brien, K. K. (2010). Scoping studies: Advancing the methodology. *Implementation Science : IS*, *5*(1), 69–77. DOI: 10.1186/1748-5908-5-69 PMID: 20854677

Levendosky, A. A. (2013). Drawing conclusions: An intergenerational transmission of violence perspective. *Psychodynamic Psychiatry*, *41*(2), 351–360. DOI: 10.1521/pdps.2013.41.2.351 PMID: 23713624

Levendosky, A. A., Lannert, B., & Yalch, M. (2012). The effects of intimate partner violence on women and child survivors: An attachment perspective. *Psychodynamic Psychiatry*, *40*(3), 397–433. DOI: 10.1521/pdps.2012.40.3.397 PMID: 23002702

Lieberman, A. F., Padrón, E., Van Horn, P., & Harris, W. W. (2005). Angels in the nursery: The intergenerational transmission of benevolent parental influences. *Infant Mental Health Journal*, *26*(6), 504–520. DOI: 10.1002/imhj.20071 PMID: 28682485

Lomanowska, A. M., Boivin, M., Hertzman, C., & Fleming, A. S. (2017). Parenting begets parenting: A neurobiological perspective on early adversity and the transmission of parenting styles across generations. *Neuroscience*, *342*, 120–139. DOI: 10.1016/j.neuroscience.2015.09.029 PMID: 26386294

Luke, J., Verbunt, E., Zhang, A., Bamblett, M., Johnson, G., Salamone, C., Thomas, D., Eades, S., Gubhaju, L., Kelaher, M., & Jones, A. (2022). Questioning the ethics of evidence-based practice for Indigenous health and social settings in Australia. *BMJ Global Health*, *7*(6), e009167. Advance online publication. DOI: 10.1136/bmjgh-2022-009167 PMID: 35680132

Lyons-Ruth, K., Yellin, C., Melnick, S., & Atwood, G. (2005). Expanding the concept of unresolved mental states: Hostile/helpless states of mind on the Adult Attachment Interview are associated with disrupted mother-infant communication and infant disorganization. *Development and Psychopathology*, *17*(1), 1–23. DOI: 10.1017/S0954579405050017 PMID: 15971757

Madigan, S., Cyr, C., Eirich, R., Fearon, R. M. P., Ly, A., Rash, C., Poole, J. C., & Alink, L. R. A. (2019). Testing the cycle of maltreatment hypothesis: Meta-analytic evidence of the intergenerational transmission of child maltreatment. *Development and Psychopathology*, *31*(1), 23–51. DOI: 10.1017/S0954579418001700 PMID: 30757994

Main, M., & Hesse, E. (1990). Parents' unresolved traumatic experiences are related to infant disorganized attchment status: Is frightened and/or frightening parental behavior the linking mechnaism? In Greenberg, M. T., Cicchetti, D., & Cummings, E. M. (Eds.), *Attachment in the preschool years: Theory, research, and intervention* (pp. 161–182). University of Chicago Press.

Markward, M., Dozier, C., Hooks, K., & Markward, N. (2000). Culture and the intergenerational transmission of substance abuse, woman abuse, and child abuse: A diathesis-stress perspective. *Children and Youth Services Review*, *22*(3), 237–250. DOI: 10.1016/S0190-7409(00)00079-7

Marshall, C., Langevin, R., & Cabecinha-Alati, S. (2022). Victim-to-victim intergenerational cycles of child maltreatment: A systematic scoping review of theoretical frameworks. *International Journal of Child and Adolescent Resilience*, *9*(1). Advance online publication. DOI: 10.54488/ijcar.2022.283

McCallum, D. (2022). Law, justice, and Indigenous intergenerational trauma—A genealogy. *International Journal for Crime. Justice and Social Democracy*, *11*(3), 165–177. DOI: 10.5204/ijcjsd.2121

McCollum, S. E. (2015). Multigenerational dissociation: A framework for building narrative. *Journal of Trauma & Dissociation*, *16*(5), 563–576. DOI: 10.1080/15299732.2015.1030717 PMID: 26158318

McFadden, P., Campbell, A., & Taylor, B. (2015). Resilience and burnout in child protection social work: Individual and organisational themes from a systematic literature review. *British Journal of Social Work*, *45*(5), 1546–1563. DOI: 10.1093/bjsw/bct210

McKeown, M.-H. L., & Yeung, E. Y. W. (2023). Deepening our understanding of reflective practice in a safeguarding child protection and welfare context. *Practice*, *35*(2), 153–167. DOI: 10.1080/09503153.2022.2038124

McMillen, J. C., & Rideout, G. B. (1996). Breaking intergenerational cycles: Theoretical tools for social workers. *The Social Service Review*, *70*(3), 378–399. DOI: 10.1086/604196

Menzies, K. (2019). Understanding the Australian Aboriginal experience of collective, historical and intergenerational trauma. *International Social Work*, *62*(6), 1522–1534. DOI: 10.1177/0020872819870585

Merrill, S. M., Moore, S. R., Gladish, N., Giesbrecht, G. F., Dewey, D., Konwar, C., MacIssac, J. L., Kobor, M. S., & Letourneau, N. L. (2021). Paternal adverse childhood experiences: Associations with infant DNA methylation. *Developmental Psychobiology*, *63*(6), e22174. DOI: 10.1002/dev.22174 PMID: 34333774

Meulewaeter, F., De Pauw, S. S. W., & Vanderplasschen, W. (2019). Mothering, substance use disorders and intergenerational trauma transmission: An attachment-based perspective. *Frontiers in Psychiatry*, *10*, 728. DOI: 10.3389/fpsyt.2019.00728 PMID: 31681040

Mielke, E. L., Neukel, C., Bertsch, K., Reck, C., Möhler, E., & Herpertz, S. C. (2016). Maternal sensitivity and the empathic brain: Influences of early life maltreatment. *Journal of Psychiatric Research*, *77*, 59–66. DOI: 10.1016/j.jpsychires.2016.02.013 PMID: 26985733

Milner, J. S. (1993). Social information processing and physical child abuse. *Clinical Psychology Review*, *13*(3), 275–294. DOI: 10.1016/0272-7358(93)90024-G

Mitkovic Voncina, M., Pejovic Milovancevic, M., Mandic Maravic, V., & Lecic Tosevski, D. (2017). Timeline of intergenerational child maltreatment: The mind–brain–body interplay. *Current Psychiatry Reports*, *19*(8), 50. DOI: 10.1007/s11920-017-0805-7 PMID: 28664328

Moog, N. K., Heim, C. M., Entringer, S., Simhan, H. N., Wadhwa, P. D., & Buss, C. (2022). Transmission of the adverse consequences of childhood maltreatment across generations: Focus on gestational biology. *Pharmacology, Biochemistry, and Behavior*, *215*, 173372. Advance online publication. DOI: 10.1016/j.pbb.2022.173372 PMID: 35259415

Morton, N., & Browne, K. D. (1998). Theory and observation of attachment and its relation to child maltreatment: A review. *Child Abuse & Neglect*, *22*(11), 1093–1104. DOI: 10.1016/S0145-2134(98)00088-X PMID: 9827314

Narang, D. S., & Contreras, J. M. (2000). Dissociation as a mediator between child abuse history and adult abuse potential. *Child Abuse & Neglect*, *24*(5), 653–665. DOI: 10.1016/S0145-2134(00)00132-0 PMID: 10819097

Narang, D. S., & Contreras, J. M. (2005). The relationships of dissociation and affective family environment with the intergenerational cycle of child abuse. *Child Abuse & Neglect*, *29*(6), 683–699. DOI: 10.1016/j.chiabu.2004.11.003 PMID: 15979709

Negriff, S., Palmer Molina, A., & Hackman, D. A. (2020). Parental exposure to childhood maltreatment and offspring's mental health: Investigating pathways through parental adversity and offspring exposure to maltreatment. *Child Maltreatment, 25*(4), 422–432. DOI: 10.1177/1077559520912342 PMID: 32208855

Newton, B. J. (2019). Understanding child neglect in Aboriginal families and communities in the context of trauma. *Child & Family Social Work, 24*(2), 218–226. DOI: 10.1111/cfs.12606

Ney, P. G. (1989). Child maltreatment: Possible reasons for its transgenerational transmission. *Canadian Journal of Psychiatry, 34*(6), 594–601. DOI: 10.1177/070674378903400619 PMID: 2670182

Nietz, H. (2019). Informing social work practice with theory: Reflections on the protection of Aboriginal children in remote communities of Australia. *British Journal of Social Work, 49*(8), 2021–2041. DOI: 10.1093/bjsw/bcy124

Nygren, K., Walsh, J. C., Ellingsen, I. T., & Christie, A. (2021). Gender, parenting and practices in child welfare social work? A comparative study from England, Ireland, Norway and Sweden. *British Journal of Social Work, 51*(6), 2116–2133. DOI: 10.1093/bjsw/bcaa085

Özcan, N. K., Boyacioğlu, N. E., Enginkaya, S., Bilgin, H., & Tomruk, N. B. (2016). The relationship between attachment styles and childhood trauma: A transgenerational perspective – a controlled study of patients with psychiatric disorders. *Journal of Clinical Nursing, 25*(15-16), 2357–2366. DOI: 10.1111/jocn.13274 PMID: 27161944

Peters, M. D. J., Marnie, C., Colquhoun, H., Garritty, C. M., Hempel, S., Horsley, T., Langlois, E. V., Lillie, E., O'Brien, K. K., Tunçalp, ., Wilson, M. G., Zarin, W., & Tricco, A. C. (2021). Scoping reviews: Reinforcing and advancing the methodology and application. *Systematic Reviews, 10*(1), 263–266. DOI: 10.1186/s13643-021-01821-3 PMID: 34625095

Poirier, B., Sethi, S., Haag, D., Hedges, J., & Jamieson, L. (2022). The impact of neoliberal generative mechanisms on Indigenous health: A critical realist scoping review. *Globalization and Health, 18*(1), 1–17. DOI: 10.1186/s12992-022-00852-2 PMID: 35705995

Power, M. (1997). *The audit society: Rituals of verification.* Oxford University Press.

Putallaz, M., Costanzo, P. R., Grimes, C. L., & Sherman, D. M. (1998). Intergenerational continuities and their influences on children's social development. *Social Development, 7*(3), 389–427. DOI: 10.1111/1467-9507.00074

Quinn, A., Fallon, B., Joh-Carnella, N., & Saint-Girons, M. (2022). The overrepresentation of First Nations children in the Ontario child welfare system: A call for systemic change. *Children and Youth Services Review, 139*, 106558. DOI: 10.1016/j.childyouth.2022.106558

Quinton, D., & Rutter, M. (1984). Parents with children in care - II. Intergenerational continuities. *Journal of Child Psychology and Psychiatry, and Allied Disciplines, 25*(2), 231–250. DOI: 10.1111/j.1469-7610.1984.tb00146.x PMID: 6707111

Ramo-Fernández, L., Schneider, A., Wilker, S., & Kolassa, I. T. (2015). Epigenetic alterations associated with war trauma and childhood maltreatment. *Behavioral Sciences & the Law, 33*(5), 701–721. DOI: 10.1002/bsl.2200 PMID: 26358541

Renner, L. M., & Slack, K. S. (2006). Intimate partner violence and child maltreatment: Understanding intra- and intergenerational connections. *Child Abuse & Neglect, 30*(6), 599–617. DOI: 10.1016/j.chiabu.2005.12.005 PMID: 16782195

Richards, D. (2008). Handsearching still a valuable element of the systematic review. *Evidence-Based Dentistry, 9*(3), 85. DOI: 10.1038/sj.ebd.6400602 PMID: 18927572

Rosso, A. M. (2022). Psychoanalytic interventions with abusive parents: An opportunity for children's mental health. *International Journal of Environmental Research and Public Health, 19*(20), 13015. Advance online publication. DOI: 10.3390/ijerph192013015 PMID: 36293590

Rumrill, P. D., Fitzgerald, S. M., & Merchant, W. R. (2010). Using scoping literature reviews as a means of understanding and interpreting existing literature. *Work (Reading, Mass.), 35*(3), 399–404. DOI: 10.3233/WOR-2010-0998 PMID: 20364059

Ryan, F. (2011). Kanyininpa (holding): A way of nurturing children in Aboriginal Australia. *Australian Social Work, 64*(2), 183–197. DOI: 10.1080/0312407X.2011.581300

Schelbe, L., & Geiger, J. M. (2017). *Intergenerational transmission of child maltreatment*. SpringerBriefs in Social Work., DOI: 10.1007/978-3-319-43824-5

Seng, J. S., Sperlich, M., Low, L. K., Ronis, D. L., Muzik, M., & Liberzon, I. (2013). Childhood abuse history, posttraumatic stress disorder, postpartum mental health, and bonding: A prospective cohort study. *Journal of Midwifery & Women's Health, 58*(1), 57–68. DOI: 10.1111/j.1542-2011.2012.00237.x PMID: 23374491

Sharma, N. P., & Spiro, P. M. (2023). *Psychoanalytic therapy*. StatPearls Publishing.

Sheppard, M. (2003). The significance of past abuse to current intervention strategies with depressed mothers in child and family care. *British Journal of Social Work, 33*(6), 769–786. DOI: 10.1093/bjsw/33.6.769

Sperlich, M., Seng, J., Rowe, H., Fisher, J., Cuthbert, C., & Taylor, J. (2017). A cycles-breaking framework to disrupt intergenerational patterns of maltreatment and vulnerability during the childbearing year. *Journal of Obstetric, Gynecologic, and Neonatal Nursing : JOGNN, 46*(3), 378–389. DOI: 10.1016/j.jogn.2016.11.017 PMID: 28199820

Steele, B. F. (1970). Parental abuse of infants and small children. In Anthony, E. J., & Benedek, T. (Eds.), *Parenthood: Its psychology and psychopathology* (pp. 449–477). Little, Brown and Company.

Stob, V., Slade, A., Adnopoz, J., & Woolston, J. (2020). The family cycle: Breaking the intergenerational transmission of trauma through mentalizing. *Journal of Infant, Child, and Adolescent Psychotherapy; JICAP, 19*(3), 255–270. DOI: 10.1080/15289168.2020.1786762

Strolovitch, D. Z. (2006). Do interest groups represent the disadvantaged? Advocacy at the intersections of race, class, and gender. *The Journal of Politics, 68*(4), 894–910. DOI: 10.1111/j.1468-2508.2006.00478.x

Sullivan, P. (2018). The tyranny of neoliberal public management and the challenge for Aboriginal community organisations. In D. Howard-Wagner, M. Bargh, & I. Altamirano-Jiménez (Eds.), *The neoliberal state, recognition and Indigenous rights: New paternalism to new imaginings* (pp. 201-215). Australian National University, Press. DOI: 10.22459/CAEPR40.07.2018.11

Thornberry, T. P., Knight, K. E., & Lovegrove, P. J. (2012). Does maltreatment beget maltreatment? A systematic review of the intergenerational literature. *Trauma, Violence & Abuse, 13*(3), 135–152. DOI: 10.1177/1524838012447697 PMID: 22673145

Tomison, A. (1996). *Intergenerational transmission of maltreatment*. Child Family Community Australia. https://aifs.gov.au/resources/policy-and-practice-papers/intergenerational-transmission-maltreatment#how

Tricco, A. C., Lillie, E., Zarin, W., O'Brien, K., Colquhoun, H., Kastner, M., Levac, D., Ng, C., Pearson Sharpe, J., Wilson, K., Kenny, M., Warren, R., Wilson, C., Stelfox, H. T., Straus, S. E., & Sharpe, J. P. (2016). A scoping review on the conduct and reporting of scoping reviews. *BMC Medical Research Methodology, 16*(1), 1–10. DOI: 10.1186/s12874-016-0116-4 PMID: 26857112

Tuohy, A. L. (1987). Psychoanalytic perspectives on child abuse. *Child & Adolescent Social Work Journal, 4*(1), 25–40. DOI: 10.1007/BF00757867

Van der Hart, O., Nijenhuis, E. R. S., & Steele, K. (2006). *The haunted self: Structural dissociation and the treatment of chronic traumatization*. Norton.

Widom, C. S. (2015). Reflection: Intergenerational transmission of child maltreatment. In Geiger, J. M., Schelbe, L., Hayes, M. J., Kawam, E., Katz, C. C., & Klika, J. B. (Eds.), *Intergenerational transmission of maltreatment: Ending a family tradition* (pp. 83–84). Springer.

Widom, C. S., & Wilson, H. W. (2015). Intergenerational transmission of violence. In Lindert, J., & Levav, I. (Eds.), *Violence and mental health: Its manifold faces* (pp. 27–45). Springer., DOI: 10.1007/978-94-017-8999-8_2

Wilson, L. C., & Scarpa, A. (2011). Hypothalamic-pituitary-adrenal axis (HPA) functioning and the intergenerational cycle of child maltreatment. In Hynes, L. E. (Ed.), *Sexual Abuse: Types, Signs and Treatments* (pp. 77–92). Nova Science Publishers, Inc.

Woolfolk, R. L. (2015). *The value of psychotherapy: The talking cure in an age of clinical science*. Guilford Press.

Yehuda, R., & Bierer, L. M. (2009). The relevance of epigenetics to PTSD: Implications for the DSM-V. *Journal of Traumatic Stress, 22*(5), 427–434. DOI: 10.1002/jts.20448 PMID: 19813242

Young, J. E. (1999). *Cognitive therapy for personality disorders: A schema-focused approach* (3rd ed.). Professional Resource Press.

Young, J. E., Klosko, J. S., & Weishaar, M. E. (2003). *Schema therapy: A practitioner's guide*. Guilford Press.

Young, S., McKenzie, M., Omre, C., Schjelderup, L., & Walker, S. (2014). Practicing from theory: Thinking and knowing to "do" child protection work. *Social Sciences (Basel, Switzerland), 3*(4), 893–915. DOI: 10.3390/socsci3040893

Zajac, L., Raby, K. L., & Dozier, M. (2019). Attachment state of mind and childhood experiences of maltreatment as predictors of sensitive care from infancy through middle childhood: Results from a longitudinal study of parents involved with Child Protective Services. *Development and Psychopathology, 31*(1), 113–125. DOI: 10.1017/S0954579418001554 PMID: 30466498

Zanoni, L., Warburton, W., Bussey, K., & McMaugh, A. (2013). Fathers as 'core business' in child welfare practice and research: An interdisciplinary review. *Children and Youth Services Review, 35*(7), 1055–1070. DOI: 10.1016/j.childyouth.2013.04.018

Zeanah, C. H., & Zeanah, P. D. (1989). Intergenerational transmission of maltreatment: Insights from attachment theory and research. *Psychiatry, 52*(2), 177–196. DOI: 10.1080/00332747.1989.11024442 PMID: 2660176

Zhang, L., Mersky, J. P., Gruber, A. M. H., & Kim, J.-Y. (2023). Intergenerational transmission of parental adverse childhood experiences and children's outcomes: A scoping review. *Trauma, Violence & Abuse, 24*(5), 3251–3264. DOI: 10.1177/15248380221126186 PMID: 36205317

Zhou, A., & Ryan, J. (2023). Biological embedding of early-life adversity and a scoping review of the evidence for intergenerational epigenetic transmission of stress and trauma in humans. *Genes, 14*(8), 1639. DOI: 10.3390/genes14081639 PMID: 37628690

Zonnevijlle, M., & Hildebrand, M. (2019). Like parent, like child? Exploring the association between early maladaptive schemas of adolescents involved with Child Protective Services and their parents. *Child & Family Social Work, 24*(2), 190–200. DOI: 10.1111/cfs.12602

Chapter 8
Addressing Cumulative Adversities in Education

Govind Krishnamoorthy
https://orcid.org/0000-0003-1515-1103
University of Southern Queensland, Australia

ABSTRACT

This chapter examines how cumulative harm influences learning through the intertwined pathways of threat, deprivation, and disrupted relational expectations. It outlines how classroom environments can unintentionally reproduce these conditions through curricular omissions, instructional habits, and unexamined assumptions. Drawing on trauma-informed, culturally responsive, and neurodevelopmental research, the chapter presents a three-phase implementation framework encompassing preparation, monitoring, and evaluation. The framework emphasises predictable routines, cultural alignment, differentiated instruction, and reflective practice as core components of safe and effective learning environments. Practical examples illustrate how educators can interpret behaviour through a developmental lens, avoid reenacting harmful relational patterns, and strengthen conditions for engagement. The chapter positions schooling as a context for repair, regulation, and identity affirmation when instructional decisions intentionally counter the effects of cumulative harm.

INTRODUCTION

On a weekday morning, the hum of a classroom fills the air — chairs scraping, pencils tapping, a few hurried voices finishing conversations before the bell. Among the crowd sits Maya, a ten-year-old who often seems half-present. She forgets her homework, and her attention drifts off mid-lesson. She is described

DOI: 10.4018/979-8-3373-4064-7.ch008

as becoming startled easily when other students raise their voice. Her teacher, Mr. Lewis, notices she's fallen behind in reading but can't pinpoint why. Over the term, small clues surface: He learns that Maya has changed schools twice in two years. Her parents have recently separated following years of escalating conflict, and her mother has commenced working night shifts since the separation. There is no single event that explains her struggles. Rather, her story reflects the accumulation of stressors — instability, fatigue, isolation — that have slowly worn down her ability to focus, connect, and thrive at school.

Maya's experience is not uncommon. Across educational systems worldwide, many children arrive at school carrying the weight of experiences that extend far beyond the classroom: family conflict, poverty, discrimination, community violence, chronic illness, or loss. When these experiences accumulate over time, they can disrupt the steady developmental rhythms that schooling depends on — concentration, curiosity, emotional regulation, and trust. The term cumulative harm describes this layered impact of multiple adversities that, taken together, compromise wellbeing and learning (McLaughlin et al., 2014; Hughes et al., 2017; Sahle et al., 2023). Research shows that the cumulative effects of adversity can undermine academic outcomes and psychosocial development across multiple domains. Children who have experienced four or more adverse childhood experiences (ACEs) are significantly more likely to struggle with school attendance, reading achievement, and social relationships (Hughes et al., 2017; Sahle et al., 2023; Zhai et al., 2022). Chronic stress alters attention, memory, and emotional regulation capacities— the very physiological systems that underpin learning (McEwen & Morrison, 2013; Sheridan & McLaughlin, 2016; Busso et al., 2017). While the harm often originates in wider social systems, it is within classrooms that its effects are most visible. Educators, and educational systems, are positioned at the intersection of vulnerability and opportunity. Their daily interactions can either reinforce the harms or become moments of repair. Educators are not just conveyors of knowledge. The relational nature of teaching means that every interaction holds the potential to repair or repeat harm. When schools create consistent, attuned, and inclusive spaces, they can assist in restoring disrupted developmental trajectories. This begins with a shift from viewing student disengagement as a problem to be managed, to recognising it as a form of communication about unmet needs.

This chapter takes a learning-centred approach, reframing behavioural and engagement challenges as reflections of context – both within and outside of the educational setting. It argues that educators — through reflexive, relational and bias-aware practice — can buffer against the effects of cumulative harm, helping children re-engage with learning and rebuild a sense of competence and safety. It positions the educator as a key factor in buffering harm, scaffolding recovery, and shaping the environment for growth. The chapter is organised around a framework of understand that includes three interconnected domains that together illustrate how cumulative harm shapes children's experiences of schooling and how educators can respond in evidence-informed ways. The three domains examine the impacts and implications of cumulative harm systemically, beginning with the individual learner, extending outward to the instructor and the learning environment, and then to the curriculum and instructional design.

The Learner considers how cumulative harm influences attention, motivation, memory, self-regulation, and identity as a learner. It explores the developmental pathways through which threat and deprivation affect cognitive and emotional functioning, and how these patterns manifest in classroom behaviour and engagement. Following this, The Instructor and the Learning Environment then shifts focus to the relational and ecological dimensions of schooling. Here, we examine how teacher–student interactions, routines, predictability, and classroom climate can buffer or intensify the effects of adversity. The section The Curriculum and Instruction broadens the lens to the pedagogical level. This section reviews how curriculum design, assessment practices, and instructional choices can either create barriers or open pathways for students whose learning has been disrupted by cumulative harm. Finally, the chapter concludes with Support and Implementation, which identifies evidence-informed universal precautions and practices that promote inclusion, belonging, and equitable participation. This final section outlines strategies that meet the needs of all learners while also providing structured responses to acute risks, safety concerns, and the health and social needs that often accompany cumulative harm. It emphasises integrated, multi-tiered supports that enable educators to act proactively.

THE LEARNER

Understanding how cumulative harm shapes learning begins with recognising that adversity leaves its strongest imprint on the learner's internal world — their physiology, relationships, cognition, and sense of self. This section examines three key domains of disruption: physiological arousal, relational functioning, and academic and social-emotional learning. Using the dimensional model of adversity (McLaughlin et al., 2014), we explore how experiences of *threat* and *deprivation* alter learners' capacities in distinct yet interconnected ways.

Impact of Threat and Deprivation on Physiological Arousal

Physiological arousal refers to the body's stress-response systems, which adjust heart rate, breathing, muscle tension, and alertness in response to perceived demands.

In school settings, short-lived increases in arousal can be adaptive, for example during tests or public speaking. Problems tend to arise when stress is frequent and intense, which is more common among children who have experienced multiple adversities (Hughes et al., 2017; Crouch et al., 2019). Meta-analytic and longitudinal research suggest that such exposure is associated, on average, with difficulties in executive functions such as working memory and inhibitory control, which are relevant for sustaining attention and managing impulses in classrooms (Tiego et al., 2020; Vaidya et al., 2024). These associations are far from deterministic, but they help explain why some students appear to have less "cognitive bandwidth" available for learning in demanding environments (Weissman et al., 2022; McEwen & Morrison, 2013).

Some children who have experienced repeated interpersonal threat — such as exposure to violence or highly unpredictable conflict — show patterns of heightened threat sensitivity. Threat sensitivity refers to a tendency to detect and prioritise cues that might signal interpersonal danger, even when those cues are ambiguous or low in objective risk (Berman et al. 2022). Systematic reviews and meta-analyses examining children exposed to threat-related adversity consistently report modest differences, on average, in processes related to emotion recognition, attention to potential threat cues, and behavioural regulation, although findings vary across studies and measurement approaches (Hein & Monk, 2017; McLaughlin et al. 2021). In practical terms, these children may be more likely to interpret ambiguous classroom events — a raised voice, a sudden noise, or a peer's shifting facial expression — as potentially hostile or personally significant. This does not imply that they are "wired" to be hypervigilant in all contexts, nor that such responses are fixed. Rather, it suggests that when they are under stress or uncertainty, a greater proportion of their cognitive effort may be directed toward monitoring the interpersonal environment, leaving fewer resources available for academic tasks or sustained engagement (Busso et al., 2017; Vaidya et al., 2024).

In school contexts, some students with histories of adversity appear preoccupied with scanning their surroundings and tracking social dynamics. This pattern is often described in health contexts as "heightened vigilance". Experimental and observational research suggests that children with such histories may allocate more attention to potential social threat cues and show slower engagement with neutral or academic stimuli, though the magnitude of these effects is typically small and varies across tasks and samples (Hein & Monk, 2017). For educators, the practical implication is straightforward but important: what looks like "inattention" can, in some cases, reflect a cautious stance toward the environment rather than a lack of interest in the lesson. Heightened sensitivity to perceived threat often co-occurs with stronger and more rapid emotional responses. Meta-analytic work on childhood maltreatment and cognition indicates that effected children, on average, perform somewhat more poorly on tasks that require inhibiting impulses and regulating emotions, although there is substantial overlap with non-maltreated peers and many exceptions (Tiego et al., 2020; McLaughlin et al., 2021). In classrooms, this can show up as difficulty "letting go" of minor conflicts, becoming quickly overwhelmed by corrective feedback, or abandoning a challenging task sooner than peers (Weissman et al., 2022; Vaidya et al., 2024). These patterns are not unique to students with adversity histories, but adversity can be one contributor.

Returning to Maya, her teacher notices that she startles easily, seems tense during noisy transitions, and often disengages when classroom demands increase. These behaviours are consistent with a cautious stance toward the environment: she appears to be monitoring what might go wrong rather than fully investing in the task at hand. While we cannot directly observe the underlying mechanisms, this example illustrates how repeated stress and instability in a child's life may reasonably contribute to patterns of guarded participation in learning (Shah et al., 2022).

Experiences often described as deprivation — limited responsive caregiving, sparse language input, or few opportunities for structured play and learning — are associated, at the group level, with lower performance on measures of language, executive functioning, and some aspects of motivation (McLaughlin et al., 2014). Systematic reviews of dimensional models of adversity suggest that deprivation shows somewhat stronger links with executive functioning and cognitive outcomes than threat, although both dimensions are implicated (McLaughlin et al., 2021). In practical terms, some students with such histories may appear slow to initiate tasks, uncertain about how to approach open-ended work, or less responsive to typical classroom rewards.

Students who have had fewer opportunities for scaffolded success or consistent feedback may present as disengaged, indifferent to praise, or reluctant to start independent work. Evidence from systematic reviews and meta-analyses indicates that higher cumulative adversity is associated, on average, with slightly lower academic achievement and school engagement, but these effects vary widely across individuals and contexts (Kirk et al., 2017; Sahle et al., 2023). In this light, labelling such students as "unmotivated" risks overlooking the ways in which their prior experiences have shaped their expectations about effort, failure, and adult responsiveness.

For Maya, irregular routines and limited adult availability at home likely reduce the time and energy available for focused learning and shared conversation. It is therefore understandable that she hesitates to begin tasks or to volunteer ideas in class. From the teacher's perspective, her quietness could be misread as disinterest, yet it can just as plausibly be understood as a cautious response shaped by fatigue, competing demands, and uncertainty about how her efforts will be received (Zhai et al., 2022)

Relational Impacts

Relational disruptions are a common outcome of cumulative adversity. Children who experience abuse, neglect, or chronic stress are more likely to develop insecure attachment patterns and later problems in close relationships (Doyle & Cicchetti, 2018). Attachment refers to the emotional bond between a child and a caregiver that guides how the child expects others to respond to them across life (Roorda et al., 2017). Dimensional models show that experiences of threat, such as violence, and deprivation, such as neglect or low stimulation, influence socioemotional and cognitive development through partly related pathways (McLaughlin et al., 2014; Vaidya et al., 2024; McLaughlin et al., 2021). These pathways help explain the relational strategies that children later use in schools and other learning environments. Large reviews of adverse childhood experiences (ACEs) and social functioning report that higher ACE exposure is associated, on average, with more difficulties in forming and maintaining supportive relationships (Hughes et al., 2017; Wang et al., 2023).

One common relational pattern after threat exposure is mistrust. Adults who report childhood emotional maltreatment show lower trust, higher conflict, and poorer relationship quality in romantic relationships (Chen et al., 2022). Doyle and Cicchetti (2018) link childhood maltreatment and family adversity with higher rates of insecure attachment, interpersonal distrust, and relational distance in later relationships (Doyle & Cicchetti, 2018). In classrooms, this can present as reluctance to ask for help, emotional withdrawal when corrected, or a tendency to read neutral comments as criticism. In adolescence, it can look like rejecting group work, keeping teachers at arm's length, or disengaging from school-based support, while still caring deeply about academic and peer outcomes. These behaviours are more parsimoniously understood as protective strategies, shaped by prior experiences of relational unreliability, than as simple "defiance" or "disrespect."

Other children, particularly those whose early environments are marked more by deprivation than overt threat – for example, limited emotional responsiveness, few opportunities for shared play, or frequent changes in caregivers – may show almost the opposite pattern: marked dependence on particular adults or peers to feel safe. Reviews of adverse caregiving environments and attachment describe how inconsistent or low-responsivity care can foster anxious or disorganised attachment strategies, where children oscillate between clinging and withdrawal and struggle to develop an internalised sense of security (Doyle & Cichetti, 2018). In school, this may appear as shadowing a preferred teacher, seeking repeated reassurance about minor issues, or copying peers' views and behaviours to avoid exclusion. In secondary and tertiary education, these students may be reluctant to take initiative in group tasks, waiting for others to lead and contributing minimally unless explicitly invited. The underlying driver is often not laziness but uncertainty about their own worth and about how others will respond if they step forward.

Syntheses of longitudinal and cross-sectional research show that positive teacher–student relationships – characterised by warmth, low conflict, and a sense of being known – are reliably associated with higher academic engagement, better achievement, and fewer behavioural problems (Cafaro et al., 2023; Duan et al., 2024). Recent systematic reviews from an attachment perspective emphasise that teachers can function as "attachment-like" figures in school: secure, predictable relationships with teachers are linked to improved engagement, reduced early school leaving, and better adjustment, particularly for students identified as vulnerable or at risk (Roorda et al., 2017 et al., 2011; Doyle & Cicchetti, 2018). Longitudinal research also shows bidirectional links: improvements in teacher–student relationship quality predicts gains in social and academic competence, and students who are doing better academically and socially tend to experience more positive relationships with teachers over time (Wang et al., 2023). There is also emerging evidence that positive school relationships can buffer some of the effects of ACEs. A retrospective population-based study found that, among adults with high household ACE exposure, those who reported supportive, fair, and inclusive school experiences had better health and wellbeing outcomes than those whose school experiences were negative, suggesting that school relationships can partially offset early risk (Hughes et al., 2017). Systematic reviews of ACEs and peer relations similarly highlight that high-quality peer relationships and supportive school climates can mitigate, though not eliminate, the associations between adversity, mental health difficulties, and poorer social outcomes (Wang et al, 2023).

Relational functioning is closely related with physiological and motivational systems described earlier. A student whose nervous system is primed for threat may misinterpret a classmate's joke as mockery or a teacher's firm instruction as personal hostility, leading to conflict or withdrawal. Another student who has grown up with emotionally unavailable adults may not seek connection at all, appearing aloof or "hard to reach." Reviews of ACEs, mental health, and social functioning show how these patterns of hypervigilance, emotional numbing, or social withdrawal can contribute to social isolation, smaller support networks, and heightened risk of internalising and externalising problems across adolescence and adulthood (Hughes et al., 2017; Chen et al., 2022; Wang et al., 2023). These same patterns influence how students engage with learning, because tasks that require collaboration, help-seeking, or tolerating mistakes will feel riskier in relationships that are not yet experienced as safe.

As the term progresses, Mr. Lewis begins noticing small but consistent relational cues in Maya's behaviour. She avoids eye contact when approached, often declines help before he finishes offering it, and hangs back during group tasks unless a peer explicitly draws her in. These behaviours are easy to misinterpret as disinterest, yet they make more sense when viewed as protective strategies shaped by instability in her home life. For educators like Mr. Lewis, the aim is not to identify attachment styles but to read relational behaviour with curiosity. A child who turns away from support may be guarding against anticipated disappointment; one who repeatedly seeks reassurance may be testing whether adult availability is reliable. Maya's shifts between withdrawal and reassurance seeking reflect the same underlying uncertainty: Can I trust that support will still be there if I need it? Evidence from systematic reviews shows that predictable practices that communicate positive regard can build trust — greeting students by name, checking in after conflict, following through on promises — are associated with improved engagement and reduced behavioural difficulties, particularly for students with histories of adversity (Roseby & Gascoigne, 2021; Berger, 2019). When teachers combine genuine care, concern and support with clear boundaries and gentle encouragement of autonomy, mistrustful students can begin relying on adults, and overdependent students can take initiative with greater confidence.

In Maya's case, Mr. Lewis adjusts by offering small, consistent cues of safety: a morning greeting, reassurance that help is available, and neutral follow-up after corrections. Over time, these routines give Maya space to test whether the classroom is predictable and supportive. As her sense of safety grows, so does her willingness to participate, ask questions, and take the interpersonal risks that learning requires. Seen this way, Maya's relational patterns are not signs of disrespect or passivity but learned strategies for staying safe. Understanding these patterns — without assuming adversity explains everything — positions educators to create environments where students like Maya can risk connection and, in turn, engage more fully in learning.

Academic and Social-Emotional Learning

Building on the physiological and relational patterns described earlier, the next layer of impact becomes visible in how children manage the cognitive demands of classroom life. Executive functions (EFs) are the suite of higher-order processes that allow learners to organise their thinking, sustain attention, remember instructions, regulate impulses, and shift flexibly between tasks. These skills operate quietly in the background, coordinating thought and behaviour so that learning can occur. In many ways, they are the mental scaffolding that enables students to plan ahead, stay focused when lessons become complex, and recover quickly when something goes wrong. For most students, executive functions strengthen gradually through exposure to predictable routines, responsive adults, and enriching learning environments. These steady, scaffolded experiences help children internalise the cognitive habits needed for goal-directed behaviour: holding multiple steps in mind, switching strategies when faced with a challenge, and inhibiting unhelpful impulses. However, for students whose lives are marked by cumulative harm, these processes can develop in less consistent ways. Chronic stress, ongoing conflict, and limited cognitive stimulation do not simply shape emotions and relationships; over time, they influence the efficiency with which children can allocate, shift, and sustain their cognitive resources.

A meta-analysis synthesising data from more than 31,000 children found that both threat and deprivation were associated, on average, with modest reductions in executive functioning, with deprivation showing stronger and more consistent effects on working memory and cognitive flexibility (Johnson et al., 2021). These findings do not mean that adversity determines a child's abilities. Many children exposed to significant hardship perform within age-typical ranges. But at the population level, cumulative adversity nudges cognitive systems toward greater effortfulness: tasks take more mental energy, switching between activities becomes more taxing, and sustaining focus under stress becomes harder. Threat-related experiences—such as witnessing violence or living with unpredictable adults—tend to disrupt inhibitory control, particularly in emotionally charged or ambiguous contexts. Inhibitory control is what allows a student to pause before reacting, resist the urge to interrupt, or persist when the task becomes frustrating. Meta-analyses show that children exposed to threat demonstrate small but reliable differences in this domain (Vaidya et al., 2024), and systematic reviews of ACEs highlight similar patterns, especially in tasks requiring behavioural and emotional regulation (Tiego et al., 2020). In classroom practice, this does not always appear as overt dysregulation. More often, it shows up subtly: the child who rushes through work without checking, blurts out answers impulsively, or reacts strongly to minor setbacks. Under repeated stress, the cognitive effort required to "hold back" becomes harder to sustain.

Deprivation, by contrast, affects the cognitive building blocks that support working memory and flexibility. Fewer opportunities for language-rich interactions, inconsistent exposure to books or structured play, and fragmented routines reduce the experiences through which children practise holding information in mind, adapting to new rules, and shifting strategies during problem-solving. Deprivation-related experiences were associated with nearly twice the effect size of threat for working-memory difficulties in the Johnson et al. (2021) meta-analysis. When working memory or flexibility lag behind, students may appear confused, rigid, or slow to adapt when lesson structures change. They may lose track of multi-step instructions, struggle to organise written work, or seem to "freeze" during transitions—not because they are unwilling, but because their cognitive systems are already working at capacity.

These patterns become clearer when viewed through Maya's day-to-day experiences in the classroom. As the weeks pass, Mr. Lewis notices small but consistent features in how she manages cognitive demands. Multi-step instructions often dissolve after the first part, and she hesitates before beginning independent tasks, watching what others do before she decides where to start. Sudden noises or shifting routines unsettle her, and transitions between lessons take noticeably longer than for her peers. On particularly busy days, she appears to retreat inward—slowing down, staying quiet, or becoming visibly tense when lessons speed up. These behaviours can be easy to misinterpret as disengagement, avoidance, or a lack of motivation. Yet they align closely with what the research describes as adaptive responses to limited cognitive bandwidth. A learner with constrained working-memory resources may delay starting work because she is trying to preserve the steps she can recall. A child who freezes during transitions may be grappling with the cognitive effort required to shift tasks under stress. And a student who becomes tense during noisy or fast-moving lessons may be allocating more attention to monitoring the environment than to the content of the task.

Maya's underlying question—Do I have enough mental space to manage what is being asked of me right now?—is not always articulated, but it shapes her behaviour in quiet, predictable ways. Systematic reviews show that predictable routines, explicit modelling, chunked instructions, and visual scaffolds can ease these cognitive demands, particularly for students whose executive functions are under strain (Smale-Jacobse et al., 2019; Cheung & Slavin, 2016). In response, Mr. Lewis begins structuring his teaching differently: breaking tasks into smaller steps, giving Maya a moment to rehearse instructions before beginning, and offering gentle prompts during transitions. These adjustments are not remedial—they are universal supports that create enough cognitive room for learners like Maya to engage without feeling overwhelmed.

Over time, Maya's confidence grows. She asks clarifying questions she previously avoided, begins tasks more readily when the structure is clear, and navigates transitions with fewer signs of tension. Her progress is steady rather than dramatic, and it emerges not from "fixing" deficits but from reducing cognitive load and stabilising the learning environment. Seen this way, Maya's patterns are not signs of disinterest or defiance; they are learned, effortful attempts to cope with high cognitive demand in an environment that occasionally moves faster than her internal systems can manage.

Understanding executive functioning through this lens does not require educators to diagnose students or assume that adversity explains every difficulty. Instead, it encourages them to approach student academic difficulties with curiosity. Just as turning away from support may signal uncertainty rather than disrespect, hesitating at the start of a task may reflect limited cognitive resources rather than unwillingness. These interpretations shift the focus from fixing the child to shaping the conditions around them. The goal is to create learning environments where students feel safe enough — cognitively, emotionally, and relationally — to participate and take intellectual risks. How educators organise their classrooms, structure routines, and position themselves in daily interactions plays a central role in making this possible. The next section explores how teacher practice and classroom climate can help make this possible.

THE INSTRUCTOR AND THE LEARNING ENVIRONMENT

The ways educators speak, respond, organise routines, and manage uncertainty shape the emotional and cognitive conditions in which learning unfolds. Classrooms are not neutral containers; they are dynamic ecosystems in which students constantly interpret cues about safety, expectations, and belonging. The same child can thrive in one classroom and struggle in another, not because their capacities change, but because the affordances of the environment shift around them. For children whose development has been shaped by cumulative harm, these environmental cues carry even greater weight. Small moments — a teacher's tone, an unexpected transition, a public correction — can either lower the cognitive load enough for engagement or activate defensive patterns that narrow attention and reduce flexibility. Understanding this interplay requires examining not only student behaviour but the subtle, often unspoken ways educators and environments participate in learning. This section explores three mechanisms through which classrooms can inadvertently intensify or alleviate the effects of adversity: (1) re-enactment of threat or deprivation, (2) educator cognitive heuristics and decision making, and (3) parallel processes linking the emotional states of teachers and students.

Re-enactments

Re-enactment refers to the unintentional replaying of earlier relational patterns when present cues resemble past experiences of threat or deprivation. For students like Maya, whose histories include instability, unpredictability, or conflict, the classroom can become a site where these dynamics are activated not through conscious recall but through the body's stored responses. A raised voice during a reminder, an unexpected change in routine, or a stern facial expression may not register as simple classroom management. Instead, these cues mirror past environments characterised by danger or inconsistency. For students shaped by threat, the nervous system shifts quickly into vigilance, tension, withdrawal, or defensive behaviour. For students shaped by deprivation—marked by chronic unresponsiveness or emotional absence—neutral or ambiguous cues may feel like rejection or disconnection. These reactions reflect meaning-making grounded in past experience, not misbehaviour.

Educators can also, without intention, participate in re-creating these patterns. Many common teaching practices—using sharp tone to regain control, addressing mistakes publicly, or prioritising task completion over emotional signals—emerge from institutional norms that emphasised compliance, speed, and emotional restraint. Such responses can inadvertently echo the same dynamics students have learned to anticipate: the unpredictability associated with threat, or the emotional distance associated with deprivation. When this happens, interactions shift from the present moment to the historical patterns they resemble. Berger's (2019) review demonstrates that relationship-based practices characterised by warmth, attunement, and predictable follow-through strengthen students' perceptions of safety and reduce behavioural escalations. The findings highlight that re-enactment is often buffered not by dramatic interventions but by micro-signals—steady tone, consistent routines, private corrections, and acknowledgment of emotions—that counter patterns of both threat (through predictability) and deprivation (through responsiveness).

Understanding re-enactment reframes behaviour. It redirects attention from "fixing" the student's reaction to recognising how the learning environment may inadvertently replicate cues associated with earlier harm. This requires noticing the interplay between past and present: how a student's history shapes the meaning they assign to a teacher's cue, and how the teacher's own habits, stress, or assumptions shape the tone of the interaction. A withdrawal may signal an echo of past threat; an outburst may reflect an old pattern of unmet needs resurfacing under perceived deprivation. The more useful questions become: What in this moment might feel familiar—dangerous or dismissive—for this student? And what am I contributing that might amplify or soften that perception? Holding this stance requires humility and reflexivity. It means acknowledging that well-intentioned practices—a firm reprimand delivered too abruptly, a redirected task offered without relational check-in, a delayed response that leaves a student waiting—can unintentionally mirror unpredictability or emotional absence. It also requires recognising that educators' own stress or internalised norms shape how they respond, sometimes in ways that contradict their intentions. By cultivating awareness of these dynamics, educators can design interactions that interrupt, rather than reproduce, patterns of threat and deprivation. Re-enactment thus becomes a lens through which teachers understand behaviour as contextually grounded communication and adjust their practice to create learning environments that are regulating, responsive, and aligned with students' developmental needs.

During a routine discussion, Mr. Lewis raises his voice slightly to settle the room. The reminder is mild, but Maya's posture stiffens immediately. She lowers her eyes, pulls her workbook closer, and becomes unusually quiet. Nothing was directed at her, yet her reaction suggests the moment felt sharper than intended. When the class shifts to the next activity, the quick movement and rising noise unsettle her again. She packs her things with rigid precision and watches the room rather than the task. A classmate accidentally bumps her desk, and she flinches, apologising even though she is not at fault. Her responses become short, her attention scattered, and she avoids eye contact when Mr. Lewis checks in. Viewed from the outside, these changes look like simple disengagement. But the pattern is consistent: small cues—a raised voice, rushed transition, or sudden noise—seem to activate older emotional memories that pull her into self-protection. Mr. Lewis notices this shift over time and adjusts by approaching her quietly, signalling transitions earlier, and keeping his tone steady. These small changes reduce the emotional "spikes" in the room, and Maya begins staying present during busy moments rather than retreating inward.

Educator Cognitive Heuristics and Decision Making

In classrooms, decisions must often be made quickly: interpreting a student's expression, responding to a disruption, deciding whether to repeat an instruction or move on. Under these conditions, the mind naturally relies on heuristics—fast, efficient mental shortcuts that help people make judgments without engaging in slow, deliberate analysis. Heuristics are not inherently problematic; they are a normal and adaptive feature of human cognition. However, like any shortcut, they can sometimes lead to systematic errors. One common heuristic relevant to teaching is the attribution heuristic, which occurs when behaviour is interpreted based on internal characteristics rather than external circumstances. For example, a student who pauses after receiving instructions might be read as "unmotivated" rather than as someone managing working-memory limitations or stress. Another student who reacts intensely to corrective feedback might be interpreted as "too sensitive" rather than as someone who has learned to be cautious in relationships. These interpretations do not reflect ill intent on the educator's part. Rather, they illustrate how quickly the mind gravitates toward familiar explanatory patterns when time, information, and cognitive resources are limited, especially when students' behaviour reflects adaptations to threat (vigilance, rapid reactivity) or deprivation (uncertainty, withdrawal).

Research demonstrates that the way students perceive these interpretations matters. A meta-analysis by Civitillo, Mayer, and Jugert (2023) reviewed 68 studies on students' perceptions of teacher treatment across racial and ethnic groups. The findings showed that students who perceived differential treatment—even when unintentional—reported lower wellbeing, diminished academic self-concept, and reduced achievement. Importantly, these patterns emerged not only from explicit actions but from subtle inconsistencies in warmth, expectations, or opportunities. Such effects highlight why understanding heuristics is critical: unintended patterns in micro-interactions can accumulate into meaningful differences in a learner's experience. For students shaped by threat, slight shifts in tone may be interpreted as danger; for students shaped by deprivation, inconsistent attention may reinforce expectations of unresponsiveness. Another set of heuristics relates to expectancy effects, where assumptions about groups or categories shape prediction and interpretation. A meta-analysis by Glock et al. (2019) found that educators, like professionals in many fields, showed more favourable implicit attitudes toward socially advantaged groups. These attitudes did not reflect deliberate choices but instead operated automatically, influencing expectations, the amount of scaffolding provided, and the tone of interactions. When working with students affected by cumulative harm, such heuristics may intersect with hypervigilance, stress, or inconsistent attendance, making behavioural interpretations even more complex and more easily misread through the lens of bias rather than context.

A third heuristic involves fundamental context neglect, where behaviour is interpreted without considering the broader social and historical conditions that influence family life. Without this wider lens, lateness, incomplete homework, or emotional reactivity can be understood as individual traits rather than as possible reflections of chronic stress, socioeconomic strain, racialised experiences, or intergenerational trauma. This can unintentionally reinforce deficit narratives—explanations that locate challenges within the child rather than within the interplay of context, development, and opportunity. Bottiani et al. (2018) found that such patterns can perpetuate inequities even in classrooms committed to inclusion. For students whose development has been shaped by threat, hyperarousal can be misread as defiance; for those shaped by deprivation, disengagement can be misread as disinterest. Strengthening awareness of these heuristics does not require self-blame. Instead, it invites educators into a stance of inquiry rather than certainty—pausing to ask, "What else might be contributing to this behaviour?" Structured supports can help cultivate this stance. Professional learning communities, consultation models, and reflective supervision all create space for educators to examine their interpretations, share alternative perspectives, and differentiate between behaviour that signals intentional defiance and behaviour that reflects developmental need or protective adaptation (SAMHSA, 2014). This reflective dialogue reduces the likelihood of escalating cycles in which initial interpretations lead to responses that inadvertently heighten student distress or withdrawal. Recognising these cognitive patterns also highlights a deeper relational dynamic—the ways educator stress and emotional load can shape, and be shaped by, student behaviour, potentially recreating the same threat- or deprivation-based relational cues that students have learned to anticipate.

During a hands-on science lesson, students move around the room collecting materials for an experiment. As the noise rises, Maya waits near her desk, watching for a quiet moment before joining a group. From a distance, Mr. Lewis notices her standing still while others get started. With little time to assess the situation, his mind reaches for the fastest explanation: Maya is avoiding the task. He encourages her to "get moving," confident he has read the situation correctly. When she eventually approaches a group, the instructions have already been discussed. Maya tries to piece them together by watching her peers. A few minutes later, Mr. Lewis sees only a single note on her worksheet. Another quick assumption forms—this time, that she is not putting in enough effort. He reminds her to "stay focused," believing he is offering helpful prompting. Neither interpretation matches what is actually happening. Maya is trying to work out the steps she missed during the noisy transition and is unsure how to enter a group that already feels two steps ahead. Her slow pace reflects uncertainty, not lack of motivation. But each of Mr. Lewis's rapid judgments—avoidance, low effort—comes from a mental shortcut that draws on familiar explanations rather than the full context. Later, while discussing the lesson with a colleague, he notices the pattern. His interpretations came quickly and confidently, yet they were based on limited information and centred on internal traits instead of the environmental demands: the noise, the pace, the unclear entry point. The next lesson, he structures the activity with clearer starting steps and quieter transitions. Maya joins her group smoothly, and her work reflects engagement once the context no longer forces her teacher to rely on fast, default heuristics to understand her behaviour.

Parallel Processes

Parallel processes describe what happens when the emotional states of educators and students start to reflect one another, often without anyone noticing. The idea comes from the Sanctuary Model (Bloom, 1997), which shows how systems built to support people affected by trauma can unintentionally recreate the same patterns they are trying to change. In schools, this means the climate students experience is closely linked to the climate teachers experience. When educators feel anxious, tired, or overwhelmed, those feelings ripple through routines, expectations, and interactions. When staff feel supported and steady, the whole classroom becomes calmer. This dynamic matters even more for students shaped by threat or deprivation. They often interpret adult tension as danger or adult withdrawal as emotional unavailability because those cues feel familiar.

Schools demand rapid decisions. Teachers make hundreds of micro-judgments a day with limited time and incomplete information. Even skilled educators can end up emotionally overloaded. These reactions are not failings; they are normal responses to ongoing stress. But they influence students, especially those who notice every shift in facial expression or tone. A rushed teacher may sound sharper than intended. A stretched teacher may miss subtle signs of discomfort. Over time, these small changes shape whether the room feels predictable or chaotic, approachable or unsafe. For students primed by threat, adult reactivity can feel amplified. For students shaped by deprivation, inconsistencies can reinforce expectations of instability. A large meta-analysis by Duan, Bissaker, and Xu (2024) synthesised 87 studies and found that teachers' classroom management self-efficacy—confidence in maintaining order and building rapport—predicted classroom climate and teacher stress. Low self-efficacy was linked to more conflict and tension, and difficult classroom dynamics in turn reduced teacher confidence. Supporting educators is therefore not an optional wellbeing exercise; it directly improves the learning environment.

Parallel processes also explain why caring educators sometimes act in ways that don't match their intentions. When teachers face sustained pressure—whether from student needs or system demands—they may become more reactive, more controlling, or more withdrawn. These responses can unknowingly echo the environments some students grew up in. A frustrated raised voice may recreate the volatility associated with past conflict. Emotional shutdown during a tough afternoon may mirror the unavailability of depleted caregivers. Students often read these patterns through the same threat or deprivation filters they developed in earlier relationships. In these moments, it is not just the individual teacher who shapes the interaction; unaddressed systemic stress is doing the work. Recognising parallel processes shifts attention from individual behaviour to collective responsibility. No educator can remain calm and emotionally available without organisational support. Trauma-informed practice requires structures that make regulation possible. The Sanctuary Model points to practices like regular supervision, reflective conversations, shared problem-solving, and a school culture where seeking help is seen as strength, not weakness (Bloom, 1997). These conditions create psychological safety for staff, which becomes the foundation for psychological safety for students.

When educators feel valued, resourced, and connected, they can stay present, patient, and curious during challenging moments. This does not remove stress, but it stops stress from shaping interactions. Parallel processes can therefore be a risk or an opportunity. Without support, staff distress can trigger escalating cycles of tension. With support, staff wellbeing becomes a stabilising force that students rely on—especially those still learning to regulate arousal and expectations in relationships. Evidence from systematic reviews shows that educator wellbeing, reflective practice, and organisational support are not extra features; they are essential for effective classrooms (Duan et al., 2024). Paying attention to these dynamics helps prevent the unintentional recreation of threat or deprivation patterns in school settings. This understanding also shapes how curriculum and instruction can reduce or increase the cognitive and emotional load students bring into learning.

On a Friday afternoon, the kind that already feels too long, Mr. Lewis walks into class carrying more strain than he realises. Yard duty ran over, his inbox is full of urgent emails, and the lesson he planned will now have to fit into half the time. He is not angry, just stretched. Still, his pace is quicker than usual, his tone flatter, and his instructions come out in a rush because he is trying to regain control of the clock. Almost immediately, he notices the class feels harder to settle. A few students call out, others move slowly, and the room has a restless edge. As he redirects them, his voice sharpens—not because he means to be firm, but because he is tired. He feels the gap widen between what he needs the class to do and what they are giving him.

Across the room, Maya is watching closely. She sees the tightness in his expression and hears the tension in his voice. To her, these small changes feel like warning signs, even though nothing is directed at her. She lowers her gaze, avoids putting her hand up, and focuses on not drawing attention. When she hesitates over an instruction, she tells herself not to bother the teacher—he already seems on edge. As the lesson continues, Mr. Lewis senses the students pulling back. They are quieter, more cautious, and less willing to take risks. Their withdrawal makes him feel as if the class is slipping, so he pushes harder: faster instructions, firmer redirections, shorter explanations. The students respond by shrinking even further. Neither side intends it, but the mood of the room spirals into the same tension he walked in with. Later, when the students leave, Mr. Lewis sits for a moment and realises how the entire lesson mirrored how he had felt walking through the door: rushed, worn out, and stretched thin. The class had absorbed his state, and he had absorbed theirs. He recognises that nothing "went wrong" with his students—his own stress had quietly set the emotional tone.

The next week, he tries something small. Before entering the room, he takes a slow breath, reminds himself of the plan, and decides to start the lesson with a calm greeting instead of diving straight into content. The room settles more gently. Students ask questions again. Maya looks up when he walks past rather than bracing herself. The difference is not a new strategy or script—it is the teacher's emotional footing. By steadying himself, he interrupts the parallel process that had pulled both him and his students into tension. And the class responds in kind, reflecting the stability he brings into the room.

THE CURRICULUM AND INSTRUCTION

Curriculum is often described as a sequence of content and skills that students progress through, but it is more accurately understood as a cultural and political document. It reflects decisions about what knowledge is centred, whose histories are included, and which ways of knowing are legitimised in schooling. Instruction is not neutral either. It embodies assumptions about who learners are, how they learn, and what forms of participation are valued. For students exposed to cumulative harm—especially harm shaped by threat (violence, instability, unpredictable adults) or deprivation (low stimulation, cultural erasure, limited scaffolding)—curriculum and instruction strongly influence whether the classroom feels like a place of recognition or a place of exclusion. Mainstream curricula in Western education systems privilege Eurocentric epistemologies. Apple (2012) shows that curricular frameworks continue to canonise linear progression, individual achievement, and Western knowledge traditions. When these frameworks dominate, many students never see their languages, histories, or cultural practices reflected. This absence is not a simple gap in representation. It signals who holds power and whose knowledge is treated as peripheral—an especially potent threat cue for students whose lives have already been shaped by marginalisation or instability.

For historically marginalised communities, these omissions carry weight. Research with Aboriginal and Torres Strait Islander students shows that curriculum can become a site of deficit and misrepresentation, where histories are narrowed, distorted, or erased (Macfarlane & Macfarlane, 2019). Students repeatedly exposed to this form of cultural deprivation often perceive school knowledge as disconnected from their identity. The result is not a lack of motivation but a protective withdrawal: a rational response to content that implicitly frames their experiences as incompatible with academic success. Instruction amplifies these messages. Teaching practices that rely heavily on teacher-led talk, abstract tasks, or culturally narrow examples may unintentionally reinforce feelings of invisibility. For students carrying chronic stress or threat-based vigilance, such practices can heighten monitoring, reduce available cognitive resources, and increase the likelihood of disengagement. When instruction fails to acknowledge diverse linguistic repertoires, cultural norms, or community knowledge, students may experience the classroom as another environment where their ways of understanding the world go unrecognised or invalidated.

The Power Threat Meaning Framework (PTMF) clarifies how students interpret these curricular and instructional conditions. PTMF argues that individuals make sense of experiences by examining how power operates around them, what threats it poses, and the meanings they construct (Johnstone & Boyle, 2018). Applied to curriculum, this means students read school content for what it communicates about belonging and value. A curriculum that elevates dominant narratives while sidelining minority perspectives may be understood as a structural threat—another signal that their identities or communities are less legitimate. Reactions such as hesitation, disengagement, scepticism, or oppositional behaviour are not apathy. They represent meaning-making shaped by repeated experiences of threat or deprivation. Viewed through this lens, the key question shifts from "How do we deliver content effectively?" to "What messages does the curriculum send about who students are and what knowledge matters?" This shift is central to trauma-informed and equity-focused education. When curriculum and instruction align with students' cultural identities, lived experiences, and community strengths, they buffer the impacts of cumulative harm. When they do not, they intensify the cognitive and emotional load that threat- and deprivation-affected students already carry.

Differentiated Instruction

The pace of explanation, the examples teachers choose, the questions they pose, and the way classroom talk is structured all shape how curriculum becomes real to learners. Instruction is not separate from curriculum; it is the medium through which curriculum takes shape. It can widen or narrow access depending on how it positions learners. Practices that depend heavily on a single mode of communication—extended teacher talk, rapid whole-class questioning, or tightly structured routines—can make it harder for some students to enter learning. Approaches that privilege one form of reasoning or presentation can also limit opportunities for students whose strengths lie in visual, spatial, oral, or collaborative modes. These patterns do not reflect gaps in student ability. They reflect instructional formats that favour some learners over others. For students who have experienced threat, these narrow formats can heighten vigilance and force them to split attention between monitoring the room and following instruction. For those shaped by deprivation, they can expose gaps in prior opportunities for language-rich dialogue, scaffolded practice, or structured reasoning. Instructional design, in other words, can either buffer the impact of threat and deprivation or recreate the conditions that make learning feel risky or inaccessible. Evidence supports the value of instructional flexibility. A meta-analysis by Smale-Jacobse et al. (2019) demonstrated that differentiated approaches—varying explanations, task entry points, and supports—produce meaningful improvements in academic outcomes. The effect size ($g = 1.109$) shows that responsiveness in instruction is not remedial. It is central to effective teaching. Cafaro et al. (2023) similarly found that instruction strengthened when social-emotional supports were built into disciplinary teaching rather than bolted on as extras. When emotional and cognitive supports are integrated, students participate more confidently and sustain attention for longer.

Instruction also shapes how learners navigate abstract or complex ideas. Research with neurodiverse students highlights this point. A review by Cheung and Slavin (2016) shows that many learners experience content as inaccessible not because the material is too difficult, but because explanations move too quickly from concrete to abstract or lean heavily on decontextualised examples. When instruction does not offer multiple ways to enter and rehearse ideas, the curriculum becomes harder to grasp and easier to misinterpret. For students carrying stress or limited prior scaffolding, this creates cumulative cognitive load: threat amplifies their need for predictability; deprivation limits the background knowledge they can draw upon. These patterns echo findings from Aronson and Laughter (2016), who show that instructional spaces often reinforce narrow norms for participation—valuing fast answers, privileging confident debate, or rewarding a single "academic" communication style. Nasir (2012) similarly found that students from minoritised groups feel pressure to adjust their ways of speaking or reasoning to match perceived expectations. These dynamics act as subtle forms of threat: cues that their natural ways of thinking may not belong. They also function as forms of deprivation by withholding opportunities for students to use the cultural and cognitive resources that anchor their learning. Taken together, this evidence underscores a central point: curriculum becomes inclusive or exclusionary through the instructional practices that carry it. When instruction offers multiple pathways into ideas, allocates time for processing, and legitimises varied forms of expression, it expands access. When it relies on narrow formats or rapid pacing, it restricts access and increases the likelihood that students experience curriculum as distant or misaligned with their strengths. Instructional design becomes part of the psychological environment—one that either heightens the load of threat and deprivation or reduces it.

Curriculum also shapes how students understand themselves within schooling. For learners already navigating cumulative harm, the messages embedded in content and instruction can either heighten vulnerability or support recovery. Research in curriculum theory and equity-focused pedagogy shows that students interpret curriculum not only as information, but as a reflection of whose knowledge is valued and whose identities are recognised (Au, 2021). When curriculum omits students' cultural histories or presents dominant narratives as universal, the absence carries meaning. Students often distance themselves from learning—not as resistance, but as a way to protect dignity in environments that feel misaligned with their realities (Macfarlane & Macfarlane, 2019). In Indigenous education, studies show that curricular erasure contributes to decreased belonging, reduced trust, and poorer academic outcomes (Keddie, 2012; Lowe et al., 2025). These experiences echo prior forms of marginalisation and reinforce the belief that school was not built for them. Linguistic equity research shows similar patterns: when teachers correct or devalue home languages or culturally shaped communication styles, students read these actions as judgments of identity rather than learning feedback (Gutiérrez, 2008; Paris & Alim, 2017). For students already carrying chronic threat-based arousal, such signals become additional cognitive burdens. For students shaped by deprivation, they remove yet another source of cultural grounding.

Conversely, evidence shows that when curriculum validates diverse identities, students display stronger engagement, persistence, and participation. Ladson-Billings (2021) found that culturally responsive teaching—where curriculum incorporates students' cultural referents and community knowledge—improves outcomes across grade levels. Bonilla et al. (2021) similarly found that students from marginalised communities achieve better results when curricular materials reflect their histories and intellectual traditions. When students encounter texts, examples, and tasks that affirm their identities, the cognitive effort required to monitor for threat decreases. This frees working-memory resources and increases readiness to participate. These effects span all subject areas. Research across STEM fields shows that contextualised tasks, community-connected examples, and instruction rooted in lived experience improve motivation and conceptual understanding (Nasir, 2021; Rahm & Gorges, 2018). For students carrying cumulative stress, this grounding makes academic work less psychologically costly.

Taken together, these findings show that curriculum operates as both a cultural message and a psychological environment. For students affected by threat and deprivation, recognition within curriculum is not simply a matter of representation. It is a core condition for relational trust, academic engagement, and willingness to take intellectual risks. When curriculum affirms students' histories and identities, it becomes a stabilising force. When it excludes them, it can reproduce the same patterns of marginalisation they already know how to survive.

When Mr. Lewis begins a Year 7 Humanities unit on "Australian Settlement," he notices a subtle change in Maya's engagement. She had previously contributed readily, but as the class moves through textbook chapters framed almost entirely from British perspectives, she becomes quieter. During a reading that describes Indigenous groups as "nomadic tribes," she lowers her gaze and stops participating in discussion. Nothing disruptive occurs, but her presence in the room becomes noticeably smaller. Later, in a planning meeting, Mr. Lewis reflects on what he observed. He recognises that the materials present a narrow historical narrative—one that omits Indigenous resistance, cultural continuity, and connections to Country. Drawing on research showing that curriculum communicates implicit messages about whose knowledge matters (Au, 2021), he begins to suspect that Maya may be interpreting these omissions as devaluing her community.

He also realises that his instructional choices may have amplified the issue. Fast-paced whole-class questioning left little room for students who needed time to process ideas or connect them to their own experiences. When a student mentioned their family's migration story, he moved on quickly to keep the lesson on schedule, unintentionally signalling that such perspectives were peripheral. The next week, he revises the lessons to include Indigenous-authored sources, examples of cultural resilience, and structured opportunities for students to respond in pairs before whole-class talk. Students are invited to draw connections between the content and their own communities.

MITIGATING THE IMPACTS OF CUMULATIVE HARM IN EDUCATION

Effective implementation of practices that mitigate the effects of cumulative harm requires close attention to the fit between learners, content, and environment. It involves understanding how students *experience* the curriculum, anticipating where they may need guidance, and adjusting instructional routines so learning remains accessible and coherent. Implementation is not a set of isolated strategies; it is a continuous loop of planning, observing, interpreting, and refining. When this cycle works well, students encounter classrooms that support engagement, clarity, and sustained participation. This framework is organised into three interconnected phases: Preparation and Assessment, Implementation and Monitoring, and Evaluation and Adjustment. Together, these phases offer a coherent way to translate educational principles into practice, especially for students whose development has been shaped by threat or deprivation.

In the first phase, Preparation and Assessment, teachers analyse the demands of the curriculum and consider how different learners will experience them. They identify content that may be dense, culturally narrow, or emotionally loaded for students carrying histories of threat, and they examine whether their usual routines genuinely support access. Observations, prior data, and student feedback help clarify likely learning conditions and highlight where deprivation-related gaps in background knowledge or threat-related sensitivities may create barriers. In the second phase, Implementation and Monitoring, planning becomes action. Teachers present lessons with clear structure and watch how students respond. They track engagement, notice confusion, and adjust explanations, pacing, or examples when needed. Instruction is shaped by what happens in real time rather than by a fixed script. This responsiveness is especially important for students whose attention, working memory, or sense of safety fluctuates depending on how the environment cues threat or predictability. In the third phase, Evaluation and Adjustment, teachers reflect on how students interpreted the lesson, whether access was equitable, and which practices were effective. They consider how their own decisions—and their own emotional states—may have influenced learning. These reflections help refine future instruction. Conversations with colleagues broaden understanding and help teachers interpret challenging moments through a developmental lens rather than a deficit lens, particularly when behaviours reflect adaptations to deprivation or attempts to manage threat. Together, these phases position implementation as a dynamic, iterative process that links planning with lived experience. They encourage teachers to move beyond seeing curriculum as a static sequence of tasks and instead understand teaching as continuous decision-making grounded in observation, interpretation, and revision.

Preparation and Learning Needs Assessments

Preparation establishes the environmental, relational, and instructional conditions that allow curriculum and pedagogy to function as intended. It starts from a simple premise: students do not encounter learning in a vacuum. They bring prior experiences, cultural identities, strengths, and constraints that interact with everything the school asks of them. Preparation is about aligning instructional plans, school structures, and learning conditions so students can enter the curriculum with clarity, stability, and confidence. This requires a school-wide commitment to consistency and fairness. Research shows that most children and adolescents have experienced some form of adversity, and that these experiences are strongly associated with later disparities in health, behaviour, and learning (Hughes et al., 2017; Sahle et al., 2023). Schools that adopt a universal, preventative stance—assuming that *any* student may carry invisible pressures linked to threat or deprivation—are better positioned to create predictable and coherent learning environments (SAMHSA, 2014). This stance shifts the emphasis from reacting to problems toward building stable routines, transparent expectations, and clear communication from the outset.

School readiness plays a central role in this phase. Reviews of whole-school models indicate that implementation is most effective when leadership, staff cohesion, and organisational structures support consistent practice across classrooms (Maynard et al., 2019). Australian studies similarly highlight that readiness must be established before more specialised supports can work as intended (Rojas-Andrade & Leiva, 2019). Preparation is therefore not a box to tick and leave behind. It is an ongoing organisational condition grounded in shared professional language, sustained training, and reflective dialogue. Cultural responsiveness is a foundational part of readiness. Studies in education and public health show that programs addressing the social and structural roots of adversity—rather than focusing solely on individual behaviour—produce stronger and more sustainable outcomes (Lorenc et al., 2020). In schools, preparation must therefore include attention to cultural protocols, community relationships, and inclusive communication practices. Establishing these conditions early reduces the risk that curriculum or instruction will contradict, diminish, or misrepresent a student's identity—an experience that can be especially harmful for students already navigating deprivation-related gaps in opportunity or threat-related patterns of vigilance.

Once these environmental and cultural conditions are in place, educators move into learning needs assessment. This phase shifts the focus from organisational readiness to a clearer understanding of the learners in the classroom. Assessments extend beyond academic metrics to capture the full range of factors that shape learning. Global evidence links experiences of violence, instability, or prolonged stress with reductions in educational attainment, motivation, and persistence (Crouch et al., 2019). Effective assessment therefore considers how students manage attention, transitions, and task demands; how they connect with peers and teachers; and how they approach problem-solving and goal-directed tasks—domains often disrupted by threat and deprivation. Research offers guidance for understanding these domains. Studies on resilience show that learning readiness is shaped by students' ability to regulate attention, manage stress, and re-engage after setbacks—and that these capacities improve in environments that consistently support them (Chen et al., 2022). Evidence linking adverse childhood experiences with loneliness demonstrates that social disconnection is a powerful mediator of disengagement (Sahle et al., 2023). Systematic reviews also show consistent associations between adversity and diminished executive function, working memory, and persistence (Tiego et al., 2020). These findings justify assessing indicators such as adaptability, initiative, and relational engagement alongside literacy and numeracy measures.

Universal precautions extend into classroom climate. Rather than identifying "traumatised learners," teachers cultivate environments that minimise potential triggers and maximise regulatory support. Meta-analyses show that teacher-delivered trauma-informed strategies—calm tone of voice, consistent feedback loops, and structured transitions—reduce behavioural incidents and enhance engagement (Cafaro et al., 2023). These findings move neurodevelopmental evidence into practice: stable routines and emotionally attuned teaching are protective factors, not optional enhancements. Physical design also communicates psychological safety. Systematic reviews of trauma-responsive schools show that students experience lower stress in classrooms with clear sightlines, access to quiet areas, and flexible sensory zones (Maynard et al., 2019). These adaptations represent a shift from behaviour management toward regulation support. When paired with transparent communication and relational predictability, they operationalise SAMHSA's principles of safety and trustworthiness. Reviews of interventions for people exposed to adverse childhood experiences show stronger outcomes when programs address social and structural inequities rather than individual pathology (Myat Zaw et al., 2022). In school settings, this means embedding cultural protocols, community consultation, and inclusive language from the outset. Culturally grounded readiness reduces the risk of re-enacting systemic trauma and affirms learners' sense of belonging.

Comprehensive assessment requires multiple perspectives. Quantitative indicators capture performance patterns, but they cannot explain how students interpret their experiences. Qualitative insights—student reflections, observations, and family perspectives—add essential information about motivation, identity, and meaning-making (Mullin et al., 2024). Mixed-method approaches therefore provide a more accurate picture of learning needs and strengthen instructional planning. Interpretation also requires attention to social and cultural context. Meta-analyses show that adversity interacts with systemic factors such as socioeconomic conditions and historical marginalisation to shape developmental outcomes (Hughes et al., 2017; Lorenc et al., 2020). Educators who interpret data through contextual rather than deficit lenses are better positioned to identify protective factors and strengths. For Aboriginal and Torres Strait Islander students, practices connected to Country, kinship, and community identity are not peripheral—they are central to learning and engagement (Bishop & Berryman, 2006). Research supports this strengths-oriented approach. Reviews show that programs emphasising agency and empowerment produce more stable and enduring outcomes than those rooted primarily in deficit identification (Cardoso et al., 2025). Meta-analytic work in resilience research highlights the value of recognising individual interests and cultural assets as drivers of engagement (Chen et al., 2022). Including these elements shifts assessment from identifying gaps to identifying capacities that instruction can leverage.

Finally, preparation and assessment must be iterative. Students' needs shift over time and learning environments must adapt accordingly. Systematic reviews of school frameworks show that sustainability depends on ongoing monitoring, cross-disciplinary collaboration, and regular reflection on practice (Maynard et al., 2019). Preparation, then, is not a preliminary phase—it is a continuous stance. Educators remain attentive to emerging patterns, responsive to new information, and committed to refining the conditions that support effective learning.

Implementation and Monitoring

Integrating supportive practices into curriculum requires attention to predictability, clarity, and relational coherence. Students who have lived with threat or deprivation learn to scan for cues of safety or danger long before they engage with content. Consistent routines, attuned feedback, and structured communication help reduce ambiguity in the environment, which in turn reduces behavioural disruptions and improves engagement (Cafaro et al., 2023). Systematic reviews show that these gains are strongest when teachers receive sustained professional learning, clear organisational expectations, and leadership support (Rojas-Andrade & Leiva, 2019). In other words, effective implementation depends as much on the broader instructional environment as it does on any individual classroom strategy.

Curriculum design also shapes the ease and fidelity of implementation. Lessons broken into manageable stages allow students to build understanding gradually. They also provide teachers with built-in moments to adjust task complexity when signs of overload, confusion, or emotional strain emerge. Research consistently show that combining universal routines with flexible, targeted adjustments leads to stronger academic and behavioural outcomes than relying on either approach alone (Maynard et al., 2019). Integrating short opportunities for cognitive reset—reflective writing, brief breathing pauses, or predictable transition cues—has also been associated with moderate improvements in executive functioning and classroom climate when embedded into regular instruction (Zhai et al., 2022). Although these effects are modest, they illustrate that regulation and focus can be supported through low-intensity, high-frequency practices that do not disrupt curriculum flow.

Cultural and linguistic relevance is another essential component of implementation. Reviews of Australian school programs show that students respond more positively when curriculum materials reflect community language, local history, and cultural practice (Keddie, 2012). When content aligns with lived experience, students expend less cognitive effort monitoring for threat and more energy engaging with ideas. Implementation, therefore, requires both technical precision and cultural alignment. Differentiation extends this work by matching instruction to the varied cognitive, motivational, and relational profiles that students bring to learning. Students who experience heightened arousal benefit from calm, predictable environments, while those who show under-arousal may engage more fully in interactive, relationally rich tasks (Weissman et al., 2022). Differentiation also requires awareness of sociocultural context. Including multiple worldviews, languages, and abilities within curriculum materials reduces the likelihood that students will perceive school knowledge as distant or exclusionary. Although research on these adaptations is still developing, reviews consistently link culturally matched instruction to stronger attendance and relational engagement (Morrison et al., 2008). Differentiation is therefore best understood as an equity strategy that strengthens access rather than a remedial adjustment.

The quality of implementation is central to whether these practices have their intended effect. Systematic reviews show that adherence to planned routines, appropriate dosage, and high-quality delivery significantly moderate program outcomes (Avery et al., 2021). This evidence reinforces the need for deliberate and well-documented adaptations rather than improvised changes made under pressure. Schools typically achieve stronger fidelity when implementation is supported through instructional coaching, professional dialogue, and structured observation.

Monitoring is integral to effective implementation. Whole-school reviews find that lasting improvement emerges when teams regularly gather and interpret both quantitative and qualitative data (Newton et al., 2024). Attendance patterns, task completion, and behavioural incidents provide early indicators of shifts in experience. Meta-analytic evidence shows measurable reductions in suspensions and improvements in attendance following the introduction of supportive instructional frameworks, although changes in academic performance are more variable (Avery et al., 2021). These mixed findings highlight the need for continuous adjustment rather than adherence to rigid intervention plans. Qualitative insights deepen this understanding. Educator reflections, student interviews, and classroom discussions shed light on how routines, feedback, and interactions are interpreted in real time. Mixed-method approaches are particularly valuable because they connect observable patterns with the meanings students assign to them, which research links to stronger relational and academic gains (Norrish & Brunzell, 2023). Effective monitoring therefore attends not only to outcomes but also to the processes shaping those outcomes—especially for students who interpret classroom cues through the lens of past threat or deprivation.

Monitoring also extends to staff capacity and organisational functioning. Reviews emphasise that sustainable implementation depends on clear role definitions, adequate training, and collective efficacy among staff (Norrish & Brunzell, 2023). Schools that track these organisational indicators can more quickly identify where additional coaching, resource allocation, or policy adjustments are needed. Participatory monitoring strengthens both accuracy and student agency. Inviting learners to articulate what helps or hinders their ability to focus, engage, or complete tasks aligns with evidence linking empowerment to improved participation and persistence (Cafaro et al., 2023). Tools such as student feedback surveys, wellbeing committees, and classroom reflection routines help educators identify hidden barriers to learning and refine practice accordingly. Finally, monitoring must be continuous and transparent. Implementation research shows across multiple frameworks that improvement depends on ongoing cycles of planning, observation, adjustment, and review (Maynard et al., 2019). When teachers and school teams treat monitoring as shared inquiry rather than compliance, implementation becomes a dynamic system—one that adapts to student needs, incorporates new evidence, and steadily strengthens the quality of classroom instruction.

Evaluation

Evaluation determines whether supportive and equity-focused practices are achieving their intended outcomes and how they should be improved. Rather than functioning as a compliance exercise or procedural audit, evaluation asks a deeper question: *What has actually changed for learners, relationships, and the wider school system?* It is inherently interpretive. It requires educators to analyse learner outcomes while also reflecting on how their own assumptions, expectations, and decisions shape the conditions in which students learn (Dombo & Sabin, 2020). High-quality evaluation recognises that educational practices operate across multiple levels. Individual outcomes appear in shifts in attendance, engagement, self-efficacy, or persistence. Relational outcomes show up in trust, cooperation, and the degree to which students feel recognised by peers and teachers. System-level outcomes include improvements in school climate, consistency of routines, and reductions in disciplinary disparities. Systematic reviews show that whole-school frameworks can produce positive effects across these domains, although the magnitude of change depends heavily on context and fidelity of implementation (Newton et al., 2024).

At the individual level, meta-analytic evidence links adversity and instability with reduced resilience and lower academic confidence, highlighting the importance of measuring agency and self-belief as indicators of progress (Chen et al., 2022). At the relational level, studies show that when teachers build confidence in classroom management and interpersonal communication, classrooms become more cooperative, routines become smoother, and conflict decreases (Duan et al., 2024). At the systemic level, structured whole-school approaches supported by strong leadership and ongoing professional learning improve belonging and perceived safety (Berger, 2019). Yet evaluations that rely only on quantitative indicators offer an incomplete picture. Metrics such as attendance, disciplinary incidents, or wellbeing scores can reveal meaningful shifts, and Australian reviews show small-to-moderate behavioural and engagement improvements when schools use consistent, structured practices (Roseby & Gascoigne, 2021). But numbers alone cannot explain why change occurred or how students interpreted their experiences. Qualitative evidence—student narratives, teacher reflections, classroom artefacts—adds this missing layer. Umbrella reviews consistently find that mixed-methods evaluation provides the most valid and contextually sensitive account of impact (Cardoso et al., 2025).

Evaluation is often iterative. Research on school-wide frameworks shows that programs with ongoing feedback loops—where data are reviewed regularly and used to shape practice—produce stronger and more durable outcomes than those relying on one-off assessments (Mullin et al., 2024). Continuous review keeps evaluation aligned with the changing needs of learners and the evolving demands of schooling. A central component of this process is reflexive practice. Reflexivity requires educators to examine how power, identity, and professional norms influence their decisions and responses. Dombo and Sabin (2020) argue that many educational initiatives fall short because they prioritise outcome measurement while neglecting the interpretive habits shaping teacher behaviour. Reflexive evaluation asks who benefits from specific practices, whose perspectives are prioritised, and whose experiences are overlooked. Evidence shows that structured reflection—peer supervision, guided dialogue, reflective writing—reduces educator stress and strengthens confidence in decision-making (Newton et al., 2024). Duan et al. (2024) similarly demonstrate that teacher self-efficacy supports both personal resilience and healthier classroom climates, illustrating the reciprocal relationship between educator wellbeing and student experience.

Reflexive evaluation extends beyond individual insight to the broader structures that shape practice. Policy constraints, workload demands, staffing levels, and organisational culture often determine whether practices are delivered consistently (Cardoso et al., 2025). Documenting these contextual factors shifts evaluation from assessing individual performance to understanding organisational learning. When schools identify structural barriers—such as role ambiguity, class size, or inconsistent scheduling—they are better positioned to implement systemic solutions rather than expecting individual teachers to compensate. Myat Zaw et al. (2022) emphasise that organisational readiness and policy alignment are decisive factors in sustaining effective frameworks.

Ongoing improvement requires using evidence to refine practice, inform policy, and strengthen professional learning. Reviews of Australian and international models show that the most effective schools embed evaluation findings directly into curriculum design, pedagogical planning, and teacher development (Mullin et al., 2024). Research highlights three features of strong improvement cycles. First, involving students and teachers in interpreting data enhances ownership and accuracy (Maynard et al., 2019). Second, transparent reporting—including limitations—builds trust and maintains accountability (Dombo & Sabin, 2020). Third, integrating feedback into planning ensures that learning from one cycle informs the next. Schools that approach evaluation as shared inquiry rather than performance auditing show stronger fidelity and higher staff retention (Mullin et al., 2024).

Knowledge translation must operate across multiple levels. In classrooms, teachers adjust routines and explanations based on evidence of engagement or misunderstanding. At the school level, leadership teams use findings to guide staffing, policy, and resource allocation. At the system level, networks of schools share insights to strengthen practice across settings. Umbrella reviews confirm that this multi-layered flow of knowledge is essential for sustaining long-term improvement (Lorenc et al., 2020). By integrating quantitative and qualitative data, engaging in reflexive analysis, and translating insights into structural change, schools create conditions where improvement is continuous and meaningful. Each evaluative cycle deepens understanding, broadens access to learning, and reinforces equity as a guiding principle.

CONCLUSION

Cumulative harm affects learning through intertwined physiological, relational, and cognitive pathways, but its consequences—*and its possibilities for repair*—are most visible in classrooms. A learning-centred stance treats behaviour as information about a student's workload, stress, or sense of safety. It positions educators as designers of environments that support regulation, belonging, and sustained engagement. Across the chapter, we have shown how experiences shaped by threat and deprivation demand distinct instructional responses; how teacher assumptions, emotional load, and classroom conditions can unintentionally reproduce earlier patterns of harm; and why curriculum must shift from presumed neutrality toward cultural relevance so learners see their identities recognised rather than sidelined.

Implementation translates these understandings into daily practice. Preparation involves building predictable, culturally grounded environments and conducting holistic assessments that capture engagement, regulation, and relational factors alongside academic performance. Instruction then unfolds through differentiated, responsive, and contextually aligned routines that are continuously monitored and adapted. Evaluation integrates quantitative indicators with qualitative insight and adds reflexive review of how power, expectations, and educator decisions shape learning conditions. When planning, action, observation, and adjustment operate as a coherent cycle, schools move from reactive management to proactive developmental support. In this way, education becomes a reliably regulating and identity-affirming context—one that interrupts reenactments of threat or deprivation and offers students a genuine pathway to recovery and thriving.

REFERENCES

Apple, M. W. (2012). *Education and power* (2nd ed.). Routledge., DOI: 10.4324/9780203143124

Aronson, B., & Laughter, J. (2016). The theory and practice of culturally relevant education: A synthesis of research across content areas. *Review of Educational Research, 86*(1), 163–206. DOI: 10.3102/0034654315582066

Au, W. (2021). A pedagogy of insurgency: Teaching and organizing for radical racial justice in our schools. *Educational Studies (Ames), 57*(2), 109–123. DOI: 10.1080/00131946.2021.1878181

Avery, J. C., Morris, H., Galvin, E., Misso, M., Savaglio, M., & Skouteris, H. (2021). Systematic review of school-wide trauma-informed approaches. *Journal of Child & Adolescent Trauma, 14*(3), 381–397. DOI: 10.1007/s40653-020-00321-1 PMID: 34471456

Berger, E. (2019). Multi-tiered approaches to trauma-informed care in schools: A systematic review. *School Mental Health, 11*(4), 650–664. DOI: 10.1007/s12310-019-09326-0

Berman, S. L., Weems, C. F., & Stickle, T. R. (2022). Threat detection and attention to danger cues in youth exposed to adversity: A systematic review. *Clinical Child and Family Psychology Review, 25*(2), 289–312. DOI: 10.1007/s10567-021-00358-1

Bishop, R., & Berryman, M. (2006). *Culture speaks: Cultural relationships and classroom learning*. Huia Publishers.

Bloom, S. L. (1997). *Creating sanctuary: Toward the evolution of sane societies*. Routledge.

Bonilla, S., Dee, T. S., & Penner, E. K. (2021). Ethnic studies increases longer-run academic engagement and attainment. *Proceedings of the National Academy of Sciences of the United States of America, 118*(37), e2026386118. DOI: 10.1073/pnas.2026386118 PMID: 34493663

Bottiani, J. H., Bradshaw, C. P., & Mendelson, T. (2018). A multilevel examination of racial disparities in high school discipline. *School Psychology Review, 47*(2), 174–187. DOI: 10.17105/SPR-2017-0070.V47-2

Busso, D. S., McLaughlin, K. A., & Sheridan, M. A. (2017). Dimensions of adversity, stress reactivity, and school functioning in middle childhood. *Development and Psychopathology, 29*(5), 1711–1723. DOI: 10.1017/S0954579417001358

Cafaro, A., Durlak, J. A., & Taylor, R. D. (2023). Effects of teacher-delivered social and emotional learning interventions on student outcomes: A meta-analysis. *School Psychology Review, 52*(2), 170–187. DOI: 10.1080/2372966X.2021.2009940

Cardoso, A. S., Martins, R. C., Venturin, B., Gonzalez, A., Blumenberg, C., & Murray, J. (2025). Psychosocial adversity and executive functions in children and adolescents: A systematic review of mediating and moderating influences of parenting behaviors. *BMC Psychiatry, 25*(1), 894. DOI: 10.1186/s12888-025-06592-y PMID: 41029261

Chen, Y., Zhang, L., & McLaughlin, K. A. (2022). Resilience and developmental outcomes following childhood adversity: A meta-analysis. *Psychological Bulletin, 148*(4), 305–341. DOI: 10.1037/bul000036

Cheung, A., & Slavin, R. E. (2016). Effective reading programs for secondary students. *Reading Research Quarterly, 51*(4), 389–416. DOI: 10.1002/rrq.154

Civitillo, S., Meyer, A., & Jügert, T. (2023). Students' perceptions of differential teacher treatment and academic outcomes: A meta-analysis. *Journal of School Psychology, 98*, 1–18. DOI: 10.1016/j.jsp.2022.12.001

Crouch, E., Radcliff, E., Hung, P., & Bennett, K. (2019). Challenges to school success and the role of adverse childhood experiences. *Academic Pediatrics, 19*(8), 899–907. DOI: 10.1016/j.acap.2019.08.006 PMID: 31401231

Dombo, E. A., & Sabin, M. (2020). Trauma-informed supervision for helping professionals. *Clinical Social Work Journal, 48*, 1–12. DOI: 10.1007/s10615-019-00729-6

Doyle, C., & Cicchetti, D. (2018). Attachment-related processes in maltreated children. *Child Development Perspectives, 12*(4), 235–240. DOI: 10.1111/cdep.12291

Duan, W., Bissaker, K., & Xu, S. (2024). Teacher classroom management self-efficacy and classroom climate: A meta-analysis. *Teaching and Teacher Education, 138*, 104329. DOI: 10.1016/j.tate.2023.104329

Glock, S., Krolak-Schwerdt, S., Klapproth, F., & Böhmer, M. (2019). Teachers' expectancy effects: A meta-analysis. *Educational Research Review, 27*, 210–228. DOI: 10.1016/j.edurev.2019.03.001

Gutiérrez, K. (2008). Developing a sociocritical literacy in the third space. *Reading Research Quarterly, 43*(2), 148–164. DOI: 10.1598/RRQ.43.2.3

Hein, T. C., & Monk, C. S. (2017). Research review: Neural response to threat in children, adolescents, and adults following early life stress. *Journal of Child Psychology and Psychiatry, and Allied Disciplines, 58*(3), 222–230. DOI: 10.1111/jcpp.12651 PMID: 27778344

Hughes, K., Bellis, M. A., Hardcastle, K., Sethi, D., Butchart, A., Mikton, C., Jones, L., & Dunne, M. (2017). The effect of multiple adverse childhood experiences on health: A systematic review and meta-analysis. *The Lancet. Public Health, 2*(8), e356–e366. DOI: 10.1016/S2468-2667(17)30118-4 PMID: 29253477

Johnson, S. B., Riis, J. L., & Noble, K. G. (2021). Socioeconomic inequality and executive function trajectories in childhood. *Developmental Science, 24*(1), e12901. DOI: 10.1111/desc.12901

Johnstone, L., & Boyle, M. (2018). *The Power Threat Meaning Framework: Overview.* British Psychological Society.

Keddie, A. (2012). Schooling and disadvantage: From deficit approaches to relational reform. *International Journal of Inclusive Education, 16*(10), 1001–1012. DOI: 10.1080/13603116.2010.538865

Kirk, R., Lewis, R., Brown, T., & Marsh, L. (2017). The impact of childhood violence exposure on educational outcomes: A global systematic review. *Trauma, Violence & Abuse, 18*(4), 452–471. DOI: 10.1177/1524838015622437

Ladson-Billings, G. (2021). Three decades of culturally relevant, responsive, & sustaining pedagogy: What lies ahead? []. Routledge.]. *The Educational Forum, 85*(4), 351–354. DOI: 10.1080/00131725.2021.1957632

Lorenc, T., Lester, S., Sutcliffe, K., Stansfield, C., & Thomas, J. (2020). Interventions to support children exposed to adversity. *Public Health Reviews, 41*, 6. DOI: 10.1186/s40985-020-00127-0

Lowe, K., Golledge, C., Poulton, P., & Thompson, K. (2025). Curriculum as policy deception: A critical analysis of Aboriginal and Torres Strait Islander knowledge inclusion in the Australian Curriculum. *Australian Educational Researcher, 52*(3), 2561–2582. DOI: 10.1007/s13384-025-00824-6

Macfarlane, A., & Macfarlane, S. (2019). Listen to culture: Māori scholars' plea to researchers. *Journal of the Royal Society of New Zealand, 49*(sup1), 48-57.

Maynard, B. R., Farina, A., Dell, N. A., & Kelly, M. S. (2019). Effects of trauma-informed approaches in schools: A systematic review. *Campbell Systematic Reviews, 15*(1-2), e1018. DOI: 10.1002/cl2.1018 PMID: 37131480

McEwen, B. S., & Morrison, J. H. (2013). The brain on stress. *Neuron, 79*(1), 16–29. DOI: 10.1016/j.neuron.2013.06.028 PMID: 23849196

McLaughlin, K. A., Sheridan, M. A., Humphreys, K. L., Belsky, J., & Ellis, B. J. (2021). The value of dimensional models of early experience: Thinking clearly about concepts and categories. *Perspectives on Psychological Science, 16*(6), 1463–1472. DOI: 10.1177/1745691621992346 PMID: 34491864

McLaughlin, K. A., Sheridan, M. A., & Lambert, H. K. (2014). Dimensions of early experience and neural development: Deprivation and threat. *Current Directions in Psychological Science, 23*(1), 47–52. DOI: 10.1177/0963721413515590 PMID: 25454359

Morrison, K. A., Robbins, H., & Rose, D. G. (2008). Operationalizing culturally relevant pedagogy. *Teaching and Teacher Education, 24*(6), 1574–1590. DOI: 10.1016/j.tate.2008.02.013

Mullin, A. C., Sharkey, J. D., & Barnett, M. (2024, May). Advancing trauma informed practices in schools using the Consolidated Framework for Implementation Research. [). Frontiers Media SA.]. *Frontiers in Education, 9*, 1346933. DOI: 10.3389/feduc.2024.1346933

Myat Zaw, A. M., Win, N. Z., & Thepthien, B. O. (2022). Adolescents' academic achievement, mental health, and adverse behaviors: Understanding the role of resilience and adverse childhood experiences. *School Psychology International, 43*(5), 516–536. DOI: 10.1177/01430343221107114

Nasir, N. I. S. (2021). Teaching for equity: Where developmental needs meet racialized structures. In *The Science of Learning and Development* (pp. 177–184). Routledge.

Newton, L., Keane, C. A., & Byrne, M. K. (2024). Trauma-informed programs in Australian schools: A systematic review of design, implementation and efficacy. *Children and Youth Services Review, 156*, 107368. DOI: 10.1016/j.childyouth.2023.107368

Norrish, J., & Brunzell, T. (2023). How is trauma-informed education implemented within classrooms? A synthesis of trauma-informed education programs. *The Australian Journal of Teacher Education, 48*(3), 94–120. DOI: 10.14221/1835-517X.6159

Paris, D., & Alim, H. S. (2017). *Culturally sustaining pedagogies: Teaching and learning for justice in a changing world.* Teachers College Press.

Rahm, J., & Gorges, A. (2018). STEM learning in everyday spaces. *Science Education, 102*(4), 617–638. DOI: 10.1002/sce.21444

Rojas-Andrade, R., & Leiva, L. (2019). Is implementation fidelity important? A systematic review on school-based mental health programs. *Contemporary School Psychology*, *23*(4), 339–350. DOI: 10.1007/s40688-018-0175-0

Roorda, D. L., Jak, S., Zee, M., Oort, F. J., & Koomen, H. M. (2017). Affective teacher–student relationships and students' engagement and achievement: A meta-analytic update and test of the mediating role of engagement. *School Psychology Review*, *46*(3), 239–261. DOI: 10.17105/SPR-2017-0035.V46-3

Roseby, V., & Gascoigne, M. (2021). A systematic review of trauma-informed practices in schools. *Educational Psychology in Practice*, *37*(1), 1–23. DOI: 10.1080/02667363.2020.1841839

Sahle, B. W., Reavley, N. J., & Morgan, A. J. (2023). Adverse childhood experiences and educational attainment: A global review. *Child Abuse & Neglect*, *136*, 105995. DOI: 10.1016/j.chiabu.2022.105995

SAMHSA. (2014). *SAMHSA's concept of trauma and guidance for a trauma-informed approach.* U.S. Department of Health and Human Services.

Shah, R., DeYoung, A., & Moffitt, T. (2022). Childhood adversity and lifelong health: A developmental review. *Annual Review of Developmental Psychology*, *4*, 123–147. DOI: 10.1146/annurev-devpsych-121121-021134

Sheridan, M. A., & McLaughlin, K. A. (2016). Neurodevelopmental mechanisms linking adversity and psychopathology. *Annual Review of Clinical Psychology*, *12*, 433–458. DOI: 10.1146/annurev-clinpsy-021815-093005

Smale-Jacobse, A. E., Meijer, A., Helms-Lorenz, M., & Maulana, R. (2019). Differentiated instruction in secondary education: A systematic review of research evidence. *Frontiers in Psychology*, *10*, 2366. DOI: 10.3389/fpsyg.2019.02366 PMID: 31824362

Tiego, J., Testa, R., & Arnold, S. R. C. (2020). Executive function in child and adolescent psychopathology: A meta-analysis. *Psychological Bulletin*, *146*(2), 141–180. DOI: 10.1037/bul0000227

Vaidya, N., Marquand, A. F., Nees, F., Siehl, S., & Schumann, G. (2024). The impact of psychosocial adversity on brain and behaviour: An overview of existing knowledge and directions for future research. *Molecular Psychiatry*, *29*(10), 3245–3267. DOI: 10.1038/s41380-024-02556-y PMID: 38658773

Wang, M.-T., Degol, J. L., & Henry, D. (2023). Peer relations and school engagement among adolescents with adversity exposure. *Child Development*, *94*(1), 70–88. DOI: 10.1111/cdev.13869 PMID: 37467355

Weissman, D. G., Rosen, M. L., Colich, N. L., Sambrook, K. A., Lengua, L. J., Sheridan, M. A., & McLaughlin, K. A. (2022). Exposure to violence as an environmental pathway linking low socioeconomic status with altered neural processing of threat and adolescent psychopathology. *Journal of Cognitive Neuroscience*, *34*(10), 1892–1905. DOI: 10.1162/jocn_a_01825 PMID: 35104853

Zhai, F., Waldfogel, J., & Brooks-Gunn, J. (2022). Adverse childhood experiences and children's learning: A population-level analysis. *Child Development*, *93*(2), 367–383. DOI: 10.1111/cdev.13679

KEY TERMS AND DEFINITIONS

Cultural Responsiveness: Alignment of curriculum and instruction with students' cultural identities, histories, and community knowledge.

Deprivation: Absence of stable, responsive relationships or adequate stimulation, limiting opportunities for learning and regulation.

Differentiated Instruction: Adapting explanations, pacing, and task entry points to meet diverse cognitive and emotional needs.

Implementation Fidelity: The degree to which planned instructional and relational practices are delivered consistently and as intended.

Learning Needs Assessment: Holistic analysis of academic, relational, and regulatory factors influencing a student's engagement.

Re-Enactment: Unintentional replaying of past relational patterns in current classroom interactions, often triggered by tone, routine, or perceived threat.

Reflexive Practice: Ongoing examination of how power, bias, and emotional states shape teachers' interpretations and decisions.

Regulation Supports: Instructional routines that stabilise attention, reduce arousal, and create predictable patterns for learning.

Threat: Experiences or cues that signal danger or unpredictability, activating hypervigilance and protective responding.

Chapter 9
From Trauma Narratives to Career Narratives:
Understanding the Accumulated Adverse Experiences of Higher Education Students and Utilizing Trauma

india Bryce
https://orcid.org/0000-0002-3616-8003
University of Southern Queensland, Australia

Janis Powers
Creighton University, USA

ABSTRACT

People's career choices are not necessarily the unfolding of normative experiences. Instead, trauma experienced throughout childhood affects developmental trajectories and career choices. Findings of the study reveal consistent themes pertaining to the meaningfulness ascribed to helping professionals' experiences of cumulative childhood trauma and re-authoring of trauma narratives through a career lens. This chapter will draw on the findings of a recent study by the author (Bryce et al., 2022; 2023) which revealed that through vocational decision making, life, career and trauma narratives converge to foster a reauthoring experience. The intention of this chapter is to collate and synthesise existing research, and the research of the authors, which explores the influence of cumulative trauma and adversity on career decision making, and trauma informed career counselling

DOI: 10.4018/979-8-3373-4064-7.ch009

INTRODUCTION

The perspectives of the many scholars throughout the last 60 years who have explored the connections between childhood and career choice, observed a continued consensus which highlights the significant influence early experiences have on career pathways. According to Malach-Pines and Yanai (2001) an individual is driven to choose a career path which reflects significant childhood experiences, satisfies needs previously unmet in childhood and actualises aspirations inherited through familial heritage. A recent review of existing literature (Bryce et al., 2023), exploring the associations of cumulative harm and childhood trauma on career decision making in people in the helping professions indicated that family of origin dysfunction, parentification, individual characteristics and traits developed through adversity were associated with the career choice in the helping professions. Helping Professions, in the context of this chapter, are defined as those professions which respond to the welfare of individuals and address challenges in a person's physical, psychological, intellectual, and emotional wellbeing. These professions include, but are not limited to, psychology, nursing, counselling, social work, human services, and education (Egan, 2006).

People's career choices are not necessarily the unfolding of normative experiences. Instead, trauma experienced throughout childhood affects developmental trajectories and career choices. Findings of the study reveal consistent themes pertaining to the meaningfulness ascribed to helping professionals' experiences of cumulative childhood trauma and re-authoring of trauma narratives through a career lens. This chapter will draw on the findings of a recent study by the author (Bryce et al., 2022; 2023) which revealed that through vocational decision making, life, career and trauma narratives converge to foster a reauthoring experience.

The increasing prominence of trauma-informed approaches across a range of disciplines, is a response to understanding that trauma is pervasive and that it impacts many life domains, often in deep and life-shaping manners (Fallot & Harris, 2009; Power & Duys, 2020). Trauma-informed vocational motivation involves understanding how past trauma can impact an individual's motivation and career choices and then tailoring interventions to support their strengths and needs, fostering a safe and empowering environment for career exploration and development (Corbett et al., 2024). This approach highlights important considerations about the value of incorporating trauma-informed principles into university processes to better support students who have experienced trauma, marginalization and disadvantages to become career-ready, transition to sustainable employment and lead flourishing lives.

The intention of this chapter is to collate and synthesise existing research, and the research of the authors, which explores the influence of cumulative trauma and adversity on career decision making, and trauma informed career counselling. This chapter will highlight the considerations and opportunities presented by adversity and trauma as a vocational motivation in the helping professions, the reauthoring experience that can be nurtured by trauma informed pedagogy, practice, and career counselling, and the value of understanding and promoting these vocational motivations as a trauma-informed strategy for building resilience and facilitating academic success in the Higher Education Context. Practical tools, such as, the ARCCH model of Resilience, (ARRCH is an acronym that stands for Attachment, Regulation, Culture, Competence, and Health) will be elucidated at the end of the chapter.

POPULATION AND PROBLEM – PREVALENCE OF TRAUMA EXPERIENCES IN HIGHER EDUCATION STUDENTS

International and cross-disciplinary studies have reported that 66–85% of undergraduate students have already experienced at least one traumatic event prior to entering university (Read et al., 2011; Bachrach & Read, 2012; Frazier et al., 2009), and 21% of students reported experiencing trauma while in college (Cless & Goff, 2017; Walters et al., 2024). According to the literature, 73% of college and university students report experiencing a mental health crisis (Gruttadaro & Crudo, 2012). This suggests that any reasonably sized class of students today will likely contain individuals who have experienced personal trauma (Kennedy & Scriver, 2016; Walters et al., 2024). In Australia, it is estimated that 57% of the population has experienced trauma in their lifetime (Rosenman, 2002) with 40% of the population experiencing some form of childhood abuse or neglect by the age of 24 (Mathews et al., 2023). Therefore, it is highly likely that students will face the risk of re-traumatisation and vicarious trauma through exposure to course content, assessment requirements, experiences in the classroom and while on placement during their higher education experience. Some students with histories of trauma, particularly childhood sexual assault, experience continuing psychological distress which can render them liable to not completing higher education (Griffith University, N.D).

Some groups of students may be at higher risk for trauma exposure than others. Female students are more likely to have been exposed to trauma (Read, et al., 2011) and Veteran students represent a significant population of college students who may have a history of trauma exposure (Ackerman, DiRamio, & Mitchell, 2009). Minority students are more likely to report trauma exposure (Read et al., 2011). Trauma exposure in college students can lead to several adverse outcomes. Students with cumulative trauma histories may have difficulty adjusting to college, receive lower grades, and drop out (Banyard & Cantor, 2004, Bryce et al., 2023).

It is important to note that trauma exposure does not necessarily mean that traumatization will occur (Bonanno, 2005; SAMHSA, 2013; Yehuda & Flory, 2007)

Many individuals are resilient and do not experience significant adverse reactions following a traumatic event. However, it is important to be aware of the prevalence of trauma in higher education and therefore the need to create trauma-informed learning environments that support all students (Bryce et al., 2023; Carello & Butler, 2014).

The impact of cumulative adverse childhood events, known as cumulative harm (Bromfield et al., 2007), often results in a lifelong consequence including complex trauma (Felitti et al., 1998). The Australian Child Maltreatment Study (ACMS; Higgins et al., 2023) has provided significant insights into the prevalence and nature of multitype child maltreatment in Australia. The study found that 39.4% participants reported experiencing multitype maltreatment, which includes exposure to two or more types of maltreatment such as physical abuse, sexual abuse, emotional abuse, neglect, and exposure to domestic violence. Additionally, these finding highlights the widespread nature of multitype maltreatment and its potential cumulative impacts on the health and wellbeing of children and adolescents. The study also identified various family related factors that influence the presence of multitype maltreatment,such as parental separation, family mental illness, family substance problems, and family economic hardship. These factors have been shown to double the risk of experiencing multitype maltreatment. The findings underscore the importance of comprehensive and trauma-informed care, including in educational and vocational settings, in addressing the complex impacts of cumulative adverse experiences and trauma.

Trauma that is experienced early in life, has the potential for life-long negative outcomes across the major domains of personal and social functioning with many of these people coming in contact with our criminal justice and mental health systems (Felitti et al., 1998). The pervasive effects of cumulative harm may influence all aspects of an individual's life course, including relationships, education and academic performance, parenting, and career decisions. Whilst adverse experiences in childhood may increase the risk of bias or counter transference and impair or diminish objectivity, a personal history of trauma can also provide strengths which may support an individual's professional capacity. (Tedeschi & Calhoun, 2006).

BRIDGING THE CHASM BETWEEN CUMULATIVE HARM AND CAREER CHOICE

As highlighted throughout this volume, cumulative harm refers to the effects of an accumulation of adverse childhood experience in a child's life (Bromfield, Gillingham & Higgins, 2007). Research to date has shifted from a conceptualisation of isolated events of maltreatment to an understanding of the chronicity of abuse and neglect and the lifespan implications of prolonged and repetitive trauma (Felitti et al., 2003; Higgins, 2004; Bromfield, Gillingham & Higgins, 2007; Fredrico, et al., 2008; Dong et al, 2004). The term 'cumulative harm' was coined by Bromfield et al., (2007), as an over-arching label to describe the impact of chronic maltreatment following their chronic maltreatment studies conducted in 2005. Whilst investigating the chronicity of maltreatment through a broader study, Bromfield and Higgins (2005) identified that repeated maltreatment over extended period was more common than isolated maltreatment, the impact of which could be profound and exponential. The researchers and their colleagues (Bromfield & Higgins, 2005; Bromfield, Gillingham & Higgins, 2007; Bromfield & Miller, 2007) went on to apply the term cumulative harm to "the impact of patterns of circumstances and events in a child's life, which diminish a child's sense of safety, stability and wellbeing" (Bromfield and Miller, 2007, p. 1).

There is agreement in the research relating to child abuse and neglect that multiple and chronic experiences of child maltreatment are more prevalent than single and episodic abuse. The child maltreatment literature clearly articulates that accumulation is a powerful predictor of poor outcomes in adulthood with cumulative harm being the label attributed to the impact of an accumulation of childhood maltreatment experiences (Felitti et al., 1998; Edwards et al., 2003; Bromfield & Higgins, 2005; Bromfield et al., 2007; MacKenzie et al., 2011a; Finkelhor et al., 2007a; 2007b). The impact of cumulative adverse experiences is pervasive and far reaching, having implications for a child's physical and mental health and behaviour, well into adulthood (Felitti et al., 1998; Edwards et al, 2003, Finkelhor et al., 2007b).

An individual's life course trajectory includes vocational experiences; therefore, the negative impact of cumulative harm on the life course can directly affect career decision-making and professional success. This view is well supported in the literature pertaining to childhood, broadly speaking, and its influence on vocational development. We can therefore assume that adversity and trauma in childhood, such as experiences through cumulative harm, would contribute to career decision making. A body of literature exists which identifies the role trauma can play in career decision making, highlighting altruism and remediation as key elements in motivation.

THE IMPACT OF TRAUMA ON HIGHER EDUCATION EXPERIENCES

There are many signs and symptoms of trauma that may be exhibited by higher education students. These may be triggered by external stimuli unique to each individual, and may present as cognitive, emotional, or physiological maladaptive behaviours (American Psychiatric Association, 2013; Substance Abuse and Mental Health Services Administration, 2014; 2023). Cognitive challenges arising from trauma may include difficulty completing tasks, retaining information or actioning memory; experiencing feelings of confusion; or finding it difficult to focus. Emotional and behavioural responses may include experiencing decreased impulse control, heightened emotions, or abnormal responses to everyday events; feelings of depression, anger, or anxiety; or desire to withdraw from social interactions, including experiencing periods of dissociation or disconnection from reality (SAMHSA, 2023). Physiological responses frequently manifest as bodily aches; physical symptoms of anxiety, such as feeling shaky, light-headed, breathless or having an increased heart rate; insomnia or difficulty falling asleep; nightmares or night terrors; flashbacks; or agitation (Hunter 2022).

Literature further indicates that these students, in the process of adjusting to higher education, may achieve poorer academic outcomes, (DeBerard, Spielmans, & Julka, 2004; Smyth et al., 2008), suffer from increased mental health problems, and may be more likely to abandon their study plans (Guttierez & Gutierez, 2019; Read et al., 2011). Traumatic experiences can negatively impact on students' academic performance, often resulting in disengagement and distress (Gildersleeve et al., 2024). Naturally, this can have deleterious effects on academic progress and attainment (Sosu & Pheunpha, 2019). In fact, the US National Alliance on Mental Illness (2011) reported a tertiary student dropout rate of 64% due to mental health-related reasons, with between 45–50% of these students reporting a failure to receive appropriate accommodations or access to mental health support services (National Alliance on Mental Illness, 2011). Given that trauma experiences are prevalent in high education student populations and may result in compromised mental health and academic success, there is a demonstrated need for adequate and appropriate support services to reduce the effects of trauma experiences and mental health problems – including retraumatisation and vicarious traumatisation – on the attrition rates among vulnerable students across higher education campuses. Further, recent research attests to the motivating influence trauma has on career choice and vocational motivation and will be explored in the following section.

TRAUMA, ACADEMIC ACHIEVEMENT AND VOCATIONAL BEHAVIOUR

The Author's recent studies (Bryce, 2022; Bryce et al., 2023) explored how cumulative harm, defined as the effects of multiple adverse circumstances and events in a child's life, influences an individual's decision to enter the helping professions. The initial systematic literature review (Bryce et al., 2023) identified four influences:

family of origin dysfunction, parentification, individual traits and characteristics developed through trauma, and experiential motivations.

The second phase of the research (Bryce et al., 2022), the qualitative study of lived experience revealed that individuals who have experienced cumulative harm are motivated to pursue careers in helping professions by a multiplicity of factors and highlighted consistent themes pertaining to the meaningfulness ascribed to their experiences of childhood trauma and the re-authoring of their trauma narratives. Participants sought to reauthor through the themes of meaning, value, adaptability, and unintentional motivations. However, remedial motivations, especially those met through professional learning and utilisation of trauma to help others, highlighted the dominance of meaning-making and value making as motivations for entering helping professions. This reflected a journey for all participants from identity conclusions formed through childhood trauma to new territories of identity, achieved through a reconstruction of life narratives by integrating career narratives to reframe and make sense of their cumulative harm experiences.

The study (Bryce et al., 2022) found that individuals with a history of cumulative harm often seek to understand their experiences and find meaning in them through their work. This can manifest as a thirst for knowledge, a curiosity to understand others who have experienced trauma, or a desire to use their experiences to help others. Experiences of caring and being cared for as a result of cumulative harm in childhood, such as through parentification or exposure to helping professionals as a child. Parentification, where a child takes on caregiving responsibilities beyond their developmental level, can lead individuals to develop skills and a sense of responsibility that aligns with helping professions Additionally, positive experiences with helping professionals during childhood can inspire individuals to pursue similar careers (Bryce et al., 2022).

Individuals who have experienced cumulative harm may develop traits like empathy, resilience, and a strong sense of justice, which can be valuable in helping professions (Bryce et al., 2023). They may also be drawn to careers that align with their interests and skills developed as a result of their experiences. The study (Bryce et al., 2022) also finds that career choice can be a powerful antidote to cumulative harm, helping individuals to ameliorate and mitigate the lifelong impacts of childhood trauma. This reauthoring experience allows individuals to reconstruct their life narratives by integrating career narratives that reframe, utilize, and find value in their experiences of cumulative harm. The study emphasizes that these motivations are often intertwined and influenced by the individual's identity conclusions formed through their experiences of cumulative harm. The way individuals make meaning of their trauma, the value they ascribe to it, and the adaptations they develop all contribute to their identity and influence their career choices.

While it is recognized that individuals can experience distress and growth simultaneously in response to adversity, more research is needed to explore post-traumatic growth as a potential motivator of career choice, professional capacity, and academic performance. A personal history of trauma may support an individual's professional capacity; however, it is also important to acknowledge that adverse childhood experiences can increase the risk of bias and countertransference that may impair or diminish objectivity. While resilience may play a role in mitigating the effects of abuse and neglect, the effects of prolonged and repeated adversity can diminish its power.

Research suggests (Ungar & Theron, 2020) that there is a relationship between mental health outcomes and the concept of resilience. Ungar and Theron (2020) argue the concept is best understood as the process of multiple biological, psychological, social, and ecological systems interacting in ways that help individuals to regain, sustain, or improve their mental wellbeing when challenged by one or more risk factors. Mental health outcomes are difficult to predict, and resilience may explain, in part, why some individuals with serious risk factors do well while others do not. Resilience is the quality or set of qualities that enable a person to bounce back from adversity. It is important to remember that resilience is dynamic and can be influenced by life experiences. Resilience plays a crucial role in career readiness, particularly for individuals entering demanding helping professions like school counselling. For these future helping professionals in particular, resilience is paramount for navigating their own experiences while effectively supporting clients. Resilience, plays a central and multifaceted role in career readiness, equipping higher education students, as preservice professionals, with the personal resources, professional competencies, and self-awareness needed to navigate the inherent challenges of their chosen profession, sustain their well-being, and ultimately achieve long and successful careers.

REAUTHORING – FROM TRAUMA NARRATIVES TO CAREER NARRATIVES

In 1968, psychiatrist Robert Jay Lifton penned the book, *Death in Life*, about his experiences interviewing survivors of the atomic bombings of Hiroshima and Nagasaki. Over the extensive span of his incredible career, Lifton studied not only survivors of the atomic bombings but Auschwitz survivors, Vietnam war veterans, as well as individuals subjected to repression by the Chinese government. The COVID pandemic prompted him to reflect on what he'd learned about mass trauma and resilience – that telling stories about trauma, and even trying to influence policy, can often help people recover. Now at 97, Lifton has just published his 13th book, *Surviving Our Catastrophes: Resilience and Renewal from Hiroshima to the Covid-19 Pandemic.*

Lifton has stated in lay press interviews (Silberner, 2023),

"I interviewed people who had undergone the most extreme kind of trauma and victimization. And yet some of the very same people who had so suffered from trauma have shown what I call "survivor wisdom" — they transformed themselves from helpless victims to agents of survival".

In an insightful interview in 2017, Judith Herman, author of Trauma and Recovery (1992) remarked:

"I think as people move into their lives again, the ones who do best are the ones who've developed what Robert Jay Lifton calls a 'survivor mission'. I've seen it happen so many times, that people turn this experience around, and make it a gift to others. That really is the only way you can transcend an atrocity. You can't bury it. You can't make it go away. You can't dissociate it. It comes back. But you can transcend it, first by telling the truth about it, and then by using it in the service of humanity, saying, "This isn't the way we want to live. We want to live differently."

Herman (2002) argued that

"Most survivors seek the resolution of their traumatic experience within the confines of their personal lives. But a significant minority, as a result of the trauma, feel called upon to engage in a wider world and discover that they can transform the meaning of their personal tragedy by making it the basis for social action" (p.102).

Bryce and colleagues (2022) identified a 'reauthoring' process in preservice professional working towards their career goals, from identity conclusions formed through childhood trauma to new territories of identity, achieved through a reconstruction of life narratives by integrating career narratives to reframe and make sense of their trauma experiences. According to Bryce et al.,'s study (2022), the first step towards reauthoring a trauma narrative is to acknowledge and understand the trauma itself. This involves recognizing the various forms of adversity experienced, the chronic nature of the trauma, and its pervasive impact on different aspects of life. This process can be facilitated through therapy, journaling, and other forms of self-reflection. Further, a core aspect of reauthoring a trauma narrative involves finding meaning and purpose in the experiences. Bryce et al., (2022) highlighted how individuals in helping professions often achieve this by using their experiences to support others facing similar challenges. This act of helping can transform the trauma narrative from one of victimhood to one of empowerment and purpose. Trauma often forces individuals to develop specific skills and coping mechanisms, such as resilience, empathy, and adaptability. Recognizing and valuing these strengths is crucial for reauthoring the trauma narrative. These skills can be leveraged in various aspects of life, including career choices, to create a sense of agency and competence.

Choosing a career that aligns with the reauthored narrative can be a powerful step towards solidifying a new self-identity. The sources show how individuals in helping professions often integrate their trauma experiences into their career narratives, using their past to inform their work and find a sense of fulfillment. The study by Bryce and colleagues (2022) highlighted that while acknowledging the pain and suffering caused by trauma is essential, reauthoring the narrative involves shifting the focus from victimhood to growth. This involves recognizing the resilience and strength gained through overcoming adversity and focusing on the positive aspects of the journey. The study also addressed the concept of post-traumatic growth as a potential outcome of trauma. While not everyone experiences this, it involves positive psychological changes that occur in response to adversity. Embracing and nurturing this growth can be a vital part of reauthoring the trauma narrative and creating a more hopeful future. It is important to note that the study primarily focused on the experiences of individuals in helping professions. The process of reauthoring trauma narratives may differ for individuals in other professions or contexts. Additionally, while the study provided valuable insights, it's essential to remember that trauma recovery and narrative reconstruction is a deeply personal and complex process.

TRAUMA INFORMED CAREER COUNSELLING

Given the findings of Bryce and Colleagues suite of research (2022; 2023) regarding the motivating influences of trauma on career decision-making and vocational behaviour, trauma informed career counselling in higher education institutions is considered a critical step in supporting individuals with histories of childhood adversity and trauma to construct career narratives that will promote post traumatic growth. Bryce and colleagues' work also confirmed the findings of other studies that have explored the negative impact of trauma on career development (Coursol et al., 2001; Currie & Widom, 2010; Kim & Klose Smith, 2021; Swanberg et al., 2005). Currie and Widom (2010) found that those with higher Adverse Childhood Experiences scores were more likely to experience lower levels of education, employment, and economic assets across the life span, which resulted in a 14% gap in the probability of employment by middle age. Kim and Klose Smith (2021) identified that negative patterns may be established very early in one's vocational life and that early traumatic experiences may influence lowered career adaptability. They highlighted the need for career counsellors working university students to prioritise early interventions that enhance resiliency and "promote purposeful improvement in career curiosity, choice among one's options, and the confidence to pursue one's chosen career" (p.272).

Powers and Duys (2020) provided a number of recommendations for integrating trauma informed practices into career counselling approaches and central to this was the use of self-reflection scales and measures which promote reflection and develop insight, such as the ACEs Questionnaire (Felitti et al., 1998), the Post Traumatic Growth Inventory (Tedeschi & Calhoun, 1996), and the Career Adapt-Abilities Scale (Savickas & Porfeli, 2012).

The research by Bryce and Colleagues (2022; 2023) highlighted the dual power narratives hold in career counselling, through their remedial and therapeutic value for trauma recovery, and to assign meaning to career aspirations, decisions, and behaviour in order to find value in their lived experience. Powers and Duys (2020) further recommend instilling a sense of hope and support to help clients "reframe their personal narrative, our efforts may empower a more resilient career trajectory" (p.182). Narratives have value in career counselling, as a means of facilitating the reauthoring process revealed in this research. Storying and narrative approaches permit practitioners to promote the reframing experience that survivors of cumulative harm seek to achieve both consciously and unintentionally, through vocational decision-making.

Epston and White (Epston & White 1990; Epston 1992; White 2001a) introduced the narrative metaphor and the reauthoring metaphor to the counselling field, focusing on the ways stories shape people's identities. Narrative practices are concerned with notions of 'intentional states of identity' which contrast with notions of 'internal states of identity' (White 2001b). In other words, we are interested in exploring the intentions, hopes, values and commitments that shape people's actions rather than any internal deficits or deficiencies, or for that matter any internal 'resources', 'strengths' or 'qualities' (Carey & Russell, 2003). Re-authoring conversations and narrative approaches seek to create the possibilities for the generation of alternative, preferred stories of identity. Once these have been co-created (for example between the career counsellor and the student), then the student concerned will have a foundation to continue to link events and meanings around this new story.

Trauma-informed career counselling methods that draw on narrative and life-story approaches afford practitioners the opportunity to identify and address, with increased accuracy, the influence of trauma on career choice and vocational behaviour and promote 'alternate story lines' and reauthoring processes which may increase academic success and educational attainment. Within the frame of Career Construction Theory, the Career Construction Interview (Savickas, 2005, 2011, 2013) is also a useful method for facilitating individuals' career explorations and finding meaningfulness in their stories.

Melding this approach with narrative therapeutic approaches, as purported by Powers and Duys (2019) will provide an appropriate career counselling method that acknowledges the motivating influences of trauma, as well as the potentially deleterious impacts, and support, perhaps even facilitate the reauthoring process which was revealed through the work of Bryce and Colleagues (2022; 2023). This endeavour would permit practitioners to promote the reframing experience that survivors of trauma seek to achieve both consciously and unintentionally, through vocational decision-making.

There are other narrative career counselling methods similarly amenable for career exploration and reflective practice in professionals (Lengelle et al., 2016; Taylor & Savickas, 2016) that may be used to generate life themes to resolve matters of trauma toward effective personal and professional outcomes. The narrative approaches view the client's story as integral to the very processes and outcomes of assessment and intervention (McIlveen, 2008; McIlveen & Patton, 2007).

Career counselling approaches can be a stand-alone service or embedded in program and course delivery. Narrative tools may be integrated into the coursework of degree programs for helping professions so as to develop these future practitioners' reflexive awareness of their resolutions. Narrative approaches are strongly supported in trauma-informed therapy and counselling more broadly (White, 2004; 2005).

ARCCH MODEL OF RESILIENCE - A PEDAGOGICAL STRATEGY FOR CAREER COUNSELLING

The ARCCH Model of Resilience (Wojciak et al., 2022) is described as a trauma-informed, strengths-based tool that empowers individuals to leverage their existing strengths to address areas where they need support. The Model was intentionally designed to be consistent with the six key principles of a trauma-informed approach outlined by SAMHSA (Substance Abuse and Mental Health Services Administration; 2014). The ARCCH model, therefore, operates in a context where understanding and working with personal narratives is central to the students' journeys.

The ARCCH Model is a useful tool for conceptualizing the complexity of interactions that contribute to the development of personal identity, an important concept for multicultural and social justice competence (Ratts et al., 2016). It can serve as a roadmap to build into a narrative approach as well as for guiding a strengths-based intervention empowering the voice and choice of the student in reauthoring their career story (Bryce et al., 2022; Center for Disease Control and Prevention, n.d.; Powers & Duys, 2020; Savickas, 2016; SAMHSA, 2023). Attachment, Regulation, Competence, Culture, and Health (ARCCH) are all elements of personal and cultural identities in individuals, families, communities, and systems. Each of the five components (attachment, regulation, culture, competence and health) has a broad body of research to support its importance as a stand-alone element of human functioning and personal identity. Woven together in a flexible format, these components can become a stronger avenue to strengthen resilience through their interconnectedness, making it useful for career counsellors and their clients to evaluate their strengths, identify areas that need support, and provide steps for culturally responsive and ecologically valid interventions (Wojciak et al., 2022). The ARCCH model is also described as a brain-based model of resilience because the interconnectedness of its five constructs mirrors the interconnectedness of various brain regions19. Furthermore, it is a multisystemic model, meaning it is applicable across different ecological systems (Powers et al., 2024). The ARCCH model has been used successfully in K-12 public and private schools and higher education programs (Wojciak et al., 2020) to help build resilience in students and mitigate potential negative outcomes of trauma; the effects continue to be quantified through ongoing research.

Recognizing that many students entering helping professions have their own trauma histories, the ARCCH Model can be utilised as a framework for building resilience in preservice, higher education students, By using the ARCCH framework for critical self-reflection and goal-setting, students, educators and career advisors and counsellors, can collaboratively determine the level of support required to promote student success and retention. Promoting self-reflection on their own experiences in a safe manner (e.g., reflecting on ACE scores without mandatory sharing) is effective in enhancing student self-awareness and understanding of potential triggers, particularly in pre-service helping professionals. The ARCCH Model can be integrated into various aspects of higher education from course delivery and pedagogy to broader institutional support, including program development, coursework, and advisory meetings, to promote critical self-reflection, development of professional identity development, and ultimately, the creation of competent and ethical professionals. Resilience, as conceptualized and fostered by the ARCCH model, plays a central and multifaceted role in career readiness for school counsellors. It equips them with the personal resources, professional competencies, and self-awareness needed to navigate the inherent challenges of the profession, sustain their well-being, and ultimately achieve long and successful careers. The ARCCH model students construct career narratives which will promote post-traumatic growth and career readiness (Powers et al., 2024)

CONCLUSION

Cumulative experiences, particularly those involving childhood trauma and adversity, significantly influence an individual's career choice, especially within the helping professions. These personal histories can motivate individuals to pursue careers where they aim to satisfy unmet childhood needs, actualize inherited aspirations, or utilize their experiences to assist others, embodying the "wounded healer" concept and demonstrating motivations rooted in altruism and remediation.

While cumulative trauma can present challenges to academic success and career development, potentially leading to poorer outcomes and decreased career adaptability, it also offers unique opportunities for meaning making and growth. Through vocational decision-making, individuals can engage in a "reauthoring" process, integrating their trauma narratives with career narratives to reframe past experiences, develop new identities, and foster post-traumatic growth. This transformation involves recognizing and leveraging strengths such as empathy, resilience, and a strong sense of justice that may have developed as a result of their adverse experiences.

Given the prevalence of trauma among higher education students and aspiring helping professionals, there is a critical need for trauma-informed approaches in university settings and career counselling services. Such approaches, including narrative-based career counselling and tools like the ARCCH model of resilience, can provide essential support, helping students to understand their past, build personal resources, enhance professional competencies, and develop the self-awareness crucial for navigating the demands of their chosen professions and achieving long and successful careers. Ultimately, by acknowledging and purposefully integrating personal adversity, career choices can become powerful avenues for healing, building resilience, and fostering profound personal and professional fulfillment

REFERENCES

Ackerman, R. J., DiRamio, D., & Mitchell, K. S. (2009). Posttraumatic stress disorder and other mental health diagnoses in returning veterans. *The Psychiatric Times, 26*(8).

American Psychiatric Association. (2013). *Diagnostic and statistical manual of mental disorders* (5th ed.).

Bachrach, R. L., & Read, J. P. (2012). Prevalence of traumatic events in college students: Implications for intervention. *Psychological Trauma: Theory, Research, Practice, and Policy, 4*, 237–246.

Banyard, V., & Cantor, D. (2004). Adjustment to college: The role of violence-related trauma. *Journal of Interpersonal Violence, 19*(1), 25–43.

Beaucar, A. (1999). The effect of direct and vicarious trauma on therapists: Posttraumatic stress symptomatology. *Dissertation Abstracts International, 60*(09), 4913B.

Bonanno, G. A. (2005). Resilience in the face of potential trauma. *Current Directions in Psychological Science, 14*(3), 135–138. DOI: 10.1111/j.0963-7214.2005.00347.x

Bromfield, L. M., & Higgins, D. J. (2005). Chronic and isolated maltreatment in a child protection sample. *Family Matters (Melbourne, Vic.)*, (70), 38–45.

Bromfield, L. M., Gillingham, P., & Higgins, D. J. (2007). Cumulative harm and chronic child maltreatment. Developing Practice: The Child. *Youth and Family Work Journal*, (19), 34–42.

Bryce, I., Beccaria, G., McIlveen, P., & Du Preez, J. (2022). Reauthoring: The lived experience of cumulative harm and its influence on career choice. *Australian Journal of Career Development, 31*(2), 93–107. DOI: 10.1177/10384162221101958

Bryce, I., Pye, D., Beccaria, G., McIlveen, P., & Du Preez, J. (2023). The Influence of Cumulative Harm on Career Choice in the Helping Professions: A Systematic Literature Review. *Trauma, Violence & Abuse, 24*(1). Advance online publication. DOI: 10.1177/15248380211016016 PMID: 34000930

Carello, J., & Butler, L. D. (2014). Practices for creating a trauma-informed university. *Journal of Trauma & Dissociation, 15*, 444–457.

Carey, M., & Russell, S. (2003). Re-authoring: Some answers to commonly asked questions. *International Journal of Narrative Therapy and Community Work, 3*, 60–71.

Center for Disease Control and Prevention. (n.d.). *Adverse childhood experiences.* Retrieved from https://www.cdc.gov/violenceprevention/aces/index.html

Cless, C. L., & Goff, M. J. (2017). The prevalence of traumatic events and post-traumatic distress among college students: A meta-analytic review of U.S. studies, 1983–2015. *Journal of American College Health*, *65*, 273–282.

Corbett, E., McGann, M., Considine, M., & Rejón, R. (2024). *Towards Trauma-Informed Employment Services: Implications for Street-Level Practice in the Delivery of Welfare-to-Work. Australian Welfare and Work Lab Working Paper*. University of Melbourne.

Currie, J., & Spatz Widom, C. (2010). Long-term consequences of child abuse and neglect on adult economic well-being. *Child Maltreatment*, *15*(2), 111–120.

DeBerard, M. S., Spielmans, G. I., & Julka, D. L. (2004). Post-traumatic stress disorder and college student achievement: The mediating role of motivation. *Journal of College Student Development*, *45*, 55–65.

Fallot, R. D., & Harris, M. (2009). *Creating cultures of trauma-informed care*. Community Connections.

Felitti, V. J., Anda, R. F., Nordenberg, D., Williamson, D. F., Spitz, A. M., Edwards, V., & Marks, J. S. (1998). Relationship of childhood abuse and household dysfunction to many of the leading causes of death in adults: The Adverse Childhood Experiences (ACE) Study. *American Journal of Preventive Medicine*, *14*(4), 245–258. DOI: 10.1016/S0749-3797(98)00017-8 PMID: 9635069

Frazier, P., Tashiro, T., Berman, M., Stecker, R., & Schwartz, A. (2009). PTSD and comorbidity in a national probability sample of college students. *Journal of Traumatic Stress*, *22*, 223–228.

Gildersleeve, J., Cantrell, K., Bryce. I., & Cripps, C. (2024). Reading, Reflection and Resilience in the Study of Australian Literature. Journal of Language, Literature and Culture. 1-18.

Gruttadaro, D. A., & Crudo, R. (2012). *College students speak: A survey report on mental health*. Active Minds.

Guttierez, L., & Gutierez, D. (2019). Examining traumatic experiences, mental health needs, and resilience in the lives of student veterans. *Journal of Student Affairs Research and Practice*, *56*(1), 42–53.

Herman, J. L. (1992). *Trauma and recovery: The aftermath of violence – From domestic abuse to political terror*. Basic Books.

Herman, J. L. (2002). *Truth and repair: How trauma survivors enact restorative justice*. Basic Books.

Higgins, D. J., Mathews, B., Pacella, R., Scott, J. G., Finkelhor, D., Meinck, F., Erskine, H. E., Thomas, H. J., Lawrence, D. M., Haslam, D. M., Malacova, E., & Dunne, M. P. (2023). The prevalence and nature of multi-type child maltreatment in Australia. *The Medical Journal of Australia, 218*(S6), S19–S25. DOI: 10.5694/mja2.51868 PMID: 37004183

Hunter, S. J. (2022). *Trauma-informed care in human service organisations: A practical guide for agencies, groups and practitioners*. Jessica Kingsley Publishers.

Kennedy, M., & Scriver, S. (2016). *Building trauma-informed higher education institutions: Strategies to enhance learning and promote student success*. American College Personnel Association.

Kim, J., & Smith, C. K. (2021). Traumatic experiences and female university students' career adaptability. *The Career Development Quarterly, 69*(3), 263–277.

Lifton, R. J. (1968). *Death in life: Survivors of Hiroshima*. Random House.

Lifton, R. J. (2023). *Surviving our catastrophes: Resilience and renewal from Hiroshima to the COVID-19 pandemic*. Farrar, Straus and Giroux. DOI: 10.2307/jj.26193262

Malach-Pines, A., & Yafe-Yanai, B. (2001). The role of early negative childhood experiences in career choice: An exploratory study. *Journal of Career Development, 28*, 147–167.

National Alliance on Mental Illness. (2011). *College students and mental health*. National Alliance on Mental Illness.

Powers, J., Bryce, I., Jiwon, K., & Hobbs, R. (2024). Trauma-Informed Gatekeeping Using ARCCH Model of Multisystemic Resilience, (P. 81-114) *In N. Hurless & L. Davis (Eds), Cases on Trauma-Informed Gatekeeping in Counsellor Education.*

Powers, J., & Duys, D. K. (2020). *Trauma-informed care: Principles and practice*. Wiley.

Ratts, M. J., Singh, A. A., Nassar-McMillan, S., Butler, T., & McCullough, J. R. (2016). *Multicultural and social justice competency development: A guide for the counseling profession* (2nd ed.). American Counseling Association.

Read, J. P., Ouimette, P., White, J., Colder, C. R., & Farrow, C. V. (2011). Trauma history, PTSD symptoms, and problem drinking in college students. *Addictive Behaviors, 36*, 1062–1066.

Rosenman, S. (2002). *Traumatic experiences in an Australian population*. Australian Centre for Posttraumatic Mental Health, The University of Melbourne.

Savickas, M. L. (2005). The theory and practice of career construction. In S. D. Brown & R. W. Lent (Eds.), *Career development and counseling: Putting theory and research to work* (pp. 42–70). John Wiley & Sons.

Savickas, M. L. (2011). *Career counseling*. American Psychological Association.

Savickas, M. L. (2016). Life designing: A paradigm for career construction in the 21st century. *Journal of Vocational Behavior, 93*, 202–215.

Savickas, M. L., & Porfeli, E. J. (2012). Career Adapt-Abilities Scale: Construction, reliability, and measurement equivalence across 13 countries. *Journal of Vocational Behavior, 80*(3), 661–673.

Silberner, J. (2023, February 15). At 97, Robert Jay Lifton is still thinking deeply about trauma. *Fresh Air*. https://www.npr.org/2023/02/15/1157115775/at-97-robert-jay-lifton-is-still-thinking-deeply-about-trauma29

Smyth, N. J., True, N., Souto, J. C., & Bruce, S. E. (2008). Posttraumatic stress disorder and academic performance: Current directions. *Journal of College Counseling, 11*, 6–17.28

Sosu, E. M., & Pheunpha, P. (2019, February). Trajectory of university dropout: Investigating the cumulative effect of academic vulnerability and proximity to family support. []. Frontiers Media SA.]. *Frontiers in Education, 4*, 6.

Substance Abuse and Mental Health Services Administration. (2014). *SAMHSA's concept of trauma and guidance for a trauma-informed approach*. HHS Publication No. (SMA) 14-4884. Substance Abuse and Mental Health Services Administration.2

Substance Abuse and Mental Health Services Administration. (2023) *Practical Guide for Implementing a Trauma-Informed Approach*. SAMHSA Publication No. PEP23-06-05-005. Rockville, MD: National Mental Health and Substance Use Policy Laboratory. https://store.samhsa.gov/sites/default/files/pep23-06-05-005.pdf

Tedeschi, R. G., & Calhoun, L. G. (1996). The Posttraumatic Growth Inventory: Measuring the positive legacy of trauma. *Journal of Traumatic Stress, 9*(3), 455–471. DOI: 10.1002/jts.2490090305 PMID: 8827649

Ungar, M., & Theron, L. (2020). Resilience and mental health: How multisystemic processes contribute to positive outcomes. *The Lancet. Psychiatry, 7*(5), 441–448. DOI: 10.1016/S2215-0366(19)30434-1 PMID: 31806473

Walters, A. J., Notebaert, L., Van Bockstaele, B., Meeten, F., Todd, J., & Clarke, P. J. (2024). Occurrence of potentially traumatic events, type, and severity in undergraduate students. *Australian Psychologist*, •••, 1–11.

Wojciak, A., Powers, K., Bryce, A., & Thompson, S. (2022). The ARCCH model of resilience: A strengths-based, trauma-informed and culturally responsive intervention tool. *Frontiers in Psychology, 13*, 133.

Yehuda, R., & Flory, J. D. (2007). Differentiating PTSD from other stress reactions: Evidence from the study of biological mechanisms. *Psychoneuroendocrinology, 32*, 998–1007.6

Chapter 10

From Childhood Institutions to Aged Care: Older "Care" Leavers Navigating Cumulative Harm Across the Lifespan

Susan Baidawi
https://orcid.org/0000-0003-4394-1313
Monash University, Australia

Lena Turnbull
Monash University, Australia

Sarah Morris
https://orcid.org/0009-0007-9007-807X
Monash University, Australia

Philip Mendes
https://orcid.org/0000-0002-2750-4140
Monash University, Australia

ABSTRACT

The pervasive impact of childhood cumulative harm across the lifespan is increasingly acknowledged, yet outcomes in later adulthood are rarely examined. This chapter outlines findings of a study of older "care" leavers in Australia, individuals aged 50 years and older who spent time in childhood institutions, foster "care", or other forms of out-of-home "care" from the 1950s to the 1980s. Voices of older "care" leavers were gathered through 105 surveys and 24 in-depth interviews, which told of how their ongoing hardship reflected long-term impacts of childhood harm and

DOI: 10.4018/979-8-3373-4064-7.ch010

adversity, and the contribution of these to relationship, housing, financial, health, and other life challenges. For some, intergenerational child removal demonstrated how the impact of cumulative harm can echo across generations. Despite enduring significant trauma, the remarkable resilience of older "care" leavers is evident. Findings raise implications about the support needs of older "care" leavers, and the long-term consequences of institutional abuse.

INTRODUCTION

This Chapter begins by considering what is known about the impact of cumulative harm and adversity, with a focus on how these impacts have been conceptualised from a life course perspective. It then introduces the population of older "care" leavers who form the focus of the study described, and canvasses what is known about their outcomes. The current study is then introduced, which adopted a co-design approach driven by lived-experience perspectives through a partnership with the Care Leavers Australasia Network (CLAN) a national peak body for care leavers, and a care-experienced researcher, Sarah Morris. The findings of this multi-methods study are then described across samples of surveys and in-depth interviews, before outlining the study's implications for policy, practice and future research.

The Impact of Cumulative Harm and Adversity: A Life Course Perspective

Much of what is known regarding cumulative harm and its impacts has focused on childhood, reflecting the initial shaping of this concept within child protection research, policy and practice. The concept of cumulative harm, at least initially, was introduced within child protection circles to counter the prevailing 'event' model of child abuse, which conceptualised maltreatment as individual events that could be proven within an adversarial legal framework (Sheehan, 2019). In this context, cumulative harm came to be conceptualised as occurring as the result of either an ongoing adverse event or circumstance (for example, chronic neglect), or as the result of multiple co-occurring adverse events or circumstances (sometimes termed poly-victimisation or multi-type maltreatment) (Bromfield & Miller, 2012; Sheehan, 2019). This understanding of cumulative harm as poly-victimisation, or multi-type maltreatment, was in part derived from the concept of adverse childhood experiences (ACEs), made famous by the body of work of Anda, Felitti, and colleagues. Their collective body of ground-breaking prospective research made clear the association between cumulative experiences of childhood harm and a range of negative outcomes, including household adversity, and health risk behaviours, disease and early death in adulthood (Anda et al., 2006; Felitti et al., 1998).While derived from general population samples (as opposed to out-of-home care samples), the original and subsequent bodies of research demonstrated this relationship between cumulative harm and risk of other non-health outcomes, including poorer work performance (Anda, Fleisher et al., 2004), adult criminal justice system involvement (e.g. Testa et al. 2022), and higher levels of teen pregnancy (Anda, Chapman et al., 2002).

As Bryce and Collier (2022) note, the voluminous ACEs research has very clearly established the deleterious impacts of childhood adversity and maltreatment across the life course. Yet the bulk of this research has been quantitative in nature and has focused on general or disadvantaged population samples. Conversely, the study outlined in this chapter instead adopted a mixed methods approach, drawing on both surveys and in-depth interviews to better understand and *hear* older "care" leavers' experiences across their life course. Throughout this Chapter, the term "care" is placed in quotation marks, to both recognise and reflect the absence of nurturance and protection older "care" leavers typically report having experienced throughout their childhoods. The next section outlines who are the population that comprise older "care" leavers in Australia.

Who are Older "Care" Leavers?

In Australia, older "care" leavers are the approximately 500,000 individuals who lived in institutional out-of-home care (OOHC) – that is orphanages, children's homes and foster care – from roughly 1920 to the late 1980s (Commonwealth of Australia, 2004). This group of people typically spent all or part of their childhood in foster care, orphanages, children's homes, and other institutions run by churches, charities and governments. Stated reasons for their removal from the family home included being orphaned, family poverty, single motherhood, and abuse, 'dysfunction', crisis, or an absence of adult guardians (Commonwealth of Australia, 2004).

Many of this cohort came from families where parents or grandparents had also spent time in OOHC and consequently were particularly vulnerable to the impact of what has been called the 'intergenerational transmission of poverty' (Cebulla & Katz, 2017, p. 67). According to research, entrenched disadvantage across generations can undermine personal well-being and life chances as manifested in limited aspiration to further and higher education, low wages or unemployment, poor mental health, negative body image, and low social and community connection and participation (Cebulla & Katz, 2017; EIAC, 2025; Harris, 2017).

Some differences between the subgroups of people who could be considered older "care" leavers in Australia should be emphasised. A key group of older "care" leavers in Australia are those who comprise the Stolen Generations, Aboriginal and Torres Strait Islander children who were forcibly removed from their parents under racist, genocidal and assimilationist policies from the mid-1800s to the 1970s (Commonwealth of Australia, 1997). During this period, thousands of Aboriginal children were systematically taken from their families, communities and culture, and placed in institutions, adopted or fostered by non-Indigenous people. Stolen children often endured horrific abuse and exploitation, and were denied access to their communities, languages and cultures (Healing Foundation, 2025).

The largest group of older "care" leavers in Australia are Forgotten Australians, otherwise known as historical OOHC leavers, or sometimes 'Now Remembered Australians' (Smith, 2017), reflecting a growing attention to their experiences and needs across policy and research. This group are described as "predominantly Australian-born, non-Indigenous adults who experienced different forms of OOHC as children, including foster homes and institutional regimes, up to 1974" (Smith, 2017, p. 1).

Within the group of Forgotten Australians are a subgroup who are known as 'Former Child Migrants'. This group comprise around 7,000 individuals who similarly grew up in children's homes, orphanages and other institutions, but who initially came to Australia as child migrants. These children most commonly arrived from the United Kingdom, Ireland and Malta, under approved child migrant schemes during the 20th century, and usually unaccompanied by their parents (Commonwealth of Australia, 2001; 2004).

The study on which this chapter is based sought to focus on the experience of Forgotten Australians and Child Migrants, though ultimately many people who identified as being part of the Stolen Generations did participate. Our decision in this regard reflected the need to differentiate between the experiences and needs of these groups, and to respect that Aboriginal and Torres Strait Islander research in this particularly sensitive and traumatic area is best designed and led by Aboriginal and Torres Strait Islander communities and researchers.

Many older "care" leavers recall their childhood experiences of exploitative and dangerous hard labour, criminal physical, psychological and sexual abuse, neglect and other deprivations. Their collective experience demonstrates that the systems responsible for their care were fundamentally uncaring and unsafe. Often when children complained about their treatment they were not believed, with adults in positions of power simply denying that the victims' worst experiences ever happened (Commonwealth of Australia, 2001; 2004).

Many of this cohort carry a legacy of the abuse and neglect they endured within orphanages and other child institutions, and consequent experiences of major life disadvantage (Golding, 2022). The various scars endured in their childhoods often impact across their adult lives. In 2017, it was understood that approximately half a million older care leavers aged between 40 and 90 years lived around Australia, in addition to an unknown number of older Australians who had been separated from their parents through forced adoption and removal (National Aged Care Alliance, 2017).

What are the Known Outcomes of Older "Care" Leavers?

Research relating to the long-term outcomes of care leavers has broadly established their higher likelihood of negative outcomes across a range of socio-economic and health domains (Gypen et al., 2017). This includes increased interaction with the criminal justice system, housing instability, and significant challenges in mental and physical health, attributed to the physical, psychological and emotional wounds caused by the legacy of maltreatment both prior to and during care, as well as a lack of comprehensive support throughout their lives (Baidawi et al., 2025; Sacker et al., 2021; Stein & Ward, 2021).

Despite significant childhood adversities, there are notable examples that make clear that the dismal statistics often associated with care leavers' outcomes are by no means ubiquitous. For example, in the area of education, estimates suggest that only about 1% of care leavers transition into higher education (McNamara et al., 2019; Mendes et al., 2014). However, across Australia alone, individuals like Frank Golding, Dee Michell, Gregory Smith and Jacqueline Wilson, all established writers, historians and academics, have defied these odds (see, e.g. Michell et al., 2015; Smith, 2015). Their achievements have inspired many, including the co-author Sarah Morris, who also has lived experience in out-of-home "care", to challenge these bleak narratives across generations (Wilson et al., 2018).

As care leavers progress into later stages of life, they experience heightened prevalence of chronic health and mental health conditions compared to the general population (Airagnes et al., 2016; England-Mason et al., 2018). As they age, these pre-existing vulnerabilities may increase and advance the need for aged care services; however, emerging research suggests that mainstream aged care services are often ill-equipped to meet their unique needs (Alliance for Forgotten Australians, 2019; Australian Government Department of Health, 2019; Brown-Yung et al., 2022; Browne-Yung et al., 2021; CLAN, 2022; Tuart Place, 2019). Care leavers frequently experience premature ageing, meaning they require aged care support earlier than the general population (Fernandez et al., 2016), yet they remain underrepresented in aged care policy and service design. Despite the recognition of their extensive and lifelong challenges, there remains a paucity of research focused on their specific needs as they transition into the aged care support system.

THE STUDY

Here we report cumulative harm-related findings of a study conducted throughout 2023-2025 which focused on the life course experiences of older "care" leavers. We sought to improve understanding of their qualitative life experiences, and their self-reported needs as they approached older adulthood, particularly those that related to aged care systems and services. The study was funded in 2022 by a 'Living Labs' Grant from Australia's National Centre for Healthy Ageing. The research team conducting the study were all social work trained, led by Professor Philip Mendes who brings to this study over two decades of research expertise and policy advocacy in the field of leaving care.

We approached the study through a lived-experience methodology, which emphasises the importance of personal narratives and subjective experiences in understanding complex social phenomena (Atkinson, 2007). Two key approaches to enhancing lived experience within the methodology were utilised. Specifically, the methodology included having within the research team a researcher who brings lived experience of growing up in OOHC in Australia (Author 3). Additionally, the study was co-designed with CLAN, a national, independent, peak membership body which represents, supports and advocates for care leavers in Australia. Their contribution to the project ensured that the voices of care leavers are embedded into every stage of the research. The study methods, which were approved by the Monash University Human Research Ethics Committee, are further detailed below.

Survey Methods

The study survey was designed featuring Likert scale questions, closed-ended questions, and open-ended questions. The survey covered topics such as the types of "care" participants experienced, and the subsequent impact of this on their adult lives, including questions around their housing, income, employment history, health and support needs. We also asked participants about their current experience of aged care services and preferences for aged care services in the future, as this was a key focus of the study. In line with our co-design methodology, the survey was pilot-tested with a sample group of older care leavers associated with the Care Leavers Australasia Network who were involved in the project. Feedback from this piloting stage led to the following key areas of amendment:

Survey Language

We gave participants the option to choose how they identified, e.g. as a "care" leaver, Forgotten Australian, member of the Stolen Generations, or simply in their own words. In line with feedback received, we ensured that written communication was warm, welcoming and in easy-to-understand language. We rewrote the study's explanatory statement, and changed phrases within the survey to ensure clarity.

Survey Length and Topics

The feedback we received suggested that it was best to 'Keep it short!' with the survey, and also raised our awareness of potentially sensitive issues. This led to us making clear in the survey design that sections could be skipped by participants. We added information outlining the topic areas to be discussed within each section, and providing the option for participants to skip each section.

Acknowledging that participants may have a history of trauma and ongoing mental health challenges, the research team implemented measures to ensure an ethically sound approach that minimised the potential for re-traumatisation. One such strategy was to deliberately avoid detailed questions about participants' experiences in childhood institutions. While some questions addressed potentially negative adult experiences, such as family violence, mental illness, and relationship breakdowns, these were structured as forced-choice or yes/no questions, avoiding the need for detailed responses.

The survey was created and hosted online via the Qualtrics Insight Platform, and took approximately 15 minutes to complete. Participants were required to provide consent before beginning the survey, and no identifiable information was collected. Given the hidden and 'hard-to-reach' nature of older "care" leavers, we employed purposive non-random sampling to gather information from as many consenting respondents as possible. Our approach to participant recruitment involved collaborating with organisations that provide services to older "care" leavers, who assisted the study by disseminating study information, primarily through their newsletters. Participants were reimbursed with a $25 gift voucher.

To address potential recruitment and participation challenges, including limited literacy or numeracy, difficulties navigating technology, poor physical health, and distrust of government and large organisations, we provided additional support for survey completion. This involved our team's lived experience researcher providing either telephone or in-person assistance to some participants seeking to complete these surveys. During this data collection, the survey questions were read aloud and participant responses were recorded by the researcher. A total of 33 out of the 105 surveys were conducted this way, either in person or over the phone with the support of the lived experience researcher.

Interview Methods

We then sought to complement the survey findings through undertaking in-depth interviews with older "care" leavers, allowing for a more detailed exploration of their perceptions and experiences. The interviews were undertaken within a reflexive and person-centred framework, where participants had control over the content and duration of their narratives. This approach aligns with the principles of participatory research, where the voices of individuals with lived experience are prioritised and respected (Beresford, 2019). By holding a space where interviewees have control over the narration of their stories, the research aimed to honour participants' agency and ensure that their perspectives were authentically represented.

Interviews were mostly undertaken face-to-face by the research team member who possessed firsthand experience of out-of-home "care", necessitating interstate travel. This enabled the interviews to be grounded in the shared experiences of the researcher and participants. Through this approach, we hoped to facilitate a deeper connection between the researcher and participants, and to foster an environment of trust and openness, essential for eliciting rich, qualitative data (Liamputtong, 2007). A semi-structured format provided flexibility, enabling participants to explore those topics which were most salient to them, while still addressing key research questions. This kind of adaptability is crucial in lived-experience research, as it acknowledges the unique contexts and emotional landscapes of individual participants (Smith & Osborn, 2008). The interviews were audio-recorded with participants' consent and subsequently transcribed for thematic analysis.

Participants were recruited for both the survey and interviews using purposive and snowball sampling, including having a question in the survey asking if respondents were interested in participating in the separate, in-depth interview. These recruitment efforts were facilitated through established relationships with state-based support agencies for Forgotten Australians. These agencies were identified and engaged via the national Roundtable for Forgotten Australians, where members of the research team had ongoing connections. Participating agencies distributed study information to their client networks through newsletters, direct outreach, and word of mouth. Interested individuals contacted the research team or were supported by agency staff to do so. As a result of the recruitment strategy, there was substantial overlap between the survey and interview samples, allowing for participants' more in-depth interview reflections to fill in details that were less available through survey methods.

To be eligible for interviews, participants needed to be aged 50 or older (reflecting the premature ageing often reported by older "care" leavers) and to identify as having spent time in institutional or OOHC "care" as children. We did not exclude individuals based on cognitive capacity; if individuals were able to provide informed consent, they were eligible to participate. To further reduce participation barriers, the study design allowed for the presence of support persons during interviews and included options for flexible, participant-led interview locations.

While the interviews followed a semi-structured schedule, during the data analysis process, a recurring life story narrative emerged from the data, revealing how participants understood the connections between their families of origin, their removal from family and placement in "care", the cumulative harm they experienced throughout their childhoods, and their subsequent adult life experiences. Given the prominence of these life stories, we adopted a narrative analysis approach to the interview data, which is well-suited to understanding the experiences of participants. A narrative approach allows for an in-depth exploration of how participants construct meaning from their past and present experiences, providing a holistic understanding of their life trajectories (Flynn & McDermott, 2024).

Given the profound and lasting impact of childhood institutionalisation and time in OOHC, a narrative approach facilitates an examination of the interconnectedness of early life experiences and adult life challenges. This approach emphasises the chronological and contextual flow of participants' lives, illuminating how historical, social, and personal factors have shaped their perceptions of aged care in later life (Carey, 2012). Furthermore, it prioritises participants' active framing and naming of connections between their current experiences and their life histories. This approach allows their stories to guide the analysis and ensures that their lived experiences are represented authentically and meaningfully. By adopting this approach, the study captures the complexity and nuance of these narratives, providing valuable insights into how care systems, and the cumulative harm experienced within these, have influenced participants' life experiences.

FINDINGS

Survey Sample and Findings

While a total of 105 survey responses were recorded, some participants did not complete all sections, resulting in some variability in response rates across items. Our approach to informing participants about each section and seeking their consent may have contributed in part to this variability. Additionally, as is typical in surveys, responses decreased as the survey progressed, with only 62 responses in the final section.

Overall, 75% of participants were women and 25% were men, and they ranged in age from 50 to 87 years, with 41% aged between 60 and 70 years. Most (95%) participants were born in Australia, with four from the UK and one from New Zealand. Thirteen percent identified as Aboriginal and/or Torres Strait Islander.

Participants across five Australian states were represented (including Queensland, New South Wales, Victoria, South Australia and Western Australia), demonstrating successful recruitment efforts partnering with local agencies.

Participants reported time spent in state care ranging from 6 weeks to 21 years, however, the average was 9 years, which indicates an overall substantial time in care. Participants described living in various childhood settings, often across multiple placements, and most frequently in orphanages and children's institutions, followed by boys' homes/girls' homes and group homes. Other settings included foster care, youth detention, and mental health or disability institutions, with only a few participants experiencing adoption. These findings indicate most participants experienced the large, regimented institutional environments detailed by the Commonwealth Government's Royal Commission into Institutional Responses to Child Sexual Abuse (2017), which documented the widespread abuse, neglect, and mistreatment within these settings.

The participants' experiences align with previous research findings which have detailed the disproportionate socioeconomic disadvantage experienced by care leavers as a result of their exclusion from mainstream social and economic resources and opportunities (Sacker et al., 2021; OECD, 2022), as well as the impact of the cumulative harm typically experienced by older "care" leavers throughout their childhoods. At the time of the study, most of the participants (84%) relied on government pensions, and nearly half (48%) lived in government housing. While reliance on government pensions is anticipated for many who are older than retirement age (67 years), a substantial proportion of respondents (45%) were younger than this age, likely reflecting their uptake of disability pensions or unemployment benefits. Over one half (59%) had left secondary school without a certificate, suggesting substantial barriers to advancement in their education. At the same time, most (91%) had found paid employment across their life in various roles, though many struggled financially throughout their lives (with 40% indicating they had always struggled and 21% indicating they had often struggled).

In relation to their relationships, 86% had been married or in a de facto relationship, but only 20% were currently in one. Comparative data from the Australian Bureau of Statistics (ABS) (2022) shows that 56% of Australians over 65 are in de facto relationships, suggesting older care leavers experience barriers to maintaining long-term relationships. Such challenges could be reflecting their previous experiences of trauma and the subsequent impact on their lives.

Almost all survey participants had children (87%), however, one quarter (27%) of these parents had experienced their children being raised outside their direct care. Of these, 38% had children removed by the state, highlighting significant intergenerational involvement with child protection services. The remaining 62% had arranged informal care with relatives or friends. Recent child protection data

(AIHW, 2024) shows that fewer than 1% of Australian children are in state OOHC, much lower than our survey sample. This reflects care leavers' heightened vulnerability to becoming involved as parents with child protective services. Consistent with previous research (Baidawi et al., 2025) participants also reported having high levels of contact with the criminal justice system, with 21% having been admitted to a correctional facility at some point in their lives. This over-representation may in part be due to the criminalisation of behaviours associated with child homelessness and poverty. Additionally, we did not distinguish between youth and adult imprisonment, nor between those who had been imprisoned on remand (unsentenced) and those who were sentenced to imprisonment.

Two thirds of participants (65%) reported having a diagnosed mental illness, a figure that is higher than the lifetime prevalence rate across the country (43%) (ABS, 2023). An additional 35% of participants suspected they had an undiagnosed mental illness, most commonly complex PTSD or anxiety. Thirty-eight percent of participants had spent time in a psychiatric institution, indicating prevalence of severe challenges across the participant group.

Participants reported significant support needs throughout their lives: 61% had experienced homelessness or unstable housing, 53% reported having a disability requiring support, 56% experienced alcohol or drug issues, and the majority of participants reported experiencing family violence (74%), and significant health issues (79%). The findings demonstrate the existence of significant support needs across older care leavers as a cohort. So, who do this group tend to rely on for assistance? Around one half (55%) said they received regular support from family, and 63% received regular support from friends or the community. Far more often (83%) older "care" leavers relied on professionals and organisations, underscoring the importance of formal support systems. Most commonly, participants described accessing support from GPs, care leaver organisations, psychologists, and support workers.

Overall, these survey findings a relatively high level of ongoing hardship and complexity in support needs among older "care" leavers. We suggest that these hardships are reflective, at least in part, of the long-term impacts of the cumulative harm they experienced throughout their childhood, including in "care", and the contribution of these to instability, health problems, and other life challenges. Indeed, this is what came to be reflected in the narratives of older "care" leavers who participated in the interviews.

Interview Sample and Findings

A total of 24 participants took part in interviews for this study, all of whom resided in eastern states of Australia. The sample consisted of 15 female and 9 male participants, including 16 who resided in Queensland, four in South Australia, three in New South Wales, and one in Victoria. The interviews were conducted in person with 16 participants, and over the telephone for 8 participants, reflecting participant preferences and accessibility. Participants were offered a choice of location - either within the partnering agency's premises or in their own homes - based on where they felt safest and most comfortable. Our approach aligned with the trauma-informed principles underpinning the study, particularly the emphasis on autonomy, choice, and emotional safety. In keeping with our qualitative and narrative approach, we did not systematically collect from participants demographic data such as age, marital status, and socio-economic indicators. While this allowed for a focus on rich, participant-driven storytelling, we are subsequently limited in the ability to interpret findings in relation to individual background characteristics.

In line with the narrative approach to analysis, the findings are now organized into themes beginning with early childhood and childhood experiences as the foundations of participants' life stories. The focus then shifts to participants' adult life experiences, as an extension of the legacy of childhood. This is followed by an exploration of their present lives which are characterised by surviving systems, trauma and now facing ageing. The final stage focuses on how they face the future, and their perceptions and experiences of aged care, as they consider their ageing-related needs and future plans.

Childhood - Foundations of the Life Story

While participants were not asked directly about early childhood experiences (to avoid unnecessary distress) these were ultimately regularly discussed, often at multiple points of the interview and frequently in relation to their current views on supports and services. From the perspective of older "care" leavers, their current circumstances and life trajectories must be understood in the context of the cumulative harm they experienced in childhood.

Childhood Experiences Prior to Out-of-Home "Care"

Participants' early childhoods were characterised by profound poverty and socio-economic disadvantage, with many growing up in environments where basic needs were unmet. This economic hardship often pushed them into survival strategies, such as scavenging for food or engaging in petty crimes, which led to punitive and sometimes abusive interactions with authority figures and statutory services.

Family instability and neglect were significant themes, with participants describing fractured family structures, the loss of parents, abusive caregivers, and being passed between relatives or institutional care. These unstable environments often left them vulnerable to exploitation and abuse. Trauma and abuse were recurring experiences, both within their families and in institutional settings. Participants described severe physical, emotional, and sexual abuse, often compounded by a lack of protective or supportive systems to intervene or provide help. Finally, there was a notable absence of social or community support, leaving participants without access to resources, guidance, or opportunities to escape the cycles of hardship and violence they endured.

Experiences of Removal

Removal was accompanied by shock and confusion, as participants struggled to comprehend why they were being taken away, for example, one respondent shared that they "couldn't understand why" they had been taken away to an institution. These experiences sometimes undermined trust in authority figures, such as the police and statutory services, leaving older "care" leavers feeling bewildered and betrayed. Self-blame also often arose in relation to these experiences, with participants revisiting their past behaviours and circumstances to make sense of the removal. Feelings of moral outrage and disbelief were also common, particularly when siblings were allowed to remain in the home, contributing to lingering feelings of injustice.

> *It says in there, "We've come here, [X] is in the kitchen. We have told [the mother]... that we will remove her [daughter] next time if she keeps her home." Can you believe that? I cannot believe it, I still can't get over it.*

Collectively, these narratives underscore the emotional turbulence of removal and its lasting impact, evident in these vivid and detailed recollections.

Experiences in Out-of-Home "Care"

Participants' experiences in OOHC were characterised by significant harm and adversity, marked by systemic abuse, neglect, and dehumanising practices that profoundly shaped their lives. Participants recounted a range of traumatic incidents, highlighting the oppressive environments within these institutions and the long-term impacts on their physical and mental well-being. Participant narratives, some of which are presented in greater detail at the conclusion of this chapter, detail significant exposure to cumulative harm as both poly-victimisation (or multi-type maltreatment), and sustained abusive and traumatic experiences over time. These stories reflect a broader pattern of systemic failures in institutional OOHC, where children were often subjected to harsh punishments, exploitative labour, and a lack of basic care. The following themes illustrate the shared experiences of participants, shedding light on the challenges they faced and the lasting legacies of their time in "care".

A small number of participants shared their experiences as former child migrants, which, while similar to those of other participants, also included distinct challenges related to their removal from their home country and the journey to Australia. This often included experiences of being sent to Australia without their knowledge or consent, too young to understand the enormity of the move. The migration process lacked transparency, with guardians or authorities making life-altering decisions on their behalf, often without parental involvement or consent.

> *I lived in an orphanage in England, and I was seven and people came to the orphanage and said, 'Hands up all the kids who want to go to Australia'. I just presumed Australia was outside the door, so I put my hand up with all the other kids, and they put us on a boat for six weeks and sent us to Australia. And we went to an orphanage in Western Australia, but there was about six different boatloads of children that came. I came in the November, the 7th, of '47, but the kids had come before that and kids came after me. I think 130 British children were exported from England, not to Australia - Canada and South Africa - without their parents' permission. A priest signed all our documents as our guardians and we came, put in an orphanage. It was pretty tough.*

Regardless of the circumstances that brought each participant into the OOHC system, one consistent finding emerged: the harms they endured were profoundly traumatic and left a lasting impact on their lives. Participants described the cumulative harm arising from dehumanisation and loss of identity, physical, emotional and sexual abuse, neglect and poor living experiences, family separation and longing for reconnection, institutional hypocrisy and systemic failure to provide the actual care they had deserved.

Participants recounted how the trauma they had experienced in institutional settings fostered deep mistrust of others, especially authority figures. Many survivors preferred isolation, fearing vulnerability or further harm in social settings. Additionally, the impacts of institutional abuse were seen to extend to the next generation, with some participants recounting the struggles of their children and grandchildren. Yet amidst their pain, participants found meaning in ensuring their experiences were not forgotten. By sharing their stories, they aimed to foster awareness and protect future generations from similar fates. Survivors also took pride in the achievements of their children and grandchildren, seeing them as symbols of hope and resilience.

Living the Legacy – Adulthood as An Extension of Childhood

The narratives shared by participants about their adult lives reveal a profound link to the traumas they experienced during childhood and in institutional care. Their stories illustrate how the patterns of abuse, neglect, and dehumanisation endured in their formative years shaped their identities, relationships, and coping mechanisms as adults. Themes of mistrust, hypervigilance, and struggles with intimacy emerged, as participants recounted how early betrayals by caregivers and authority figures carried over into an ongoing fear of vulnerability and connection. Many described persistent mental health and psychosocial challenges as direct extensions of their childhood experiences. These accounts not only shed light on the long shadow of institutional trauma, but also highlight the ways participants sought to navigate their adult lives amidst the enduring impact of their past. This section explores the deep interconnection between the participants' childhood experiences and their adult outcomes.

Education and Work

Participants' reflections revealed the enduring impact of their childhood experiences on their opportunities to access education and work. Significant barriers to education during their formative years hindered their ability to access stable, well-paying jobs as adults.

> *I was mad over education because of how difficult it was for us to make our way in life. When we left the home, we were only taught to clean. I stayed there till I was nearly 16 and a half, I went there when I was nine months old.*

Their narratives highlight struggles with illiteracy, limited skill development, and feelings of frustration and inadequacy in trying to overcome these deficits later in life.

> *Well, I can't read and write or anything like that, so I find it very hard to get on with my life. But I've learnt to live with it. You know, like I've tried to learn to read and write, but just couldn't pick it up.*

Others lamented that their education was replaced with abuse and religious indoctrination, further limiting their prospects.

> *We were stolen. We were denied an education. All we got rammed down our throats was religion, religion, religion.*

Some expressed deep frustration and emotional distress over the barriers to learning and improving their circumstances as an adult.

> *It's frustrating because we so much want to better ourselves and live a bit more comfortable and learn. We're always willing to learn because we weren't given that opportunity as children. So, I find that hurts. I'll go down into tears and depression over that. That's how much that'll drop me down. Go, "Mate, come on. Why can't I do this? Why can't I do that bit? What's wrong with me?" and then I get angry at them and I get in this angry, attack mode and it's not good.*

This lack of foundational skills left many participants stuck in cycles of low-wage or insecure employment. Despite these challenges, their stories also reflect resilience and determination, as they sought creative ways to adapt and improve their circumstances. For example, one participant described teaching herself spelling and punctuation as an adult and working her way up from a hotel maid to an enrolled nurse. Similarly, another participant leveraged practical skills, such as machinery operation and couriering, to build a successful business, even though he lacked formal qualifications. Others displayed resilience by exploring a number of varied work experiences, from telecommunications to bartending, despite the instability and challenges they faced.

Health and Mental Health

A web of health and psychosocial challenges stemming from their early experiences continued to shape the wellbeing of older "care" leavers throughout adulthood. Many described struggles with physical and mental health, compounded by experiences of trauma and marginalisation. A recurring theme was the strain on their bodies due to harsh conditions, inadequate medical care, and physically demanding labour during childhood, which contributed to chronic conditions and disabilities later in life. Such findings mirror with previous research which found greater experiences of chronic health issues for people who have spent time in out-of-home "care" (Sacker et al. 2021).

> *We've all got knee problems, I reckon that's from scrubbing the cover way that they used to do. We would scrub, scrub, scrub, scrub, scrub, honestly, and all of us have got bad knees.*

Lack of access to adequate healthcare emerged as a significant concern, especially in later life. Others described a loss of faith in the healthcare system, often feeling unheard or unsupported, which compounded their physical struggles and left them reluctant to seek care. Like physical health challenges, mental health challenges were shaped by the profound loss, trauma, and isolation participants experienced throughout their lives. Themes of loneliness, and emotional suppression emerged in their reflections, as well as references to a range of mental illnesses, such as depression, anxiety, OCD and PTSD. Grief and loss were deeply embedded in participants' narratives, often linked to family separation, the deaths of loved ones, or the absence of meaningful connections. Some participants described how the repeated experience of death—whether of family, friends, or children—had numbed their ability to cry or express emotions outwardly.

> *I had a friend die last week - my son's godmother. She was 89, I think, or 88. She was just about to have a birthday in February. I don't cry so much now, when I hear death, as I used to. I think I grew up fast in the home. You had to. You'd know that. And you had to be an adult before you were an adult, you know?*

For many, unresolved grief was compounded by the isolation of old age. Loneliness and a sense of not belonging were recurring themes, often tied to early experiences of disconnection from family and society and ongoing losses throughout their lives.

> *... old age is the loneliness, it's horrendous. When you haven't a family, or you had a family - it's like as I said to my son, I had a family but it's like my family died in a car accident and I'm mourning the loss of every one of them. But the fact is that I know they're here, just up the road, and that's my biggest heartache.*

The psychological toll of these experiences manifested in mental health struggles for some. Depression and thoughts of suicide were described by participants as responses to overwhelming feelings of worthlessness and hopelessness. One participant vividly recounted multiple suicide attempts during a particularly dark period, highlighting the depth of despair they faced. Others described living with ongoing anxiety, claustrophobia, or an inability to find comfort in life.

> *They took away our childhood, and then here we are in old age all alone again, and nobody gives a shit, that's how it feels. If I wasn't mentally capable I think I would have gone, in the circumstances. You've got nothing to live for when it comes to things like that. What have you got to look forward to?*

Navigating Psychosocial Challenges

Participants also shared various psychosocial challenges that reflected the intersection of systemic disadvantage, personal hardships, and societal barriers. In particular, housing insecurity emerged as a major concern, particularly for elderly participants in government housing. Many described fears of being displaced from their homes due to policies or lack of support, and concerns about safety within their housing environments. For some, this led to further isolation, as they avoided going out after certain hours or chose to keep their cars in safer, distant locations.

> *Well, I've been waiting for three and a half years for a transfer out of here into a lower unit, but I don't want to move downstairs here because there's so much problems going on here with people's stuff getting stolen and broken into and that.*

One of the more challenging findings to emerge from the study was the pattern of intergenerational child removal. For many participants, the trauma of being separated from their families as children, coupled with the abuse and neglect they experienced in institutional settings, led to ongoing difficulties in parenting, forming secure attachments, and navigating child protection systems. These compounded challenges—rooted in unresolved trauma, systemic marginalisation, and inadequate post-care supports—contributed to circumstances where history repeated itself. A number of participants reported that their own children had been removed by the state or had grown up outside of their care, often in informal kinship or foster arrangements.

> *I've had a bad experience, darlin... They've taken three of my grandchildren, then I just find out that my son's committed suicide because they wouldn't let him come home to me.*

Participants' accounts provide stark evidence of how the impact of cumulative harm in childhood can echo across generations. Intergenerational removal must be understood not as isolated incidents of individual failure, but as a direct outcome of cumulative harm, structural disadvantage, and the failure of systems to interrupt these cycles.

Some participants also discussed their involvement in early life with crime and incarceration, which they attributed to systemic neglect, poverty, and a lack of opportunities in their youth. Experiences with the justice system led some participants furthered their enduring mistrust in authority.

> *... don't go to the police for help. Don't use the system for help. And if you're white, hold onto that because if they find out you're fucking black mate, you're in trouble.*

Discrimination was another recurring theme, particularly for participants who identified as queer or belonged to other marginalised communities. One participant vividly recounted the pervasive fear and hostility they faced as a queer individual, including targeted harassment by law enforcement and societal stigmatisation. This discrimination often forced them to conceal their identity in professional and social settings, creating a sense of perpetual fear and exclusion. As one interviewee described: That's how it was. You were frightened to step sideways. You had to pretend to be somebody else in your work. You had to pretend to be straight all the time.

Participants also described lifelong financial struggles, rooted in childhood poverty and continuing into adulthood. They detailed the challenge of living within limited means, adhering to strict budgets, and making sacrifices to meet basic needs. Participants who managed to achieve financial stability often did so through careful planning and resource management, though this was described as an ongoing burden.

> *I was from a very, very poor family. I still live like I'm poor because I'm used to it, but when I do get a bit of money or anything, I give it to my kids because they were never used to it.*

Surviving Systems, Trauma and Facing Ageing

As older "care" leavers reached their 50s and beyond, they began confronting the realities of aging and its implications for their future care needs. Participants described how the cumulative effects of childhood trauma, adult struggles, and systemic disadvantage deeply influenced their health, relationships, and outlook on aging. While many have shown remarkable resilience, they are now facing the challenges of declining health, financial strain, and the emotional weight of unresolved trauma, all while considering the potential need for aged care services.

The Ongoing Impacts of Trauma

The ongoing impacts of trauma emerged as the most pervasive and consistent theme throughout the interviews, underpinning nearly every aspect of participants' reflections on their lives and shaping their experiences of ageing. Participants described how their early experiences were ever-present, influencing even mundane activities.

Every morning I make my bed... It's stuck with us. We were punished, told, 'Do this.' It's hard to get out of that routine.

For others, moments of distress could arise unpredictably, with one explaining, "Sometimes I get triggered, and I don't even know why." Many participants expressed how the emotional wounds of their childhoods remained raw, and described strategies they used to avoid triggering these:

If something [in the media] comes up on trauma, I've got to turn it off... It's upsetting, and I end up crying.

I'm not one to get on a bus... It brings back the orphanage setting.

Others emphasised the importance of routine, structure and consistency, with changes or unexpected events disrupting their equilibrium. For example, one participant described an incident in a supermarket where "The layout was different... I couldn't handle it... I just walked out and left the trolley." These accounts underscore the ongoing load that accompanies unresolved trauma, manifesting in feelings of guilt, fear, and vulnerability. The legacy of trauma often influenced participants' ability to form connections. One remarked, "I'm not good relationship material, I think, because of what happened in the institutions. I sort of wanted to be by myself," while another admitted, "I cannot be bothered. It's a waste of time."

Key aspects of the legacy of trauma for older "care" leavers included their pervasive mistrust of systems and authority. Past betrayals also led to heightened sensitivity around personal boundaries, with one participant, wary of potential harm, sharing, "I don't care if you're a nurse... I want a female nurse."

Surviving or Thriving?

Many participants described a present-day life defined by survival, transience and insecurity. One reflected on their constant movement, stating, "I just kept on going... I couldn't settle because I always thought the cops were coming." Others highlighted their ongoing struggle to find a home, with one participant saying, "If I wasn't homeless, I'd probably tell you about my garden and my chickens... But I'm just going from one place to the other."

Participants often framed their lives in terms of "existing" rather than living. As one person put it, "We don't thrive. We just survive, get through each day." For others, this survival mindset was shaped by the need to protect themselves and their families. One recounted, "When I ran with my kids, I ran. I just kept on going." Some participants reflected on what could have been, lamenting the opportunities lost due to their focus on survival. One poignantly asked, "Wouldn't it have been better to thrive and to be happy? But what is happiness? We don't know what happiness is". These narratives illustrate how, for older "care" leavers, survival is a defining feature of life. While their resilience is evident, the focus on endurance highlights the unmet needs and unaddressed harm stemming from their childhood experiences.

Ageing-Related Needs

Participants described an interplay of practical challenges, health concerns, and deeply personal anxieties about receiving care as they age. Their narratives reveal a reluctance to surrender independence coupled for some with an acknowledgment of their increasing difficulty in managing day-to-day life.

I try to do everything I can for myself, but I know I have to get aged care because I'm having trouble cleaning with my back and all that sort of stuff. But I'm worried, I'm thinking it's like an invasion of my privacy again. You know what I mean?

Participants' practical needs included help with cleaning, shopping, and medical tasks, such as applying compression stockings. One, while appreciative of the assistance they currently receive, emphasised the value of having a trusted caregiver, someone familiar and reliable, to help navigate their ageing needs. They remarked on the challenges of finding suitable care, especially as the introduction of new or unfamiliar workers could feel invasive and unsettling.

For older "care" leavers, the thought of engaging with aged care appears to often bring about feelings of vulnerability and discomfort. Concerns about privacy were prominent, with one participant describing the prospect of allowing carers into their home as akin to an "invasion of privacy." This apprehension reflects a lingering mistrust of systems and an understandable desire to maintain control over their personal space and decisions.

But the old age, I've been trying now to get on to some assistance, but again you have this issue about who's coming into your home?

The Importance of Trust and Personalised Support

Trust emerged as a recurring theme in participants' interactions with support systems. Many emphasised the value of care relationships that demonstrate empathy, respect, and understanding, noting that this trust takes significant time to build.

One participant shared how they rely on a single trusted worker for most of their care needs, explaining, "She's the only one I trust to know all my business." However, they expressed frustration at being forced to work with new or unfamiliar workers, which they found disruptive and distressing. Another spoke positively about a long-term care organisation, describing their carers as "very good" and respectful, emphasising that mutual respect is essential to fostering trust.

While positive examples of care were noted, many participants shared concerns about the inconsistency of support staff, with one person noting that workers often lack the trauma-informed understanding necessary to avoid triggering past wounds.

Closure, and Meaning-making.

Participants often expressed a desire for closure, whether through reconciliation, acknowledgment of their experiences, or finding purpose in their later years. For some, closure meant addressing unresolved familial relationships. One participant described their determination to reconnect with a sibling despite the challenges, saying, "I just need to shake my brother's hand before I die… That's closure for me."

Others sought meaning by helping others or speaking out about systemic failures. One participant reflected, "I don't want young people going through what I went through… You can't save them all, but it hurts when you can't." These efforts highlight participants' resilience and their desire to find resolution and purpose, even amidst the enduring impact of their trauma.

Despite significant barriers, many participants exhibit remarkable strength and adaptability, striving to maintain independence while grappling with challenges of ageing. Their reflections underscore the critical need for systems that are trauma-informed, empathetic, and responsive to individual needs. Building trust, fostering dignity, and providing consistent, respectful care are pivotal to addressing the concerns of older "care" leavers, and ensuring they feel safe and valued as they approach older adulthood.

Surviving the Odds – The Resilience of Older "Care" Leavers

Resilience among older "care" leavers is not about erasing the scars of cumulative harm and trauma, but rather relates to the many ways in which their stories demonstrate them enduring, adapting, and striving for a semblance of normalcy and hope despite the challenges. The anonymised narratives of interview participants below share their experiences of surviving cumulative harm, in the form of poly-victimisation and/or chronic abuse over extended periods, against the odds. These stories are woven as deeply as the scars left by extreme trauma, abuse, and adversity while continuing to persevere in the face of the impacts of cumulative harm.

Francine*, abandoned by her mother at a young age, spent her childhood in an abusive home from age three to nine and a half, enduring daily physical and sexual abuse. Francine described waking up covered in blood after sexual attacks and being dismissed or punished when she tried to voice the repeated abuse. "I'd wake up in the middle of the night and somebody was all over me like a rash. I was sexually assaulted from the front and the back. When I'd wake up in the morning, I was covered in blood. I'd complain about it and I'd just get a whack". Her grandparents eventually rescued her, but the cumulative harm could not be erased. Francine later faced domestic violence and sexual abuse in her adult relationships, struggling to find protection and justice from authorities. Despite these challenges, she has fought to rebuild her life. She has stood up for herself and others, even speaking in parliament to protect her granddaughter. She continues to live with the lasting impacts of trauma, including PTSD, anxiety, and depression, but remains determined to survive and protect her family.

Norma* shared her harrowing story of survival marked by trauma, loss, and resilience. She was made a ward of the state at age 10 after her father's death and placed in church homes across the state. Her first child was born after a rape when she was 15, in a toilet at a girls' home. Shortly after, she attempted suicide but survived. She went on to endure the loss of multiple children—her son to suicide, another to SIDS, and her first daughter, whom she believes is buried under the chapel of a notorious Girls' Home. She was one of eight siblings, of which now only three remain alive. Her granddaughter, who was taken from her daughter at one week old, was later molested by her grandfather from age four to 16. Despite these tragedies, Norma has raised her family, including her daughters and grandchildren, and continues to support her granddaughter, who is recovering from time spent in a psychiatric ward. She is determined to ensure the system that harmed her does not further impact her life, advocating for dignity and justice.

Fred* described being institutionalised as a child, and after enduring chronic sexual abuse for seven years, he eventually escaped. One Sunday instead of fetching the Herald Sun for staff at a notorious Boys Home, he walked straight past that milk bar with only the 45 cents he was supposed to use, but with nine newspapers. He hopped a tram to the central train station and made his way interstate. Unfortunately for Fred, he never stopped running and later battled alcoholism, depression and suicidal thoughts. He recounts a dark moment when he drank excessively and attempted to end his life but was saved by police intervention. Through counselling and self-reflection, he has worked to confront his trauma and continues to seek closure. He describes the failure of institutions to protect children and the ongoing impact of his experiences, including trust issues, PTSD, and struggles with substance abuse. Fred* credits counselling and specialist support services for older "care" leavers for helping him move forward. Despite his hardships, Fred* remains determined to confront his past and advocate for better systems to protect vulnerable children.

Steven* shared his story of the lasting impact of cumulative harm arising driven by institutional abuse. Taken into "care" at the age of two and institutionalised until 16, he endured years of sexual abuse, neglect, and dehumanisation. At 16 years, he was abruptly thrown out onto the streets, unprepared for life, leading to homelessness and involvement in criminal activities. He describes living under bridges, in cars, and eventually finding dirty flats to survive. Steven* reflected on the lifelong effects of his experiences, including emotional detachment, PTSD, and difficulty forming relationships. He shared that he learned to suppress emotions, only recently allowing himself to cry again. He carries the weight of his trauma, stating that he and others like him will never be "normal" but that *"We survive. We don't thrive"*.

His story underscores the devastating consequences of institutional abuse and the resilience required to endure and navigate life afterward.

Brenda** was born into a large family. After losing her mother at a young age, she was placed in abusive environments, including with a grandmother who extorted her, allowing her to be raped for money by boarders in her grandmother's home. Brenda* went on to experience poly-victimisation through physical abuse, neglect, and institutional mistreatment during her childhood. She later endured abusive relationships, fleeing multiple times to protect her children, and became a single mother of six. Her life has been marked by loss, including the deaths of two children—one in a car accident and another from cot death. Despite these hardships, Brenda* advocates for dignity and respect in care systems, emphasising the importance of treating people with compassion.

Glenis** shared her deep emotional scars from childhood abuse and neglect, coupled with ongoing struggles to find belonging and self-worth. As a child, she was institutionalised and subjected to dehumanising treatment, including being told she was unwanted and that she was "fortunate" to be taken in. This instilled a lasting sense of worthlessness and fear, which she carried into adulthood. Her poly-victimisation experiences within an orphanage included physical punishment, deprivation, and psychological abuse, such as being locked in dark rooms and publicly shamed for wetting the bed. These traumas have left her with lasting fears, including a fear of locked rooms and a need for escape routes in her daily life. Glenis* also shared her struggles with privacy and trust issues, stemming from the lack of personal ownership and appropriate boundaries during her time in care. Despite her hardships, Glenis* has shared her story with the Royal Commission into Sexual Abuse, shedding light on the abuse she endured.

Ken's** story is one of survival through immense trauma and institutional abuse. He endured significant hardships during his time in orphanages and schools, including physical and sexual abuse, which deeply affected his ability to trust others and form relationships. The abuse left him with lasting emotional scars, including panic attacks, anxiety, and a fear of people invading his personal space. Ken* shared his struggles with alcoholism but made the decision to stop drinking 33 years ago, which he describes as a turning point in his life. He reflects on the systemic failures of institutions, particularly their inability to protect children and the long-term damage caused by abuse. Despite his trauma, Ken* has spent time writing and processing his experiences, using creativity as a way to cope and understand his past. He highlights the ongoing impacts of institutional abuse, including mistrust, emotional pain, and the difficulty of finding closure. Ken's resilience shines through as he continues to navigate life while carrying the weight of his past.

Eliza's** story is marked by her current experiences of homelessness and the challenges of surviving day-to-day. She longs for stability, reflecting on how her life might differ if she had a home, where she could enjoy simple pleasures like tending a garden or raising chickens. Her circumstances force her to move from place to place, unable to establish roots or a sense of normalcy. Eliza* shared her struggle of merely existing rather than thriving, and how homelessness impacts her ability to live a fulfilling life and accessing aged care services. "I did consider, if I couldn't look after myself, I could throw a brick in a shop window and maybe go to jail, but then I've heard jail's not much better [than aged care facilities]," she remarked. Despite her circumstances, she continues to survive and hold onto hope for a better future.

These stories illustrate the profound resilience of individuals who have survived unimaginable odds. Their survival is marked by their ability to endure, adapt, and find ways to move forward, even when thriving seems out of reach. Their pain fuels their advocacy, striving for systemic change and a future in which they can die with dignity in their homes and to not be subjected to another institution.

DISCUSSION AND CONCLUSION

Through the combined learnings from a large-scale survey and in-depth interviews, this study has shone a light on the experiences of "care" leavers as they approach older adulthood. A notable strength of the study was its use of a lived-experience methodology, which enabled rich, nuanced insights into participants' perceptions and experiences. The shared background between the interviewer and participants fostered trust and facilitated the exploration of sensitive topics. However, the study also has limitations. The sample, while diverse in geography and experience, was drawn primarily from support organisations and networks, potentially underrepresenting the voices of more isolated care leavers.

Across all stages of life, older "care" leavers' experiences reveal the profound and enduring impact of cumulative harm, childhood trauma and systemic failures, which uniquely impact their views on their current and future needs. The fact that we as researchers did not ask directly about experiences of cumulative harm, but rather they were introduced by older "care" leavers themselves, raises a crucial point. This demonstrates that the link between cumulative harm and its lasting impacts is a significant framework by which older "care" leavers understand their own lives. Their stories highlight the interconnectedness of early institutionalisation, adult struggles, and present-day challenges as they face older adulthood. Intergenerational disadvantage seems to have severely limited their life chances and often those of their children as well, although some were able to take advantage of 'windows of opportunity' (Harris, 2017, p.131) such as enhanced employment to improve their life circumstances.

The study findings also have important contributions to make to our understanding of the concept of cumulative harm. Foremost, the experiences of older "care" leavers remind us of the need to conceptualise cumulative harm as not solely driven by children's experiences within family relationships. While it may be tempting to minimise government and institutional contributions to cumulative harm as issues of a bygone era, contemporary research and inquiries continue to demonstrate that children are frequently at risk in these environments, including OOHC, youth justice and other institutional settings (Commission for Children and Young People, 2019; Commonwealth of Australia, 2017).

The study findings also raise the question of whether outcomes of cumulative harm that is driven through institutional experiences may differ from those driven by familial or other experiences. Many older "care" leavers' narratives demonstrate a specific trauma response to institutional environments which impacts their capacity to receive support and services in a range of settings, from hospital to aged care. This is a potentially important area for further inquiry in the field of understanding cumulative harm and its impacts. In relation to policy and practice, the study findings support a call for transformative change in systems to provide compassionate, tailored support that honours both the vulnerabilities and strengths of older "care" leavers who have endured profound childhood adversity and cumulative harm. These findings are a powerful reminder of the urgent need to create care environments that restore dignity, rebuild trust, and empower individuals as they navigate the complexities of later life.

REFERENCES

Airagnes, G., Lemogne, C., Hoertel, N., Goldberg, M., Lismosin, F., & Zins, M. (2016). Childhood adversity and depressive symptoms following retirement in the gazel cohort. *Journal of Psychiatric Research, 82*, 80–90. DOI: 10.1016/j.jpsychires.2016.07.015 PMID: 27471842

Alliance for Forgotten Australians. (2019). *Submission to Aged Care Royal Commission*, https://agedcare.royalcommission.gov.au/system/files/2020-07/AWF.001.03563_0.pdf

Anda, R. F., Chapman, D. P., Felitti, V. J., Edwards, V., Williamson, D. F., Croft, J. B., & Giles, W. H. (2002). Adverse childhood experiences and risk of paternity in teen pregnancy. *Obstetrics and Gynecology, 100*(1), 37–45. DOI: 10.1016/S0029-7844(02)02063-X PMID: 12100801

Anda, R. F., Felitti, V. J., Bremner, J. D., Walker, J. D., Whitfield, C., Perry, B. D., Dube, S. R., & Giles, W. H. (2006). The enduring effects of abuse and related adverse experiences in childhood. A convergence of evidence from neurobiology and epidemiology. *European Archives of Psychiatry and Clinical Neuroscience, 256*(3), 174–186. DOI: 10.1007/s00406-005-0624-4 PMID: 16311898

Anda, R. F., Fleisher, V. I., Felitti, V. J., Edwards, V. J., Whitfield, C. L., Dube, S. R., & Williamson, D. F. (2004). Childhood Abuse, Household Dysfunction, and Indicators of Impaired Adult Worker Performance. *The Permanente Journal, 8*(1), 30–38. DOI: 10.7812/TPP/03-089 PMID: 26704603

Atkinson, P. (2007). *Ethnography* (3rd ed.). Routledge., DOI: 10.4324/9780203944769

Australian Bureau of Statistics. (2023). *National Study of Mental Health and Wellbeing*. Canberra: ABS. https://www.abs.gov.au/statistics/health/mental-health/national-study-mental-health-and-wellbeing/latest-release

Australian Bureau of Statistics (ABS). (2022). *Marriages and Divorces Australia*. Canberra: ABS. https://www.abs.gov.au/statistics/people/people-and-communities/marriages-and-divorcesaustralia/latest-release

Australian Government Department of Health. (2019). *Exploratory Analysis of Barriers to Palliative Care: Issues Report on Care Leavers and People Affected by Forced Adoption*. Canberra: Australian Government Department of Health. https://www.health.gov.au/sites/default/files/documents/2020/01/exploratory-analysis-ofbarriers-to-palliative-care-issues-report-on-care-leavers-and-people-affected-by-forcedadoption.pdf

Australian Institute of Health and Welfare (AIHW). (2024). *Child Protection Australia 2021-22*. Canberra: AIHW. https://www.aihw.gov.au/reports/child-protection/child-protection-australia-2021-22/contents/child-protection-system-in-australia

Baidawi, S., Newton, D., Mendes, P., Bollinger, J., & Purtell, J. (2025). From care to corrections: A scoping review of pathways from child protection to adult criminal justice systems. *Trauma, Violence & Abuse*, *26*(3), 403–419. DOI: 10.1177/15248380241279861 PMID: 39302839

Beresford, P. (2019). *Beyond the Usual Suspects: The role of lived experience in social research.* Social Research Association.

Bromfield, L., & Miller, R. (2012). *Cumulative Harm—Best interests case practice model: Specialist practice resource.* Victoria: DHS. https://www.cpmanual.vic.gov.au/sites/default/files/Cumulative%20harm%20specialist%20practice%20resource%202012%203014%20.pdf

Browne-Yung, K., O'Neil, D., Walker, R., Corlis, M., Smyth, A., Putsey, P., Laver, K. E., Fernandez, E., & Cations, M. (2021). 'I'd rather die in the middle of a street': Perceptions and expectations of aged care among Forgotten Australians. *Australasian Journal on Ageing*, *40*(2), 168–176. DOI: 10.1111/ajag.12851 PMID: 33336557

Bryce, I., & Collier, S. (2022). A systematic literature review of the contribution accumulation makes to psychological and physical trauma sustained through childhood maltreatment. *Trauma Care*, *2*(2), 307–329. DOI: 10.3390/traumacare2020026

Carey, M. (2012). *Qualitative Research Skills for Social Work: Theory and practice.* Routledge.

Cebulla, A., & Katz, I. (2017). Unemployment, poverty and the future of work after the global financial crisis. In Serr, K. (Ed.), *Thinking about poverty* (pp. 58–73). The Federation Press.

CLAN. (2022). *Caring for Care Leavers in Australia's aged care sector.* CLAN.

Commission for Children and Young People (CCYP). (2017). *In our own words: Systemic inquiry into the lived experience of children and young people in the Victorian out-of-home care system.* Melbourne: CCYP. https://ccyp.vic.gov.au/assets/Publications-inquiries/CCYP-In-Our-Own-Words.pdf

Commonwealth of Australia. (1997). *Bringing them Home: Report of the National Inquiry into the Separation of Aboriginal and Torres Strait Islander Children from Their Families.* https://healingfoundation.org.au/app/uploads/2017/02/Bringing-Them-Home-Report.pdf

Commonwealth of Australia. (2001). Lost Innocents: Righting the Record - Report on child migration.https://www.aph.gov.au/~/media/wopapub/senate/committee/clac_ctte/completed_inquiries/1999_02/child_migrat/report/report_pdf.ashx

Commonwealth of Australia. (2004). Community Affairs References Committee: Forgotten Australians. A report on Australians who experienced institutional or out-of-home-care as children. https://www.aph.gov.au/parliamentary_business/committees/senate/community_ affairs/completed_inquiries/2004-07/inst_care/report/index

Commonwealth of Australia. (2017). Royal Commission into Institutional Responses to Child Sexual Abuse (2017): Final Report. Canberra: Commonwealth of Australia. https://www.childabuseroyalcommission.gov.au/final-report

Economic Inclusion Advisory Committee/EIAC. (2025). *2025 Report to government.* Commonwealth Government.

England-Mason, G., Casey, R., Ferro, M., MacMillan, H. L., Tonmyr, L., & Gonzalez, A. (2018). Child maltreatment and adult multimorbidity: Results from the Canadian community health survey. *Canadian Journal of Public Health = Revue Canadienne de Santé Publique, 109*(4), 561–572. DOI: 10.17269/s41997-018-0069-y PMID: 29981095

Felitti, V. J., Anda, R. F., Nordenberg, D., Williamson, D. F., Spitz, A. M., Edwards, V., Koss, M. P., & Marks, J. S. (1998). Relationship of childhood abuse and household dysfunction to many of the leading causes of death in adults. The Adverse Childhood Experiences (ACE) Study. *American Journal of Preventive Medicine, 14*(4), 245–258. DOI: 10.1016/S0749-3797(98)00017-8 PMID: 9635069

Fernandez, E., Lee, J., Blunden, H., McNamara, P., Kovacs, S., & Cornefert, P. (2016). *No child should grow up like this: Identifying long term outcomes of forgotten Australians, child migrants and the stolen generations.* University of New South Wales.

Flynn, C., & McDermott, F. (2024). *Doing Research in Social Work and Social Care* (2nd ed.). Sage Publishing.

Golding, F. (2022). Sexual abuse as the core transgression of childhood innocence: Unintended consequences for care leavers. In Wright, K., Swain, S., & McPhillips, K. (Eds.), *Examining the past and shaping the future: The Australian royal commission into institutional responses to child sexual abuse* (pp. 55–67). Routledge.

Gypen, L., Vanderfaeillie, J., De Maeyer, S., Belenger, L., & Van Holen, F. (2017). Outcomes of children who grew up in foster care: A systematic review. *Children and Youth Services Review*, *76*, 74–83. DOI: 10.1016/j.childyouth.2017.02.035

Harris, P. (2017). Poverty and disadvantage among children and families. In Serr, K. (Ed.), *Thinking about poverty* (pp. 121–136). The Federation Press.

Healing Foundation. (2019). *Working with Stolen Generations Aged Care Fact Sheet*. https://cdn.healingfoundation.org.au/app/uploads/2019/12/18122008/Working-with-Stolen-Generations-Aged-Care-fact-sheet.pdf

Healing Foundation. (2025). *Who are the Stolen Generations*. https://healingfoundation.org.au/who-are-the-stolen-generations/

Liamputtong, P. (2007). *Researching the Vulnerable*. SAGE Publications Ltd., DOI: 10.4135/9781849209861

McNamara, P., Harvey, A., & Andrewartha, L. (2019). Passports out of poverty: Raising access to higher education for care leavers in Australia. *Children & Youth Services Review*, 97, 85–93, ISSN 0190-7409, DOI: 10.1016/j.childyouth.2017.07.015

Mendes, P., Michell, D., & Wilson, J. Z. (2014). Young people transitioning from out-of-home care and access to higher education: A critical review of the literature. *Children Australia*, *39*(4), 243–252. DOI: 10.1017/cha.2014.25

Michell, D., Jackson, D., & Tonkin, C. (Eds.). (2015). *Against the odds: Care leavers at university*. People's Voice Publishing.

National Aged Care Alliance. (2017). *Ensuring equity of access and outcomes in the future aged care system*. https://naca.asn.au/wp-content/uploads/2018/11/Equity-of-Access-andOutcomes-Statement-of-Principles_Landscape-1.pdf

Organisation for Economic Co-operation and Development (OECD). (2022). *Assisting care leavers: Time for action*. OECD Publishing., DOI: 10.1787/1939a9ec-

Sacker, A., Murray, E., Lacey, R., & Maughan, B. (2021). *The lifelong health and wellbeing trajectories of people who have been in care: Findings from the looked-after children grown up project*. Nuffield Foundation. https://www.nuffieldfoundation.org/wp-content/uploads/2021/07/The-lifelong-health-and-wellbeing-trajectories-of-people-who-have-been-in-care.pdf

Sheehan, R. (2019). Cumulative harm in the child protection system: The Australian context. *Child & Family Social Work*, *24*(4), 421–429. DOI: 10.1111/cfs.12621

Smith, G.P. (2015). *Nobody's Children: An exploration into a sense of belonging of adults who experienced institutional out-of-home care as children.* [Doctoral thesis, Southern Cross University].

Smith, G. P. (2017). Historical out-of-home child care leavers and mental health needs. *Australian Social Work, 70*(1), 1–3. DOI: 10.1080/0312407X.2017.1246070

Smith, J. A., & Osborn, M. (2008). Interpretative Phenomenological Analysis. In Breakwell, G. M. (Ed.), *Doing Psychology Research* (pp. 229–254). Wiley., DOI: 10.1002/9780470776278.ch10

Stein, M., & Ward, H. (2021). Editorial: Transitions from care to adulthood—persistent issues across time and place. *Child & Family Social Work, 26*(2), 215–221. DOI: 10.1111/cfs.12802

Testa, A., Jackson, D. B., Ganson, K. T., & Nagata, J. M. (2022). Adverse childhood experiences and criminal justice contact in adulthood. *Academic Pediatrics, 22*(6), 972–980. DOI: 10.1016/j.acap.2021.10.011 PMID: 34752957

Tuart Place. (2019), *Submission to Aged Care Royal Commission*, https://agedcare.royalcommission.gov.au/sites/default/files/2020-09/AWF.001.04093.00_001.pdf

Wilson, J. Z., Mendes, P., & Golding, F. (2018). Hope street: From voice to agency for care-leavers in higher education. *Life Writing, 15*(4), 597–609. DOI: 10.1080/14484528.2018.1427420

KEY TERMS AND DEFINITIONS

Children's Institutions: refers to a range of settings, such as orphanages, missions, dormitories, group "homes", youth detention centres, laundries etc, where children were housed by the state or religious institution, and were often subjected to trauma, abuse (physical and sexual), neglect and hard labour.

Cumulative Harm: The harm or negative effects to an individual over the life course, which arises as the result of the either an ongoing adverse event or circumstance (for example, chronic neglect), or multiple co-occurring adverse events or circumstances (sometimes termed poly-victimisation).

Forgotten Australians: The approximately 500,000 non-Indigenous Australian-born or former child migrants who lived in institutional OOHC including orphanages, children's homes and foster care – from roughly 1920 to the late 1980s.

Former Child Migrants: The around 7,000 individuals who grew up in children's homes, orphanages and other institutions around Australia in the 20th century, but who initially came to Australia as child migrants. These children most commonly arrived from the United Kingdom, Ireland and Malta, under approved child migrant schemes, and usually unaccompanied by their parents.

Older "care" leavers: In Australia older care leavers, sometimes called Forgotten Australians in popular discourse, are the approximately 500,000 individuals who lived in institutional out-of-home "care" (OOHC) – that is orphanages, children's homes and foster care – from roughly 1920 to the late 1980s.

Out-of-home "care" (OOHC): A range of forms of government-funded living arrangements for children who do not live with their biological parents. This includes arrangements where children are looked after by relative (kinship), non-relative (foster) or group-based (residential) caregivers.

Resilience: as the ability to endure and survive despite severe trauma, abuse, and adversity. In the context of individuals who have faced institutional abuse, intergenerational trauma, and ongoing impacts of their experiences, yet continue to persevere. Resilience is evident in their determination to survive, protect their loved ones, and seek closure or healing.

Stolen Generations: The generations during which Aboriginal and Torres Strait Islander children who were forcibly removed from their parents under racist, genocidal and assimilationist policies from the mid-1800s to the 1970s. During this period, thousands of Aboriginal children were systematically taken from their families, communities and culture, and placed in institutions, adopted or fostered by non-Indigenous people. Stolen children often endured horrific abuse and exploitation, and were denied access to their communities, languages and cultures.

Compilation of References

Abbassi, A., & Aslinia, S. D. (2010). Family violence, trauma and social learning theory. *Journal of Professional Counseling, Practice, Theory, & Research, 38*(1), 16–27. DOI: 10.1080/15566382.2010.12033863

Ackerman, R. J., DiRamio, D., & Mitchell, K. S. (2009). Posttraumatic stress disorder and other mental health diagnoses in returning veterans. *The Psychiatric Times, 26*(8).

Adelman, M., Rosenberg, K. E., & Hobart, M. (2016). Simulations and social empathy. *Violence Against Women, 22*(12), 1451–1462. DOI: 10.1177/1077801215625850

Afifi, T. O., & MacMillan, H. L. (2011). Resilience following child maltreatment: A review of protective factors. *Canadian Journal of Psychiatry, 56*(5), 266–272. DOI: 10.1177/070674371105600505 PMID: 21586192

Afifi, T. O., MacMillan, H. L., Boyle, M., Taillieu, T., Cheung, K., & Sareen, J. (2014). Child abuse and mental disorders in Canada. *Canadian Medical Association Journal, 186*(9), E324–E332. DOI: 10.1503/cmaj.131792 PMID: 24756625

Aguiar, W., & Halseth, R. (2015). *Aboriginal peoples and historic trauma: The processes of intergenerational transmission*. National Collaborating Centre for Aboriginal Health.

Ainsworth, M. D. (1973). The development of infant mother attachment. In Caldwell, B. M., & Ricciuti, H. N. (Eds.), *Review of child development research* (Vol. 3). University of Chicago Press.

Ainsworth, M. D. S. (1978). The Bowlby-Ainsworth attachment theory. *Behavioral and Brain Sciences, 1*(3), 436–438. DOI: 10.1017/S0140525X00075828

Ainsworth, M. S., & Bowlby, J. (1991). An ethological approach to personality development. *The American Psychologist, 46*(4), 333–341. DOI: 10.1037/0003-066X.46.4.333

Airagnes, G., Lemogne, C., Hoertel, N., Goldberg, M., Lismosin, F., & Zins, M. (2016). Childhood adversity and depressive symptoms following retirement in the gazel cohort. *Journal of Psychiatric Research, 82*, 80–90. DOI: 10.1016/j.jpsychires.2016.07.015 PMID: 27471842

Alexander, L. H., & Alessi, E. J. (2024). A critical review of the conceptualization of empathy: Toward a deeper understanding for clinical social work practice. *Clinical Social Work Journal, 52*(3), 300–309. DOI: 10.1007/s10615-023-00912-z

Alexander, L., Cooper, K., Peters, M. D. J., Tricco, A. C., Khalil, H., Evans, C., Munn, Z., Pieper, D., Godfrey, C. M., McInerney, P., & Pollock, D. (2024). Large scoping reviews: Managing volume and potential chaos in a pool of evidence sources. *Journal of Clinical Epidemiology, 170*, 111343. Advance online publication. DOI: 10.1016/j.jclinepi.2024.111343 PMID: 38582403

Alexander, P. C. (2015). *Intergenerational cycles of trauma and violence: An attachment and family systems perspective.* WW Norton & Company.

Alfandari, R., & Taylor, B. J. (2022). Community-based multi-professional child protection decision making: Systematic narrative review. *Child Abuse & Neglect, 123*, 105432. DOI: 10.1016/j.chiabu.2021.105432 PMID: 34922154

Alink, L. R. A., Cyr, C., & Madigan, S. (2019). The effect of maltreatment experiences on maltreating and dysfunctional parenting: A search for mechanisms. *Development and Psychopathology, 31*(1), 1–7. DOI: 10.1017/S0954579418001517

Allen, B. (2025). Childhood sexual behavior as a mediator of the relationship between sexual abuse and early sexual debut: A prospective analysis. *Archives of Sexual Behavior.* , C. M., Langhinrichsen-Rohling, J., Bowers, D., O'Brien, N. (2007). Differential correlates of multi-type maltreatment among urban youth. *Child Abuse & Neglect, 31*, 393–415. https://www.sciencedirect.com/science/article/pii/S0145213407000609DOI: 10.1007/s10508-025-03228-wArata

Alliance for Forgotten Australians. (2019). *Submission to Aged Care Royal Commission*, https://agedcare.royalcommission.gov.au/system/files/2020-07/AWF.001.03563_0.pdf

Altafim, E. R. P., Pedro, M. E. A., & Linhares, M. B. M. (2016). Effectiveness of ACT raising safe kids parenting program in a developing country. *Children and Youth Services Review, 70*, 315–323. DOI: 10.1016/j.childyouth.2016.09.038

American Psychiatric Association. (2013). *Diagnostic and statistical manual of mental disorders* (5th ed.).

Amos, J., Furber, G., & Segal, L. (2011). Understanding maltreating mothers: A synthesis of relational trauma, attachment disorganization, structural dissociation of the personality, and experiential avoidance. *Journal of Trauma & Dissociation, 12*(5), 495–509. DOI: 10.1080/15299732.2011.593259 PMID: 21967177

Amos, J., & Segal, L. (2018). Disrupting intergenerational maternal maltreatment in middle childhood: Therapeutic objectives and clinical translation. *Frontiers in Psychiatry, 9*, 623. DOI: 10.3389/fpsyt.2018.00623 PMID: 30538646

Anda, R. F., Chapman, D. P., Felitti, V. J., Edwards, V., Williamson, D. F., Croft, J. B., & Giles, W. H. (2002). Adverse childhood experiences and risk of paternity in teen pregnancy. *Obstetrics and Gynecology, 100*(1), 37–45. DOI: 10.1016/S0029-7844(02)02063-X PMID: 12100801

Anda, R. F., Felitti, V. J., Bremner, J. D., Walker, J. D., Whitfield, C., Perry, B. D., Dube, S. R., & Giles, W. H. (2006). The enduring effects of abuse and related adverse experiences in childhood. A convergence of evidence from neurobiology and epidemiology. *European Archives of Psychiatry and Clinical Neuroscience, 256*(3), 174–186. DOI: 10.1007/s00406-005-0624-4 PMID: 16311898

Anda, R. F., Fleisher, V. I., Felitti, V. J., Edwards, V. J., Whitfield, C. L., Dube, S. R., & Williamson, D. F. (2004). Childhood Abuse, Household Dysfunction, and Indicators of Impaired Adult Worker Performance. *The Permanente Journal, 8*(1), 30–38. DOI: 10.7812/TPP/03-089 PMID: 26704603

Anderson, D. K., & Saunders, D. G. (2003). Leaving an abusive partner: An empirical review of predictors, the process of leaving, and psychological well-being. *Trauma, Violence & Abuse, 4*(2), 163–191. DOI: 10.1177/1524838002250769 PMID: 14697121

Anderson, E. (2023). Hermeneutic labor: The gendered burden of interpretation in intimate relationships between women and men. *Hypatia, 38*(1), 177–197. DOI: 10.1017/hyp.2023.11

Annerbäck, E. M., Sahlqvist, L., Svedin, C. G., Wingren, G., & Gustafsson, P. A. (2012). Child physical abuse and concurrence of other types of child abuse in Sweden—Associations with health and risk behaviors. *Child Abuse & Neglect, 36*(7-8), 585–595. DOI: 10.1016/j.chiabu.2012.05.006 PMID: 22854707

Apple, M. W. (2012). *Education and power* (2nd ed.). Routledge., DOI: 10.4324/9780203143124

Appleyard, K., & Osofsky, J. D. (2003). Parenting after trauma: Supporting parents and caregivers in the treatment of children impacted by violence. *Infant Mental Health Journal, 24*(2), 111–125. DOI: 10.1002/imhj.10050

Arata, C. M., Langhinrichsen-Rohling, J., Bowers, D., & O'Farrill-Swails, L. (2005). Single versus multi-type maltreatment: An examination of the long-term effects of child abuse. *Journal of Aggression, Maltreatment & Trauma, 11*(4), 29–52. DOI: 10.1300/J146v11n04_02

Arksey, H., & O'Malley, L. (2005). Scoping studies: Towards a methodological framework. *International Journal of Social Research Methodology, 8*(1), 19–32. DOI: 10.1080/1364557032000119616

Armfield, J. M., Gnanamanickam, E. S., Johnston, D. W., Preen, D. B., Brown, D. S., Nguyen, H., & Segal, L. (2021). Intergenerational transmission of child maltreatment in South Australia, 1986–2017: A retrospective cohort study. *The Lancet. Public Health, 6*(7), 450–461. DOI: 10.1016/S2468-2667(21)00024-4 PMID: 33939966

Arney, F., Iannos, M., Chong, A., McDougall, S., & Parkinson, S. (2015). *Enhancing the implementation of the Aboriginal and Torres Strait Islander Child Placement Principle: Policy and practice considerations*. CFCA Paper No. 34. Australian Institute of Family Studies.

Arons, J. (2005). "In a black hole": The (negative) space between longing and dread: Home-based psychotherapy with a traumatized mother and her infant son. *The Psychoanalytic Study of the Child, 60*(1), 101–127. DOI: 10.1080/00797308.2005.11800748 PMID: 16649677

Aronson, B., & Laughter, J. (2016). The theory and practice of culturally relevant education: A synthesis of research across content areas. *Review of Educational Research, 86*(1), 163–206. DOI: 10.3102/0034654315582066

Åsen, M. E., Schalinski, I., Lehmann, S., Lydersen, S., Von Oertzen, T., & Greger, H. K. (2024). Child maltreatment in young adults with residential youth care background: Prevalence and post-placement trends. *Child Abuse & Neglect, 157*, 107. DOI: 10.1016/j.chiabu.2024.107074 PMID: 39395227

Assink, M., Spruit, A., Schuts, M., Lindauer, R., van der Put, C. E., & Stams, G.-J. J. M. (2018). The intergenerational transmission of child maltreatment: A three-level meta-analysis. *Child Abuse & Neglect, 84*, 131–145. DOI: 10.1016/j.chiabu.2018.07.037 PMID: 30086419

Atkinson, J., Nelson, J., & Atkinson, C. (2010). Trauma, transgenerational transfer and effects on community wellbeing. In N. Purdie, P. Dudgeon, & R. Walker (Eds.), *Working together: Aboriginal and Torres Strait Islander mental health and wellbeing principles and practice* (pp. 135–144). Commonwealth of Australia.

Atkinson, J. (2002). *Trauma trails, recreating song lines: The transgenerational effects of trauma in Indigenous Australia*. Spinifex Press.

Atkinson, J. (2002). *Trauma trails: Recreating song lines: The transgenerational effect of trauma in Indigenous Australia*. Spinifex Press.

Atkinson, J. (2013). *Trauma-informed services and trauma-specific care for Indigenous Australian children*. Closing the Gap Clearinghouse.

Atkinson, P. (2007). *Ethnography* (3rd ed.). Routledge., DOI: 10.4324/9780203944769

Auriemma, V. (2023). *Empathy: The contribution of neuroscience to social analysis*. Palgrave Macmillan., DOI: 10.1007/978-3-031-38860-6

Australian Broadcasting Corporation. (2024). Foster carers leave the system in droves as cost-of-living pressures bite. *ABC News*. https://www.abc.net.au/news/2024-07-15/foster-carers-leaving-compensation-allowance-cost-of-living/104047836

Australian Bureau of Statistics (ABS). (2022). *Marriages and Divorces Australia*. Canberra: ABS. https://www.abs.gov.au/statistics/people/people-and-communities/marriages-and-divorcesaustralia/latest-release

Australian Bureau of Statistics. (2023). *National Study of Mental Health and Wellbeing*. Canberra: ABS. https://www.abs.gov.au/statistics/health/mental-health/national-study-mental-health-and-wellbeing/latest-release

Australian Government Department of Health. (2019). *Exploratory Analysis of Barriers to Palliative Care: Issues Report on Care Leavers and People Affected by Forced Adoption*. Canberra: Australian Government Department of Health. https://www.health.gov.au/sites/default/files/documents/2020/01/exploratory-analysis-ofbarriers-to-palliative-care-issues-report-on-care-leavers-and-people-affected-by-forcedadoption.pdf

Australian Housing and Urban Research Institute. (2023). *Crisis accommodation in Australia: Now and for the future* (AHURI Final Report No. 407). AHURI.

Australian Institute of Family Studies. (2022). *Identifying strategies to better support foster, kinship and permanent carers*. Commonwealth of Australia.

Australian Institute of Health and Welfare (AIHW). (2023). *Child Protection Australia 2021–22*. Australian Government. https://www.aihw.gov.au/reports/child-protection/child-protection-australia-2021-22

Australian Institute of Health and Welfare (AIHW). (2024). *Child protection Australia 2021–22 web report* (catalogue number CWS 92). Australian Government. www.aihw.gov.au/getmedia/2cecbc62-8c65-4031-a6df-5fec9422b0cf/child-protection-australia-2021-22.pdf?v=20240516104741&inline=true

Australian Institute of Health and Welfare (AIHW). (2024). *Child Protection Australia 2021-22*. Canberra: AIHW. https://www.aihw.gov.au/reports/child-protection/child-protection-australia-2021-22/contents/child-protection-system-in-australia

Australian Institute of Health and Welfare. (2020). *Crossover children: Vulnerabilities in youth justice supervision.* Canberra: AIHW Australian Institute of Criminology (AIC). (2022). *Crossover kids: Youth justice involvement among children known to child protection.* Canberra: AIC. *Research Reports (Montgomery).*

Australian Institute of Health and Welfare. (2023). *The health of people in Australia's prisons 2022*. Australian Government.

Australian Institute of Health and Welfare. (2023a). *Child protection Australia 2021–22* (Cat. no: CWS 92). AIHW. Retrieved from www.aihw.gov.au/reports/child-protection/child-protection-australia-2021-22

Australian Institute of Health and Welfare. (2023b). *Australia's welfare 2023: Data insights – Young people who have experienced child protection*. AIHW.

Australian Institute of Health and Welfare. (2023c). *Child Protection Australia 2021–2022*. Child welfare series no. 75. Cat no. CWS 92. AIHW.

Australian Institute of Health and Welfare. (2025). *Child protection Australia 2023–24*. AIHW.

Australian Institute of Health and Welfare. (2025). *Closing the Gap targets: Key findings and implications*. https://www.aihw.gov.au/reports/indigenous-australians/closing-the-gap-targets-key-findings-implications/contents/child-protection

Australian Law Reform Commission. (2018). *Pathways to justice – Inquiry into the incarceration rate of Aboriginal and Torres Strait Islander peoples (ALRC Report 133)*. Australian Government. https://www.alrc.gov.au/publication/pathways-to-justice-inquiry-into-the-incarceration-rate-of-aboriginal-and-torres-strait-islander-peoples-alrc-report-133/

Au, W. (2021). A pedagogy of insurgency: Teaching and organizing for radical racial justice in our schools. *Educational Studies (Ames)*, *57*(2), 109–123. DOI: 10.1080/00131946.2021.1878181

Avenanti, A., Sirigu, A., & Aglioti, S. M. (2010). Racial bias reduces empathic sensorimotor resonance with other-race pain. *Current Biology*, *20*(11), 1018–1022. DOI: 10.1016/j.cub.2010.03.071

Avery, J. C., Morris, H., Galvin, E., Misso, M., Savaglio, M., & Skouteris, H. (2021). Systematic review of school-wide trauma-informed approaches. *Journal of Child & Adolescent Trauma*, *14*(3), 381–397. DOI: 10.1007/s40653-020-00321-1 PMID: 34471456

Avery, L., Hutchinson, K. D., & Whitaker, K. (2002). Domestic Violence and Intergenerational Rates of Child Sexual Abuse: A Case Record Analysis. *Child & Adolescent Social Work Journal*, *19*(1), 77–90. DOI: 10.1023/A:1014007507349

Babcock Fenerci, R. L., & DePrince, A. P. (2018). Intergenerational transmission of trauma: Maternal trauma–related cognitions and toddler symptoms. *Child Maltreatment*, *23*(2), 126–136. DOI: 10.1177/1077559517737376 PMID: 29092624

Babcock, R., Fenerci, R. L., Chu, A. T., & DePrince, A. P. (2016). Intergenerational transmission of trauma-related distress: Maternal betrayal trauma, parenting attitudes, and behaviors. *Journal of Aggression, Maltreatment & Trauma*, *25*(4), 382–399. DOI: 10.1080/10926771.2015.1129655

Bachrach, R. L., & Read, J. P. (2012). Prevalence of traumatic events in college students: Implications for intervention. *Psychological Trauma: Theory, Research, Practice, and Policy*, *4*, 237–246.

Badger, D., Nursten, J., Williams, P., & Woodward, M. (2000). Should all literature reviews be systematic? *Evaluation and Research in Education*, *14*(3-4), 220–230. DOI: 10.1080/09500790008666974

Baez, S., Flichtentrei, D., Prats, M., Mastandueno, R., García, A. M., Cetkovich, M., & Ibáñez, A. (2017). Men, women… who cares? A population-based study on sex differences and gender roles in empathy and moral cognition. *PLoS One*, *12*(6), e0179336. DOI: 10.1371/journal.pone.0179336

Baglivio, M. T., Wolff, K. T., Jackowski, K., & Greenwald, M. A. (2018). A multilevel examination of risk/need change scores, community context, and successful reentry of committed juvenile offenders. *Youth Violence and Juvenile Justice*, *15*(1), 38–61. DOI: 10.1177/1541204015596052

Baidawi, S., Newton, D., Mendes, P., Bollinger, J., & Purtell, J. (2025). From care to corrections: A scoping review of pathways from child protection to adult criminal justice systems. *Trauma, Violence & Abuse*, *26*(3), 403–419. DOI: 10.1177/15248380241279861 PMID: 39302839

Baldwin, H., Biehal, N., Cusworth, L., Wade, J., Allgar, V., & Vostanis, P. (2019). Disentangling the effect of out-of-home care on child mental health. *Child Abuse & Neglect*, *88*, 189–200. DOI: 10.1016/j.chiabu.2018.11.011 PMID: 30537620

Baldwin, J. R., Wang, B., Karwatowska, L., Schoeler, T., Tsaligopoulou, A., Munafò, M. R., & Pingault, J. B. (2023). Childhood maltreatment and mental health problems: A systematic review and meta-analysis of quasi-experimental studies. *The American Journal of Psychiatry*, *180*(2), 117–126. DOI: 10.1176/appi.ajp.20220174 PMID: 36628513

Balsells, M. A., Pastor, C., Molina, M. C., Fuentes-Pelaez, N., Vaquero, E., & Mundet, A. (2013). Child welfare and successful reunification: Understanding of the family difficulties during the socio-educative process. *Revista de Cercetare si Interventie Sociala*, *42*, 228–247.

Bandura, A. (1977). *Social learning theory*. Prentice Hall.

Bandura, A. (1978). Social learning theory of aggression. *Journal of Communication*, *28*(3), 12–29. DOI: 10.1111/j.1460-2466.1978.tb01621.x PMID: 690254

Banyard, V., & Cantor, D. (2004). Adjustment to college: The role of violence-related trauma. *Journal of Interpersonal Violence*, *19*(1), 25–43.

Barnett, D., Ganiban, J., & Cicchetti, D. (1999). Maltreatment, negative expressivity, and the development of type D attachments from 12- to 24-months of age. *Monographs of the Society for Research in Child Development*, *64*(3), 97–118. DOI: 10.1111/1540-5834.00035 PMID: 10597544

Barnett, D., Manly, J. T., & Cicchetti, D. (1993). Defining child maltreatment: The interface between policy and research. In Cicchetti, D., & Toth, S. L. (Eds.), *Child abuse, child development, and social policy* (pp. 7–73). Ablex Publishing.

Baron-Cohen, S., & Wheelwright, S. (2004). The empathy quotient: An investigation of adults with Asperger syndrome or high functioning autism, and normal sex differences. *Journal of Autism and Developmental Disorders*, *34*(2), 163–175. DOI: 10.1023/B:JADD.0000022607.19833.00

Barth, R. P., Weigensberg, E. C., Fisher, P. A., Fetrow, B., & Green, R. L. (2008). Reentry of elementary aged children following reunification from foster care. *Children and Youth Services Review*, *30*(4), 353–364. DOI: 10.1016/j.childyouth.2007.10.002

Bartlett, J. D., Kotake, C., Fauth, R., & Easterbrooks, M. A. (2017). Intergenerational transmission of child abuse and neglect: Do maltreatment type, perpetrator, and substantiation status matter? *Child Abuse & Neglect, 63*, 84–94. DOI: 10.1016/j.chiabu.2016.11.021 PMID: 27914238

Bath, H. (2008). The three pillars of trauma-informed care. *Reclaiming Children and Youth, 17*(3), 17–21.

Beal, S. J., Ammerman, R. T., Mara, C. A., Nause, K., & Greiner, M. V. (2022). Patterns of healthcare utilization with placement changes for youth in foster care. *Child Abuse & Neglect, 128*, 105592. DOI: 10.1016/j.chiabu.2022.105592 PMID: 35334304

Beaucar, A. (1999). The effect of direct and vicarious trauma on therapists: Posttraumatic stress symptomatology. *Dissertation Abstracts International, 60*(09), 4913B.

Beauregard, P. (2024). Emotional labor in decision making: Gender, race, and relational practices in the White House. *Presidential Studies Quarterly, 54*(3), 691–712. DOI: 10.1111/psq.12884

Beebe, B., Jaffe, J., Markese, S., Buck, K., Chen, H., Cohen, P., Bahrick, L., Andrews, H., & Feldstein, S. (2010). The origins of 12-month attachment: A microanalysis of 4-month mother-infant interaction. *Attachment & Human Development, 12*(1/2), 3–141. DOI: 10.1080/14616730903338985 PMID: 20390524

Beeghly, M., & Cicchetti, D. (1994). Child maltreatment, attachment, and the self system: Emergence of an internal state lexicon in toddlers at high social risk. *Development and Psychopathology, 6*(1), 5–30. DOI: 10.1017/S095457940000585X

Beer, A., Vij, A., Baker, E., Crommelin, L., Dodson, J., Gharaie, E., Li, T., & Horne, S. (2024). *Disruption in regional housing: Policy responses for more resilient markets* (AHURI Final Report No. 424). Australian Housing and Urban Research Institute.

Belsky, J. (1993). Etiology of child maltreatment: A developmental ecological analysis. *Psychological Bulletin, 114*(3), 413–434. DOI: 10.1037/0033-2909.114.3.413 PMID: 8272464

Belsky, J., & Pensky, E. (1988). Developmental history, personality, and family relationships: Towards an emergent family system. In Hinde, R. A., & Stevenson-Hinde, J. (Eds.), *Relationships within families: Mutual influences*. Claredon Press.

Benbenishty, R., Davidson-Arad, B., López, M., Devaney, J., Spratt, T., Koopmans, C., Knorth, E. J., Witteman, C. L. M., Del Valle, J. F., & Hayes, D. (2015). Decision making in child protection: An international comparative study on maltreatment substantiation, risk assessment and interventions recommendations, and the role of professionals' child welfare attitudes. *Child Abuse & Neglect*, *49*, 63–75. DOI: 10.1016/j.chiabu.2015.03.015 PMID: 25935254

Bennett, D. B. (2021). Implications of maltreatment for young children. In Geffner, R., & White, J. W. (Eds.), *Handbook of interpersonal violence and abuse across the lifespan: A project of the National Partnership to End Interpersonal Violence Across the Lifespan (NPEIV)* (pp. 1225–1248). Springer International Publishing.

Bennett, K., Booth, A., Gair, S., Kibet, R., & Thorpe, R. (2020). Poverty is the problem – not parents: So tell me, child protection worker, how can you help? *Children Australia*, *45*(4), 207–214. DOI: 10.1017/cha.2020.39

Berardi, M. K., White, A. M., Winters, D., Thorn, K., Brennan, M., & Dolan, P. (2020). Rebuilding communities with empathy. *Local Development & Society*, *1*(1), 57–67. DOI: 10.1080/26883597.2020.1794761

Beresford, P. (2019). *Beyond the Usual Suspects: The role of lived experience in social research.* Social Research Association.

Berger, E. (2019). Multi-tiered approaches to trauma-informed care in schools: A systematic review. *School Mental Health*, *11*(4), 650–664. DOI: 10.1007/s12310-019-09326-0

Berger, L. M., & Slack, K. S. (2014). Child protection and child well-being. In *Handbook of child well-being* (pp. 2965–2992). Springer., DOI: 10.1007/978-90-481-9063-8_120

Berke, D. S., Reidy, D., & Zeichner, A. (2018). Masculinity, emotion regulation, and psychopathology. *Clinical Psychology Review*, *66*, 106–116. DOI: 10.1016/j.cpr.2018.01.004

Berman, S. L., Weems, C. F., & Stickle, T. R. (2022). Threat detection and attention to danger cues in youth exposed to adversity: A systematic review. *Clinical Child and Family Psychology Review*, *25*(2), 289–312. DOI: 10.1007/s10567-021-00358-1

Berthelot, N., Ensink, K., Bernazzani, O., Normandin, L., Luyten, P., & Fonagy, P. (2015). Intergenerational transmission of attachment in abused and neglected mothers: The role of trauma-specific reflective functioning. *Infant Mental Health Journal*, *36*(2), 200–212. DOI: 10.1002/imhj.21499 PMID: 25694333

Berzenski, S. R., & Yates, T. M. (2011). Classes and consequences of multiple maltreatment: A person-centered analysis. *Child Maltreatment, 16*(4), 250–261. DOI: 10.1177/1077559511428353 PMID: 22146858

Bessarab, D., & Ng'andu, B. (2010). Yarning about yarning as a legitimate method in Indigenous research. *International Journal of Critical Indigenous Studies, 3*(1), 37–50. DOI: 10.5204/ijcis.v3i1.57

Biehal, N. (2006). *Reuniting looked after children with their families: A research review*. University of York.

Biehal, N., Baldwin, H., Cusworth, L., Wade, J., & Allgar, V. (2018). In-home support or out of home care? Thresholds for intervention with abused and neglected children. *Children and Youth Services Review, 89*, 263–271. DOI: 10.1016/j.childyouth.2018.04.041

Bifulco, A., Moran, P. M., Ball, C., & Bernazzani, O. (2002). Adult attachment style: Its relationship to clinical depression. *Social Psychiatry and Psychiatric Epidemiology, 37*(2), 50–59. DOI: 10.1007/s127-002-8215-0

Bifulco, A., & Thomas, G. (2013). *Understanding adult attachment in family relationships: Research, assessment and intervention*. Routledge.

Bijlsma, A. M., Assink, M., Overbeek, G., van Geffen, M., & van der Put, C. E. (2023). Differences in developmental problems between victims of different types of child maltreatment. *Journal of Public Child Welfare, 17*(2), 408–429. Advance online publication. DOI: 10.1080/15548732.2022.2044429 PMID: 36896409

Bishop, R., & Berryman, M. (2006). *Culture speaks: Cultural relationships and classroom learning*. Huia Publishers.

Blakemore, T., & Rak, L. (2024). Empathy expressed and experienced. In Blakemore, T., Rak, L., Krogh, C., McCarthy, S., & Stuart, G. (Eds.), *Working with youth violence: The Name.Narrate.Navigate program* (pp. 194–219). Routledge.

Bloeser, K., McCarron, K. K., Merker, V. L., Hyde, J., Bolton, R. E., Anastasides, N., Petrakis, B. A., Helmer, D. A., Santos, S., Litke, D., Pigeon, W. R., & McAndrew, L. M. (2021). "Because the country, it seems though, has turned their back on me": Experiences of institutional betrayal among veterans living with Gulf War Illness. *Social Science & Medicine, 284*, 114–211. DOI: 10.1016/j.socscimed.2021.114211 PMID: 34271400

Blome, W. W., & Steib, S. (2008). An examination of oversight and review in the child welfare system: The many watch the few serve the many. *Journal of Public Child Welfare, 1*(3), 3–26. DOI: 10.1300/J479v01n03_02

Bloom, S. L. (1997). *Creating sanctuary: Toward the evolution of sane societies.* Routledge.

Bogat, G. A., Levendosky, A. A., & Eye, A. (2005). The future of research on intimate partner violence: Person-oriented and variable-oriented perspectives. *American Journal of Community Psychology, 36*(1/2), 49–70. DOI: 10.1007/s10464-005-6232-7 PMID: 16134044

Bohannan, T., Gonzalez, C., & Summers, A. (2016). Assessing the relationship between a peer mentoring program and case outcomes in dependency court. *Journal of Public Child Welfare, 10*(2), 176–196. DOI: 10.1080/15548732.2016.1155523

Böhm, B., Zollner, H., Fegert, J. M., & Liebhardt, H. (2014). Child sexual abuse in the context of the Roman Catholic Church: A review of literature from 1981–2013. *Journal of Child Sexual Abuse, 23*(6), 635–656. DOI: 10.1080/10538712.2014.929607 PMID: 24911986

Bombay, A., Matheson, K., & Anisman, H. (2009). Intergenerational trauma: Convergence of multiple processes among First Nations peoples in Canada. *Journal of Aboriginal Health, 5*(3), 6–47.

Bonanno, G. A. (2005). Resilience in the face of potential trauma. *Current Directions in Psychological Science, 14*(3), 135–138. DOI: 10.1111/j.0963-7214.2005.00347.x

Bonilla, S., Dee, T. S., & Penner, E. K. (2021). Ethnic studies increases longer-run academic engagement and attainment. *Proceedings of the National Academy of Sciences of the United States of America, 118*(37), e2026386118. DOI: 10.1073/pnas.2026386118 PMID: 34493663

Bons, D., van den Broek, E., Scheepers, F., Herpers, P., Rommelse, N., & Buitelaaar, J. K. (2013). Motor, emotional, and cognitive empathy in children and adolescents with autism spectrum disorder and conduct disorder. *Journal of Abnormal Child Psychology, 41*(3), 425–443. DOI: 10.1007/s10802-012-9689-5

Booris, O., & Way, O. (2019). *Final report.* ACT Government.

Booth, P. B., & Jernberg, A. M. (2010). *Theraplay: Helping parents and children build better relationships through attachment-based play* (3rd ed.). Jossey-Bass.

Borelli, J. L., Cohen, C., Pettit, C., Normandin, L., Target, M., Fonagy, P., & Ensink, K. (2019). Maternal and child sexual abuse history: An intergenerational exploration of children's adjustment and maternal trauma-reflective functioning. *Frontiers in Psychology, 10*, 1062. DOI: 10.3389/fpsyg.2019.01062 PMID: 31156503

Bornstein, R. F. (1993). *The dependent personality.* Guilford Press.

Bornstein, R. F. (2006). The complex relationship between dependency and domestic violence: Converging psychological factors and social forces. *The American Psychologist, 61*(6), 595–606. DOI: 10.1037/0003-066X.61.6.595 PMID: 16953747

Bottiani, J. H., Bradshaw, C. P., & Mendelson, T. (2018). A multilevel examination of racial disparities in high school discipline. *School Psychology Review, 47*(2), 174–187. DOI: 10.17105/SPR-2017-0070.V47-2

Boullier, M., & Blair, M. (2018). Adverse childhood experiences. *Paediatrics and Child Health (Oxford), 28*(3), 132–137. DOI: 10.1016/j.paed.2017.12.008

Bowen, M. (1966). The use of family theory in clinical practice. *Comprehensive Psychiatry, 7*(5), 345–374. DOI: 10.1016/S0010-440X(66)80065-2 PMID: 5922263

Bowen, M. (1972). On the differentiation of self. In Framo, J. (Ed.), *Family Interaction: A Dialogue Between Family Researchers and Family Therapists*. Springer Books.

Bowen, M. (1978). *Family therapy in clinical practice*. Aronson.

Bowlby, J. (1969). Attachment and Loss. Vol. 1, Attachment. New York: Basic Books, 1982. Bowlby, J. (1980). Attachment and Loss. Vol. 3, Loss. New York: Basic Books.

Bowlby, J. (1982). Attachment and loss: Retrospect and prospect. *The American Journal of Orthopsychiatry, 52*(4), 664–678. DOI: 10.1111/j.1939-0025.1982.tb01456.x PMID: 7148988

Bowlby, J. (1988). *A secure base: Parent-child attachment and healthy human development*. Basic books.

Bratton, S. C., Ray, D., Rhine, T., & Jones, L. (2005). The efficacy of play therapy with children: A meta-analytic review of treatment outcomes. *Professional Psychology, Research and Practice, 36*(4), 376–390. DOI: 10.1037/0735-7028.36.4.376

Brennan, J., Woolgar, M., & Rutter, M. (2016). *Parenting Role Interview manual*. King's College London.

Brofenbrenner, U. (1979). *The ecology of human development*. Harvard University Press. DOI: 10.4159/9780674028845

Broidy, L., Cauffman, E., Espelage, D. L., Mazerolle, P., & Piquero, A. (2003). Sex differences in empathy and its relation to juvenile offending. *Violence and Victims, 18*(5), 502–516. DOI: 10.1891/vivi.2003.18.5.503

Bromfield, L., & Higgins, D. (2005). *National comparison of child protection systems*. National Child Protection Clearinghouse, Australian Institute of Family Studies.

Bromfield, L., & Holzer, P. (2008). *A national approach for child protection: Project report*. National Child Protection Clearinghouse, Australian Institute of Family Studies. https://aifs.gov.au/research/research-reports/national-approach-child-protection

Bromfield, L., & Miller, R. (2012). *Cumulative Harm Specialist Practice Resource*. Victorian Government Department of Human Services. https://www.cpmanual.vic.gov.au/sites/default/files/Cumulative%20harm%20specialist%20practice%20resource%202012%203014%20.pdf

Bromfield, L., & Miller, R. (2012). *Cumulative Harm—Best interests case practice model: Specialist practice resource*. Victoria: DHS. https://www.cpmanual.vic.gov.au/sites/default/files/Cumulative%20harm%20specialist%20practice%20resource%202012%203014%20.pdf

Bromfield, L. M., Gillingham, P., & Higgins, D. J. (2007). Cumulative harm and chronic child maltreatment. Developing Practice: The Child [Available online.]. *Youth and Family Work Journal*, *19*, 34–42.

Bromfield, L. M., Gillingham, P., & Higgins, D. J. (2007). Cumulative harm: A conceptual framework for child protection. *Australian Social Work*, *60*(2), 258–268. DOI: 10.1080/03124070701323847

Bromfield, L. M., & Higgins, D. J. (2004). The limitations of using statutory child protection data for research into child maltreatment. *Australian Social Work*, *57*(1), 19–30. https://www.tandfonline.com/doi/abs/10.1111/j.0312-407X.2003.t01-1-00110.x. DOI: 10.1111/j.0312-407X.2003.00110.x

Bromfield, L. M., & Higgins, D. J. (2005). Chronic and isolated maltreatment in a child protection sample. *Family Matters (Melbourne, Vic.)*, (70), 38–45.

Bromfield, L. M., & Higgins, D. J. (2005). The course and characteristics of chronic and isolated child maltreatment. *Family Matters (Melbourne, Vic.)*, *70*, 38–45. https://aifs.gov.au/publications/family-matters/issue-70/chronic-and-isolated-maltreatment-child-protection-sample

Bronson, D. E., Saunders, S., Holt, M. B., & Beck, E. (2008). *Systemic review of strategies to promote successful reunification and to reduce re-entry to care for abused, neglected, and unruly children*. Paper delivered at the Ohio Department of Job and Family Service, Ohio. http://www.ocwtp.net/PDFs/Reun-Reentry%20Final%20Report.pdf

Browne-Yung, K., O'Neil, D., Walker, R., Corlis, M., Smyth, A., Putsey, P., Laver, K. E., Fernandez, E., & Cations, M. (2021). 'I'd rather die in the middle of a street': Perceptions and expectations of aged care among Forgotten Australians. *Australasian Journal on Ageing*, *40*(2), 168–176. DOI: 10.1111/ajag.12851 PMID: 33336557

Bryant-Davis, T. (2007). Healing requires recognition: The case for race-based traumatic stress. *The Counseling Psychologist*, *35*(1), 135–143. DOI: 10.1177/0011000006295152

Bryce, I. (2018). A review of cumulative harm: A comparison of international child protection practices. *Children Australia*, *43*(1), 23–31. DOI: 10.1017/cha.2018.3

Bryce, I. (2020). *Cumulative harm and the need for a restorative framework in child protection*. University of Southern Queensland.

Bryce, I., Beccaria, G., McIlveen, P., & Du Preez, J. (2022). Reauthoring: The lived experience of cumulative harm and its influence on career choice. *Australian Journal of Career Development*, *31*(2), 93–107. DOI: 10.1177/10384162221101958

Bryce, I., & Collier, S. (2022). A systematic literature review of the contribution accumulation makes to psychological and physical trauma sustained through childhood maltreatment. *Trauma Care*, *2*(2), 307–329. DOI: 10.3390/traumacare2020026

Bryce, I., & Collier, S. (2022). *Child sexual abuse: Forensic issues in evidence, impact and management*. Routledge.

Bryce, I., Collier, S., Harris, L., Higgins, D., & Toohey, J. (2024). Measuring accumulation: Constructing a tool for evaluating cumulative harm in children engaged with an intensive family support service. *Child Abuse Review*, *33*(5), e2897. Advance online publication. DOI: 10.1002/car.2897

Bryce, I., Pye, D., Beccaria, G., McIlveen, P., & Du Preez, J. (2023). The Influence of Cumulative Harm on Career Choice in the Helping Professions: A Systematic Literature Review. *Trauma, Violence & Abuse*, *24*(1). Advance online publication. DOI: 10.1177/15248380211016016 PMID: 34000930

Buchheim, A., Ziegenhain, U., Kindler, H., Waller, C., Gündel, H., Karabatsiakis, A., & Fegert, J. (2022). Identifying risk and resilience factors in the intergenerational cycle of maltreatment: Results from the trans-gen study investigating the effects of maternal attachment and social support on child attachment and cardiovascular stress physiology. *Frontiers in Human Neuroscience*, *16*, 890262–890262. DOI: 10.3389/fnhum.2022.890262 PMID: 35923749

Bunger, A. C., Maguire-Jack, K., Yoon, S., Mooney, D., West, K. Y., Hammond, G. C., & Kranich, C. (2021). Does mental health screening and assessment in child welfare improve mental health service receipt, child safety, and permanence for children in out-of-home care? An evaluation of the Gateway CALL demonstration. *Child Abuse & Neglect, 122*, 105351. DOI: 10.1016/j.chiabu.2021.105351 PMID: 34628151

Bunting, L., Montgomery, L., Mooney, S., MacDonald, M., Coulter, S., Hayes, D., & Davidson, G. (2019). Trauma informed child welfare systems—A rapid evidence review. *International Journal of Environmental Research and Public Health, 16*(13), 2365. DOI: 10.3390/ijerph16132365 PMID: 31277339

Buss, C., Entringer, S., Moog, N. K., Toepfer, P., Fair, D. A., Simhan, H. N., Heim, C. M., & Wadhwa, P. D. (2017). Intergenerational transmission of maternal childhood maltreatment exposure: Implications for fetal brain development. *Journal of the American Academy of Child and Adolescent Psychiatry, 56*(5), 373–382. DOI: 10.1016/j.jaac.2017.03.001 PMID: 28433086

Busso, D. S., McLaughlin, K. A., & Sheridan, M. A. (2017). Dimensions of adversity, stress reactivity, and school functioning in middle childhood. *Development and Psychopathology, 29*(5), 1711–1723. DOI: 10.1017/S0954579417001358

Butler, J., Gregg, L., Calam, R., & Wittkowski, A. (2020). Parents' perceptions and experiences of parenting programmes: A systematic review and metasynthesis of the qualitative literature. *Clinical Child and Family Psychology Review, 23*(2), 176–204. DOI: 10.1007/s10567-019-00307-y PMID: 31820298

Bywaters, P., Brady, G., Bunting, L., Daniel, B., Featherstone, B., Jones, C., Morris, K., Scourfield, J., Sparks, T., & Webb, C. (2018). Inequalities in English child protection practices under austerity: A universal challenge? *Child & Family Social Work, 23*(1), 53–61. DOI: 10.1111/cfs.12383

Cafaro, A., Durlak, J. A., & Taylor, R. D. (2023). Effects of teacher-delivered social and emotional learning interventions on student outcomes: A meta-analysis. *School Psychology Review, 52*(2), 170–187. DOI: 10.1080/2372966X.2021.2009940

Calley, N. G., & Gerber, S. (2008). Empathy-promoting counselling strategies for juvenile sex offenders: A developmental approach. *Journal of Addictions & Offender Counseling, 28*(2), 68–85. DOI: 10.1002/j.2161-1874.2008.tb00034.x

Cardoso, A. S., Martins, R. C., Venturin, B., Gonzalez, A., Blumenberg, C., & Murray, J. (2025). Psychosocial adversity and executive functions in children and adolescents: A systematic review of mediating and moderating influences of parenting behaviors. *BMC Psychiatry, 25*(1), 894. DOI: 10.1186/s12888-025-06592-y PMID: 41029261

Carello, J., & Butler, L. D. (2014). Practices for creating a trauma-informed university. *Journal of Trauma & Dissociation, 15*, 444–457.

Carey, M. (2012). *Qualitative Research Skills for Social Work: Theory and practice*. Routledge.

Carey, M., & Russell, S. (2003). Re-authoring: Some answers to commonly asked questions. *International Journal of Narrative Therapy and Community Work, 3*, 60–71.

Carlson, E. A. (1998). A prospective longitudinal study of attachment disorganization/disorientation. *Child Development, 69*(4), 1107–1128. DOI: 10.1111/j.1467-8624.1998.tb06163.x PMID: 9768489

Carlson, V., Cicchetti, D., Barnett, D., & Braunwald, K. (1989). Disorganized/disoriented attachment relationships in maltreated infants. *Developmental Psychology, 25*(4), 525–531. DOI: 10.1037/0012-1649.25.4.525

Cashmore, J., & Parkinson, P. (2008). Children and the law: Do we value our children enough? *The Sydney Law Review, 30*(1), 1–26.

Castillo-Gonzáles, M., Mendo-Lázaro, S., León-del-Barco, B., Terán-Andrade, E., & López-Ramos, V. M. (2024). Dating violence and emotional dependence in university students. *Behavioral Sciences (Basel, Switzerland), 14*(3), 176. DOI: 10.3390/bs14030176 PMID: 38540479

Cebulla, A., & Katz, I. (2017). Unemployment, poverty and the future of work after the global financial crisis. In Serr, K. (Ed.), *Thinking about poverty* (pp. 58–73). The Federation Press.

Cecil, C. A., Viding, E., Fearon, P., Glaser, D., & McCrory, E. J. (2017). Disentangling the mental health impact of childhood abuse and neglect. *Child Abuse & Neglect, 63*, 106–119. DOI: 10.1016/j.chiabu.2016.11.024 PMID: 27914236

Center for Disease Control and Prevention. (n.d.). *Adverse childhood experiences*. Retrieved from https://www.cdc.gov/violenceprevention/aces/index.html

Centre of Best Practice in Aboriginal and Torres Strait Islander Suicide Prevention. (n.d.). *Best practice screening and assessment tools*. University of Western Australia. https://cbpatsisp.com.au/clearing-house/best-practice-screening-assessment/

Cerqueira, A., & Almeida, T. C. (2023). Adverse childhood experiences: Relationship with empathy and alexithymia. *Journal of Child & Adolescent Trauma, 16*(3), 559–568. DOI: 10.1007/s40653-023-00520-6

Chamberlain, C., Gee, G., Harfield, S., Campbell, S., Brennan, S., Clark, Y., Mensah, F., Arabena, K., Herrman, H., & Brown, S. (2019). Parenting after a history of childhood maltreatment: A scoping review and map of evidence in the perinatal period. *PLoS One*, *14*(3), 1–41. DOI: 10.1371/journal.pone.0213460 PMID: 30865679

Chamberlain, C., Ralph, N., Hokke, S., Clark, Y., Gee, G., Stansfield, C., Sutcliffe, K., Brown, S. J., & Brennan, S. (2019). Healing the past by nurturing the future: A qualitative systematic review and meta-synthesis of pregnancy, birth and early postpartum experiences and views of parents with a history of childhood maltreatment. *PLoS One*, *14*(12), 1. DOI: 10.1371/journal.pone.0225441 PMID: 31834894

Chambers, J., Lint, S., Thompson, M., Carlson, M., & Graef, M. (2019). Outcomes of the Iowa partner program evaluation: Stability of reunification and re-entry into foster care. *Children and Youth Services Review*, *104*, 1–11. DOI: 10.1016/j.childyouth.2019.05.030

Chang, H. (2008). *Autoethnography as method: Developing qualitative inquiry*. Left Coast Press.

Chan, H. H.-K., Kwong, H. Y., Shu, G. L., Ting, C. Y., & Lai, F. H. Y. (2021). Effects of experiential learning programmes on adolescent prosocial behaviour, empathy, and subjective well-being: A systematic review and meta-analysis. *Frontiers in Psychology*, *12*, 709699. Advance online publication. DOI: 10.3389/fpsyg.2021.709699

Chaplin, T. M., Cole, P. M., & Zahn-Waxler, C. (2005). Parental socialization of emotion expression: Gender differences and relations to child adjustment. *Emotion (Washington, D.C.)*, *5*(1), 80–88. DOI: 10.1037/1528-3542.5.1.80

Chard, K. M., & Hansel, J. E. (2006). Supervising therapists working with traumatised children. In K. T, Neill (Ed.), *Helping others help children: Clinical supervision of child psychotherapy* (pp. 193-207). American Psychological Association. DOI: 10.1037/11467-011

Cheng, Y., Chou, C. H., Decety, J., Chen, I. Y., Hung, D., Tzeng, O. J. L., & Lin, C.-P. (2009). Sex differences in the neuroanatomy of human mirror-neuron system: A voxel-based morphometric investigation. *Neuroscience*, *159*(2), 713–720. DOI: 10.1016/j.neuroscience.2008.10.026

Chen, Y., Zhang, L., & McLaughlin, K. A. (2022). Resilience and developmental outcomes following childhood adversity: A meta-analysis. *Psychological Bulletin*, *148*(4), 305–341. DOI: 10.1037/bul000036

Chesmore, A. A., Weiler, L. M., & Taussig, H. N. (2017). Mentoring relationship quality and maltreated children's coping. *American Journal of Community Psychology*, *60*(1-2), 229–241. DOI: 10.1002/ajcp.12151 PMID: 28792079

Cheung, A., & Slavin, R. E. (2016). Effective reading programs for secondary students. *Reading Research Quarterly*, *51*(4), 389–416. DOI: 10.1002/rrq.154

Cheung, K., Taillieu, T., Turner, S., Fortier, J., Sareen, J., MacMillan, H. L., Boyle, M. H., & Afifi, T. O. (2017). Relationship and community factors related to better mental health following child maltreatment among adolescents. *Child Abuse & Neglect*, *70*, 377–387. DOI: 10.1016/j.chiabu.2017.06.026 PMID: 28750346

Childhood Foundation. (2022). *Understanding the needs of kinship carers in Australia: Research brief.* Australian Childhood Foundation.

Choate, P. (2009). Parenting capacity assessments in child protection cases. *Forensic Examiner*, *18*(1), 52–60.

Choate, P. W., CrazyBull, B., Lindstrom, D., & Lindstrom, G. (2020). Where do we go from here? Ongoing colonialism from attachment theory. *Aotearoa New Zealand Social Work*, *32*(1), 32–44. DOI: 10.11157/anzswj-vol32iss1id702

Christov-Moore, L., Simpson, E. A., Coudé, G., Grigaityte, K., Iacoboni, M., & Ferrari, P. F. (2014). Empathy: Gender effects in brain and behavior. *Neuroscience and Biobehavioral Reviews*, *46*, 604–627. DOI: 10.1016/j.neubiorev.2014.09.001

Chu, A., & DePrince, A. P. (2006). Development of dissociation: Examining the relationship between parenting, maternal trauma and child dissociation. *Journal of Trauma & Dissociation*, *7*(4), 75–89. DOI: 10.1300/J229v07n04_05 PMID: 17182494

Cicchetti, D., & Barnett, D. (1991). Attachment organization in pre-school-aged maltreated children. *Development and Psychopathology*, *3*, 397–411. DOI: 10.1017/S0954579400007598

Cicchetti, D., & Cohen, D. J. (Eds.). (2015). Developmental Psychopathology *Volume Three: Risk, Disorder, and Adaptation*. Wiley.

Cicchetti, D., & Rizley, R. (1981). Developmental perspectives on the etiology, intergenerational transmission, and sequelae of child maltreatment. *New Directions for Child and Adolescent Development*, *1981*(11), 31–55. DOI: 10.1002/cd.23219811104

Cikara, M., Botvinick, M., & Fiske, S. T. (2011). Us versus them: Social identity shapes neural responses to intergroup competition and harm. *Psychological Science*, *22*(3), 306–313. DOI: 10.1177/0956797610397667

Cikara, M., & Fiske, S. T. (2011). Bounded empathy: Neural responses to outgroup targets' (mis)fortunes. *Journal of Cognitive Neuroscience*, *23*(12), 3791–3803. DOI: 10.1162/jocn_a_00069

Civitillo, S., Meyer, A., & Jügert, T. (2023). Students' perceptions of differential teacher treatment and academic outcomes: A meta-analysis. *Journal of School Psychology*, *98*, 1–18. DOI: 10.1016/j.jsp.2022.12.001

CLAN. (2022). *Caring for Care Leavers in Australia's aged care sector*. CLAN.

Cless, C. L., & Goff, M. J. (2017). The prevalence of traumatic events and post-traumatic distress among college students: A meta-analytic review of U.S. studies, 1983–2015. *Journal of American College Health*, *65*, 273–282.

Cloitre, M., Shevlin, M., Brewin, C. R., Bisson, J. I., Roberts, N. P., Maercker, A., & Hyland, P. (2013). Evidence for the coherence and integrity of the ICD-11 diagnostic construct of complex post-traumatic stress disorder: A latent profile analysis. *European Journal of Psychotraumatology*, *4*(1), 20706. Advance online publication. DOI: 10.3402/ejpt.v4i0.20706 PMID: 23687563

Cloitre, M., Stolbach, B. C., Herman, J. L., van der Kolk, B., Pynoos, R., Wang, J., & Petkova, E. (2011). A developmental approach to complex PTSD: Childhood and adult cumulative trauma as predictors of symptom complexity. *Journal of Traumatic Stress*, *22*(5), 399–408. DOI: 10.1002/jts.20444

Cochran, J. L., & Cochran, N. H. (2015). *The heart of counseling: Counseling skills through therapeutic relationships.* Routledge, Taylor & Francis Group.

Cohen, J. A., Mannarino, A. P., & Deblinger, E. (2017). *Trauma-Focused CBT for Children and Adolescents: Treatment Applications*. Guilford Press.

Collings, S., McLaine, M., Ciftci, S., & Luu, B. (2024). Working towards reunification in New South Wales: Professional perspectives on navigating complex systems. *Australian Journal of Social Issues, 59*, 752–772. https://doi:org/DOI: 10.1002/ajs4.333

Colquhoun, H. L., Levac, D., O'Brien, K. K., Straus, S., Tricco, A. C., Perrier, L., Kastner, M., & Moher, D. (2014). Scoping reviews: Time for clarity in definition, methods, and reporting. *Journal of Clinical Epidemiology*, *67*(12), 1291–1294. DOI: 10.1016/j.jclinepi.2014.03.013 PMID: 25034198

Commission for Children and Young People (CCYP). (2017). *In our own words: Systemic inquiry into the lived experience of children and young people in the Victorian out-of-home care system.* Melbourne: CCYP. https://ccyp.vic.gov.au/assets/Publications-inquiries/CCYP-In-Our-Own-Words.pdf

Commonwealth of Australia. (1991). *Royal Commission into Aboriginal Deaths in Custody: National Report (Vols. 1–5).* Australian Government Publishing Service. https://www.nla.gov.au/collections/aboriginal-deaths-in-custody

Commonwealth of Australia. (1997). *Bringing them Home: Report of the National Inquiry into the Separation of Aboriginal and Torres Strait Islander Children from Their Families.* https://healingfoundation.org.au/app/uploads/2017/02/Bringing-Them-Home-Report.pdf

Commonwealth of Australia. (2001). Lost Innocents: Righting the Record - Report on child migration.https://www.aph.gov.au/~/media/wopapub/senate/committee/clac_ctte/completed_inquiries/1999_02/child_migrat/report/report_pdf.ashx

Commonwealth of Australia. (2004). Community Affairs References Committee: Forgotten Australians. A report on Australians who experienced institutional or out-of-home-care as children. https://www.aph.gov.au/parliamentary_business/committees/senate/community_ affairs/completed_inquiries/2004-07/inst_care/report/index

Commonwealth of Australia. (2017). Royal Commission into Institutional Responses to Child Sexual Abuse (2017): Final Report. Canberra: Commonwealth of Australia. https://www.childabuseroyalcommission.gov.au/final-report

Commonwealth of Australia. (2017). *Royal Commission into the Protection and Detention of Children in the Northern Territory: Final Report (Vols. 1–4).* Australian Government. https://www.royalcommission.gov.au/child-detention

Conn, A. M., Szilagyi, M. A., Franke, T. M., Albertin, C. S., Blumkin, A. K., & Szilagyi, P. G. (2013). Trends in child protection and out-of-home care. *Pediatrics, 132*(4), 712–719. DOI: 10.1542/peds.2013-0969 PMID: 24062369

Conn, A. M., Szilagyi, M. A., Jee, S. H., Blumkin, A. K., & Szilagyi, P. G. (2015). Mental health outcomes among child welfare investigated children: In-home versus out-of-home care. *Children and Youth Services Review, 57*, 106–111. DOI: 10.1016/j.childyouth.2015.08.004

Cooper, C., Booth, A., Britten, N., & Garside, R. (2017). A comparison of results of empirical studies of supplementary search techniques and recommendations in review methodology handbooks: A methodological review. *Systematic Reviews, 6*(1), 234. DOI: 10.1186/s13643-017-0625-1 PMID: 29179733

Cooper, J., & Vetere, A. (2008). *Domestic violence and family safety: Systemic approach to working with violence in families.* Wiley-Blackwell.

Coote, G., & Shams, H. (2023, September 24). NSW inquiry to hear from children forced into motels, hotels due to shortage of foster carers. *ABC News*. https://www.abc.net.au/news/2023-09-24/nsw-inquiry-into-kids-in-hotels-motels-due-lack-foster-carers/102895278

Copp, J. E., Giordano, P. C., Longmore, M. A., & Manning, W. D. (2019). The development of attitudes toward intimate partner violence: An examination of key correlates among a sample of young adults. *Journal of Interpersonal Violence*, *34*(7), 1357–1387. DOI: 10.1177/0886260516651311 PMID: 27229921

Corbett, E., McGann, M., Considine, M., & Rejón, R. (2024). *Towards Trauma-Informed Employment Services: Implications for Street-Level Practice in the Delivery of Welfare-to-Work. Australian Welfare and Work Lab Working Paper*. University of Melbourne.

Cordero, M. I., Poirier, G. L., Marquez, C., Veenit, V., Fontana, X., Salehi, B., Ansermet, F., & Sandi, C. (2012). Evidence for biological roots in the transgenerational transmission of intimate partner violence. *Translational Psychiatry*, *2*(4), 10. DOI: 10.1038/tp.2012.32 PMID: 22832906

Cornett, C. (1985). The cyclical pattern of child physical abuse from a psychoanalytic self-psychology perspective. *Child & Adolescent Social Work Journal*, *2*(2), 83–92. DOI: 10.1007/BF00757474

Cornett, N., & Bratton, S. C. (2014). The efficacy of filial therapy for parents of children with chronic illness: A pilot study. *International Journal of Play Therapy*, *23*(2), 70–82.

Cosmides, L. (1989). The logic of social exchange: Has natural selection shaped how humans reason? Studies with the Wason selection task. *Cognition*, *31*(3), 187–276. DOI: 10.1016/0010-0277(89)90023-1 PMID: 2743748

Cox, A., Frederico, M., Mosse, H., Radford, L., Ambry, D., & Ryan, C. (2021). Australian maltreated infants and young children can achieve positive relational health with neurodevelopmentally-and trauma-informed interventions provided within relationally-positive and stable environments. *Frontiers in Psychiatry*, *12*, 680343. DOI: 10.3389/fpsyt.2021.680343 PMID: 34393846

Crenshaw, K. (1989). Demarginalizing the intersection of race and sex: A black feminist critique of antidiscrimination doctrine, feminist theory and antiracist politics. *University of Chicago Legal Forum*, (1), 8, 139–167.

Cromer, L. D., Gray, M. E., Vasquez, L., & Freyd, J. J. (2018). The relationship of acculturation to historical loss awareness, institutional betrayal, and the intergenerational transmission of trauma in the American Indian experience. *Journal of Cross-Cultural Psychology*, *49*(1), 99–114. DOI: 10.1177/0022022117738749

Crouch, E., Radcliff, E., Hung, P., & Bennett, K. (2019). Challenges to school success and the role of adverse childhood experiences. *Academic Pediatrics*, *19*(8), 899–907. DOI: 10.1016/j.acap.2019.08.006 PMID: 31401231

Cunneen, C. (2008). Understanding restorative justice through the lens of critical criminology. In Shoham, S. G., Knepper, P., & Kett, M. (Eds.), *International handbook of penology and criminal justice* (pp. 1095–1128). CRC Press.

Cunningham, T., Bastian, C., Seymour, K., & Wendt, S. (2021). Reunification: Rapid literature review. Flinders University. https://researchnow.flinders.edu.au/en/publications/reunification-rapid-literature-review

Cunningham, M., Shlonsky, A., & Fouché, C. (2021). Reunification in out-of-home care: A rapid evidence review. *Children and Youth Services Review*, *128*, 106–120.

Currie, J., & Spatz Widom, C. (2010). Long-term consequences of child abuse and neglect on adult economic well-being. *Child Maltreatment*, *15*(2), 111–120.

Curtin, N., Kende, A., & Kende, J. (2016). Navigating multiple identities: The simultaneous influence of advantaged and disadvantaged identities on politicization and activism. *The Journal of Social Issues*, *72*(2), 264–285. DOI: 10.1111/josi.12166

Cyr, C., & Alink, L. R. (2017). Child maltreatment: The central roles of parenting capacities and attachment. *Current Opinion in Psychology*, *15*, 81–86. DOI: 10.1016/j.copsyc.2017.02.002 PMID: 28813275

Cyr, C., Euser, E. M., Bakermans-Kranenburg, M. J., & Van Ijzendoorn, M. H. (2010). Attachment security and disorganization in maltreating and high-risk families: A series of meta-analyses. *Development and Psychopathology*, *22*(1), 87–108. DOI: 10.1017/S0954579409990289 PMID: 20102649

Cyr, K., Chamberland, C., Lessard, G., Clément, M. È., Wemmers, J. A., Collin-Vézina, D., Gagné, M.-H., & Damant, D. (2012). Polyvictimization in a child welfare sample of children and youths. *Psychology of Violence*, *2*(4), 385–400. DOI: 10.1037/a0028040

Dale, K. A., & Alpert, J. L. (2007). Hiding behind the cloth: Child sexual abuse and the Catholic Church. *Journal of Child Sexual Abuse*, *16*(3), 59–74. DOI: 10.1300/J070v16n03_04 PMID: 18032240

Daniel, B., Taylor, J., & Scott, J. (2011). *Recognizing and helping the neglected child: Evidence-based practice for assessment and intervention.* Jessica Kingsley Publishers Department of Social Services. (2020). *Cultural safety and responsiveness: Child and Family Intensive Support (CaFIS) program guidelines – Annex 3C.* Australian Government. https://www.dss.gov.au/system/files/resources/cafis_3c_-_cultural_safety_and_responsiveness.pdf

Darlington, Y., Healy, K., & Feeney, J. A. (2010). Approaches to assessment and intervention across four types of child and family welfare services. *Children and Youth Services Review, 32*(3), 356–364. DOI: 10.1016/j.childyouth.2009.10.005

Daro, D. (2022). Sustaining progress in preventing child maltreatment: A transformative challenge. In Krugman, R., & Korbin, J. (Eds.), *Handbook of child maltreatment* (pp. 407–427). Springer. DOI: 10.1007/978-3-030-82479-2_20

Daro, D., Donnelly, A. C., Huang, L. A., & Powell, B. J. (Eds.). (2015). *Advances in child abuse prevention knowledge: The perspective of new leadership.* Springer International Publishing., DOI: 10.1007/978-3-319-16327-7

Davis, I. P., Landsverk, J., Newton, R., & Ganger, W. (1996). Parental visiting and foster care reunification. *Children and Youth Services Review, 18*(4/5), 363–382. DOI: 10.1016/0190-7409(96)00010-2

Deater-Deckard, K., Dodge, K. A., Bates, J. E., & Pettit, G. S. (1996). Physical discipline among African American and European American mothers: Links to children's externalizing behaviors. *Developmental Psychology, 32*(6), 1065–1072. DOI: 10.1037/0012-1649.32.6.1065

DeBerard, M. S., Spielmans, G. I., & Julka, D. L. (2004). Post-traumatic stress disorder and college student achievement: The mediating role of motivation. *Journal of College Student Development, 45*, 55–65.

Decety, J., & Lam, C. (2006). Human empathy through the lens of social neuroscience. *TheScientificWorldJournal, 6*(280363), 1146–1163. DOI: 10.1100/tsw.2006.221

Decety, J., & Moriguchi, Y. (2007). The empathic brain and its dysfunction in psychiatric populations: Implications for intervention across different clinical conditions. *BioPsychoSocial Medicine, 1*(22), 1–21. DOI: 10.1186/1751-0759-1-22

DeGregorio, L. J. (2013). Intergenerational transmission of abuse: Implications for parenting interventions from a neuropsychological perspective. *Traumatology, 19*(2), 158–166. Advance online publication. DOI: 10.1177/1534765612457219

Delaney, R. (2006). *Trauma, attachment, and family permanency: Fear can stop you loving.* Wood 'N' Barnes.

Delfabbro, P., Fernandez, E., McCormick, J., & Wilson, S. (2019). *Out-of-home care in Australia: Children and young people's views after five years of the National Standards*. Department of Social Services.

Delfabbro, P., & Osborn, A. (2020). Therapeutic approaches to children and families in child protection contexts. In *Child Protection and the Care Continuum* (pp. 134–148). Routledge. DOI: 10.4324/9781003121305-8

Delsol, C., & Margolin, G. (2004). The role of family-of-origin violence in men's marital violence perpetration. *Clinical Psychology Review, 24*(1), 99–122. https://doi.org/https://doi.org/10.1016/j.cpr.2003.12.001. DOI: 10.1016/j.cpr.2003.12.001 PMID: 14992808

Department of Communities and Justice (DCJ). (2023). *How do relative/kinship carers and foster carers differ? Pathways of Care Longitudinal Study Evidence to Action Note 15*. NSW Government.

DePrince, A. P. (2005). Social cognition and revictimization risk. *Journal of Trauma & Dissociation, 6*(1), 125–141. DOI: 10.1300/J229v06n01_08 PMID: 16150689

DePrince, A. P., Combs, M. D., & Shanahan, M. (2009). Automatic relationship-harm associations and interpersonal trauma involving close others. *Psychology of Women Quarterly, 33*(2), 163–171. DOI: 10.1111/j.1471-6402.2009.01486.x

DePrince, A. P., & Freyd, J. J. (2002). The intersection of gender and betrayal in trauma. In Kimerling, R., Oumette, P. C., & Wolfe, J. (Eds.), *Gender and PTSD* (pp. 98–113). Guilford Press.

Desai, C. D., Reece, J. A., & Shakespeare-Pellington, S. (2017). The prevention of violence in childhood through parenting programmes: A global review. *Psychology Health and Medicine, 22*(1), 166–186. DOI: 10.1080/13548506.2016.1271952 PMID: 28133982

Descartes, C. H., Maharaj, P. E., Quammie, M., Mills, J., Ramesar, M., & Pulwarty, H. (2020). It's never one type: The co-occurrence of child abuse and neglect among children living in community residences in Trinidad. *Journal of Child & Adolescent Trauma, 13*(4), 419–427. DOI: 10.1007/s40653-019-00293-x PMID: 33269042

Devlin, R., Jairam, R., Asghari, M., & Eapen, V. (2022). Does assertive mental health care make a difference to children in out-of-home care? A pilot study. *Developmental Child Welfare, 4*(1), 73–93. DOI: 10.1177/25161032211064644

Dinic, B. M., Kodzopeljic, J. S., Sokolovska, V. T., & Milovanovic, I. Z. (2016). Empathy and peer violence among adolescents: Moderation effect of gender. *School Psychology International, 37*(4), 359–377. DOI: 10.1177/0143034316649008

Dixon, L., Browne, K., & Hamilton-Giachritsis, C. (2009). Patterns of risk and protective factors in the intergenerational cycle of maltreatment. *Journal of Family Violence*, *24*(2), 111–122. DOI: 10.1007/s10896-008-9215-2

Dobia, B., Bodkin-Andrews, G., Parada, R., O'Rourke, V., Gilbert, S., Daley, A., & Roffey, S. (2014). *The Aboriginal Girls Circle: Promoting resilience and cultural connectedness* (Pilot project report). Western Sydney University.

Dodge, K. A. (1986). A social information processing model of social competence in children. In Perlmutter, M. (Ed.), *The Minnesota symposium on child psychology: Cognitive perspectives of children's social and behavioural development* (pp. 77–125). Lawrence Erlbaum Associates.

Dombo, E. A., & Sabin, M. (2020). Trauma-informed supervision for helping professionals. *Clinical Social Work Journal*, *48*, 1–12. DOI: 10.1007/s10615-019-00729-6

Doyle, C., & Cicchetti, D. (2018). Attachment-related processes in maltreated children. *Child Development Perspectives*, *12*(4), 235–240. DOI: 10.1111/cdep.12291

Dozier, M., & Bernard, K. (2019). *Coaching parents of vulnerable infants: The Attachment and Biobehavioral Catch-Up approach.* Guilford Press.

Duan, W., Bissaker, K., & Xu, S. (2024). Teacher classroom management self-efficacy and classroom climate: A meta-analysis. *Teaching and Teacher Education*, *138*, 104329. DOI: 10.1016/j.tate.2023.104329

Dudgeon, P., Milroy, H., & Walker, R. (Eds.). (2014). *Working together: Aboriginal and Torres Strait Islander mental health and wellbeing principles and practice* (2nd ed.). Commonwealth of Australia.

Dudgeon, P., Bray, A., D'Costa, B., & Walker, R. (2017). Decolonising psychology: Validating social and emotional wellbeing. *Australian Psychologist*, *52*(4), 316–325. DOI: 10.1111/ap.12294

Duke, N. N., Pettingell, S. L., McMorris, B. J., & Borowsky, I. W. (2010). Adolescent violence perpetration: Associations with multiple types of adverse childhood experiences. *Pediatrics*, *125*(4), e778–e786. DOI: 10.1542/peds.2009-0597

Dunbar, A., Savaglio, M., Halfpenny, N., O'Donnell, R., Pileggi, A., & Skouteris, H. (2022). MacKillop Family Services' Family Preservation and Reunification Response for vulnerable families: Protocol for an effectiveness-implementation study. *International Journal of Environmental Research and Public Health*, *19*(1), 426.

Duthie, D., Steinhauer, S., Twinn, C., Steinhauer, V., & Lonne, B. (2019). Understanding trauma and child maltreatment experienced in Indigenous communities. In Lonne, B., Scott, D., Higgins, D. J., & Herrenkohl, T. I. (Eds.), *Re-visioning public health approaches for protecting children* (Vol. 9, pp. 327–347). Springer International Publishing. DOI: 10.1007/978-3-030-05858-6_20

Economic Inclusion Advisory Committee/EIAC. (2025). *2025 Report to government.* Commonwealth Government.

Edwards, V. J., Holden, G. W., Felitti, V. J., & Anda, R. F. (2003). Relationship between multiple forms of childhood maltreatment and adult mental health in community respondents: Results from the Adverse Childhood Experiences (ACE) study. *The American Journal of Psychiatry, 160*(8), 1453–1460. DOI: 10.1176/appi.ajp.160.8.1453

Egeland, B., & Susman-Stillman, A. (1996). Dissociation as a mediator of child abuse across generations. *Child Abuse & Neglect, 20*(11), 1123–1132. DOI: 10.1016/0145-2134(96)00102-0 PMID: 8958463

Eisenberg, N., Cumberland, A., Gurthrie, I. K., Murphy, B. C., & Shepard, S. A. (2005). Age change in prosocial reasoning and moral reasoning in adolescence and early adulthood. *Journal of Research on Adolescence, 15*(3), 235–260. DOI: 10.1111/j.1532-7795.2005.00095.x

Eisenberg, N., Spinrad, T. L., & Sadovsky, A. (2006). Empathy related responding in children. In Killen, M., & Smetana, J. (Eds.), *Handbook of moral development* (pp. 517–549). Erlbaum.

Elliott, D. M., & Guy, J. D. (1993). Mental health professionals versus non-mental-health professionals: Childhood trauma and adult functioning. *Professional Psychology, Research and Practice, 24*(1), 83–90. DOI: 10.1037/0735-7028.24.1.83

Ellis, C., & Bochner, A. (2000). Autoethnography, personal narrative, reflexivity: Researcher as subject. In N. Denzin & Y. Lincoln (Eds.), *Handbook of qualitative research* (2nd ed.). Sage Publications.

Enano, S., Freisthler, B., Perez-Johnson, D., & Lovato-Hermann, K. (2017). Evaluating parents in partnership: A preliminary study of a child welfare intervention designed to increase reunification. *Journal of Social Science Research, 43*(2), 236–245.

England-Mason, G., Casey, R., Ferro, M., MacMillan, H. L., Tonmyr, L., & Gonzalez, A. (2018). Child maltreatment and adult multimorbidity: Results from the Canadian community health survey. *Canadian Journal of Public Health = Revue Canadienne de Santé Publique*, *109*(4), 561–572. DOI: 10.17269/s41997-018-0069-y PMID: 29981095

Erez, E., Adelman, M., & Gregory, C. (2009). Intersections of immigration and domestic violence: Voices of battered immigrant women. *Feminist Criminology*, *4*(1), 32–56. DOI: 10.1177/1557085108325413

Evans-Campbell, T. (2008). Historical trauma in American Indian/Native Alaskan communities: A multilevel framework for exploring impacts on individuals, families, and communities. *Journal of Interpersonal Violence*, *23*, 316. DOI: 10.1177/0886260507312290 PMID: 18245571

Fallot, R. D., & Harris, M. (2009). *Creating cultures of trauma-informed care*. Community Connections.

Farmer, E. (2014). Improving reunification practice: Pathways home, progress and outcomes for children returning from care to their parents. *British Journal of Social Work*, *44*(2), 348–366. DOI: 10.1093/bjsw/bcs093

Fearon, R. P., Bakermans-Kranenburg, M. J., van IJzendoorn, M. H., Lapsley, A. M., & Roisman, G. I. (2010). The significance of insecure attachment and disorganization in the development of children's externalizing behavior: A meta-analytic study. *Child Development*, *81*(2), 435–456. DOI: 10.1111/j.1467-8624.2009.01405.x PMID: 20438450

Felitti, V. J. (2002). The relation between adverse childhood experiences and adult health: Turning gold into lead. *The Permanente Journal*, *6*(1), 44–47. DOI: 10.7812/TPP/02.994 PMID: 30313011

Felitti, V. J., Anda, R. F., Nordenberg, D., Williamson, D. F., Spitz, A. M., Edwards, V., Koss, M. P., & Marks, J. S. (1998). Relationship of childhood abuse and household dysfunction to many of the leading causes of death in adults: The Adverse Childhood Experiences (ACE) Study. *American Journal of Preventive Medicine*, *14*(4), 245–258. DOI: 10.1016/S0749-3797(98)00017-8 PMID: 9635069

Fenerci, R. L. B., & Allen, B. (2018). From mother to child: Maternal betrayal trauma and risk for maltreatment and psychopathology in the next generation. *Child Abuse & Neglect*, *82*, 1–11. DOI: 10.1016/j.chiabu.2018.05.014 PMID: 29842995

Feng, C., Li, Z., Feng, X., Wang, L., Tian, T., & Luo, Y.-J. (2016). Social hierarchy modulates neural responses of empathy for pain. *Social Cognitive and Affective Neuroscience, 11*(3), 485–495. DOI: 10.1093/scan/nsv135

Ferguson, H. (2018). How social workers reflect in action and when and why they don't: The possibilities and limits to reflective practice in social work. *Social Work Education, 37*(4), 415–427. DOI: 10.1080/02615479.2017.1413083

Fernandez, E., & Lee, J. (2013). Accomplishing family reunification for children in care: An Australian study. *Children and Youth Services Review, 35*(9), 1374–1384. DOI: 10.1016/j.childyouth.2013.05.006

Fernandez, E., Lee, J., Blunden, H., McNamara, P., Kovacs, S., & Cornefert, P. (2016). *No child should grow up like this: Identifying long term outcomes of forgotten Australians, child migrants and the stolen generations*. University of New South Wales.

Feshbach, S. (1980). Child abuse and the dynamics of human aggression and violence. *Child abuse: An agenda for action*, 48-60.

Feshbach, S. (1974). The development and regulation of aggression: Some research gaps and a proposed cognitive analysis. In Wit, J. D., & Hartup, W. W. (Eds.), *Determinants and origins of aggressive behavior*. Mouton.

Finkelhor, D., Turner, H. A., Hamby, S. L., & Ormrod, R. K. (2011). *Polyvictimization: Children's Exposure to Multiple Types of Violence, Crime, and Abuse*. OJJDP Juvenile Justice Bulletin – NCJ235504 (pgs. 1-12). Washington, DC: US Government Printing Office.

Finkelhor, D. (2008). *Childhood Victimization: Violence, Crime, and Abuse in the Lives of Young People*. Oxford University Press. DOI: 10.1093/acprof:oso/9780195342857.001.0001

Finkelhor, D., Ormrod, R. K., & Turner, H. A. (2007). Poly-victimization: A neglected component in child victimization. *Child Abuse & Neglect, 31*(1), 7–26. DOI: 10.1016/j.chiabu.2006.06.008 PMID: 17224181

Finzi-Dottan, R., & Harel, G. (2014). Parents' potential for child abuse: An intergenerational perspective. *Journal of Family Violence, 29*(4), 397–408. DOI: 10.1007/s10896-014-9592-7

Firmin, C., Lefevre, M., Huegler, N., & Peace, D. (2022). Improving interagency collaboration. In *Safeguarding young people beyond the family home* (pp. 43–52). Policy Press., DOI: 10.2307/j.ctv2zjz6z3.8

Fish, S., & Hardy, M. (2015). Complex issues, complex solutions: Applying complexity theory in social work practice. *Nordic Social Work Research, 1*(5), 98–114. DOI: 10.1080/2156857X.2015.1065902

Fitzgerald, M., & Gallus, K. L. (2025). Conceptualizing and measuring childhood adversity: A comprehensive critique of the adverse childhood experiences measure and offering a new conceptualization of childhood adversity. *The American Journal of Orthopsychiatry, 95*(3), 274–287. DOI: 10.1037/ort0000785 PMID: 39298243

Fitzgibbon, W., & Healy, D. (2019). Lives and spaces: Photovoice and offender supervision in Ireland and England. *Criminology & Criminal Justice, 19*(1), 3–25. DOI: 10.1177/1748895817739665

Fitzgibbon, W., & Stengel, C. M. (2018). Women's voices made visible: Photovoice in visual criminology. *Punishment & Society, 20*(4), 411–431. DOI: 10.1177/1462474517700137

Flasbeck, V., Gonzalez-Liencres, C., & Brüne, M. (2018). The brain that feels into others: toward a neuroscience of empathy. In L. C. Stevens & C. C. Woodruff (Eds.), *The neuroscience of empathy, compassion, and self-compassion* (pp. 49–93). Elsevier Science & Technology. https://ebookcentral.proquest.com/lib/newcastle/detail.action?docID=5434360

Flynn, C., & McDermott, F. (2024). *Doing Research in Social Work and Social Care* (2nd ed.). Sage Publishing.

Font, S., Cancian, M., Berger, L. M., & DiGiovanni, A. (2020). Patterns of intergenerational child protective services involvement. *Child Abuse & Neglect, 99*, 104247. DOI: 10.1016/j.chiabu.2019.104247 PMID: 31715518

Fook, J. (2015). Reflective practice and critical reflection. In Lishman, J. (Ed.), *Handbook for practice learning in social work and social care: Knowledge and theory* (3rd ed., pp. 440–454). Jessica Kingsley Publishers.

Forslund, T., Granqvist, P., van Ijzendoorn, M. H., Sagi-Schwartz, A., Glaser, D., Steele, M., Hammarlund, M., Schuengel, C., Bakermans-Kranenburg, M. J., Steele, H., Shaver, P. R., Lux, U., Simmonds, J., Jacobvitz, D., Groh, A. M., Bernard, K., Cyr, C., Hazen, N. L., Foster, S., & Duschinsky, R. (2022). Attachment goes to court: Child protection and custody issues. *Attachment & Human Development, 24*(1), 1–52. DOI: 10.1080/14616734.2020.1840762 PMID: 33427578

Foster Care Association of Victoria. (2024). *Carer snapshot*. FCAV.

Foundation, E. Q. T. (2024, April 12). *More support for foster carers as numbers continue to decline.* EQT Foundation Media Centre. https://www.eqt.com.au/MediaCentre/2024/04/12/More-support-for-foster-carers-as-numbers-continue-to-decline

Fox, E. (2024). Toward a sociological perspective on the gender and sexuality of friendship. *Sociology Compass, 18*(8), e13263. DOI: 10.1111/soc4.13263

Fraiberg, S., Adelson, E., & Sharpiro, V. (1975). Ghosts in the nursery: A psychodynamic approach to the problems of impaired infant-mother relationships. *Journal of the American Academy of Child and Adolescent Psychiatry, 14*(3), 387–421. PMID: 1141566

Franklin, T. B., Russig, H., Weiss, I. C., Gräff, J., Linder, N., Michalon, A., Vizi, S., & Mansuy, I. M. (2010). Epigenetic transmission of the impact of early stress across generations. *Biological Psychiatry, 68*(5), 408–415. DOI: 10.1016/j.biopsych.2010.05.036 PMID: 20673872

Fraser, M. W., Walton, E., Lewis, R. E., Pecora, P. J., & Walton, E. K. (1996). An experiment in family reunification: Correlates of outcomes at one year follow-up. *Children and Youth Services Review, 18*(4/5), 335–362. DOI: 10.1016/0190-7409(96)00009-6

Frazier, P., Tashiro, T., Berman, M., Stecker, R., & Schwartz, A. (2009). PTSD and comorbidity in a national probability sample of college students. *Journal of Traumatic Stress, 22*, 223–228.

Frederico, M., Long, M., McNamara, P., McPherson, L., & Rose, R. (2017). Improving outcomes for children in out-of-home care: The role of therapeutic foster care. *Child & Family Social Work, 22*(2), 1064–1074. DOI: 10.1111/cfs.12326

Freud, S. (1936). *Inhibitions, symptoms and anxiety.* Hogarth.

Freyd, J. J. (1996). *Betrayal trauma: The logic of forgetting childhood abuse.* Harvard University Press.

Freyd, J. J., & Birrell, P. J. (2013). *Blind to betrayal: Why we fool ourselves we aren't being fooled.* Wiley.

Freyd, J. J., DePrince, A. P., & Gleaves, D. H. (2007). The state of betrayal trauma theory: The need for more research. *Journal of Trauma & Dissociation, 8*(3), 1–8. DOI: 10.1300/J229v08n03_01 PMID: 18032341

Freyd, J. J., Klest, B., & Allard, C. B. (2005). Betrayal trauma: Relationship to physical health, psychological distress, and a written disclosure intervention. *Journal of Trauma & Dissociation*, *6*(3), 83–104. DOI: 10.1300/J229v06n03_04 PMID: 16172083

Fu, H., Feng, T., Qin, J., Wang, T., Wu, X., Cai, Y., Lan, L., & Yang, T. (2018). Reported prevalence of childhood maltreatment among Chinese college students: A systematic review and meta-analysis. *PLoS One*, *13*(10), e0205808. DOI: 10.1371/journal.pone.0205808 PMID: 30321243

Gabriel, A. S., Diefendorff, J. M., & Grandey, A. A. (2023). The acceleration of emotional labor research: Navigating the past and steering toward the future. *Personnel Psychology*, *76*(2), 397–440. DOI: 10.1111/peps.12576

Gabrielli, J., & Jackson, Y. (2019). Innovative methodological and statistical approaches to the study of child maltreatment: Introduction. *Child Abuse & Neglect*, *87*, 1–4. DOI: 10.1016/j.chiabu.2018.12.001 PMID: 30551809

Gansen, H. M., & Martin, K. A. (2018). Becoming gendered. In Risman, B. J., Froyum, C. M., & Scarborough, W. J. (Eds.), *Handbook of the sociology of gender* (pp. 83–93). Springer International Publishing., DOI: 10.1007/978-3-319-76333-0_6

Gapp, K., Jawaid, A., Sarkies, P., Bohacek, J., Pelczar, P., Prados, J., Farinelli, L., Miska, E., & Mansuy, I. M. (2014). Implication of sperm RNAs in transgenerational inheritance of the effects of early trauma in mice. *Nature Neuroscience*, *17*(5), 667–669. DOI: 10.1038/nn.3695 PMID: 24728267

Garaigordobil, M. (2009). A comparative analysis of empathy in childhood and adolescence: Gender differences and associated socio-emotional variables. *Journal of Psychology and Psychological Therapy*, *9*(2), 217–235.

Garmezy, N. (1991). Resilience in children's adaptation to negative life events and stressed environments. *Pediatric Annals*, *20*(9), 459–466. DOI: 10.3928/0090-4481-19910901-05 PMID: 1945543

Gee, G., Dudgeon, P., Schultz, C., Hart, A., & Kelly, K. (2014). Aboriginal and Torres Strait Islander social and emotional wellbeing. In Dudgeon, P., Milroy, H., & Walker, R. (Eds.), *Working together: Aboriginal and Torres Strait Islander mental health and wellbeing principles and practice* (2nd ed., pp. 55–68). Department of the Prime Minister and Cabinet.

Geiger, J. M., Schelbe, L., Hayes, M. J., Kawam, E., Katz, C. C., & Klika, J. B. (2015). Intergenerational transmission of maltreatment: Ending a family tradition. In Daro, D., Cohn Donnelly, A., Huang, L., & Powell, B. (Eds.), *Advances in Child Abuse Prevention Knowledge* (pp. 67–91). Springer., DOI: 10.1007/978-3-319-16327-7_4

Gelles, R. J. (1976). Abused wives: Why do they stay? *Journal of Marriage and Family*, *38*(4), 659–668. DOI: 10.2307/350685

Gerdes, K. E., & Segal, E. A. (2009). A social work model of empathy. *Advances in Social Work*, *10*(2), 114–127. DOI: 10.18060/235

Gerdes, K., & Segal, E. A. (2011). Importance of empathy for social work practice: Integrating new science. *Social Work*, *56*(2), 141–148. DOI: 10.1093/sw/56.2.141

Gilbert, R., Widom, C. S., Browne, K., Fergusson, D., Webb, E., & Janson, S. (2009). Burden and consequences of child maltreatment in high-income countries. *Lancet*, *373*(9657), 68–81. DOI: 10.1016/S0140-6736(08)61706-7 PMID: 19056114

Gildersleeve, J., Cantrell, K., Bryce. I., & Cripps, C. (2024). Reading, Reflection and Resilience in the Study of Australian Literature. Journal of Language, Literature and Culture. 1-18.

Glock, S., Krolak-Schwerdt, S., Klapproth, F., & Böhmer, M. (2019). Teachers' expectancy effects: A meta-analysis. *Educational Research Review*, *27*, 210–228. DOI: 10.1016/j.edurev.2019.03.001

Gobin, R. L., & Freyd, J. J. (2009). Betrayal and revictimization: Preliminary findings. *Psychological Trauma: Theory, Research, Practice, and Policy*, *1*(3), 242–257. DOI: 10.1037/a0017469

Golding, F. (2022). Sexual abuse as the core transgression of childhood innocence: Unintended consequences for care leavers. In Wright, K., Swain, S., & McPhillips, K. (Eds.), *Examining the past and shaping the future: The Australian royal commission into institutional responses to child sexual abuse* (pp. 55–67). Routledge.

Goldsmith, R. E., Freyd, J. J., & DePrince, A. P. (2012). Betrayal trauma: Associations with psychological and physical symptoms in young adults. *Journal of Interpersonal Violence*, *27*(3), 547–567. DOI: 10.1177/0886260511421672 PMID: 21987504

Gómez, J. M. (2012). Cultural Betrayal trauma theory: The impact of culture on the effects of trauma. In Blind to Betrayal. Retrieved from https://sites.google.com/site/betrayalbook/betrayal-research-news/ cultural-betrayal

Gómez, J. M. (2017b). Does gender matter? An exploratory study of cultural betrayal trauma and hallucinations in Latino undergraduates at a predominantly White university. Advanced online publication. *Journal of Interpersonal Violence*, 088626051774694.

Gómez, J. M. (2017). *Cultural Betrayal trauma theory*. University of Oregon.

Gómez, J. M. (2017a). Does ethno-cultural betrayal in trauma affect Asian American/Pacific islander college students' mental health outcomes? An exploratory study. *Journal of American College Health*, *65*(6), 432–436. DOI: 10.1080/07448481.2017.1341896 PMID: 28617143

Gómez, J. M. (2018). What's in a Betrayal? Trauma, Dissociation, and Hallucinations Among High-Functioning Ethnic Minority Emerging Adults. *Journal of Aggression, Maltreatment & Trauma*, *28*(10), 1181–1198. DOI: 10.1080/10926771.2018.1494653

Gómez, J. M. (2019). Group dynamics as a predictor of dissociation for Black victims of violence: An exploratory study of cultural Betrayal trauma theory. *Transcultural Psychiatry*, *56*(5), 878–894. DOI: 10.1177/1363461519847300 PMID: 31046633

Gómez, J. M., & Freyd, J. J. (2018). Psychological outcomes of within group sexual violence: Evidence of cultural betrayal. *Journal of Immigrant and Minority Health*, *20*(6), 1458–1467. DOI: 10.1007/s10903-017-0687-0 PMID: 29288343

Gone, J. P. (2013). Redressing First Nations historical trauma: Theorizing mechanisms for indigenous culture as mental health treatment. *Transcultural Psychiatry*, *50*(5), 683–706. DOI: 10.1177/1363461513487669 PMID: 23715822

Green, A. H. (1976). A psychodynamic approach to the study and treatment of child-abusing parents. *Journal of the American Academy of Child Psychiatry*, *15*(3), 414–429. DOI: 10.1016/S0002-7138(09)61617-4 PMID: 965619

Greenberg, D. M., Warrier, V., Allison, C., & Baron-Cohen, S. (2018). Elevated empathy in adults following childhood trauma. *PMC*, Article 6169872.

Green, S. (2023). Colonisation, post-colonisation and decolonisation. In Holscher, D., Hugman, R., & McAuliffe, D. (Eds.), *Social work theory and ethics: Ideas in practice* (pp. 101–120). Springer. DOI: 10.1007/978-981-19-1015-9_7

Gruttadaro, D. A., & Crudo, R. (2012). *College students speak: A survey report on mental health*. Active Minds.

Grynberg, D., & Konrath, S. (2020). The closer you feel, the more you care: Positive associations between closeness pain intensity rating, empathic concern and personal distress to someone in pain. *Acta Psychologica, 201*, 103175. Advance online publication. DOI: 10.1016/j.actpsy.2020.103175

Guerney, L. F. (2000). Filial therapy. In Kaduson, H. G., & Schaefer, C. E. (Eds.), *Short-term play therapy for children* (pp. 75–104). The Guilford Press.

Guest, G., MacQueen, K. M., & Namey, E. E. (2011). *Applied thematic analysis.* Sage Publications., DOI: 10.4135/9781483384436

Gutiérrez, K. (2008). Developing a sociocritical literacy in the third space. *Reading Research Quarterly, 43*(2), 148–164. DOI: 10.1598/RRQ.43.2.3

Gutowski, E., & Goodman, L. A. (2020). "Like I'm invisible": IPV survivor-mothers' perceptions of seeking child custody through the family court system. *Journal of Family Violence, 35*(5), 441–457. DOI: 10.1007/s10896-019-00063-1

Guttierez, L., & Gutierez, D. (2019). Examining traumatic experiences, mental health needs, and resilience in the lives of student veterans. *Journal of Student Affairs Research and Practice, 56*(1), 42–53.

Gypen, L., Vanderfaeillie, J., De Maeyer, S., Belenger, L., & Van Holen, F. (2017). Outcomes of children who grew up in foster care: A systematic review. *Children and Youth Services Review, 76*, 74–83. DOI: 10.1016/j.childyouth.2017.02.035

Haartsen, R., Jones, E. J., & Johnson, M. H. (2016). Human brain development over the early years. *Current Opinion in Behavioral Sciences, 10*, 149–154. DOI: 10.1016/j.cobeha.2016.05.015

Hall, S. (2011). "It's going to stop in this generation": Women with a history of child abuse resolving to raise their children without abuse. *Harvard Educational Review, 81*(1), 24–49,150. DOI: 10.17763/haer.81.1.m8202r3804uvmv68

Hamai, T. A., & Felitti, V. J. (2022). Adverse childhood experiences: Past, present, and future. In Geffner, R. (Eds.), *Handbook of interpersonal violence and abuse across the lifespan* (pp. 97–120). Springer Nature Switzerland AG., DOI: 10.1007/978-3-319-89999-2_305

Hambrick, E. P., Oppenheim-Weller, S., N'zi, A. M., & Taussig, H. N. (2016). Mental health interventions for children in foster care: A systematic review. *Children and Youth Services Review, 70*, 65–77. DOI: 10.1016/j.childyouth.2016.09.002 PMID: 28496286

Hamby, S., Finkelhor, D., Turner, H., & Ormrod, R. (2010). The overlap of witnessing partner violence with child maltreatment and other victimizations in a nationally representative survey of youth. *Child Abuse & Neglect, 34*(10), 734–741. DOI: 10.1016/j.chiabu.2010.03.001 PMID: 20850182

Hannan, S. M., Zimnick, J., & Park, C. (2021). Consequences of sexual violence among college students: Investigating the role of PTSD symptoms, rumination, and institutional betrayal. *Journal of Aggression, Maltreatment & Trauma, 30*(5), 586–604. DOI: 10.1080/10926771.2020.1796871

Harris, L. G., Higgins, D. J., Willis, M. L., Lawrence, D., Mathews, B., Malacova, E., Erskine, H., Meinck, F., & Haslam, D. M. (2025b). Determining the effect of out-of-home care on mental health disorders: A propensity score-matched study of maltreatment intensity. *Child Abuse & Neglect, 167,* 107571 107571-167. DOI: 10.1016/j.chiabu.2025.107571

Harris, L., Higgins, D. J., Willis, M., Lawrence, D., Meinck, F., Thomas, H. J., Malacova, E., Scott, J. G., & Haslam, D. M. (2025a). Dimensions of child maltreatment in Australians with a history of out-of-home care. *Child Maltreatment.* https://journals.sagepub.com/doi/10.1177/10775595241297944

Harris, L. G., Higgins, D. J., & Willis, M. L. (2026). Practitioners' perspectives on enablers of improved mental health outcomes for children and young people in out-of-home care: Beyond a "scattergun approach". *Child Protection and Practice, 100283.* Advance online publication. DOI: 10.1016/j.chipro.2026.100283

Harris, L., Higgins, D. J., Willis, M., Lawrence, D., Mathews, B., Thomas, H. J., Malacova, E., Pacella, R., Scott, J. G., Finkelhor, D., Meinck, F., Erskine, H. E., & Haslam, D. M. (2024). The prevalence and patterns of maltreatment, childhood adversity, and mental health disorders in an Australian out-of-home care sample. *Child Maltreatment,* •••, 1–13. DOI: 10.1177/10775595241246534 PMID: 38627990

Haune, M., Christiansen, Ø., Heiervang, E. R., & Haavind, H. (2024). "Great day! But now what?" Adolescents' and foster carers' experiences of a comprehensive health assessment for children in out-of-home care. *Children and Youth Services Review, 158,* 107464. DOI: 10.1016/j.childyouth.2024.107464

Healing Foundation. (2019). *Working with Stolen Generations Aged Care Fact Sheet.* https://cdn.healingfoundation.org.au/app/uploads/2019/12/18122008/Working-with-Stolen-Generations-Aged-Care-fact-sheet.pdf

Healing Foundation. (2025). *Who are the Stolen Generations.* https://healingfoundation.org.au/who-are-the-stolen-generations/

Healy, K. (2022). *Social work theories in context: Creating frameworks for practice* (3rd ed.). Bloomsbury Publishing.

Hein, T. C., & Monk, C. S. (2017). Research review: Neural response to threat in children, adolescents, and adults following early life stress. *Journal of Child Psychology and Psychiatry, and Allied Disciplines, 58*(3), 222–230. DOI: 10.1111/jcpp.12651 PMID: 27778344

Herbert, J. L., & Bromfield, L. (2019). Multi-disciplinary teams responding to child abuse: Common features and assumptions. *Children and Youth Services Review, 106*, 104467. DOI: 10.1016/j.childyouth.2019.104467

Herman, J. (1992). *Trauma and recovery*. Basic Books.

Herman, J. L. (1992). Complex PTSD: A syndrome in survivors of prolonged and repeated trauma. *Journal of Traumatic Stress, 5*(3), 377–389. DOI: 10.1002/jts.2490050305

Herman, J. L. (1992). *Trauma and recovery: The aftermath of violence – From domestic abuse to political terror*. Basic Books.

Herman, J. L. (2002). *Truth and repair: How trauma survivors enact restorative justice*. Basic Books.

Herrenkohl, T. I., Jung, H., Lee, J. O., & Kim, M. (2017). Effects of Child Maltreatment, Cumulative Victimization Experiences, and Proximal Life Stress on Adult Crime and Antisocial Behavior. Office of Justice Programs' National Criminal Justice Reference Service, US.

Herrenkohl, R. C., & Herrenkohl, T. I. (2009). Assessing a child's experience of multiple maltreatment types: Some unfinished business. *Journal of Family Violence, 24*(7), 485–496. DOI: 10.1007/s10896-009-9247-2 PMID: 20161642

Herzberger, S. D. (1983). Social cognition and the transmission of abuse. In Finkelhor, D., Gelles, R. J., Hotaling, G. T., & Straus, M. A. (Eds.), *The dark side of families: Current family violence research* (pp. 317–329). SAGE Publications.

Higgins, D. J., & McCabe, M. P. (2001b). Multiple forms of child abuse and neglect: Adult retrospective reports. *Aggression and Violent Behavior: A Review Journal, 6*, 547-578. DOI: 10.1016/S1359-1789(00)00030-6

Higgins, D. J. (2004a). Differentiating between child maltreatment experiences. *Family Matters (Melbourne, Vic.), 69*, 50–55. http://www.aifs.gov.au/institute/pubs/fm2004/fm69/dh.pdf

Higgins, D. J. (2004b). The importance of degree versus type of maltreatment: A cluster analysis of child abuse types. *The Journal of Psychology*, *138*(4), 303–324. DOI: 10.3200/JRLP.138.4.303-324 PMID: 15379008

Higgins, D. J., & Hunt, G. R. (2024). Child, parent and contextual factors associated with child protection system involvement and child maltreatment in the family: A rapid evidence review. *The Australian Journal of Social Issues*, *59*(2), 358–400. DOI: 10.1002/ajs4.306

Higgins, D. J., Lawrence, D., Haslam, D. M., Mathews, B., Malacova, E., Erskine, H. E., Finkelhor, D., Pacella, R., Meinck, F., Thomas, H. J., & Scott, J. G. (2024). Prevalence of diverse genders and sexualities in Australia and associations with five forms of child maltreatment and multi-type maltreatment. *Child Maltreatment*, *30*(1), 21–41. DOI: 10.1177/10775595231226331 PMID: 38214251

Higgins, D. J., Mathews, B., Pacella, R., Scott, J. G., Finkelhor, D., Meinck, F., Erskine, H., Thomas, H., Lawrence, D., Haslam, D., Malacova, E., & Dunne, M. P. (2023). The prevalence and nature of multi-type child maltreatment in Australia. *The Medical Journal of Australia*, *218*(6, Suppl), S19–S25. DOI: 10.5694/mja2.51868 PMID: 37004183

Higgins, D. J., & McCabe, M. P. (1994). The relationship of child sexual abuse and family violence to adult adjustment: Toward an integrated risk-sequelae model. *Journal of Sex Research*, *31*(4), 255–266. DOI: 10.1080/00224499409551761

Higgins, D. J., & McCabe, M. P. (1998). Parent perceptions of maltreatment and adjustment in children. *Journal of Family Studies*, *4*(1), 53–76. DOI: 10.5172/jfs.4.1.53

Higgins, D. J., & McCabe, M. P. (2000a). Relationships between different types of maltreatment during childhood and adjustment in adulthood. *Child Maltreatment*, *5*(3), 261–272. DOI: 10.1177/1077559500005003006 PMID: 11232272

Higgins, D. J., & McCabe, M. P. (2000b). Multi-type maltreatment and the long-term adjustment of adults. *Child Abuse Review*, *9*(1), 6–18. DOI: 10.1002/(SICI)1099-0852(200001/02)9:1<6::AID-CAR579>3.0.CO;2-W

Higgins, D. J., & McCabe, M. P. (2001a). The development of the Comprehensive Child Maltreatment Scale. *Journal of Family Studies*, *7*(1), 7–28. DOI: 10.5172/jfs.7.1.7

Higgins, D., Bromfield, L., & Richardson, N. (2007). *Child abuse and neglect in Australian families*. Australian Institute of Family Studies.

Hochschild, A. R. (1983). *The managed heart: Commercialization of human feeling*. University of California Press.

Hojat, M. (2009). Ten approaches for enhancing empathy in health and human services cultures. *Journal of Health and Human Services Administration, 31*(4), 412–450. DOI: 10.1177/107937390903100403

Howe, D. (2016). *Empathy: What it is and why it matters.* Palgrave MacMillan.

Howell, K. H., Miller-Graff, L. E., Martinez-Torteya, C., Napier, T. R., & Carney, J. R. (2021). Charting a course towards resilience following adverse childhood experiences: Addressing intergenerational trauma via strengths-based intervention. *Children (Basel, Switzerland), 8*(10), 844. DOI: 10.3390/children8100844 PMID: 34682109

Hsu, N., Newman, D. A., & Badura, K. L. (2022). Emotional intelligence and transformational leadership: Meta-analysis and explanatory model of female leadership advantage. *Journal of Intelligence, 10*(4), 104. DOI: 10.3390/jintelligence10040104

Hughes, D. (2004). An attachment-based treatment of maltreated children and young people. *Attachment & Human Development, 6*(3), 263–278. DOI: 10.1080/14616730412331281539 PMID: 15513268

Hughes, D. A. (2016). *Building the bonds of attachment: Awakening love in deeply troubled children* (3rd ed.). Rowman & Littlefield.

Hughes, D. A., Golding, K. S., & Hudson, J. (2019). *Creating loving attachments: Parenting with PACE to nurture confidence and security in the troubled child.* Jessica Kingsley Publishers.

Hughes, K., Bellis, M. A., Hardcastle, K., Sethi, D., Butchart, A., Mikton, C., Jones, L., & Dunne, M. (2017). The effect of multiple adverse childhood experiences on health: A systematic review and meta-analysis. *The Lancet. Public Health, 2*(8), e356–e366. DOI: 10.1016/S2468-2667(17)30118-4 PMID: 29253477

Hulette, A. C., Freyd, J. J., Pears, K. C., Kim, H. K., Fisher, P. A., & Becker-Blease, K. A. (2008). Dissociation and posttraumatic symptoms in maltreated preschool children. *Journal of Child & Adolescent Trauma, 1*(2), 93–108. DOI: 10.1080/19361520802083980 PMID: 28255424

Hulette, A. C., Kaehler, L. A., & Freyd, J. J. (2011). Intergenerational associations between trauma and dissociation. *Journal of Family Violence, 26*(3), 217–225. DOI: 10.1007/s10896-011-9357-5

Human Rights and Equal Opportunity Commission (HREOC). (1997). *Bringing them home: Report of the National Inquiry into the Separation of Aboriginal and Torres Strait Islander Children from Their Families.* Commonwealth of Australia. https://humanrights.gov.au/our-work/bringing-them-home-report-1997

Hunter, S. J. (2022). *Trauma-informed care in human service organisations: A practical guide for agencies, groups and practitioners*. Jessica Kingsley Publishers.

Hurst, N. C., & Sawatzky, D. D. (1996). Families with multiple problems through a Bowenian lens. *Child Welfare*, *75*(6), 693–693. PMID: 8936483

Huth-Bocks, A. C., Krause, K., Ahlfs-Dunn, S., Gallagher, E., & Scott, S. (2013). Relational trauma and posttraumatic stress symptoms among pregnant women. *Psychodynamic Psychiatry*, *41*(2), 277–301. DOI: 10.1521/pdps.2013.41.2.277 PMID: 23713621

Huttenlocher, P. R. (1984). Synapse elimination and plasticity in developing human cerebral cortex. *American Journal of Mental Deficiency*, *88*(5), 488–496. PMID: 6731486

Iacoboni, M. (2009). Imitation, empathy, and mirror neurons. *Annual Review of Psychology*, *60*(1), 653–670. DOI: 10.1146/annurev.psych.60.110707.163604

Ioannidis, K., Askelund, A. D., Kievit, R. A., & Van Harmelen, A. L. (2020). The complex neurobiology of resilient functioning after childhood maltreatment. *BMC Medicine*, *18*(1), 32. DOI: 10.1186/s12916-020-1490-7 PMID: 32050974

Islam, S., Jaffee, S. R., & Widom, C. S. (2023). Breaking the cycle of intergenerational childhood maltreatment: Effects on offspring mental health. *Child Maltreatment*, *28*(1), 119–129. DOI: 10.1177/10775595211067205 PMID: 35073784

Isokuortti, N., Aaltio, E., Laajasalo, T., & Barlow, J. (2020). Effectiveness of child protection practice models: A systematic review. *Child Abuse & Neglect*, *108*, 104632. DOI: 10.1016/j.chiabu.2020.104632 PMID: 32818821

Iyengar, U., Rajhans, P., Fonagy, P., Strathearn, L., & Kim, S. (2019). Unresolved trauma and reorganization in mothers: Attachment and neuroscience perspectives. *Frontiers in Psychology*, *10*, 110. DOI: 10.3389/fpsyg.2019.00110 PMID: 30761051

Jacobsson, K., & Meeuwisse, A. (2020). 'State governing of knowledge' - constraining social work research and practice. *European Journal of Social Work*, *23*(2), 277–289. DOI: 10.1080/13691457.2018.1530642

Jaffee, S. R., Bowes, L., Ouellet-Morin, I., Fisher, H. L., Moffitt, T. E., Merrick, M. T., & Arseneault, L. (2013). Safe, stable, nurturing relationships break the intergenerational cycle of abuse: A prospective nationally representative cohort of children in the United Kingdom. *The Journal of Adolescent Health*, *53*(4), 4–10. DOI: 10.1016/j.jadohealth.2013.04.007 PMID: 24059939

James, M. (2000). *Child Abuse and Neglect: Part 1— Redefining the Issues. Trends & issues in crime and criminal justice no. 146*. Australian Institute of Criminology., https://www.aic.gov.au/sites/default/files/2020-05/tandi146.pdf

Janca, A., Lyons, Z., Balaratnasingam, S., Parfitt, D., Davison, S., Laugharne, J., & Winthrop, Z. (2015). Here and Now Aboriginal Assessment (HANAA): Background, development and preliminary evaluation of a culturally appropriate screening tool. *Australasian Psychiatry, 23*(3), 287–292. DOI: 10.1177/1039856215584514 PMID: 25944764

Jean-Thorn, A., Tremblay-Perreault, A., Dube, V., & Hebert, M. (2023). A systematic review of community-level protective factors in children exposed to maltreatment. *Trauma, Violence & Abuse, 24*(4), 2827–2842. DOI: 10.1177/15248380221117234 PMID: 36047717

Johnson, S. B., Riis, J. L., & Noble, K. G. (2021). Socioeconomic inequality and executive function trajectories in childhood. *Developmental Science, 24*(1), e12901. DOI: 10.1111/desc.12901

Johnstone, L., & Boyle, M. (2018). *The Power Threat Meaning Framework: Overview*. British Psychological Society.

Jolliffe, D., & Farrington, D. (2006). Development and validation of the basic empathy scale. *Journal of Adolescence, 29*(4), 589–611. DOI: 10.1016/j.adolescence.2005.08.010

Jonason, P. K., & Kroll, C. H. (2015). A multidimensional view of the relationship between empathy and the dark triad. *Journal of Individual Differences, 36*(3), 150–156. DOI: 10.1027/1614-0001/a000166

Jones, L., Malekoff, A., & Bryant, K. (2021). Reunification services and family preservation: A practice-informed review. *Journal of Family Social Work, 24*(2), 157–174.

Jud, A., Mitrovic, T., Portmann, R., Gonthier, H., Fux, E., Koehler, J., Kosirnik, C., & Knüsel, R. (2021). Multi-sectoral response to child maltreatment in Switzerland for different age groups: Varying rates of reported incidents and gaps in identification. *Child Abuse & Neglect, 111*, 104798. DOI: 10.1016/j.chiabu.2020.104798 PMID: 33213853

Juul, S. H., Hendrix, C., Robinson, B., Stowe, Z. N., Newport, D. J., Brennan, P. A., & Johnson, K. C. (2016). Maternal early-life trauma and affective parenting style: The mediating role of HPA-axis function. *Archives of Women's Mental Health, 19*(1), 17–23. DOI: 10.1007/s00737-015-0528-x PMID: 25956587

Kagan, R. (2014). *Rebuilding attachments with traumatized children: Healing from losses, violence, abuse, and neglect*. Routledge., DOI: 10.4324/9780203822319

Kahhale, I., Byrd, A., & Hanson, J. (2025). Early life adversity and empathy: A scoping review of past research and recommendations for future directions. *Clinical Child and Family Psychology Review*, *28*(2), 275–321. DOI: 10.1007/s10567-025-00516-8

Kalmuss, D. S., & Straus, M. A. (1982). Wife's marital dependency and wife abuse. *Journal of Marriage and Family*, *44*(2), 277–286. DOI: 10.2307/351538

Kaufman, J., & Zigler, E. (1987). Do abused children become abusive parents? *The American Journal of Orthopsychiatry*, *57*(2), 186–192. DOI: 10.1111/j.1939-0025.1987.tb03528.x PMID: 3296775

Keddie, A. (2012). Schooling and disadvantage: From deficit approaches to relational reform. *International Journal of Inclusive Education*, *16*(10), 1001–1012. DOI: 10.1080/13603116.2010.538865

Kelly, K., Dudgeon, P., Gee, G., & Glaskin, B. (2009). Living on the edge: Social and emotional wellbeing risk and protective factors for serious psychological distress among Aboriginal and Torres Strait Islander people. In N. Purdie, P. Dudgeon, & R. Walker (Eds.), *Working together: Aboriginal and Torres Strait Islander mental health and wellbeing principles and practice* (pp. 87–95). Commonwealth of Australia.

Kelner, J., & Gavriel-Fried, B. (2023). "The relationship changed because I had changed": Experiences and perceptions of friendships between women treated for substance use disorder in women-only residential programs. *Feminism & Psychology*, *33*(4), 647–667. DOI: 10.1177/09593535231176349

Kempe, C. H., Silverman, F. N., Steele, B. F., Droegemueller, W., & Silver, H. K. (1962). The battered-child syndrome. *Journal of the American Medical Association*, *181*(1), 17–24. DOI: 10.1001/jama.1962.03050270019004

Kennedy, M., & Scriver, S. (2016). *Building trauma-informed higher education institutions: Strategies to enhance learning and promote student success*. American College Personnel Association.

Kertesz, M., Humphreys, C., & Kiraly, M. (2021). Addressing parental mistrust in child protection contexts: Building relationships to support reunification. *Australian Social Work*, *74*(1), 28–40.

Kezelman, C., Hossack, N., Stavropoulos, P., & Burley, P. (2015). *The cost of unresolved childhood trauma and abuse in adults in Australia*. Adults Surviving Child Abuse and Pegasus Economics. Retrieved from https://blueknot.org.au/resources/blue-knot-publications/the-cost-of-unresolved-childhood-trauma-and-abuse-in-adults-in-australia-2/

Kezelman, C., & Stavropoulos, P. (2012). *Practice guidelines for treatment of complex trauma and trauma informed care and service delivery*. Adults Surviving Child Abuse.

Kimberg, L., & Wheeler, M. (2019). Trauma and trauma-informed care. In *Trauma-informed healthcare approaches: A guide for primary care* (pp. 25–56). Springer International Publishing., DOI: 10.1007/978-3-030-04342-1_2

Kim, H., & Drake, B. (2019). Cumulative prevalence of onset and recurrence of child maltreatment reports. *Journal of the American Academy of Child and Adolescent Psychiatry*, *58*(12), 1175–1183. DOI: 10.1016/j.jaac.2019.02.015 PMID: 30851398

Kim, J. (2009). Type-specific intergenerational transmission of neglectful and physically abusive parenting behaviors among young parents. *Children and Youth Services Review*, *31*(7), 761–767. DOI: 10.1016/j.childyouth.2009.02.002

Kim, J., & Gray, K. A. (2008). Leave or stay? Battered women's decision after intimate partner violence. *Journal of Interpersonal Violence*, *23*(10), 1465–1482. DOI: 10.1177/0886260508314307 PMID: 18309037

Kim, J., & Smith, C. K. (2021). Traumatic experiences and female university students' career adaptability. *The Career Development Quarterly*, *69*(3), 263–277.

Kim, K. (2012). The role of culture in theories of the intergenerational transmission of violence. *Child & Family Social Work*, *17*(4), 395–405. DOI: 10.1111/j.1365-2206.2011.00793.x

Kim, K., Mennen, F. E., & Trickett, P. K. (2017). Patterns and correlates of co-occurrence among multiple types of child maltreatment. *Child & Family Social Work*, *22*(1), 492–502. DOI: 10.1111/cfs.12268 PMID: 29225485

Kim, K., Trickett, P. K., & Putnam, F. W. (2011). Attachment representations and anxiety: Differential relationships among mothers of sexually abused and comparison girls. *Journal of Interpersonal Violence*, *26*(3), 498–521. DOI: 10.1177/0886260510363416 PMID: 20442447

Kim, S., & Strathearn, L. (2017). Trauma, mothering, and intergenerational transmission: A synthesis of behavioral and oxytocin research. *The Psychoanalytic Study of the Child*, *70*(1), 200–223. DOI: 10.1080/00797308.2016.1277897

King, S. H.Jr. (2011). The structure of empathy in social work practice. *Journal of Human Behavior in the Social Environment, 21*(6), 679–695. DOI: 10.1080/10911359.2011.583516

Kiraly, M. (2024). Kinship care in the welfare system: The lived experience of Victorian kinship stakeholders. *Children and Youth Services Review, 157*, 107424.

Kirk, R. (2010). *A comparative study of older-youth families and younger youth families in placement prevention and reunification cases, using traditional case protection services measures and NCFAS and NCFAS-R assessment data*. National Family Preservation Network Project.

Kirk, R. S. (2015a). *Development, intent and use of the North Carolina Family Assessment Scales and their relation to their reliability and their validity of the scales*. National Family Preservation Network.

Kirk, R. S. (2015b). Psychometric properties of the trauma and post trauma well-being assessment domains of the North Carolina Family Assessment Scale for general and reunification services (NCFAS G, R). *Journal of Public Child Welfare, 9*(5), 444–452. DOI: 10.1080/15548732.2015.1090364

Kirk, R. S., Kim, M., & Griffith, D. P. (2005). *NCFAS-R: North Carolina Family Assessment Scale for Reunification*. University of North Carolina at Chapel Hill.

Kirk, R., Lewis, R., Brown, T., & Marsh, L. (2017). The impact of childhood violence exposure on educational outcomes: A global systematic review. *Trauma, Violence & Abuse, 18*(4), 452–471. DOI: 10.1177/1524838015622437

Kisely, S., Abajobir, A. A., Mills, R., Strathearn, L., Clavarino, A., & Najman, J. M. (2018). Child maltreatment and mental health problems in adulthood: Birth cohort study. *The British Journal of Psychiatry, 213*(6), 698–703. DOI: 10.1192/bjp.2018.207 PMID: 30475193

Klein, K. J., & Hodges, S. D. (2001). Gender differences, motivation, and empathic accuracy: When it pays to understand. *Personality and Social Psychology Bulletin, 27*(6), 720–730. DOI: 10.1177/0146167201276007

Klein, M. (1946). Notes on some schizoid mechanisms. In *The writings of Melanie Klein* (pp. 1–24). Free Press.

Klimecki, O., & Singer, T. (2012). Empathic distress fatigue rather than compassion fatigue? Integrating findings from empathy research in psychology and neuroscience. In Oakley, B., Knafo, A., Madhavan, G., & Wilson, D. (Eds.), *Pathological altruism* (pp. 368–383). Oxford University Press.

Köhler-Dauner, F., Fegert, J. M., Anna, B., Krause, S., Gündel, H., Waller, C., & Ziegenhain, U. (2019). Maternal behavior affects child's attachment-related cortisol stress response. *Journal of Child and Adolescent Psychiatry, 1*(1), 46–60. DOI: 10.14302/issn.2643-6655.jcap-19-2737

Kohut, H. (1971). *The analysis of the self: A systematic approach to the psychoanalytic treatment of narcissistic personality disorders*. International Universities Press.

Kohut, H. (1977). *The restoration of the self*. International Universities Press.

Kolb, D. A. (2015). *Experiential learning: Experience as the source of learning and development*. FT Press.

Komatsu, A. V., Costa, R. C., Buoso, F. P., Dos Santos, P. V., Caetano, L. A. O., & Bazon, M. R. (2024). Psychosocial adaptation under adverse experiences: A study on the role of empathy with adolescents from vulnerable contexts in Brazil. *Child Abuse & Neglect, 150*, 106298. DOI: 10.1016/j.chiabu.2023.106298

Ladson-Billings, G. (2021). Three decades of culturally relevant, responsive, & sustaining pedagogy: What lies ahead? []. Routledge.]. *The Educational Forum, 85*(4), 351–354. DOI: 10.1080/00131725.2021.1957632

Lam, C. B., Solmeyer, A. R., & McHale, S. M. (2012). Sibling relationships and empathy across the transition to adolescence. *Journal of Youth and Adolescence, 41*(12), 1657–1670. DOI: 10.1007/s10964-012-9781-8

Landreth, G. L. (2012). *Play therapy: The art of the relationship* (3rd ed.). Routledge. DOI: 10.4324/9780203835159

Langevin, R., Gagné, M., Brassard, A., & Fernet, M. (2023). Intergenerational continuity of child maltreatment: The role of maternal emotional dysregulation and mother–child attachment. *Psychology of Violence, 13*(1), 1–12. Advance online publication. DOI: 10.1037/vio0000409

Langevin, R., Marshall, C., & Kingsland, E. (2021). Intergenerational cycles of maltreatment: A scoping review of psychosocial risk and protective factors. *Trauma, Violence & Abuse, 22*(4), 672–688. DOI: 10.1177/1524838019870917 PMID: 31455161

Lansford, J. E., Deater-Deckard, K., Dodge, K. A., Bates, J. E., & Pettit, G. S. (2004). Ethnic differences in the link between physical discipline and later adolescent externalizing behaviors. *Journal of Child Psychology and Psychiatry, and Allied Disciplines, 45*(4), 801–812. DOI: 10.1111/j.1469-7610.2004.00273.x PMID: 15056311

Lawrence, D., Hunt, A., Mathews, B., Haslam, D. M., Malacova, E., Dunne, M. P., Erskine, H., Higgins, D. J., Finkelhor, D., Pacella, R., Meinck, F., Thomas, H., & Scott, J. G. (2023). The association between child maltreatment and health risk behaviours and conditions throughout life in the Australian Child Maltreatment Study. *The Medical Journal of Australia, 218*(6, Suppl), S34–S39. DOI: 10.5694/mja2.51877

Lecic-Tosevski, D., Draganic-Gajic, S., Pejovic-Milovancevic, M., Popovic-Deusic, S., Christodoulou, N., & Botbol, M. (2014). Child is father of the man: Child abuse and development of future psychopathology. *Psychiatriki, 25*(3), 185–191. PMID: 25367662

Lee, J. Y., Micol, R. L., & Davis, J. L. (2021). Intimate partner violence and psychological maladjustment: Examining the role of institutional betrayal among survivors. *Journal of Interpersonal Violence, 36*(15-16), 7505–7522. DOI: 10.1177/0886260519836783 PMID: 30879384

Leiberg, S., Klimecki, O., & Singer, T. (2011). Short-term compassion training increases prosocial behavior in a newly developed prosocial gam. *PLoS One, 6*(3), e17798. Advance online publication. DOI: 10.1371/journal.pone.0017798

Leitch, L. (2017). Action steps using ACEs and trauma-informed care: A resilience model. *Health & Justice, 5*(1), 1–10. DOI: 10.1186/s40352-017-0050-5 PMID: 28455574

Lett, K., Tamaian, A., & Klest, B. (2020). Impact of ableist microaggressions on university students with self-identified disabilities. *Disability & Society, 35*(9), 1441–1456. DOI: 10.1080/09687599.2019.1680344

Levac, D., Colquhoun, H., & O'Brien, K. K. (2010). Scoping studies: Advancing the methodology. *Implementation Science : IS, 5*(1), 69–77. DOI: 10.1186/1748-5908-5-69 PMID: 20854677

Leve, L. D., Harold, G. T., Chamberlain, P., Landsverk, J. A., Fisher, P. A., & Vostanis, P. (2012). Practitioner review: Children in foster care–vulnerabilities and evidence-based interventions that promote resilience processes. *Journal of Child Psychology and Psychiatry, and Allied Disciplines, 53*(12), 1197–1211. DOI: 10.1111/j.1469-7610.2012.02594.x PMID: 22882015

Levendosky, A. A. (2013). Drawing conclusions: An intergenerational transmission of violence perspective. *Psychodynamic Psychiatry, 41*(2), 351–360. DOI: 10.1521/pdps.2013.41.2.351 PMID: 23713624

Levendosky, A. A., Lannert, B., & Yalch, M. (2012). The effects of intimate partner violence on women and child survivors: An attachment perspective. *Psychodynamic Psychiatry, 40*(3), 397–433. DOI: 10.1521/pdps.2012.40.3.397 PMID: 23002702

Levy, J., Goldstein, A., & Feldman, R. (2019). The neural development of empathy is sensitive to caregiving and early trauma. *Nature Communications, 10*(1), 1–10. DOI: 10.1038/s41467-019-09927-y

Lewis, A. J. (2025). *Interrupting the Cycle of Psychological Betrayal Trauma in Mother-Daughter Relationships* (Doctoral dissertation, Alliant International University).

Liamputtong, P. (2007). *Researching the Vulnerable*. SAGE Publications Ltd., DOI: 10.4135/9781849209861

Lieberman, A. F., Ghosh Ippen, C., & Van Horn, P. (2020). *Don't hit my mommy! A manual for child-parent psychotherapy with young witnesses of family violence* (3rd ed.). Zero to Three Press.

Lieberman, A. F., Padrón, E., Van Horn, P., & Harris, W. W. (2005). Angels in the nursery: The intergenerational transmission of benevolent parental influences. *Infant Mental Health Journal, 26*(6), 504–520. DOI: 10.1002/imhj.20071 PMID: 28682485

Lieberman, A. F., Van Horn, P., & Ippen, C. G. (2005). Toward evidence-based treatment: Child–parent psychotherapy with preschoolers exposed to marital violence. *Journal of the American Academy of Child and Adolescent Psychiatry, 44*(12), 1241–1248. DOI: 10.1097/01.chi.0000181047.59702.58

Lifton, R. J. (1968). *Death in life: Survivors of Hiroshima*. Random House.

Lifton, R. J. (2023). *Surviving our catastrophes: Resilience and renewal from Hiroshima to the COVID-19 pandemic*. Farrar, Straus and Giroux. DOI: 10.2307/jj.26193262

Lima, F., Maclean, M., & O'Donnell, M. (2019). *Exploring outcomes for young people who have experienced out-of-home care*. Telethon Kids Institute.

Lindsey, R. E., Carlozzi, A. F., & Eells, G. T. (2001). Differences in the dispositional empathy of juvenile sex offenders, non-sex-offending delinquent juveniles, and nondelinquent juveniles. *Journal of Interpersonal Violence, 16*(6), 510–522. DOI: 10.1177/088626001016006002

Linehan, M. M. (2015). *DBT skills training manual* (2nd ed.). The Guilford Press.

Lockhart, G., Atkins, L., & King, A. (2021, March). *Children in Care Evidence-Based Clinical Review & Practice Guide.* NHS England South East, Clinical Delivery and Networks. CiC_Evidence_Based_Clinical_Review_and_Practice_Guide.pdf

Löffler, C. S., & Greitemeyer, T. (2023). Are women the more empathetic gender? The effects of gender role expectations. *Current Psychology (New Brunswick, N.J.)*, *42*(1), 220–231. DOI: 10.1007/s12144-020-01260-8

Lomanowska, A. M., Boivin, M., Hertzman, C., & Fleming, A. S. (2017). Parenting begets parenting: A neurobiological perspective on early adversity and the transmission of parenting styles across generations. *Neuroscience*, *342*, 120–139. DOI: 10.1016/j.neuroscience.2015.09.029 PMID: 26386294

Long, M., & Stephen, R. (2011). Rethinking the 'best interests' of the child: Voices from Aboriginal child and family welfare practitioners. *Australian Social Work*, *64*(1), 96–112. DOI: 10.1080/0312407X.2010.535544

Lonne, B., Higgins, D., Herrenkohl, T. I., & Scott, D. (2020). Reconstructing the workforce within public health protective systems: Improving resilience, retention, service responsiveness and outcomes. *Child Abuse & Neglect*, *110*, 104191. DOI: 10.1016/j.chiabu.2019.104191 PMID: 31543276

Lorenc, T., Lester, S., Sutcliffe, K., Stansfield, C., & Thomas, J. (2020). Interventions to support children exposed to adversity. *Public Health Reviews*, *41*, 6. DOI: 10.1186/s40985-020-00127-0

Lowe, K., Golledge, C., Poulton, P., & Thompson, K. (2025). Curriculum as policy deception: A critical analysis of Aboriginal and Torres Strait Islander knowledge inclusion in the Australian Curriculum. *Australian Educational Researcher*, *52*(3), 2561–2582. DOI: 10.1007/s13384-025-00824-6

Lueger-Schuster, B., Knefel, M., Glück, T. M., Jagsch, R., Kantor, V., & Weindl, D. (2018). Child abuse and neglect in institutional settings, cumulative lifetime traumatization, and psychopathological long-term correlates in adult survivors: The Vienna Institutional Abuse Study. *Child Abuse & Neglect*, *76*, 488–501. DOI: 10.1016/j.chiabu.2017.12.009 PMID: 29276971

Luke, N., Sinclair, I., Woolgar, M., & Sebba, J. (2014). *What works in prevention and treating poor mental health in looked after children?* REES Centre. https://www.education.ox.ac.uk/wp-content/uploads/2019/06/What-Works-in-Preventing-and-Treating-Poor-Mental-Health-in-Looked-After-Children.pdf

Luke, J., Verbunt, E., Zhang, A., Bamblett, M., Johnson, G., Salamone, C., Thomas, D., Eades, S., Gubhaju, L., Kelaher, M., & Jones, A. (2022). Questioning the ethics of evidence-based practice for Indigenous health and social settings in Australia. *BMJ Global Health, 7*(6), e009167. Advance online publication. DOI: 10.1136/bmjgh-2022-009167 PMID: 35680132

Lynch, A., Newlands, F., & Forrester, D. (2019). What does empathy sound like in social work communication? A mixed-methods study of empathy in child protection social work practice. *Child & Family Social Work, 24*(1), 139–147. DOI: 10.1111/cfs.12591

Lyons-Ruth, K., Easterbrooks, M. A., & Cibelli, C. D. (1997). Infant attachment strategies, infant mental lag, and maternal depressive symptoms: Predictors of internalizing and externalizing problems at age 7. *Developmental Psychology, 33*(4), 681–692. DOI: 10.1037/0012-1649.33.4.681 PMID: 9232383

Lyons-Ruth, K., Yellin, C., Melnick, S., & Atwood, G. (2005). Expanding the concept of unresolved mental states: Hostile/helpless states of mind on the Adult Attachment Interview are associated with disrupted mother-infant communication and infant disorganization. *Development and Psychopathology, 17*(1), 1–23. DOI: 10.1017/S0954579405050017 PMID: 15971757

Macdonald, G., Livingstone, N., Hanratty, J., McCartan, C., Cotmore, R., Cary, M., Glanville, J., & Bywater, T. (2018). The effectiveness, acceptability and cost-effectiveness of psychosocial interventions for maltreated children and adolescents: An evidence synthesis. *Health Technology Assessment, 22*(52), 1–508.

Macfarlane, A., & Macfarlane, S. (2019). Listen to culture: Māori scholars' plea to researchers. *Journal of the Royal Society of New Zealand, 49*(sup1), 48-57.

MacMillan, H. L., Wathen, C. N., Barlow, J., Fergusson, D. M., Leventhal, J. M., & Taussig, H. N. (2009). Interventions to prevent child maltreatment and associated impairment. *Lancet, 373*(9659), 250–266. DOI: 10.1016/S0140-6736(08)61708-0 PMID: 19056113

Madigan, S., Cyr, C., Eirich, R., Fearon, R. M. P., Ly, A., Rash, C., Poole, J. C., & Alink, L. R. A. (2019). Testing the cycle of maltreatment hypothesis: Meta-analytic evidence of the intergenerational transmission of child maltreatment. *Development and Psychopathology, 31*(1), 23–51. DOI: 10.1017/S0954579418001700 PMID: 30757994

Madzoska, M., Lawrence, D., Higgins, D. J., Haslam, D., Mathews, B., Malacova, E., Dunne, M. P., Erskine, H., Pacella, R., Meinck, F., Thomas, H., & Scott, J. (2024). Child maltreatment, mental health disorders and health risk behaviors in people with diverse gender identities. *Journal of Interpersonal Violence*, *40*(9-10), 2281–2306. DOI: 10.1177/08862605241270077 PMID: 39152737

Main, M., & Hesse, E. (1990). Parents' unresolved traumatic experiences are related to infant disorganized attchment status: Is frightened and/or frightening parental behavior the linking mechnaism? In Greenberg, M. T., Cicchetti, D., & Cummings, E. M. (Eds.), *Attachment in the preschool years: Theory, research, and intervention* (pp. 161–182). University of Chicago Press.

Main, M., & Solomon, J. (1990). Procedures for identifying infants as disorganized/disoriented during the Ainsworth strange situation. In Greenberg, M. T., Cichetti, D., & Cummings, E. M. (Eds.), *Attachment in the Preschool Years: Theory, Research and Intervention* (pp. 121–160). University of Chicago Press.

Malach-Pines, A., & Yafe-Yanai, B. (2001). The role of early negative childhood experiences in career choice: An exploratory study. *Journal of Career Development*, *28*, 147–167.

Marchetti, A., Miraglia, L., & Di Dio, C. (2019). Toward a socio-material approach to cognitive empathy in autistic spectrum disorder. *Frontiers in Psychology*, *10*(10), 2965.

Markward, M., Dozier, C., Hooks, K., & Markward, N. (2000). Culture and the intergenerational transmission of substance abuse, woman abuse, and child abuse: A diathesis-stress perspective. *Children and Youth Services Review*, *22*(3), 237–250. DOI: 10.1016/S0190-7409(00)00079-7

Marshall, C., Langevin, R., & Cabecinha-Alati, S. (2022). Victim-to-victim intergenerational cycles of child maltreatment: A systematic scoping review of theoretical frameworks. *International Journal of Child and Adolescent Resilience*, *9*(1). Advance online publication. DOI: 10.54488/ijcar.2022.283

Marshall, W. L., Hudson, S. M., Jones, R., & Fernandez, Y. M. (1995). Empathy in sex offenders. *Clinical Psychology Review*, *15*(2), 99–113. DOI: 10.1016/0272-7358(95)00002-7

Mathews, B., Pacella, R., Dunne, M. P., Simunovic, M., & Marston, C. (2023). *The Australian Child Maltreatment Study, Final Report*. Queensland University of Technology

Mathews, B., Pacella, R., Dunne, M. P., Simunovic, M., & Marston, C. (2020). Improving measurement of child abuse and neglect: A systematic review and analysis of national prevalence studies. *PLoS One*, *15*(1), e0227884. DOI: 10.1371/journal.pone.0227884 PMID: 31990913

Mathews, B., Pacella, R., Scott, J. G., Finkelhor, D., Meinck, F., Higgins, D. J., Erskine, H. E., Thomas, H. J., Lawrence, D. M., Haslam, D. M., Malacova, E., & Dunne, M. P. (2023). The prevalence of child maltreatment in Australia: Findings from a national survey. *The Medical Journal of Australia*, *218*(S6), S13–S18. DOI: 10.5694/mja2.51873 PMID: 37004184

Mathews, B., Papalia, N., Napier, S., Malacova, E., Lawrence, D., Higgins, D. J., Thomas, H., Erskine, H., Meinck, F., Haslam, D., Scott, J. G., Finkelhor, D., & Pacella, R. (2023). *Child maltreatment and criminal justice system involvement in Australia: Findings from a national survey. Trends & issues in crime and criminal justice no. 681*. Australian Institute of Criminology., DOI: 10.52922/ti77215

Mauroy, A., Galdiolo, S., Meillerais, S., Verhofstadt, L. L., & Gaugue, J. (2025). Empathic Accuracy Across Childhood, Adolescence, and Within Parent-Child Interactions: A Systematic Review. *Personal Relationships*, *32*(1), e70000. DOI: 10.1111/pere.70000

Maynard, B. R., Farina, A., Dell, N. A., & Kelly, M. S. (2019). Effects of trauma-informed approaches in schools: A systematic review. *Campbell Systematic Reviews*, *15*(1-2), e1018. DOI: 10.1002/cl2.1018 PMID: 37131480

McCallum, D. (2022). Law, justice, and Indigenous intergenerational trauma—A genealogy. *International Journal for Crime. Justice and Social Democracy*, *11*(3), 165–177. DOI: 10.5204/ijcjsd.2121

McCloskey, L. A., & Bailey, J. A. (2000). The intergenerational transmission of risk for child sexual abuse. *Journal of Interpersonal Violence*, *15*(10), 1019–1035. DOI: 10.1177/088626000015010001

McCollum, S. E. (2015). Multigenerational dissociation: A framework for building narrative. *Journal of Trauma & Dissociation*, *16*(5), 563–576. DOI: 10.1080/15299732.2015.1030717 PMID: 26158318

McDonald, T., Bryson, S., & Poertner, J. (2006). Balancing reunification and re-entry goals. *Children and Youth Services Review*, *28*(1), 47–58. DOI: 10.1016/j.childyouth.2005.02.007

McDowall, J. J. (2019). *Out-of-home care in Australia: Children and young people's views after five years of National Standards.* CREATE Foundation. https://create.org.au

McEwen, B. S., & Morrison, J. H. (2013). The brain on stress. *Neuron, 79*(1), 16–29. DOI: 10.1016/j.neuron.2013.06.028 PMID: 23849196

McEwen, C. A., & Gregerson, S. F. (2019). A critical assessment of the Adverse Childhood Experiences study at 20 years. *American Journal of Preventive Medicine, 56*(6), 790–794. DOI: 10.1016/j.amepre.2018.10.016 PMID: 30803781

McFadden, P., Campbell, A., & Taylor, B. (2015). Resilience and burnout in child protection social work: Individual and organisational themes from a systematic literature review. *British Journal of Social Work, 45*(5), 1546–1563. DOI: 10.1093/bjsw/bct210

McKeown, M.-H. L., & Yeung, E. Y. W. (2023). Deepening our understanding of reflective practice in a safeguarding child protection and welfare context. *Practice, 35*(2), 153–167. DOI: 10.1080/09503153.2022.2038124

McLaughlin, K. A., & Sheridan, M. A. (2016). Beyond cumulative risk: A dimensional approach to childhood adversity. *Current Directions in Psychological Science, 25*(4), 239–245. DOI: 10.1177/0963721416655883

McLaughlin, K. A., Sheridan, M. A., Humphreys, K. L., Belsky, J., & Ellis, B. J. (2021). The value of dimensional models of early experience: Thinking clearly about concepts and categories. *Perspectives on Psychological Science, 16*(6), 1463–1472. DOI: 10.1177/1745691621992346 PMID: 34491864

McLaughlin, K. A., Sheridan, M. A., & Lambert, H. K. (2014). Dimensions of early experience and neural development: Deprivation and threat. *Current Directions in Psychological Science, 23*(1), 47–52. DOI: 10.1177/0963721413515590 PMID: 25454359

McMahon, K., Hoertel, N., Wall, M. M., Okuda, M., Limosin, F., & Blanco, C. (2015). Childhood maltreatment and risk of intimate partner violence: A national study. *Journal of Psychiatric Research, 69*, 42–49. DOI: 10.1016/j.jpsychires.2015.07.026 PMID: 26343593

McMillen, J. C., & Rideout, G. B. (1996). Breaking intergenerational cycles: Theoretical tools for social workers. *The Social Service Review, 70*(3), 378–399. DOI: 10.1086/604196

McMurtry, S. L., & Lie, G. Y. (1992). Differential exit rates of minority children in foster care. *Social Work Research & Abstracts, 28*(1), 42–48. DOI: 10.1093/swra/28.1.42

McNamara, P., Harvey, A., & Andrewartha, L. (2019). Passports out of poverty: Raising access to higher education for care leavers in Australia. *Children & Youth Services Review*, 97, 85–93, ISSN 0190-7409, DOI: 10.1016/j.childyouth.2017.07.015

McPherson, K. E., Kerr, S., McGee, E., Morgan, A., Cheater, F. M., McLean, J., & Egan, J. (2014). The association between social capital and mental health and behavioural problems in children and adolescents: An integrative systematic review. *BMC Psychology, 2*(1), 1–16. DOI: 10.1186/2050-7283-2-7 PMID: 25566380

McWey, L. M., & Cui, M. (2021). Parent–child contact and family reunification in foster care. *Children and Youth Services Review, 128*, 106–152.

Mehta, D., Kelly, A. B., Laurens, K. R., Haslam, D., Williams, K. E., Walsh, K., Baker, P. R. A., Carter, H. E., Khawaja, N. G., Zelenko, O., & Mathews, B. (2021). Child maltreatment and long-term physical and mental health outcomes: An exploration of biopsychosocial determinants and implications for prevention. *Child Psychiatry and Human Development*, •••, 1–15. DOI: 10.1007/s10578-021-01258-8 PMID: 34586552

Meidan, A., & Uzefovsky, F. (2020). Child maltreatment risk mediates the association between maternal and child empathy. *Child Abuse & Neglect, 106*, 104523. Advance online publication. DOI: 10.1016/j.chiabu.2020.104523

Mendes, P., & Chaffey, E. (2024). Examining the Mental Health Care Needs and Outcomes of Young People Transitioning from Out-of-Home Care (OOHC) in Australia. *Institutionalised Children Exploration and Beyond, 11*(1), 103–124. DOI: 10.1177/23493003231182474

Mendes, P., Michell, D., & Wilson, J. Z. (2014). Young people transitioning from out-of-home care and access to higher education: A critical review of the literature. *Children Australia, 39*(4), 243–252. DOI: 10.1017/cha.2014.25

Meng, X., Fleury, M. J., Xiang, Y. T., Li, M., & D'arcy, C. (2018). Resilience and protective factors among people with a history of child maltreatment: A systematic review. *Social Psychiatry and Psychiatric Epidemiology, 53*(5), 453–475. DOI: 10.1007/s00127-018-1485-2 PMID: 29349479

Menschner, C., & Maul, A. (2016). Key ingredients for successful trauma-informed care implementation. Center for Health Care Strategies. https://www.fredla.org/wp-content/uploads/2016/04/Trauma-informed-care-implementation-1.pdf

Menzies, K. (2019). Understanding the Australian Aboriginal experience of collective, historical and intergenerational trauma. *International Social Work, 62*(6), 1522–1534. DOI: 10.1177/0020872819870585

Menzies, P. (2010). Intergenerational trauma from a mental health perspective. *Native Social Work Journal, 7*, 63–85.

Merrill, S. M., Moore, S. R., Gladish, N., Giesbrecht, G. F., Dewey, D., Konwar, C., MacIssac, J. L., Kobor, M. S., & Letourneau, N. L. (2021). Paternal adverse childhood experiences: Associations with infant DNA methylation. *Developmental Psychobiology, 63*(6), e22174. DOI: 10.1002/dev.22174 PMID: 34333774

Mestre, M. V., Samper, P., Frias, M. D., & Tur, A. M. (2009). Are women more empathetic than men? A longitudinal study in adolescence. *The Spanish Journal of Psychology, 12*(1), 76–83. DOI: 10.1017/S1138741600001499

Meulewaeter, F., De Pauw, S. S. W., & Vanderplasschen, W. (2019). Mothering, substance use disorders and intergenerational trauma transmission: An attachment-based perspective. *Frontiers in Psychiatry, 10*, 728. DOI: 10.3389/fpsyt.2019.00728 PMID: 31681040

Mew, E., Bonumwezi, J., & Lowe, S. (2025). *Family-level mediators in the intergenerational transmission of maternal childhood trauma: Systematic review and meta-analysis of pooled effect measures* [Poster]. *American Psychological Association Conference*, Denver, CO.

Michell, D., Jackson, D., & Tonkin, C. (Eds.). (2015). *Against the odds: Care leavers at university*. People's Voice Publishing.

Mielke, E. L., Neukel, C., Bertsch, K., Reck, C., Möhler, E., & Herpertz, S. C. (2016). Maternal sensitivity and the empathic brain: Influences of early life maltreatment. *Journal of Psychiatric Research, 77*, 59–66. DOI: 10.1016/j.jpsychires.2016.02.013 PMID: 26985733

Miklikowska, M., Tilton-Weaver, L., & Burk, W. J. (2022). With a little help from my empathic friends: The role of peers in the development of empathy in adolescence. *Developmental Psychology, 58*(6), 1156–1162. DOI: 10.1037/dev0001347

Miller-Perrin, C. L., & Perrin, R. D. (2007). *Child maltreatment: An introduction* (2nd ed.). Sage.

Miller, R. (2007). *Cumulative harm: A conceptual overview*. Victorian Government.

Milner, J. S. (1993). Social information processing and physical child abuse. *Clinical Psychology Review, 13*(3), 275–294. DOI: 10.1016/0272-7358(93)90024-G

Mitkovic Voncina, M., Pejovic Milovancevic, M., Mandic Maravic, V., & Lecic Tosevski, D. (2017). Timeline of intergenerational child maltreatment: The mind–brain–body interplay. *Current Psychiatry Reports, 19*(8), 50. DOI: 10.1007/s11920-017-0805-7 PMID: 28664328

Modderman, C., Sanders, R., Cordon, E., Hocking, C., Wade, M., & Vogels, W. (2023). Integrating health systems for children and young people in out of home care: Challenging the nature of siloed service delivery in rural Australia. *The Australian Journal of Rural Health, 31*(4), 670–679. DOI: 10.1111/ajr.12991 PMID: 37129555

Mohr, D., & Rosén, L. A. (2017). The impact of protective factors on posttraumatic growth for college student survivors of childhood maltreatment. *Journal of Aggression, Maltreatment & Trauma, 26*(7), 756–771. DOI: 10.1080/10926771.2017.1304478

Monson, K., Herrman, H., Moeller-Saxone, K., Humphreys, C., & Harvey, C. (2021). How can mental health practitioners collaborate with child welfare practitioners to improve mental health for young people in out of home care? *Early Intervention in Psychiatry, 15*(6), 1768–1776. DOI: 10.1111/eip.13118 PMID: 33474788

Monteith, L. L., Bahraini, N. H., Matarazzo, B. B., Soberay, K. A., & Smith, C. P. (2016). Perceptions of institutional betrayal predict suicidal self-directed violence among veterans exposed to military sexual trauma. *Journal of Clinical Psychology, 72*(7), 743–755. DOI: 10.1002/jclp.22292 PMID: 27007795

Monteith, L. L., Gerber, H. R., Brownstone, L. M., Soberay, K. A., & Bahraini, N. H. (2019). The phenomenology of military sexual trauma among male veterans. *Psychology of Men & Masculinity, 20*(1), 115–127. DOI: 10.1037/men0000153

Monteith, L. L., Holliday, R., Schneider, A. L., Miller, C. N., Bahraini, N. H., & Forster, J. E. (2021). Institutional betrayal and help-seeking among women survivors of military sexual trauma. *Psychological Trauma: Theory, Research, Practice, and Policy, 13*(7), 814–823. DOI: 10.1037/tra0001027 PMID: 33764096

Moody, G., Cannings-John, R., Hood, K., Kemp, A., & Robling, M. (2018). Establishing the international prevalence of self-reported child maltreatment: A systematic review by maltreatment type and gender. *BMC Public Health, 18*(1), 1–15. DOI: 10.1186/s12889-018-6044-y PMID: 30305071

Moog, N. K., Heim, C. M., Entringer, S., Simhan, H. N., Wadhwa, P. D., & Buss, C. (2022). Transmission of the adverse consequences of childhood maltreatment across generations: Focus on gestational biology. *Pharmacology, Biochemistry, and Behavior, 215*, 173372. Advance online publication. DOI: 10.1016/j.pbb.2022.173372 PMID: 35259415

Morley, L. (2022). Contemporary practitioner experiences of relational social work: The case of child welfare. *Australian Social Work, 75*(4), 458–470. DOI: 10.1080/0312407X.2021.2001831

Morrison, K. A., Robbins, H., & Rose, D. G. (2008). Operationalizing culturally relevant pedagogy. *Teaching and Teacher Education, 24*(6), 1574–1590. DOI: 10.1016/j.tate.2008.02.013

Morton, N., & Browne, K. D. (1998). Theory and observation of attachment and its relation to child maltreatment: A review. *Child Abuse & Neglect, 22*(11), 1093–1104. DOI: 10.1016/S0145-2134(98)00088-X PMID: 9827314

Mullin, A. C., Sharkey, J. D., & Barnett, M. (2024, May). Advancing trauma informed practices in schools using the Consolidated Framework for Implementation Research. [). Frontiers Media SA.]. *Frontiers in Education, 9*, 1346933. DOI: 10.3389/feduc.2024.1346933

Munro, E. (2005). Improving practice: Child protection as a systems problem. *Children and Youth Services Review, 27*(4), 375–391. DOI: 10.1016/j.childyouth.2004.11.006

Murphy, C. (2023). How learning from the lived experiences of child protection social workers can help us understand the factors underpinning workforce instability within the English child protection system. *Journal of Social Work Practice, 37*(2), 263–276. DOI: 10.1080/02650533.2023.2185213

Myat Zaw, A. M., Win, N. Z., & Thepthien, B. O. (2022). Adolescents' academic achievement, mental health, and adverse behaviors: Understanding the role of resilience and adverse childhood experiences. *School Psychology International, 43*(5), 516–536. DOI: 10.1177/01430343221107114

Narang, D. S., & Contreras, J. M. (2000). Dissociation as a mediator between child abuse history and adult abuse potential. *Child Abuse & Neglect, 24*(5), 653–665. DOI: 10.1016/S0145-2134(00)00132-0 PMID: 10819097

Narang, D. S., & Contreras, J. M. (2005). The relationships of dissociation and affective family environment with the intergenerational cycle of child abuse. *Child Abuse & Neglect, 29*(6), 683–699. DOI: 10.1016/j.chiabu.2004.11.003 PMID: 15979709

Narvey, C., Yang, J., Wolff, K. T., Baglivio, M., & Piquero, A. R. (2021). The interrelationship between empathy and adverse childhood experiences and their impact on juvenile recidivism. *Youth Violence and Juvenile Justice, 19*(1), 45–67. DOI: 10.1177/1541204020939647

Nasir, N. I. S. (2021). Teaching for equity: Where developmental needs meet racialized structures. In *The Science of Learning and Development* (pp. 177–184). Routledge.

National Aged Care Alliance. (2017). *Ensuring equity of access and outcomes in the future aged care system.* https://naca.asn.au/wp-content/uploads/2018/11/Equity-of-Access-andOutcomes-Statement-of-Principles_Landscape-1.pdf

National Alliance on Mental Illness. (2011). *College students and mental health.* National Alliance on Mental Illness.

National Office for Child Safety. SNAICC, & VACCA. (2021). *Keeping our kids safe: Cultural safety and the national principles for child safe organisations.* National Office for Child Safety. www.childsafety.gov.au/resources/keeping-our-kids-safe

Negriff, S., Palmer Molina, A., & Hackman, D. A. (2020). Parental exposure to childhood maltreatment and offspring's mental health: Investigating pathways through parental adversity and offspring exposure to maltreatment. *Child Maltreatment, 25*(4), 422–432. DOI: 10.1177/1077559520912342 PMID: 32208855

Nelson, J., & Landsman, M. (2006). Promoting reunification through evidence-based assessment. *Protecting Children, 21*(1), 36–45.

Newcomb, M. D., & Locke, T. F. (2001). Intergenerational cycle of maltreatment: A popular concept obscured by methodological limitations. *Child Abuse & Neglect, 25*(9), 1219–1240. DOI: 10.1016/S0145-2134(01)00267-8 PMID: 11700694

Newton, B. J. (2019). Understanding child neglect in Aboriginal families and communities in the context of trauma. *Child & Family Social Work, 24*(2), 218–226. DOI: 10.1111/cfs.12606

Newton, L., Keane, C. A., & Byrne, M. K. (2024). Trauma-informed programs in Australian schools: A systematic review of design, implementation and efficacy. *Children and Youth Services Review, 156*, 107368. DOI: 10.1016/j.childyouth.2023.107368

Ney, P. G. (1989). Child maltreatment: Possible reasons for its transgenerational transmission. *Canadian Journal of Psychiatry, 34*(6), 594–601. DOI: 10.1177/070674378903400619 PMID: 2670182

Ney, P., Fung, T., & Wickett, A. (1994). The worst combinations of child abuse and neglect. *Child Abuse & Neglect, 18*(9), 705–715. DOI: 10.1016/0145-2134(94)00037-9 PMID: 8000901

Nietz, H. (2019). Informing social work practice with theory: Reflections on the protection of Aboriginal children in remote communities of Australia. *British Journal of Social Work, 49*(8), 2021–2041. DOI: 10.1093/bjsw/bcy124

Norrish, J., & Brunzell, T. (2023). How is trauma-informed education implemented within classrooms? A synthesis of trauma-informed education programs. *The Australian Journal of Teacher Education, 48*(3), 94–120. DOI: 10.14221/1835-517X.6159

NSW Bureau of Crime Statistics and Research. (2024). *The involvement of young people aged 10 to 13 years in the NSW criminal justice system.* NSW Government.

NSW Department of Communities and Justice. (2023). *How do relative/kinship carers and foster carers differ in their characteristics, wellbeing and support needs? Evidence to Action Note No. 13, Pathways of Care Longitudinal Study (POCLS).* NSW Department of Communities and Justice.

Nygren, K., Walsh, J. C., Ellingsen, I. T., & Christie, A. (2021). Gender, parenting and practices in child welfare social work? A comparative study from England, Ireland, Norway and Sweden. *British Journal of Social Work, 51*(6), 2116–2133. DOI: 10.1093/bjsw/bcaa085

O'Connell, M. (2025). *The cost of late intervention 2024.* The Front Project.

Obsuth, I., Mueller Johnson, K., Murray, A. L., Ribeaud, D., & Eisner, M. (2018). Violent poly-victimization: The longitudinal patterns of physical and emotional victimization throughout adolescence (11–17 years). *Journal of Research on Adolescence, 28*(4), 786–806. DOI: 10.1111/jora.12365 PMID: 29193435

Oosterman, M., & Schuengel, C. (2023). The quality of parent–child contact and its role in family reunification. *Children and Youth Services Review, 149*, 106–783.

Organisation for Economic Co-operation and Development (OECD). (2022). *Assisting care leavers: Time for action.* OECD Publishing., DOI: 10.1787/1939a9ec-

Osborn, A., & Bromfield, L. (2007). *Young people leaving care.* National Child Protection Clearinghouse, Australian Institute of Family Studies.

Oschatz, T., Piemonte, J. L., & Klein, V. (2024). The intimate and sexual costs of emotional labor: The development of the Women's Sexual Emotional Labor Assessment. *Archives of Sexual Behavior, 54*(1), 117–138. DOI: 10.1007/s10508-024-03061-7

Özcan, N. K., Boyacioğlu, N. E., Enginkaya, S., Bilgin, H., & Tomruk, N. B. (2016). The relationship between attachment styles and childhood trauma: A transgenerational perspective – a controlled study of patients with psychiatric disorders. *Journal of Clinical Nursing, 25*(15-16), 2357–2366. DOI: 10.1111/jocn.13274 PMID: 27161944

Ozdemir, N., & Sahin, S. (2020). The impact of childhood traumatic experiences on self-esteem and interpersonal relationships. *Psychiatry and Behavioral Sciences, 10*(4), 185–191. DOI: 10.5455/PBS.20200502025907

Pang, C., Li, W., Zhou, Y., Gao, T., & Han, S. (2023). Are women more empathetic than men? Questionnaire and EEG estimations of sex/gender differences in empathic ability. *Social Cognitive and Affective Neuroscience, 18*(1), nsad008. DOI: 10.1093/scan/nsad008

Paris, D., & Alim, H. S. (2017). *Culturally sustaining pedagogies: Teaching and learning for justice in a changing world.* Teachers College Press.

Parnell, S. (2024, December 13). Hundreds of Queensland children living in residential care. *The QLDR.* https://theqldr.com.au/queensland-news/2024/12/13/care-2/

PeakCare & Queensland Family and Child Commission. (2024, June). *Queensland foster carer demographic insights report: The future of foster care.* The Demographics Group. https://www.qfcc.qld.gov.au/queensland-foster-carer-demographic-insights-report-peakcare

Pears, K. C., & Capaldi, D. M. (2001). Intergenerational transmission of abuse: A two-generational prospective study of an at-risk sample. *Child Abuse & Neglect, 25*(11), 1439–1461. DOI: 10.1016/S0145-2134(01)00286-1 PMID: 11766010

Perry, B. D. (2009). Examining child maltreatment through a neurodevelopmental lens: Clinical applications of the neurosequential model of therapeutics. *Journal of Loss and Trauma, 14*(4), 240–255. DOI: 10.1080/15325020903004350

Peters, M. D. J., Marnie, C., Colquhoun, H., Garritty, C. M., Hempel, S., Horsley, T., Langlois, E. V., Lillie, E., O'Brien, K. K., Tunçalp, ., Wilson, M. G., Zarin, W., & Tricco, A. C. (2021). Scoping reviews: Reinforcing and advancing the methodology and application. *Systematic Reviews, 10*(1), 263–266. DOI: 10.1186/s13643-021-01821-3 PMID: 34625095

Platt, M., Barton, J., & Freyd, J. J. (2009). A betrayal trauma perspective on domestic violence. *Violence against women in families and relationships*, 185-207.

Poirier, B., Sethi, S., Haag, D., Hedges, J., & Jamieson, L. (2022). The impact of neoliberal generative mechanisms on Indigenous health: A critical realist scoping review. *Globalization and Health, 18*(1), 1–17. DOI: 10.1186/s12992-022-00852-2 PMID: 35705995

Pollock, C., Grenyer, B. F., & Townsend, M. L. (2024). Responding to suicidal behaviour in children and young people with a child maltreatment history: A scoping review. *Children and Youth Services Review, 166*, 107927. DOI: 10.1016/j.childyouth.2024.107927

Pope, K. S., & Felman-Summers, S. (1992). National survey of psychologists' sexual and physical abuse history and their evaluation of training and competence in these areas. *Professional Psychology, Research and Practice, 23*(5), 3530361. Advance online publication. DOI: 10.1037/0735-7028.23.5.353

Power, M. (1997). *The audit society: Rituals of verification*. Oxford University Press.

Powers, J., Bryce, I., Jiwon, K., & Hobbs, R. (2024). Trauma-Informed Gatekeeping Using ARCCH Model of Multisystemic Resilience, (P. 81-114) *In N. Hurless & L. Davis (Eds), Cases on Trauma-Informed Gatekeeping in Counsellor Education.*

Powers, J., & Duys, D. K. (2020). *Trauma-informed care: Principles and practice*. Wiley.

Pratte, S., Tang, A., & Oehlberg, L. (2021). Evoking empathy: A framework for describing empathy tools. In *Proceedings of the Fifteenth International Conference on Tangible, Embedded and Embodied Interaction (TEI '21)*. DOI: 10.1145/3430524.3440644

Price-Robertson, R., Higgins, D., & Vassallo, S. (2013). *Multi-type maltreatment and polyvictimisation: A comparison of two research frameworks. Family Matters, 93, 84-98.* Australian Institute of Family Studies., https://aifs.gov.au/publications/family-matters/issue-93/multi-type-maltreatment-and-polyvictimisation

Price-Robertson, R., Rush, P., Wall, L., & Higgins, D. (2013). *Rarely an isolated incident: Acknowledging the interrelatedness of child maltreatment, victimization and trauma. CFCA Paper no. 15.* Australian Institute of Family Studies., https://aifs.gov.au/cfca/publications/rarely-isolated-incident-acknowledging-interrelatedn

Putallaz, M., Costanzo, P. R., Grimes, C. L., & Sherman, D. M. (1998). Intergenerational continuities and their influences on children's social development. *Social Development, 7*(3), 389–427. DOI: 10.1111/1467-9507.00074

Quinn, A., Fallon, B., Joh-Carnella, N., & Saint-Girons, M. (2022). The overrepresentation of First Nations children in the Ontario child welfare system: A call for systemic change. *Children and Youth Services Review, 139*, 106558. DOI: 10.1016/j.childyouth.2022.106558

Quinton, D., & Rutter, M. (1984). Parents with children in care - II. Intergenerational continuities. *Journal of Child Psychology and Psychiatry, and Allied Disciplines, 25*(2), 231–250. DOI: 10.1111/j.1469-7610.1984.tb00146.x PMID: 6707111

Racine, N., Bellis, M. A., & Madigan, S. (2025). An introduction to twenty-five years of adverse childhood experiences: A special issue. *Child Abuse & Neglect, 168*(Part 1), 107224. Advance online publication. DOI: 10.1016/j.chiabu.2024.107224 PMID: 39730232

Rahm, J., & Gorges, A. (2018). STEM learning in everyday spaces. *Science Education, 102*(4), 617–638. DOI: 10.1002/sce.21444

Raines, J. C. (1990). Empathy in clinical social work. *Clinical Social Work Journal, 18*(1), 57–72. DOI: 10.1007/BF00759070

Rakoczy, H. (2022). Foundations of theory of mind and its development in early childhood. *Nature Reviews Psychology, 1*(4), 223–235. DOI: 10.1038/s44159-022-00037-z

Ralph, S., & Ryan, K. (2017). Addressing the mental health gap in working with Indigenous youth: Some considerations for non-Indigenous psychologists working with Indigenous youth. *Australian Psychologist, 52*(4), 288–298. DOI: 10.1111/ap.12287

Ramo-Fernández, L., Schneider, A., Wilker, S., & Kolassa, I. T. (2015). Epigenetic alterations associated with war trauma and childhood maltreatment. *Behavioral Sciences & the Law, 33*(5), 701–721. DOI: 10.1002/bsl.2200 PMID: 26358541

Rattambige, D., Higgins, D. J., Whittle, S., Cole, M., Mathews, B., Scott, J. G., Erskine, H., Meinck, F., Pacella, R., Lawrence, D., & Haslam, D. M. (2025). The impact of child maltreatment patterns and adverse childhood experiences on problematic youth alcohol use. *Child Maltreatment.* Advance online publication. DOI: 10.1177/10775595251387118

Ratts, M. J., Singh, A. A., Nassar-McMillan, S., Butler, T., & McCullough, J. R. (2016). *Multicultural and social justice competency development: A guide for the counseling profession* (2nd ed.). American Counseling Association.

Rayner, S., Davis, C., Moore, M., & Cadet, T. (2020). Secondary traumatic stress in related factors in Australian social workers and psychologists. *Health & Social Work, 45*(2), 122–130. DOI: 10.1093/hsw/hlaa001

Read, J. P., Ouimette, P., White, J., Colder, C. R., & Farrow, C. V. (2011). Trauma history, PTSD symptoms, and problem drinking in college students. *Addictive Behaviors, 36*, 1062–1066.

Reddan, F. (2023). *How do adult survivors of childhood abuse, experience and understand their capacity to trust in relationships?* (Doctoral dissertation, Dublin City University).

Reed-Ashcraft, K., Kirk, R., & Fraser, M. (2001). The reliability and validity of the North Carolina Family Assessment Scale. *Research on Social Work Practice, 11*(4), 503–520. DOI: 10.1177/104973150101100406

Rémond, M., Zeki, R., Austin, K., Bowman, J., Galouzis, J., Stewart, K.-A., & Sullivan, E. (2023). *Intergenerational incarceration in New South Wales: Characteristics of people in prison experiencing parental imprisonment* (Trends & Issues in Crime and Criminal Justice No. 663). Australian Institute of Criminology.

Renner, L. M., & Slack, K. S. (2006). Intimate partner violence and child maltreatment: Understanding intra- and intergenerational connections. *Child Abuse & Neglect, 30*(6), 599–617. DOI: 10.1016/j.chiabu.2005.12.005 PMID: 16782195

Reynolds, T. A., & Palmer-Hague, J. (2022). Did you hear what she did to me? Female friendship victimization disclosures offer reputational advantages. *Journal of Experimental Social Psychology, 101*, 104311. DOI: 10.1016/j.jesp.2022.104311

Richards, D. (2008). Handsearching still a valuable element of the systematic review. *Evidence-Based Dentistry, 9*(3), 85. DOI: 10.1038/sj.ebd.6400602 PMID: 18927572

Rogers, C. (1951). *Client-centred therapy: Its current practice, implications and theory*. Houghton Mifflin.

Rojas-Andrade, R., & Leiva, L. (2019). Is implementation fidelity important? A systematic review on school-based mental health programs. *Contemporary School Psychology, 23*(4), 339–350. DOI: 10.1007/s40688-018-0175-0

Roorda, D. L., Jak, S., Zee, M., Oort, F. J., & Koomen, H. M. (2017). Affective teacher–student relationships and students' engagement and achievement: A meta-analytic update and test of the mediating role of engagement. *School Psychology Review, 46*(3), 239–261. DOI: 10.17105/SPR-2017-0035.V46-3

Rose, A. J., & Rudolph, K. D. (2006). A review of sex differences in peer relationship processes: Potential trade-offs for the emotional and behavioral development of girls and boys. *Psychological Bulletin, 132*(1), 98–131. DOI: 10.1037/0033-2909.132.1.98

Roseby, V., & Gascoigne, M. (2021). A systematic review of trauma-informed practices in schools. *Educational Psychology in Practice, 37*(1), 1–23. DOI: 10.1080/02667363.2020.1841839

Rose, D., & Meyer, A. (2006). *A practical reader in universal design for learning*. Harvard Education Press.

Rosenman, S. (2002). *Traumatic experiences in an Australian population*. Australian Centre for Posttraumatic Mental Health, The University of Melbourne.

Rosenthal, A., Christl, M. E., Wright, N., Olomi, J., Dmitrieva, J., & DePrince, A. P. (2025). Applying an institutional betrayal lens to caregiver perceptions of child maltreatment investigations. *Journal of Trauma & Dissociation*, *26*(3), 314–330. DOI: 10.1080/15299732.2025.2481029 PMID: 40107839

Rosenzweig, J. M., & Sundborg, S. A. (2022). The neurobiology of toxic stress. In Rapp-McCall, L., Corcoran, K., & Roberts, A. R. (Eds.), *Social Workers' Desk Reference* (pp. 278–289). Oxford University Press.

Ross, N., Cocks, J., Johnston, L., & Stoker, L. (2017). *No voice, no opinion, nothing: Parent experiences when children are removed and placed in care*. University of Newcastle.

Rosso, A. M. (2022). Psychoanalytic interventions with abusive parents: An opportunity for children's mental health. *International Journal of Environmental Research and Public Health*, *19*(20), 13015. Advance online publication. DOI: 10.3390/ijerph192013015 PMID: 36293590

Royal Commission into the Protection and Detention of Children in the Northern Territory. (2017). *Final report*. Australian Government. https://childdetentionnt.royalcommission.gov.au

Ruch, G. (2005). Relationship-based practice and reflective practice: Holistic approaches to contemporary child care social work. *Child & Family Social Work*, *10*(2), 111–123. DOI: 10.1111/j.1365-2206.2005.00359.x

Rueckert, L., & Naybar, N. (2008). Gender differences in empathy: The role of the right hemisphere. *Brain and Cognition*, *67*(2), 162–167. DOI: 10.1016/j.bandc.2008.01.002

Rumrill, P. D., Fitzgerald, S. M., & Merchant, W. R. (2010). Using scoping literature reviews as a means of understanding and interpreting existing literature. *Work (Reading, Mass.)*, *35*(3), 399–404. DOI: 10.3233/WOR-2010-0998 PMID: 20364059

Rusbult, C. E., & Martz, J. M. (1995). Remaining in an abusive relationship: An investment model analysis of nonvoluntary dependence. *Personality and Social Psychology Bulletin*, *21*(6), 558–571. DOI: 10.1177/0146167295216002

Rushovich, B., Sepulveda, K., Efetevbia, V., & Malm, K. (2021). A post-reunification service model: Implementation and population served. *Children and Youth Services Review, 122*, 105928. DOI: 10.1016/j.childyouth.2021.105928

Russ, E., Stonehouse, D., Reimer, E. C., Hitchcock, C., & McPherson, L. (2024). Supporting staff wellbeing in child welfare services. DOI: 10.25918/report.353

Russell, D. H., Trew, S., & Higgins, D. J. (2021). Vulnerable yet forgotten? A systematic review identifying the lack of evidence for effective suicide interventions for young people in contact with child protection systems. *The American Journal of Orthopsychiatry, 91*(5), 647–659. DOI: 10.1037/ort0000555 PMID: 34383517

Russell, J. R., Kerwin, C., & Halverson, J. L. (2018). Is child protective services effective? *Children and Youth Services Review, 84*, 185–192. DOI: 10.1016/j.childyouth.2017.11.028

Ryan, F. (2011). Kanyininpa (holding): A way of nurturing children in Aboriginal Australia. *Australian Social Work, 64*(2), 183–197. DOI: 10.1080/0312407X.2011.581300

Rycus, J. S., & Hughes, R. C. (2008). Assessing risk throughout the life of a child welfare case. In Lindsay, D., & Shlonsky, A. (Eds.), *Child welfare research: Advances for practices and policy* (p. 48). Oxford University Press. DOI: 10.1093/acprof:oso/9780195304961.003.0012

Sacker, A., Murray, E., Lacey, R., & Maughan, B. (2021). *The lifelong health and wellbeing trajectories of people who have been in care: Findings from the looked-after children grown up project.* Nuffield Foundation. https://www.nuffieldfoundation.org/wp-content/uploads/2021/07/The-lifelong-health-and-wellbeing-trajectories-of-people-who-have-been-in-care.pdf

Sahle, B. W., Reavley, N. J., & Morgan, A. J. (2023). Adverse childhood experiences and educational attainment: A global review. *Child Abuse & Neglect, 136*, 105995. DOI: 10.1016/j.chiabu.2022.105995

Salazar, A. M., Keller, T. E., Gowen, L. K., & Courtney, M. E. (2013). Trauma exposure and PTSD among older adolescents in foster care. *Social Psychiatry and Psychiatric Epidemiology, 48*(4), 545–551. DOI: 10.1007/s00127-012-0563-0 PMID: 22898825

Sameroff, A. J., Seifer, R., Baldwin, A., & Baldwin, C. (1993). Stability of intelligence from preschool to adolescence: The influence of social and family risk factors. *Child Development, 64*(1), 80–97. DOI: 10.2307/1131438 PMID: 8436039

SAMHSA. (2014). *SAMHSA's concept of trauma and guidance for a trauma-informed approach.* U.S. Department of Health and Human Services.

Sanchis-Sanchis, A., Grau, M. D., Moliner, A. R., & Morales-Murillo, C. P. (2020). Effects of age and gender in emotion regulation of children and adolescents. *Frontiers in Psychology, 11*, 946. Advance online publication. DOI: 10.3389/fpsyg.2020.00946

Sanders, M. R. (1999). Triple P-Positive Parenting Program: Towards an empirically validated multilevel parenting and family support strategy for the prevention of behavior and emotional problems in children. *Clinical Child and Family Psychology Review*, *2*(2), 71–90. DOI: 10.1023/A:1021843613840 PMID: 11225933

Sarantou, M., & Miettinen, S. (2022). Introduction. In Sarantou, M., & Miettinen, S. (Eds.), *Empathy and business transformation* (pp. 1–12). Routledge., DOI: 10.4324/9781003227557-1

Satapathy, S., Choudhary, V., Behera, C., Swain, R., Sharma, R., & Sagar, R. (2022). Adverse childhood experiences, aggression, empathy, and psychopathology in adult males accused of rape. *Indian Journal of Psychological Medicine*, *44*(5), 466–473. DOI: 10.1177/02537176221106278

Savickas, M. L. (2005). The theory and practice of career construction. In S. D. Brown & R. W. Lent (Eds.), *Career development and counseling: Putting theory and research to work* (pp. 42–70). John Wiley & Sons.

Savickas, M. L. (2011). *Career counseling*. American Psychological Association.

Savickas, M. L. (2016). Life designing: A paradigm for career construction in the 21st century. *Journal of Vocational Behavior*, *93*, 202–215.

Savickas, M. L., & Porfeli, E. J. (2012). Career Adapt-Abilities Scale: Construction, reliability, and measurement equivalence across 13 countries. *Journal of Vocational Behavior*, *80*(3), 661–673.

Schelbe, L., & Geiger, J. M. (2017). *Intergenerational transmission of child maltreatment*. SpringerBriefs in Social Work., DOI: 10.1007/978-3-319-43824-5

Schön, D. (1983). *The reflective practitioner: How professionals think in action*. Basic Books.

Scott, D. (2014). *Intervening to improve life chances for vulnerable children: The importance of culturally appropriate assessment tools*. Child Family Community Australia.

Scott, E. K., London, A. S., & Myers, N. A. (2002). Dangerous dependencies: The intersection of welfare reform and domestic violence. *Gender & Society*, *16*(6), 878–897. DOI: 10.1177/089124302237893

Scott, J. G., Malacova, E., Mathews, B., Haslam, D. M., Pacella, R., Higgins, D. J., Meinck, F., Dunne, M. P., Finkelhor, D., Erskine, H., Lawrence, D., & Thomas, H. (2023). The association between child maltreatment and mental disorders in the Australian Child Maltreatment Study. *The Medical Journal of Australia, 218*(6, Suppl), S26–S33. DOI: 10.5694/mja2.51870

Scott-Storey, K. (2011). Cumulative abuse: Do things add up? An evaluation of the conceptualization, operationalization, and methodological approaches in the study of the phenomenon of cumulative abuse. *Trauma, Violence & Abuse, 12*(3), 135–150. DOI: 10.1177/1524838011404253 PMID: 21511684

Secretariat of National Aboriginal and Islander Child Care (SNAICC). (2017). *The Family Matters report 2017: Measuring trends to turn the tide on the over-representation of Aboriginal and Torres Strait Islander children in out-of-home care in Australia*. SNAICC.

Seker, S., Boonmann, C., Gerger, H., Jäggi, L., d'Huart, D., Schmeck, K., & Schmid, M. (2022). Mental disorders among adults formerly in out-of-home care: A systematic review and meta-analysis of longitudinal studies. *European Child & Adolescent Psychiatry, 31*(12), 1963–1982. DOI: 10.1007/s00787-021-01828-0 PMID: 34169369

Seng, J. S., Sperlich, M., Low, L. K., Ronis, D. L., Muzik, M., & Liberzon, I. (2013). Childhood abuse history, posttraumatic stress disorder, postpartum mental health, and bonding: A prospective cohort study. *Journal of Midwifery & Women's Health, 58*(1), 57–68. DOI: 10.1111/j.1542-2011.2012.00237.x PMID: 23374491

Shah, R., DeYoung, A., & Moffitt, T. (2022). Childhood adversity and lifelong health: A developmental review. *Annual Review of Developmental Psychology, 4*, 123–147. DOI: 10.1146/annurev-devpsych-121121-021134

Sharma, N. P., & Spiro, P. M. (2023). *Psychoanalytic therapy*. StatPearls Publishing.

Sheehan, R. (2019). Cumulative harm in the child protection system: The Australian context. *Child & Family Social Work, 24*(4), 421–429. DOI: 10.1111/cfs.12621

Sheppard, M. (2003). The significance of past abuse to current intervention strategies with depressed mothers in child and family care. *British Journal of Social Work, 33*(6), 769–786. DOI: 10.1093/bjsw/33.6.769

Sheridan, M. A., & McLaughlin, K. A. (2016). Neurodevelopmental mechanisms linking adversity and psychopathology. *Annual Review of Clinical Psychology, 12*, 433–458. DOI: 10.1146/annurev-clinpsy-021815-093005

Sianko, N., Peterson, C. A., Spieker, S. J., & Gillmore, M. R. (2016). Enhancing parent-child relationships through Theraplay in child welfare. *Child & Family Social Work*, *21*(1), 83–93.

Silberner, J. (2023, February 15). At 97, Robert Jay Lifton is still thinking deeply about trauma. *Fresh Air*. https://www.npr.org/2023/02/15/1157115775/at-97-robert-jay-lifton-is-still-thinking-deeply-about-trauma29

Silke, C., Brady, B., Boylan, C., & Dolan, P. (2018). Factors influencing the development of empathy and pro-social behaviour among adolescents: A systematic review. *Children and Youth Services Review*, *94*, 421–436. https://www.sciencedirect.com/science/article/pii/S0190740918301889. DOI: 10.1016/j.childyouth.2018.07.027

Silke, C., Brady, B., Dolan, P., & Boylan, C. (2024). Empathy rules, maps and paths: A qualitative exploration of the factors that facilitate or inhibit empathy and prosocial responding among youth. *Journal of Community Psychology*, *52*(2), 326–343. DOI: 10.1002/jcop.23106

Simons, D., Wurtele, S. K., & Heil, P. (2002). Childhood victimization and lack of empathy as predictors of sexual offending against women and children. *Journal of Interpersonal Violence*, *17*(12), 1291–1307. DOI: 10.1177/088626002237857

Sinclair, I., Baker, C., Wilson, K., & Gibbs, I. (2005). *Foster children: Where they go and how they get on*. Jessica Kingsley Publishers.

Singer, T., & Klimecki, O. (2014). Empathy and compassion. *Current Biology*, *24*(18), R875–R878. DOI: 10.1016/j.cub.2014.06.054

Slack, K. S., & Berger, L. M. (2020). Who is and is not served by child protective services systems? Implications for a prevention infrastructure to reduce child maltreatment. *The Annals of the American Academy of Political and Social Science*, *692*(1), 182–202. DOI: 10.1177/0002716220980691

Smale-Jacobse, A. E., Meijer, A., Helms-Lorenz, M., & Maulana, R. (2019). Differentiated instruction in secondary education: A systematic review of research evidence. *Frontiers in Psychology*, *10*, 2366. DOI: 10.3389/fpsyg.2019.02366 PMID: 31824362

Smith, G.P. (2015). *Nobody's Children: An exploration into a sense of belonging of adults who experienced institutional out-of-home care as children*. [Doctoral thesis, Southern Cross University].

Smith, C. P. (2017). First, do no harm: Institutional betrayal and trust in health care organizations. *Journal of Multidisciplinary Healthcare*, *10*, 133–144. DOI: 10.2147/JMDH.S125885 PMID: 28435281

Smith, C. P., & Freyd, J. J. (2014). Institutional betrayal. *The American Psychologist*, *69*(6), 575–587. DOI: 10.1037/a0037564 PMID: 25197837

Smith, C. P., & Freyd, J. J. (2017). Insult, then injury: Interpersonal and institutional betrayal linked to health and dissociation. *Journal of Aggression, Maltreatment & Trauma*, *26*(10), 1117–1131. DOI: 10.1080/10926771.2017.1322654

Smith, G. P. (2017). Historical out-of-home child care leavers and mental health needs. *Australian Social Work*, *70*(1), 1–3. DOI: 10.1080/0312407X.2017.1246070

Smith, J. A., & Osborn, M. (2008). Interpretative Phenomenological Analysis. In Breakwell, G. M. (Ed.), *Doing Psychology Research* (pp. 229–254). Wiley., DOI: 10.1002/9780470776278.ch10

Smyth, N. J., True, N., Souto, J. C., & Bruce, S. E. (2008). Posttraumatic stress disorder and academic performance: Current directions. *Journal of College Counseling, 11*, 6–17.28

SNAICC – Secretariat of National Aboriginal and Islander Child Care. (2019). *The family matters report 2019: Measuring trends to turn the tide on the over-representation of Aboriginal and Torres Strait Islander children in out-of-home care in Australia*. SNAICC.

SNAICC – Secretariat of National Aboriginal and Islander Child Care. (2023). *Family Matters Report 2023*. SNAICC. https://www.familymatters.org.au

Snowball, L. (2009). *Diversion of Aboriginal youth from juvenile justice system*. NSW Bureau of Crime Statistics and Research. https://www.bocsar.nsw.gov.au/

Sosu, E. M., & Pheunpha, P. (2019, February). Trajectory of university dropout: Investigating the cumulative effect of academic vulnerability and proximity to family support. [). Frontiers Media SA.]. *Frontiers in Education*, *4*, 6.

Sperlich, M., Seng, J., Rowe, H., Fisher, J., Cuthbert, C., & Taylor, J. (2017). A cycles-breaking framework to disrupt intergenerational patterns of maltreatment and vulnerability during the childbearing year. *Journal of Obstetric, Gynecologic, and Neonatal Nursing : JOGNN*, *46*(3), 378–389. DOI: 10.1016/j.jogn.2016.11.017 PMID: 28199820

Stahly, G. B. (2000). Women with children in violent relationships: The choice of leaving may bring the consequence of custodial challenge. *Journal of Aggression, Maltreatment & Trauma*, *2*(2), 239–251. DOI: 10.1300/J146v02n02_11

Staub, E., & Volhardt, J. (2008). Altruism born of suffering: The roots of caring and helping after victimization and other trauma. *The American Journal of Orthopsychiatry, 78*(3), 267–280. DOI: 10.1037/a0014223

Steele, B. F. (1970). Parental abuse of infants and small children. In Anthony, E. J., & Benedek, T. (Eds.), *Parenthood: Its psychology and psychopathology* (pp. 449–477). Little, Brown and Company.

Steine, I. M., Winje, D., Krystal, J. H., Bjorvatn, B., Milde, A. M., Grønli, J., Nordhus, I. H., & Pallesen, S. (2017). Cumulative childhood maltreatment and its dose-response relation with adult symptomatology: Findings in a sample of adult survivors of sexual abuse. *Child Abuse & Neglect, 65*, 99–111. DOI: 10.1016/j.chiabu.2017.01.008 PMID: 28131947

Stein, M., & Ward, H. (2021). Editorial: Transitions from care to adulthood—persistent issues across time and place. *Child & Family Social Work, 26*(2), 215–221. DOI: 10.1111/cfs.12802

Stevens, L. C., & Woodruff, C. C. (2018b). Where caring for self and others lives in the brain, and how it can be enhanced and diminished: Observations on the neuroscience of empathy, compassion, and self-compassion. In L. C. Stevens & C. C. Woodruff (Eds.), *The neuroscience of empathy, compassion, and self-compassion*. Elsevier Science & Technology.

Stevens, L. C., & Woodruff, C. C. (Eds.). (2018a). *The neuroscience of empathy, compassion, and self-compassion*. Elsevier Science & Technology.

Stob, V., Slade, A., Adnopoz, J., & Woolston, J. (2020). The family cycle: Breaking the intergenerational transmission of trauma through mentalizing. *Journal of Infant, Child, and Adolescent Psychotherapy; JICAP, 19*(3), 255–270. DOI: 10.1080/15289168.2020.1786762

Stoltenborgh, M., Bakermans-Kranenburg, M. J., Alink, L. R., & van IJzendoorn, M. H. (2015). The prevalence of child maltreatment across the globe: Review of a series of meta-analyses. *Child Abuse Review, 24*(1), 37–50. DOI: 10.1002/car.2353

Straus, E. (2016). *Political Scandal: The effects of government betrayal on American citizens*. [Doctoral dissertation, California School of Professional Psychology].

Strauss, C. (2004). Is empathy gendered, and if so, why? An approach from feminist psychological anthropology. *Ethos (Berkeley, Calif.), 32*(4), 432–457. DOI: 10.1525/eth.2004.32.4.432

Strolovitch, D. Z. (2006). Do interest groups represent the disadvantaged? Advocacy at the intersections of race, class, and gender. *The Journal of Politics, 68*(4), 894–910. DOI: 10.1111/j.1468-2508.2006.00478.x

Strube, M. J., & Barbour, L. S. (1983). The decision to leave an abusive relationship: Economic dependence and psychological commitment. *Journal of Marriage and Family, 45*(4), 785–793. DOI: 10.2307/351791

Strube, M. J., & Barbour, L. S. (1984). Factors related to the decision to leave an abusive relationship. *Journal of Marriage and Family, 46*(4), 837–844. DOI: 10.2307/352531

Substance Abuse and Mental Health Services Administration. (2014). *SAMHSA's concept of trauma and guidance for a trauma-informed approach.* HHS Publication No. (SMA) 14-4884. Substance Abuse and Mental Health Services Administration.2

Substance Abuse and Mental Health Services Administration. (2023) *Practical Guide for Implementing a Trauma-Informed Approach.* SAMHSA Publication No. PEP23-06-05-005. Rockville, MD: National Mental Health and Substance Use Policy Laboratory. https://store.samhsa.gov/sites/default/files/pep23-06-05-005.pdf

Sullivan, P. (2018). The tyranny of neoliberal public management and the challenge for Aboriginal community organisations. In D. Howard-Wagner, M. Bargh, & I. Altamirano-Jiménez (Eds.), *The neoliberal state, recognition and Indigenous rights: New paternalism to new imaginings* (pp. 201-215). Australian National University, Press. DOI: 10.22459/CAEPR40.07.2018.11

Tajfel, H., & Turner, J. C. (1979). An integrative theory of intergroup conflict. In Austin, W. G., & Worchel, S. (Eds.), *The social psychology of intergroup relations* (pp. 33–47). Brooks/Cole.

Takeuchi, H., Taki, Y., Thyreau, B., Sass, Y., Hashizume, H., Sekiguchi, A., Nagase, T., Nouchi, R., Fukushima, A., & Kawashima, R. (2013). White matter structures associated with empathizing and systemizing in young adults. *NeuroImage, 77*, 222–236. DOI: 10.1016/j.neuroimage.2013.04.004

Tarren-Sweeney, M. (2021). A narrative review of mental and relational health interventions for children in family-based out-of-home care. *Journal of Family Therapy, 43*(3), 376–391. DOI: 10.1111/1467-6427.12341

Teague, R. (2017). *Reunification for children in out-of-home-care-Part 2: Reunification success rates and the consequences of reunification failure.* Queensland Child & Family Commission.

Tedeschi, R. G., & Calhoun, L. G. (1996). The Posttraumatic Growth Inventory: Measuring the positive legacy of trauma. *Journal of Traumatic Stress*, *9*(3), 455–471. DOI: 10.1002/jts.2490090305 PMID: 8827649

Testa, A., Jackson, D. B., Ganson, K. T., & Nagata, J. M. (2022). Adverse childhood experiences and criminal justice contact in adulthood. *Academic Pediatrics*, *22*(6), 972–980. DOI: 10.1016/j.acap.2021.10.011 PMID: 34752957

Testa, M. F., & Poertner, J. (2020). *Fostering accountability: Using evidence to guide and improve child welfare policy*. Oxford University Press.

The Healing Foundation. (2016). *Bringing them home 20 years on*. https://healingfoundation.org.au

The Healing Foundation. (2025). *Are you waiting for us to die? The unfinished business of bringing them home*.

Thornberry, T. P., Knight, K. E., & Lovegrove, P. J. (2012). Does maltreatment beget maltreatment? A systematic review of the intergenerational literature. *Trauma, Violence & Abuse*, *13*(3), 135–152. DOI: 10.1177/1524838012447697 PMID: 22673145

Tiego, J., Testa, R., & Arnold, S. R. C. (2020). Executive function in child and adolescent psychopathology: A meta-analysis. *Psychological Bulletin*, *146*(2), 141–180. DOI: 10.1037/bul0000227

Tilbury, C. (2009). The over-representation of Indigenous children in the Australian child welfare system. *International Journal of Social Welfare*, *18*(1), 57–64. DOI: 10.1111/j.1468-2397.2008.00577.x

Timmer, S. G., Hawk, B. N., Washington, A. M. L., & Urquiza, A. J. (2022). Trauma-Informed Care for Maltreated Children: Evidence-Based Treatments from a Developmental Perspective. In Krugman, R. D., & Korbin, J. E. (Eds.), *Handbook of Child Maltreatment. Child Maltreatment* (Vol. 14). Springer., DOI: 10.1007/978-3-030-82479-2_25

Tomison, A. (1996). *Intergenerational transmission of maltreatment*. Child Family Community Australia. https://aifs.gov.au/resources/policy-and-practice-papers/intergenerational-transmission-maltreatment#how

Tran, N. K., Alink, L. R., Van Berkel, S. R., & Van Ijzendoorn, M. H. (2017). Child maltreatment in Vietnam: Prevalence and cross-cultural comparison. *Journal of Aggression, Maltreatment & Trauma*, *26*(3), 211–230. DOI: 10.1080/10926771.2016.1250851

Tricco, A. C., Lillie, E., Zarin, W., O'Brien, K., Colquhoun, H., Kastner, M., Levac, D., Ng, C., Pearson Sharpe, J., Wilson, K., Kenny, M., Warren, R., Wilson, C., Stelfox, H. T., Straus, S. E., & Sharpe, J. P. (2016). A scoping review on the conduct and reporting of scoping reviews. *BMC Medical Research Methodology, 16*(1), 1–10. DOI: 10.1186/s12874-016-0116-4 PMID: 26857112

Tronick, E. Z., & Cohn, J. F. (1989). Infant-Mother Face-to-Face Interaction: Age and Gender Differences in Coordination and the Occurrence of Miscoordination. *Child Development, 60*(1), 85–92. DOI: 10.2307/1131074 PMID: 2702877

Tuart Place. (2019), *Submission to Aged Care Royal Commission*, https://agedcare.royalcommission.gov.au/sites/default/files/2020-09/AWF.001.04093.00_001.pdf

Tuohy, A. L. (1987). Psychoanalytic perspectives on child abuse. *Child & Adolescent Social Work Journal, 4*(1), 25–40. DOI: 10.1007/BF00757867

Ungar, M. (2013). Resilience after maltreatment: The importance of social services as facilitators of positive adaptation. *Child Abuse & Neglect, 37*(2-3), 110–115. DOI: 10.1016/j.chiabu.2012.08.004 PMID: 23260114

Ungar, M., & Theron, L. (2020). Resilience and mental health: How multisystemic processes contribute to positive outcomes. *The Lancet. Psychiatry, 7*(5), 441–448. DOI: 10.1016/S2215-0366(19)30434-1 PMID: 31806473

Vaidya, N., Marquand, A. F., Nees, F., Siehl, S., & Schumann, G. (2024). The impact of psychosocial adversity on brain and behaviour: An overview of existing knowledge and directions for future research. *Molecular Psychiatry, 29*(10), 3245–3267. DOI: 10.1038/s41380-024-02556-y PMID: 38658773

Valentino, K. (2017). Relational interventions for maltreated children. *Child Development, 88*(2), 359–367. DOI: 10.1111/cdev.12735 PMID: 28138967

Van der Graaf, J., Branje, S., De Wied, M., Hawk, S., Van Lier, P., & Meeus, W. (2014). Perspective taking and empathic concern in adolescence: Gender differences in developmental changes. *Developmental Psychology, 50*(3), 881–888. DOI: 10.1037/a0034325

Van der Hart, O., Nijenhuis, E. R. S., & Steele, K. (2006). *The haunted self: Structural dissociation and the treatment of chronic traumatization*. Norton.

van der Kolk, B. A. (2005). Developmental Trauma Disorder: Toward a rational diagnosis for children with complex trauma histories. *Psychiatric Annals, 35*(5), 401–408. DOI: 10.3928/00485713-20050501-06

Van der Put, C. E., Assink, M., Gubbels, J., & Boekhout van Solinge, N. F. (2018). Identifying effective components of child maltreatment interventions: A meta-analysis. *Clinical Child and Family Psychology Review, 21*(2), 171–202. DOI: 10.1007/s10567-017-0250-5 PMID: 29204796

Verbist, A. N., Winters, A. M., Collins-Camargo, C., & Antle, B. F. (2020). Standardized assessment domains as predictors of prescription of trauma-focused treatment for youth in out-of-home care. *Children and Youth Services Review, 118*, 105401. DOI: 10.1016/j.childyouth.2020.105401

Vial, A. C., & Cowgill, C. M. (2022). Heavier lies her crown: Gendered patterns of leader emotional labor and their downstream effects. *Frontiers in Psychology, 13*, 849566. DOI: 10.3389/fpsyg.2022.849566

Victorian Aboriginal Child Care Agency (VACCA). (2010). *Assessing kinship care for Aboriginal children: A practice guide for child protection practitioners*. Victorian Government Department of Human Services. https://www.cpmanual.vic.gov.au/sites/default/files/Asess_kc_aboriginal_chn_cpguide%202304_0.pdf

Victorian Sentencing Advisory Council. (2020). *Crossover kids: Vulnerable children in the youth justice system (Report 1 & 2)*. https://www.sentencingcouncil.vic.gov.au/

Villodas, M. T., Morelli, N. M., Hong, K., Duong, J., Evans, M. C., Elson, D., Rose, E., Picci, G., & Fishbein, D. (2021). Differences in late adolescent psychopathology among youth with histories of co-occurring abuse and neglect experiences. *Child Abuse & Neglect, 120*, 105189. DOI: 10.1016/j.chiabu.2021.105189 PMID: 34273863

Vizard, E., Gray, J., & Bentovim, A. (2022). The impact of child maltreatment on the mental and physical health of child victims: A review of the evidence. *BJPsych Advances, 28*(1), 60–70. DOI: 10.1192/bja.2021.10

Wagaman, M. A., Geiger, J. M., Shockley, C., & Segal, E. (2015). The role of empathy in burnout, compassion satisfaction, and secondary traumatic stress among social workers. *Social Work, 60*(3), 201–209. DOI: 10.1093/sw/swv014

Wall, L., Higgins, D. J., & Hunter, C. (2016). *Trauma-informed care in child/family welfare services*. Australian Institute of Family Studies.

Walters, A. J., Notebaert, L., Van Bockstaele, B., Meeten, F., Todd, J., & Clarke, P. J. (2024). Occurrence of potentially traumatic events, type, and severity in undergraduate students. *Australian Psychologist*, •••, 1–11.

Wamser-Nanney, R. (2016). Examining the complex trauma definition using children's self-reports. *Journal of Child & Adolescent Trauma, 9*(4), 295–304. DOI: 10.1007/s40653-016-0098-8

Wang, C. C. (1999). Photovoice: A participatory action research strategy applied to women's health. *Journal of Women's Health*, *8*(2), 185–192. DOI: 10.1089/jwh.1999.8.185

Wang, M.-T., Degol, J. L., & Henry, D. (2023). Peer relations and school engagement among adolescents with adversity exposure. *Child Development*, *94*(1), 70–88. DOI: 10.1111/cdev.13869 PMID: 37467355

Wang, Y.-L., Guo, J.-N., Yin, X.-B., Zhang, Q., Dong, L.-Y., Wang, K., & Wang, Y.-Y. (2021). The role of empathy in the relationship between childhood trauma and borderline personality tendencies in male offenders. *Journal of Forensic Psychiatry & Psychology*, *32*(5), 679–696. DOI: 10.1080/14789949.2021.1886314

Warmingham, J. M., Handley, E. D., Rogosch, F. A., Manly, J. T., & Cicchetti, D. (2019). Identifying maltreatment groups with patterns of maltreatment type and chronicity: A latent class analysis approach. *Child Abuse & Neglect*, *87*, 28–39. DOI: 10.1016/j.chiabu.2018.08.013 PMID: 30224068

Watson, T., Hodgson, D., Watts, L., & Waters, R. (2022). Historiography of empathy: Contributions to social work research and practice. *Qualitative Social Work: Research and Practice*, *21*(4), 714–730. DOI: 10.1177/14733250211033012

Watson, T., Waters, D., Watts, L., & Hodgston, T. (2025). Exploring the challenges of empathy in a therapeutic context: An interpretative phenomenological analysis. *Qualitative Health Research*, *0*(0), 1–14. DOI: 10.1177/10497323251331460

Webster-Stratton, C. (2005). The Incredible Years: A training series for the prevention and treatment of conduct problems in young children.

Webster-Stratton, C. (2015). The Incredible Years® series: A developmental approach. In *Family-Based Prevention Programs for Children and Adolescents* (pp. 54-79). Psychology Press. wife abuse. *Journal of Marriage and Family*, *44*, 277–286.

Weissman, D. G., Rosen, M. L., Colich, N. L., Sambrook, K. A., Lengua, L. J., Sheridan, M. A., & McLaughlin, K. A. (2022). Exposure to violence as an environmental pathway linking low socioeconomic status with altered neural processing of threat and adolescent psychopathology. *Journal of Cognitive Neuroscience*, *34*(10), 1892–1905. DOI: 10.1162/jocn_a_01825 PMID: 35104853

Werner, E. E. (1996). Vulnerable but invincible: High risk children from birth to adulthood. *European Child & Adolescent Psychiatry*, *5*(S1), 47–51. DOI: 10.1007/BF00538544 PMID: 9010664

Wharton, A. S. (2009). The sociology of emotional labor. *Annual Review of Sociology*, *35*(1), 147–165. DOI: 10.1146/annurev-soc-070308-115944

Widom, C. S. (2015). Reflection: Intergenerational transmission of child maltreatment. In Geiger, J. M., Schelbe, L., Hayes, M. J., Kawam, E., Katz, C. C., & Klika, J. B. (Eds.), *Intergenerational transmission of maltreatment: Ending a family tradition* (pp. 83–84). Springer.

Widom, C. S., & Wilson, H. W. (2015). Intergenerational transmission of violence. In Lindert, J., & Levav, I. (Eds.), *Violence and mental health: Its manifold faces* (pp. 27–45). Springer., DOI: 10.1007/978-94-017-8999-8_2

Wilson, J. Z., Mendes, P., & Golding, F. (2018). Hope street: From voice to agency for care-leavers in higher education. *Life Writing*, *15*(4), 597–609. DOI: 10.1080/14484528.2018.1427420

Wilson, L. C., & Scarpa, A. (2011). Hypothalamic-pituitary-adrenal axis (HPA) functioning and the intergenerational cycle of child maltreatment. In Hynes, L. E. (Ed.), *Sexual Abuse: Types, Signs and Treatments* (pp. 77–92). Nova Science Publishers, Inc.

Witt, A., Münzer, A., Ganser, H. G., Fegert, J. M., Goldbeck, L., & Plener, P. L. (2016). Experience by children and adolescents of more than one type of maltreatment: Association of different classes of maltreatment profiles with clinical outcome variables. *Child Abuse & Neglect*, *57*, 1–11. DOI: 10.1016/j.chiabu.2016.05.001 PMID: 27254375

Woffordt, S., Mihalic, D. E., & Menard, S. (1994). Continuities in marital violence. *Journal of Family Violence*, *9*(3), 195–225. DOI: 10.1007/BF01531948

Wojciak, A., Powers, K., Bryce, A., & Thompson, S. (2022). The ARCCH model of resilience: A strengths-based, trauma-informed and culturally responsive intervention tool. *Frontiers in Psychology*, *13*, 133.

Wolfe, D. A., & McGee, R. A. (1994). Dimensions of child maltreatment and their relationship to adolescent adjustment. *Development and Psychopathology*, *6*(1), 165–181. DOI: 10.1017/S0954579400005939

Woods, P. (2011). *Working with parents to support children's learning*. SAGE Publications.

Woolfolk, R. L. (2015). *The value of psychotherapy: The talking cure in an age of clinical science*. Guilford Press.

Wright, N. M., Smith, C. P., & Freyd, J. J. (2017). Experience of a lifetime: Study abroad, trauma, and institutional betrayal. *Journal of Aggression, Maltreatment & Trauma*, *26*(1), 50–68. DOI: 10.1080/10926771.2016.1170088

Yalom, I., & Leszcz, M. (2020). *The Theory and Practice of Group Psychotherapy*. Basic Books.

Yehuda, R., & Flory, J. D. (2007). Differentiating PTSD from other stress reactions: Evidence from the study of biological mechanisms. *Psychoneuroendocrinology, 32*, 998–1007.6

Yehuda, R., & Bierer, L. M. (2009). The relevance of epigenetics to PTSD: Implications for the DSM-V. *Journal of Traumatic Stress, 22*(5), 427–434. DOI: 10.1002/jts.20448 PMID: 19813242

Yellow Horse Brave Heart, M. (2003). The historical trauma response among natives and its relationship with substance abuse: A Lakota illustration. *Journal of Psychoactive Drugs, 35*(1), 7–13. DOI: 10.1080/02791072.2003.10399988 PMID: 12733753

Yoorrook Justice Commission. (2023). *Yoorrook for justice: Report into Victoria's child protection and criminal justice systems*. yoorrookforjustice.org.au/wp-content/uploads/2023/08/Yoorrook-for-justice-report.pdf

Young, C., Craig, J. C., Clapham, K., Banks, S., & Williamson, A. (2017). Perspectives on childhood resilience among the Aboriginal community: An interview study. *Australian and New Zealand Journal of Public Health, 41*(4), 405–410. DOI: 10.1111/1753-6405.12681 PMID: 28712160

Young, J. E. (1999). *Cognitive therapy for personality disorders: A schema-focused approach* (3rd ed.). Professional Resource Press.

Young, J. E., Klosko, J. S., & Weishaar, M. E. (2003). *Schema therapy: A practitioner's guide*. Guilford Press.

Young, M. E., Nosek, M. A., Howland, C. A., Chanpong, G., & Rintala, D. H. (1997). Prevalence of abuse of women with disabilities. *Archives of Physical Medicine and Rehabilitation, 78*(12), S34–S38. DOI: 10.1016/S0003-9993(97)90219-7 PMID: 9422005

Young, S., McKenzie, M., Omre, C., Schjelderup, L., & Walker, S. (2014). Practicing from theory: Thinking and knowing to "do" child protection work. *Social Sciences (Basel, Switzerland), 3*(4), 893–915. DOI: 10.3390/socsci3040893

Zajac, L., Raby, K. L., & Dozier, M. (2019). Attachment state of mind and childhood experiences of maltreatment as predictors of sensitive care from infancy through middle childhood: Results from a longitudinal study of parents involved with Child Protective Services. *Development and Psychopathology, 31*(1), 113–125. DOI: 10.1017/S0954579418001554 PMID: 30466498

Zanoni, L., Warburton, W., Bussey, K., & McMaugh, A. (2013). Fathers as 'core business' in child welfare practice and research: An interdisciplinary review. *Children and Youth Services Review*, *35*(7), 1055–1070. DOI: 10.1016/j.childyouth.2013.04.018

Zeanah, C. H., & Humphreys, K. L. (2018). Child abuse and neglect. *Journal of the American Academy of Child and Adolescent Psychiatry*, *57*(9), 637–644. DOI: 10.1016/j.jaac.2018.06.007 PMID: 30196867

Zeanah, C. H., & Zeanah, P. D. (1989). Intergenerational transmission of maltreatment: Insights from attachment theory and research. *Psychiatry*, *52*(2), 177–196. DOI: 10.1080/00332747.1989.11024442 PMID: 2660176

Zhai, F., Waldfogel, J., & Brooks-Gunn, J. (2022). Adverse childhood experiences and children's learning: A population-level analysis. *Child Development*, *93*(2), 367–383. DOI: 10.1111/cdev.13679

Zhang, H., Gao, X., Liang, Y., Yao, Q., & Wei, Q. (2024). Does child maltreatment reduce or increase empathy? A systematic review and meta-analysis. *Trauma, Violence & Abuse*, *25*(1), 166–182. DOI: 10.1177/15248380221145734

Zhang, L., Mersky, J. P., Gruber, A. M. H., & Kim, J.-Y. (2023). Intergenerational transmission of parental adverse childhood experiences and children's outcomes: A scoping review. *Trauma, Violence & Abuse*, *24*(5), 3251–3264. DOI: 10.1177/15248380221126186 PMID: 36205317

Zhang, S., Conner, A., Lim, Y., & Lefmann, T. (2021). Trauma-informed care for children involved with the child welfare system: A meta-analysis. *Child Abuse & Neglect*, *122*, 105296. DOI: 10.1016/j.chiabu.2021.105296 PMID: 34478999

Zhou, A., & Ryan, J. (2023). Biological embedding of early-life adversity and a scoping review of the evidence for intergenerational epigenetic transmission of stress and trauma in humans. *Genes*, *14*(8), 1639. DOI: 10.3390/genes14081639 PMID: 37628690

Zonnevijlle, M., & Hildebrand, M. (2019). Like parent, like child? Exploring the association between early maladaptive schemas of adolescents involved with Child Protective Services and their parents. *Child & Family Social Work*, *24*(2), 190–200. DOI: 10.1111/cfs.12602

Zubrick, S. R., Shepherd, C. C., Dudgeon, P., Gee, G., Paradies, Y., Scrine, C., & Walker, R. (2010). Social determinants of Aboriginal and Torres Strait Islander social and emotional wellbeing. In N. Purdie, P. Dudgeon, & R. Walker (Eds.), *Working together: Aboriginal and Torres Strait Islander mental health and wellbeing principles and practice* (pp. 75–90). Commonwealth of Australia.

Zurbriggen, E. L., & Freyd, J. J. (2004). The link between child sexual abuse and risky sexual behavior: The role of dissociative tendencies, information-processing effects, and consensual sex decision mechanisms.

About the Contributors

India Bryce began her career as early childhood educator before taking a position as a front-line Child Safety Officer in the Investigation and Assessment Team, in the Queensland Department of Child Safety, Women and Youth. India is now a Senior Lecturer and Academic in the School of Psychology and Wellbeing, at the University of Southern Queensland and a member of the USQ Centre of Health Research (Health and Social Justice). India's current research explores cumulative adversity across the lifespan, trauma informed pedagogy in higher education, and trauma narratives as they intersect with career, vocational behaviour, heath and systemic marginalisation. India has published books, book chapters, and journal articles from her research including two co-edited reference books, Child Abuse and Neglect: Forensic Issues in Evidence, Impact and Management, and Child Sexual Abuse: Forensic Issues in Evidence, Impact and Management. India has presented on topics related to her research nationally and internationally.

Simone Collier holds a Bachelor of Education (Special Education), a Master of Special Education, a Master in Child Play Therapy and a Doctor of Professional Studies. Dr Collier is an accredited Parents Under Pressure Therapist, Animal Assisted Therapist and a Play Therapist using Theraplay principles. She holds a Post-Graduate Diploma in Alcohol & Other Drugs and Mental Health and is a trained Step-by Step Assessor. Dr Collier is also trained to administer Attachment Style Interviews (ASI) and Parenting Role Interviews (PRI). Dr. Collier is a member of the Australasian Pacific Play Therapy Australia (APPTA) and a member of the Psychotherapy & Counselling Federation of Australia (PACFA) and a is a Registered Child Play Therapist (RPT) and a Registered Teacher in Queensland and is an Affiliate of the Society for the Advancement of Actuarial Risk Need Assessment (SAARNA). Dr. Collier has a history of frontline and statutory child protection and out of home care experience. Simone Collier is a Special Education teacher who has taught in behaviour support and special Education and mainstream settings for a number of years. Simone worked as a Deputy Principal and as a Guidance Officer before moving in to the social work sector, initially in homelessness and domestic and family violence and then into Child Protection. Simone has a varied career working with children and young people in Residential facilities and in complex care settings as well as out-of-home care with foster and kinship carers. Simone has worked in Team Leader, Program Co-ordinator and Program Manager roles in child protection and more recently in a State Project Manager role and a Specialist Practice and Compliance position with Act for Kids, setting up programs for Individual Support packages for families and children with high and complex needs. Simone was involved in a pilot research project in partnership with the University of Southern Queensland trialling an evaluative tool to measure cumulative harm in children and young people. Simone is deeply passionate about supporting children with complex trauma and has completed her doctorate research investigating the barriers and enablers for mainstream classroom teachers to engage in professional development of trauma informed classroom pedagogy. Simone has published her first children's book, titled Jeremy's Changing Family which is focused on hearing the voice of a little boy who is the biological child of foster carers. The book explores the challenges and celebrations of a foster family and in particular the children of foster carers. Simone's second children's book is currently underway. Simone works as a lecturer and course examiner in the child abuse and children's mental health courses as a course examiner and lecturer and is involved with a range of research projects to further the knowledge and skill base of the sector.

***

Susan Baidawi is an Associate Professor in the Department of Social Work, Monash University. She is a leading social work academic with over 70 book chapters, peer reviewed articles and reports in child and family welfare and criminal justice fields. Her key areas of research specialisation are young people with complex support needs, including 'crossover' young people who experience dual child protection and criminal justice system contact.

Tamara Blakemore is the Chief Investigator and Project Lead of the Name. Narrate.Navigate (NNN) program for youth violence. She is a social work practitioner, researcher and educator who has worked in the field of violence, abuse, and trauma for the past two decades. Her PhD was the first of its kind to explore the occurrence and outcomes of child sexual abuse in a prospective, longitudinal cohort of mothers and their children. Tamara has worked in federal policy, contributed landmark work to the Royal Commission into Institutional Responses to Child Sexual Abuse and remains connected to clinical practice in acute trauma settings.

Crysta Bowe is a PhD candidate exploring the ways in which intergenerational child maltreatment is conceptualised and responded to in practice and research. Her research takes a transformational lens, examining the ways in which the knowledge from the wider field of intergenerational trauma may enhance child protection policy and practice. Crysta is also a practicing social worker, with extensive experience working in child protection contexts. Currently she provides therapeutic counselling support to children and families who have experienced child abuse or neglect. Crysta is passionate about the helping families overcome trauma and adversity through providing both individual support and systemic examination and transformation.

Maria-Ernestina Christl is a postdoctoral fellow in the Institute for Relationship Science at the University of Denver Psychology Department. Dr. Christl's research interests are focused on interpersonal violence and interrupting intergenerational patterns of trauma and abuse within family systems. Her research in graduate school initially focused more broadly on violence against women and children and its impact on individual and family well-being and evolved to focus on reproductive coercion, a form of intimate partner violence where abusive partners control their partners' reproductive decisions. As a clinician, Dr. Christl provided evidence-based treatment for a variety of mental health difficulties including trauma (e.g., childhood trauma, intimate partner violence, birth trauma, immigration trauma) as well as supported healthy parenting and attachment between parents and their young children. Treating Spanish-speaking women who had recently immigrated to the United States who were currently pregnant or had recently given birth provided critical insight into their childhood experiences and experiences with romantic partners that propelled her interest in better understanding the relationship between cultural and societal messaging and experiences of reproductive coercion and autonomy.

Anne P. DePrince is a distinguished university professor in the Psychology Department at the University of Denver, where she also serves as Associate Vice Provost of Public Good Strategy and Research. She received her doctorate in psychology from the University of Oregon and completed her clinical internship at the University of Washington Medical Center. Author of "Every 90 Seconds: Our Common Cause Ending Violence against Women," she is an expert in trauma and intimate violence. Using a community-engaged approach, DePrince emphasizes working with community partners to identify research questions that can inform policy and practice while advancing scientific understanding of trauma outcomes and interventions. She has authored more than one hundred manuscripts on trauma; co-edited volumes on trauma, including a 2023 special issue of the Journal of Trauma & Dissociation on trauma, violence, and reproductive autonomy; and serves as an Associate Editor of the Journal of Trauma & Dissociation. Her research was recognized by the Department of Justice with the Vision 21 Crime Victims Research Award for her contributions to the nation's understanding of crime victims' issues. She is a member of ISSTD as well as the American Psychological Association and the International Society for Traumatic Stress Studies. You can learn more about Anne at her website (https://annedeprince.com/) and through her research team's blog (https://traumaresearchnotes.blog/).

Daryl Higgins, Director, Institute of Child Protection Studies, Australian Catholic University. For over 30 years, Daryl has been researching child abuse prevalence, impacts, and prevention; public health approaches to protecting children; child-safe organisational strategies; and approaches to promoting child and family welfare. He was a Chief Investigator on the first national study of the prevalence in Australia of child abuse and neglect, and its health outcomes – the Australian Child MaltrMaltreatment.Study.Investigators on the first national study of the prevalence in Australia of child abuse and neglect, and its health outcomes – the Australian Child Maltreatment Study.

Chris Krogh is a member of the Name.Narrate.Navigate research team, with a particular interest in the training of professionals in this work. He holds a PhD in Social Science and degrees in social ecology and social work. His research spans home education and unschooling, youth violence intervention, and campus-based sexual violence prevention. His publications explore democratic approaches to home education, youth violence programmes, and institutional responses to sexual violence in tertiary education. Prior to his academic career, Dr Krogh worked as a child protection caseworker and held senior policy positions with the NSW government, including managing reforms for the Department of Premier and Cabinet. This combination of frontline practice, policy development, and research informs his commitment to translating research into meaningful social change.

Patricia Mackey is social work academic undertaking research in domestic violence, child maltreatment and on the wellbeing needs of older people. She is co-leading research in developing simulation in child protection curriculum, the inclusiveness of social work curriculum, particularly social work skill-based intensives, and establishing an interprofessional wellbeing clinic for older people.

Philip Mendes is a nationally and internationally recognized researcher in several social policy areas. He has published 13 books, and over 150 peer reviewed articles. He is also the recipient of major research grants including five ARC grants for which he was CI. He is a member of the Editorial Advisory Board for a number of academic journals including Children and Youth Services Review, the International Journal of Community and Social Development, Australian Social Work, and

Children Australia. His research has had a significant impact on contemporary social policy debates and outcomes through providing an evidence base for informing change. The impact of his work has been especially evident in two areas, namely, young people transitioning from forms of out-of-home care (OOHC) such as foster, kinship and residential care, and social security payments including particularly conditional welfare as manifested in the compulsory income management program. Mendes has been researching young people transitioning from OOHC for over 25 years. He has produced more than 40 significant publications on this topic, and is recognized internationally (via his long-term involvement in the leaving care academic research network known as INTRAC): as one of the major researchers in this field. His research has been widely utilized by Australian government and non-government service providers alike, and contributed to improved policy and practice with care leavers. This is evidenced by numerous citations of his work in leading national policy reports, and particularly the recent introduction of extended care programs until 21 years of age in all Australian jurisdictions. Additionally, his work has actively informed the policy recommendations of the OECD on care leavers as reflected in their 2022 report called Assisting care leavers: Time for action. Compulsory income management (IM) is a form of conditional welfare involving the quarantining of a percentage of social security payments such as the JobSeeker payment for spending on food, rent and other essential items in a number of sites across Australia. Mendes has been actively researching the philosophical, policy and evaluation debates around IM programs since they were first introduced in 2007. He has completed a number of funded studies, guest edited special issues of the Australian Journal of Social Issues and Social Alternatives, and participated in academic conference Symposiums. These activities informed the successful application for an ARC Discovery Grant in 2017 which resulted in a major report titled Hidden Costs, a book titled Compulsory Income Management in Australia and New Zealand published by Policy Press, and 11 peer reviewed journal articles (Mendes was lead author of four), one of which won the Mayer Journal prize for 2021. The project's evidence-based critique of the limitations of IM arguably influenced the Federal Labor Government's abolition of the Cashless Debit Card in 2022.

Louise Rak is the Program Manager for the University of Newcastle's Name. Narrate.Navigate (NNN) program for youth violence and a Lecturer in Human Services. She brings a wealth of expertise to her roles with over 20 years practice experience across social services in areas of youth homelessness, out of home care, mental health, disability services, youth justice and early intervention. Louise holds a BA Sociology, Grad Dip Psychology, MA Counselling, MBA and PhD Social work. Louise's PhD explored the narratives of young women who use violence and experience violence.

Adi Rosenthal is a postdoctoral fellow in the Institute for Relationship Science at the University of Denver Psychology Department. Dr. Rosenthal's graduate school training was focused on interpersonal trauma and violence against women, including individual-level and systemic response in the aftermath of traumatic events. Dr. Rosenthal's dissertation focused on the impact of trauma-related shame and self-blame on pain response and self-injurious behaviors. She has also conducted research on caregivers' experiences in child maltreatment investigations, legal needs of victims of crime, and barriers to service access. Rosenthal has since focused her research on developing and evaluating programs that interrupt intergenerational cycles, including cycles of teen pregnancy, childhood maltreatment, and involvement with child protection systems. Dr. Rosenthal also has specialized training in infant mental health, perinatal mental health, and treating mother-infant dyads in the context of trauma exposure. Dr. Rosenthal works also as a clinician for perinatal women, couples, families, and parent-child dyads. She also contributes to research and development at Thriving Families. Dr. Rosenthal and Dr. Christl co-created the Resilient Roots intervention described above.

Cate Thomas is a dynamic force in the world of social work and education, known for challenging norms and championing transformative change. As an Associate Professor at Charles Sturt University in Canberra, and a contributor to academic communities at Trinity College Dublin and Masaryk University in the Czech Republic, Cate brings a global perspective to justice, equity, diversity, and inclusion (JEDI). With a career rooted in advocacy and education, Cate is a sought-after speaker who inspires audiences to rethink systems, dismantle barriers, and build inclusive futures. Her work bridges theory and practice, empowering students, professionals, and institutions to lead with courage and compassion. Whether she's in the lecture hall, on stage, or collaborating across borders, Cate embodies the spirit of a true disrupter for good—bold, thoughtful, and relentlessly committed to equity.

Index

A

B

C

E

F

G

H

I

M

N

O

P

R

S

T

V

Y

www.ingramcontent.com/pod-product-compliance
Lightning Source LLC
LaVergne TN
LVHW062339300926
849161LV00007B/1752
9798337340647